The
Psychopharmacologists

Interviews by Dr David Healy

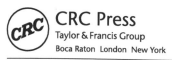

CRC Press
Taylor & Francis Group
Boca Raton London New York

CRC Press is an imprint of the
Taylor & Francis Group, an **informa** business
A CHAPMAN & HALL BOOK

First published 1996 by Chapman & Hall

Published 2019 by CRC Press
Taylor & Francis Group
6000 Broken Sound Parkway NW, Suite 300
Boca Raton, FL 33487-2742

© 2001 by Taylor & Francis Group, LLC
CRC Press is an imprint of Taylor & Francis Group, an Informa business

First issued in paperback 2019

No claim to original U.S. Government works

ISBN 13: 978-0-367-44775-5 (pbk)
ISBN 13: 978-1-86036-008-4 (hbk)

Visit the Taylor & Francis Web site at
http://www.taylorandfrancis.com

and the CRC Press Web site at
http://www.crcpress.com

Distributed in the USA by
Oxford University Press Inc.

British Library Cataloguing in Publication Data
A catalogue record for this book is available from the British Library

Library of Congress Cataloging-in-Publication Data
A catalog record for this book is available from the Library of Congress

Contents

Contributors

Jules Augst
Department of Psychiatry, Psychiatrische Universiteäts Klinik Zurich, Postfach 68, CH-8029, Zurich 8, Switzerland.

Julius Axelrod
Laboratory of Cell Biology, National Institute of Mental Health, Building 36, 9000 Rockville Pyke, Bethesda, Maryland 20892, USA

Frank Ayd
1130 East Cold Spring Lane, Baltimore, Maryland 21239-3931, USA

Thomas A. Ban
1177 Yonge Street, Toronto, Ontario M4T 2Y4, Canada

George Beaumont
11 Dorchester Road, Hazel Grove, Stockport, Cheshire SK7 5HE, UK

Floyd Bloom
Department of Neuropharmacology, The Scripps Research Institute, 10666 North Terney Pines Road, La Hella, California 92037, USA

Alan Broadhurst
Vicarage Grove, The Park, Great Barton, near Bury St Edmonds, Suffolk IP31 2SU, UK

Arvid Carlsson
Department of Pharmacology, University of Gothenburg, Mediconaregatan 7, S-41390 Gothenburg, Sweden

Gordon Claridge
Magdalen College, Oxford OX1 4AU, UK

Jonathan Cole
57 Ellery Street, Cambridge, Massachusetts 02138, USA

Alec Coppen
5 Walnut Close, Downs Road, Epsom, Surrey, UK

Alex Delini-Stula
Roche International Clinical Research Center, Parc Club des Tanneries, BP 83, F-673 82 Lingoisheim, France

Silvio Garattini
Director, Institue de Ricerche Farmacologiche 'Mario Negri', Via Eritrea 62, 20157 Milan, Italy

Hanns Hippius
Am Forst 4-A, 82166 Grafelfing, Germany

John Hughes
Director, Park-Davies Neuroscience Centre, Addenbrooke's Hospital, Hill Road, Cambridge CB2 2QB, UK

Donald F. Klein
1016 Fifth Avenue, New York NY 10028, USA

Malcolm Lader
Institute of Psychiatry, Clinical Psychopharmacology Section, De Crespigny Park, Denmark Hill, London SE5 8AF, UK

Heinz Lehmann
1212 Pine Avenue, Montreal, Quebec H39 1A9, Canada

Brian Leonard
Department of Pharmacology, University College, Galway, Republic of Ireland

Herbert Meltzer
Department of Psychiatry, Hanna Pavilion, 2040 Abingden Road, Cleveland, Ohio 44104, USA

Pierre Pichot
24 rue de Fosses, Saint Jacques 75005 Paris, France

Merton Sandler
Department of Chemical Pathology, Queen Charlotte's Maternity Hospital, Goldhawk Road, London W6 0XG, UK

Hannah Steinberg
Health Research Centre, School of Psychiatry, Middlesex University, Queensway, Enfield EN3 4SF, UK

Herman van Praag
Professor and Chairman, Academic Psychiatric Centre, University of Limburg, PO Box 616, 6200 MD Maastricht, The Netherlands

Peter Waldmeier
K-125,607, Ciba-Geigy Limited, Basle, Switzerland

Preface

The impetus to put this book together came from a number of sources. One was a need to do some research for a history of the period (see References). During the course of this, it became clear that others might also be interested in the raw material of the interviews and might have quite differing interpretations. The precipitating event was a train ride with George Beaumont from London to Guildford. This only takes an hour or so; just as the train pulled out, for whatever reason, I told George I'd been thinking about doing this and his story about how he targeted clomipramine for OCD was one of the ones I'd be interested to have. We looked at each other, I whipped out a tape recorder and we began the first interview. There are a number of interviews in the book that are almost *verbatim* as they were first recorded. George's is one of these. Another was Silvio Garattini's, which was done in the dark in the back of a taxi while travelling from Heathrow into London. Once a few had been done, the project just grew.

There were a few things I was keen to chase, which didn't come out. One of these was an idea that science operates more often because of clashes of personality than anyone suspects. A good example involved the race for absolute zero, which happened between groups in England and Holland at the turn of the century. The English lost out because the two people who needed to cooperate with each other in order to produce a result, Ramsay and Dewar, weren't prepared to talk to each other. The psychoanalytic story, similarly, is a story of people coming to particular viewpoints almost to spite someone else rather than because of the intrinsic merits of their position. Now this may have to do with ambition and priority issues but you also have to check and see that things are not happening because of who stole whose wife, for instance. Indeed one of the wives put it to me that I might find out more about the history of psychopharmacology by interviewing the wives rather than the 'great men' themselves. There's something to be said for this. You can often gauge the real reaction to a person or an event from a spouse where the participant in the event has to inhibit their feelings because the game is ongoing.

Part of the reason this kind of material didn't actually emerge may have been that the people I've interviewed came out on top, so they have less need to recall these things. There was a reluctance or at least a caution about speaking ill of others. Nevertheless there are clashes buried in the interviews that can be traced by looking at who fails to cite whom, even when they worked in the same institution. And there have been very visible clashes, as in the discovery of the opioid peptides, recounted by John Hughes, and the story of the evaluation of lithium, which got fairly personalized. There have also been clashes around the foundation of ECNP, BAP and CINP, which seem to have involved the clash of personality styles.

Personality styles – or historical forces as expressed through personalities? Another motive to do these interviews was that at the time I was the Secretary for the British Association for Psychopharmacology and I thought it would be a good idea to chase the origins of the BAP. Now at just this time, the Presidency of the BAP had become a hot political issue. For 20 years the question of who was going to be the next President had been a fix but in 1994, it was bitterly contested, with all sorts of personalized comments flying around and skullduggery that came close to being actionable.

On one level, the issues were pitched as a battle between the fixers, who wanted to stitch things up behind the scenes, and those who wanted a transparent democracy. To my surprise, I found myself on the fixer side of the argument. This I think was because these things never come as single issues. Open democracy as I saw it was being linked to a particular view of how science operates, the classical idea that we should be systematically testing models, as opposed to a pragmatic 'let's fish' model. On this level the fishing model is much more open and democratic while the purist model can be something of a stitch-up – at least as I saw it then. Historically, psychopharmacology has been a pragmatic exercise, whereas neuroscience, which is springing forth, Athena-like from it, is classically principled. Add in the personality end of it and you have the historical dilemma of trying to decide how much of history is down to personalities – would we have had the Second World War without Hitler; would the Northern Ireland problem have been as bad without Paisley? Given that I was arguing for a position that in many respects was alien to me, I was left wondering how much we become the pawns of historical forces, which produce a situation in which people who would otherwise have a lot in common end up divided by deep animosities.

I took these issues with me into many of the interviews – where are societies like the British Association and the American College for Neuropsychopharmacology situated today? What's going to happen them? The ACNP has thrown off a Society for Clinical Psychopharmacology and it's not clear how the BAP will evolve. In some ways, societies like the ACNP and BAP can act as the miner's canary for changes in the scientific atmosphere because they are relatively pure scientific societies, rather than semi-trade unions like the American Psychiatric Association or the Royal College of Psychiatrists. ACNP/BAP are shaped by completely different dynamics to the APA/RCP. Committee behaviour anywhere in my experience involves illusory intimacies between people who when the going gets difficult are usually more concerned to ensure that no one shouts too loud in case the neighbours are listening than they are about anything else. But because the preserve of professional turf is not on the agenda for BAP, in practice what happens is much less likely to be dictated by the actions of people who may be almost openly referred to as blustering bullies but whose behaviour cannot be or is not contained.

Another reason for trying to put a history together can be to try to make sense of what has happened in one's own life. Having trained in medicine, I got involved in psychopharmacology research, partly for the not-very-elevated reason that it seemed a good idea in order to be able to get some control over the kind of jobs I might want. The only research happening in Ireland in 1980 that seemed in any way relevant was with Brian Leonard – looking at what psychotropic drugs did to 5-HT reup-take. At the time, it seemed that working on these drugs was one of the few serious ways into the brain and the mind and the inter-relationships between brain and behaviour.

In my case, however, this led away from the now highly topical area of amine reuptake to work on circadian rhythms in affective disorders. I happen to think that a circadian model is much more persuasive than the amine theories ever were. There are coherent competing hypotheses to choose between – so it should be of interest to the purists but on the contrary the whole area has remained a backwater. The other area I've been involved in has been giving drugs to healthy human volunteers to test what effects these have on mental functioning with a view to working backwards from that to how the brain works – but the whole area is closing down it seems. It's difficult to get ethical committees or funding agencies to agree to projects even though the agents in question may have little more effect than, say, coffee. This seems to represent an important 'loss of nerve' and trying to trace the origins of this has been another reason to examine the history. To paraphrase Oscar Wilde, if one area of research you're involved in gets eclipsed, that's bad luck but if two do, you have to wonder what's going on.

Fairly early in my 5-HT uptake career, it seemed to me that far from being descriptions of any reality, the amine theories were simply a case of the politically correct language – the language that had triumphed because you've got to have some view about what the drugs are doing. The psychodynamic theories were at a major disadvantage even though they were much more complex and subtle theories because they couldn't account for one of the obvious features of modern practice, which is that psychotropic drugs work. Even simplistic biological theories were better placed from that point of view. There have been tremendous advances and we may be on the verge of even greater advances but, hitherto, it seems to me the role of monamine language in discourse has been to add a certain artistic verisimillitude to proceedings rather than to convey reliable information (Healy, 1987). The Glossary explains the few technical terms in this book.

Another view which developed during a four-year stint in Cambridge was that the industry was carving up the field in a way that people weren't aware of and they were marketing concepts rather than just drugs. They were marketing panic disorder and OCD rather than alprazolam and clomipramine. At a BAP meeting I decided to come up front and give a talk on how the nosological systems we have, DSM-III etc., have gained acceptance in part because they suit the purposes of the pharmaceutical industry rather than because of any necessary correspondence with reality. I went through the history of how people had come to think that clomipramine might be useful for OCD. I hadn't been aware that George Beaumont was in the audience. He of course was the person from Ciba-Geigy who had 'engineered' the marketing of clomipramine for OCD. He smiled at me and said 'well, you got that about right'. This rather directly led to the first interview.

But whereas I had thought at first that the marketing of concepts by the industry was a dubious exercise, the issues now seem much more complex. I think we've got to the situation where the industry can indeed pick out entities. Currently, for instance, what is happening is that social phobia is being marketed in order to sell the new RIMAs and the concept of delusional disorders will, in due course, be used to sell the next generation of atypical neuroleptics. But, arguably, what's happening is helpful because conditions like delusional disorders, social phobia and OCD are now recognized as being a lot more common than it was even quite recently thought they were and I'm sure that current estimates are more accurate. Psychiatric diagnoses are a social construction. There's no way to get around this fact. It would be the case whether or not we had drugs. Before the psychopharmacological era, the analysts defined mental illness in terms that suited their financial and professional interests. The knowledge we have always coincides to some extent with the interests of certain groups (Healy, 1996).

Anyway, having begun with the history of the BAP, I wanted to branch out because it was clear that the pioneers in the field weren't getting any younger and that if they were ever going to be interviewed it had to be now or never. It had also become clear at this point that it wasn't hard to get to interview people, which came as something of a surprise. I had written critically, for instance, about panic disorder and clozapine and yet Don Klein and Herb Meltzer were prepared to be interviewed.

I tend to think the best of people and the interviews were all friendly – it's perhaps worth noting that I regard myself as a very bad judge of personality and a poor reader of motives. The groundrules were that the interviewees had freedom to edit out whatever they were unhappy with or add in afterwards things that were missing. After a first editing done by me, aimed at eliminating the duplications and redundancies of speech where these were excessive (aimed mainly at presenting the interviewer as vaguely coherent), the great majority of interviews remained almost completely unchanged apart from correcting for spelling, etc.

One worry I had was the question of being seduced by the glamour of being a member of the club – like most people I wanted to be part of someone's gang; preferably the winning gang. At the same time, in reaction against that, I didn't want to go to the opposite extreme. From a practical point of view, interviewing was a matter of trying to find the right balance – how to push the person a bit further than he or she might have intended to go but without pushing them so far that they pulled out of the exercise completely. The only person who pulled out was Philip Bradley who generally feels that raking up the past is not a good idea.

The selection of subjects was based on a consensus that emerged from discussions with a number of colleagues as to who had done most to shape the field. There were double the number of potential interviewees, however, and the final selection depended on whom I could access with reasonable convenience – who would be attending particular meetings and would fit the mix of people from the industry, from the basic sciences and from clinical practice, that I wanted. I also wanted the discovery of the antidepressants and the antipsychotics to be covered and I wanted to end up with an even distribution of American, British and European endeavour. The book perhaps lacks contributions from the critics of the industry and biological psychiatry, such as Peter Breggin, or those who have had their difficulties on certain issues, such as Ian Oswald. It also lacks the 'behind the scenes' powerbrokers – whether this is because scientific achievement is incompatible with politics is a moot question. Finally, it lacks, and this is a significant omission, an input from the regulators.

The idea in conducting the interviews, broadly speaking, was to keep them fairly simple. To try and interview people who were involved in actually establishing that the drugs worked or how they worked or people who were involved in trying to create the marketing campaigns for various drugs. After tackling that bit for each interviewee the plan was simple – it was to move on to a common group of questions like 'how do you feel people perceive the risks associated with drugs?' and 'what do you think of the SSRIs or the "Listening to Prozac" phenomenon?' or 'what do drugs reveal about the nature of mental illness?' So there's a group of questions, most interviewees have been asked, which it is hoped provide unifying themes through the book. One advantage I experienced with an interview format was that it was much easier to see where a particular view fitted into an overall world view – to get some feel for the person behind the theory. This left me feeling that the usual scientific means of communication – the lecture, the symposium, the refereed article – can be terribly inadequate. They almost force a polarization of opinions and the launching of pre-emptive strikes.

I think in some respects I am probably coming from much the same position as many people who will read the book from outside psychopharmacology. As a grant-holder for a cognitive therapy of delusions study, I'm clearly not committed exclusively to pharmacotherapy. I remain uncertain as to whether the drugs work as well as they are claimed to do, or whether their apparent superiority to psychotherapy stems in part from the fact that our methods of assessment favour drug treatments. Or, indeed, whether perhaps drug treatments could work even better than often appears to be the case in clinical practice and that we should instead be assessing whether the therapists who give them are capable of pharmacotherapy or whether drug therapy is reduced in their hands to a technical and lifeless act. I also think current practice is over-paternalistic and I would favour some move toward earlier over-the-counter availability of many of the agents in current use.

What do these interviews show? That things are very complex. If the reader is anything like me they'll find themselves agreeing fully with what's being said by both Tom Ban and Heinz Lehmann, for instance, which leaves a problem because in a sense they are saying almost the opposite to each other. The same thing comes through with John Hughes and Peter Waldmeier.

One of the themes that crossed interviews was that we have what is almost the natural closing of an epoch. Many of the companies are moving out of the field of classical antidepressants and neuroleptics and are looking at neurodegeneration. Information technology is leading to concepts like managed care and to a feedback of information on outcomes to those engaged in bringing about those outcomes – there is a closing of the loop here that is new and will have major consequences; this in turn may involve new structures and indeed entirely new professions.

Another theme concerns the nature of psychopharmacology. Looking at the history of an area, the classicists want to hear about the great men who worked at the great places but history in psychopharmacology is about the development of instruments and about commodities like chlorpromazine and chlomipramine. To date, psychopharmacology hasn't been the kind of science that has proceeded by conjecturing and refuting or by classic experiments. It has tended to be an enterprise where people have stumbled on observations and built theories *post hoc*. A small dose of a drug like ketamine or LSD can completely change one's personal world; at the same time it blows most of the scientific models we have out of the water – technology quite clearly comes first and theory later, it seems to me. Psychopharmacology has also been something that's happened very much in peripheral centres. Whether that is changing with the development of neuroscience is an important question – it's doubtful if a science can fully develop without being taken over by places like Harvard or Cambridge, who of course then tend to think they've invented it.

Also apparent, is the hostility that can sometimes exist between treatment camps. Where does this come from – shouldn't we all be delighted if we can get people well, by whatever means? There are a number of complex issues here. One is the fact that drug therapy is something that's done to you and the actual prescribing of drugs is not something that people can do for themselves. They could do it for themselves up to 50 years ago. They can still do it themselves in many parts of the world or in this part of it when they go into health food shops and that's maybe part of the reason for the appeal of health food shops. You can go in and alter your internal balance if you take a little bit of this and a little of bit of that etc. That's the way people treated medicines up to the Second World War. The emergence of more specific treatments for specific diseases has changed all that. We've set up a whole range of arrangements whereby groups like the FDA now regulate the market and the actual prescribing of drugs has been restricted to physicians. I think this issue of taking control out of people's hands is a real problem and guaranteeing the professional status of one group by conferring prescription rights on them is another. As I mentioned, the view from the regulators is unfortunately missing.

The FDA, in fact, are central to a number of themes in the book. Their policies probably facilitated the switch from dimensional to categorical models of mental illness that took place between 1960 and 1980 – categorical models fit more easily into the regulatory framework we now have for drug development. On this score one of the pressing issues at the moment is the disease concept itself – is premature ejaculation for instance a disease? It causes a lot of distress and drugs can put it right. Is obesity a disease? These issues come up in a number of different interviews but could have been pressed further.

The issue of resistance to the mechanical implications of drugs also arises – the implication that drug treatment is putting right a piece of the machinery that has gone wrong. This is present in a number of interviews but most dramatically in the case of Herman van Praag who received death threats because of his association with biological psychiatry. The fact that drug therapy and ECT have seemed to imply something like demon-worship for many people is a topic that needs further exploring. There is also the issue – stemming partly from the overuse of the minor tranquillizers – that people feel there are big, evil drug companies out there somewhere who are going to get past their defences and hook them on compounds that they won't be able to get off.

Finally, even for the advocates of pharmacotherapy, there is the Faustian pact involved in drug treatment. This comes out in the story of the introduction of anaesthesia, when a great many people seem to have felt that it was morally wrong to use anaesthesia to take away the pain that the creator had actually designed to go with childbirth, injuries or illnesses. But a further problem was that anaesthetic agents in their own right can kill, raising the question of whether it is ethically right to do something which you know exposes patients to risk? Is it ethically right to take the life of one person in order to save the lives of 99? With drug treatment there is an inevitable ethical calculus that cannot be avoided because no drug is absolutely safe. Modern medicine is founded on this ambiguity and the issue of drug-induced injury is becoming increasingly salient. It's one thing for nature to brain damage a child through whooping cough but quite another to inflict brain damage through vaccination, even though fewer children overall will suffer as a consequence. These issues are touched on in a number of interviews. The field is extremely complex: the idea of good guys and bad guys is very difficult to sustain. There's a feeling abroad at the moment, however, that what science does is it finds some loose threads at the end of the jumper and pulls them. It's going to find that it is able to unravel all of the jumper but the worry is that having done that we won't be able to re-knit it. These interviews don't reflect such perceptions. They reflect a confidence in the capabilities of science, which I suspect has something to do with the fact that the period was something of an heroic era. When we look back, the years between 1954 and 1980, with the introduction of the first psychotropic drugs, will, I believe, rank with the period between 1890 and 1914 when the dynamic therapies were introduced, as a key epoch in the history of psychiatry.

David Healy, Bangor, UK

References

Healy, D. (1987) The structure of psychopharmacological revolutions. *Psychiatric Developments*, **5**, 349–76.

Healy, D. (1996) Psychopharmacology in the New Medical State, in *Psychotropic Drug Development. Social, Economic and Pharmacological Aspects* (D. Healy and D.P. Doogan, eds), Chapman & Hall, London.

Healy, D. (1997) *The Antidepressant Era*. Harvard University Press, Cambridge, MA.

Acknowledgements

In addition to the willingness of interviewees to be interviewed, the production of this book has depended greatly on secretarial input from Beverly Evans and Jacqueline Thomas. I have also been helped with constructive feedback from a number of readers, including Tony Roberts, Tom McMonagle, Marie Savage, Dinah Catell and Ned Shorter. Publication of this book was assisted by an educational grant from Lundbeck (UK) and three of the interviews were made possible by travel grants from Lundbeck (UK) and Astra (UK).

Glossary

CINP – Collegium Internationale Neuropsychopharmacologium. This was founded in 1957 and held its inaugural meeting in 1958. A number of the interviews in the book explore the impulses and the sequence of events that led to its foundation. Information on the origins of the CINP can also be found in:

Ban, T.A. and Hippius, H. (eds) (1988) *Thirty Years CINP*, Springer-Verlag, Berlin.

Ban, T.A. and Hippius, H. (eds) (1988) *Psychopharmacology in Perspective.* A personal account by the founders of the Collegium Internationale Neuropsychopharmacologium. Springer-Verlag, Berlin.

Ban, T.A. and Hippius, H. (eds) (1994) *Towards CINP.* From the Paris Colloquium to the Milan Symposium, J.M. Productions, Brentwood, Tennessee.

ACNP – American College of Neuropsychopharmacology. This was founded in 1960. The proceedings of the foundation meeting are recorded almost *verbatim* in a fascinating volume entitled *In The Beginning: the origin of the American College of Neuropharmacology* (1990), Am. Coll. Neuropharmacol. A number of the interviews in the book refer to the foundation and subsequent development of ACNP

APA – American Psychiatric Association. In contrast to the ACNP, which is a scientific society whose membership comprises clinicians, a range of neuroscientists and pharmacologists and both clinicians and neuroscientists from within the pharmaceutical industry, the APA is a professional body whose existence is predicated on the interests of the psychiatric profession. The dynamics of both bodies therefore differ.

BAP – British Association for Psychopharmacology. The BAP was only established in 1974 – rather late as national psychopharmacology associations go. One of the reasons for the first interviews in this series was to trace the origins of the BAP. Relevant interviews and my assessment of what happened can be found in the interviews in this book with Merton Sandler and George Beaumont and also in:

Wheatley, D. and Healy, D. (1994) The foundation of the British Associ-
ation for Psychopharmacology, *Journal of Psychopharmacology*, **8**, 268–78.
Healy, D. (1996) A History of British Psychopharmacology, in *One
Hundred and Fifty Years of British Psychiatry*, vol. 2 (eds G.E. Berrios and
H. Freeman), Athlone Press, London.

RCP – Royal College of Psychiatrists. The Royal College of Psychiatrists
was only founded in 1971 but it had a previous existence in the form of
the Royal Medico-Psychological Association, which was established in
1841. The RCP is to the BAP as the APA is to ACNP. A great deal of
the history of the RCP/RMPA can be found in: Berrios, G.E. and
Freeman, H. (1991) *One Hundred and Fifty Years of British Psychiatry*,
Gaskell, London. Interviews with many of the best-known names in
British psychiatry, including figures relevant to this volume such as Max
Hamilton and Michael Shepherd, can be found in:
Wilkinson, G. (ed.) (1993) *Talking about Psychiatry*, Gaskell, London.

AEP – Association of European Psychiatrists. With the development of
'Europe', there have in recent years been moves to develop European-
wide scientific forums and professional associations. The AEP is the
European equivalent of the APA and the RCP. Its origins are touched on
in the interview with Pierre Pichot.

ECNP – European College of Neuropsychopharmacology. The ECNP
is to AEP as ACNP is to the APA, etc. except that at present ECNP is
probably more clinically orientated than ACNP or BAP. The impetus to
the development of ECNP came from Per Bech, Alex Delini-Stula and
others. The politics of ECNP have been anything but smooth to date.
 See interview with Alex Delini-Stula, and:
Healy, D. (1993) One hundred years of psychopharmacology, *Journal of
Psychopharmacology*, **7**, 207–14.

Psychiatric institutions
Quite separate from the APA and the RCP there are psychiatric
institutions geared toward research in both America and Britain. The best
known of these in America are the National Institute for Mental Health
(NIMH), along with the National Institute for Drug Abuse (NIDA) and
the National Institute for Alcohol Abuse (NIAAA). In Britain, there is the
Institute of Psychiatry which is at the Maudsley Hospital.

The neurotransmitters
Monoamines: these include catecholamines and indoleamines;
Catecholamines: these are noradrenaline, adrenaline and dopamine;
Indoleamines: serotonin, also called 5-hydroxytryptamine or 5-HT;
Peptides: the brain contains a vast number of peptides, many of which
appear to function as neurotransmitters – see interviews with John Hughes
and Arvid Carlsson.

The instruments
Spectrometer: fluorimeter; spectrofluorimeter; spectrophotofluorimeter –
the development of these is covered in Kanigel (1993), see below;
Chromatography: there are thin-layer forms (TLC) and high pressure
forms (HPLC);
Radio-labelling: this permits radioautography, radioligand binding or
receptor binding and other techniques. Radio-labelled imipramine is
sometimes referred to as tritiated imipramine;
Scanning: available techniques now include computerized axial tomography or CAT scans, positron emission tomography or PET scans, single
positron emission tomography or SPECT scans and magnetic resonance
imaging or MRI scans.

The communicators
We live in a golden age of popular science writing. Not only have there,
recently, been excellent popularizers of science, but equally this is an age
in which clinicians and other scientists have sought to communicate
directly with the public. This seems peculiarly apposite for both psychiatry
and the neurosciences, in that, unlike astrophysics or cosmology, the world
that is being investigated is we ourselves and informing the public, not
only informs the public, but also increases the pool of people who may
be able to contribute towards offering solutions to problems.

There are some excellent books from neuroscientists or about neurosci-
ence, which outline more about the role of neurotransmission and the
development of instrumentation; these include:
Changeux, J-P. (1985) *Neuronal Man. The Biology of Mind.* Random House,
New York.
Kanigel, R. (1993) *Apprentice to Genius. The Making of a Scientific Dynasty,*
Johns Hopkins University Press, Baltimore.
Levi-Montalcini, R. (1988) *In Praise of Imperfection,* Basic Books, New
York.
Richter, D. (1989) *A Life in Research,* A Stuart Phillips Publication,
London.
Rose, S. (1993) *The Making of Memory. From Molecules to Mind,* Bantam
Press, London.

In terms of contributions to drug discovery the seminal volume is:
Ayd, F. Jr. and Blackwell, B. (1970) *Discoveries in Biological Psychiatry,*
Lippincott, Philadelphia, PA. This includes pieces by figures mentioned
in these pages such as Joel Elkes, Pierre Deniker, Nate Kline, Roland
Kuhn, John Cade, Paul Janssen and Frank Berger among others.

Other accounts can be found in:
Shepherd, M. (1982) *Psychiatrists on Psychiatry.* Cambridge University
Press, Cambridge.

This includes pieces by Pierre Pichot, Seymour Kety and Eric

Stromgren. Ayd, F. J. (1991) The early history of modern psychopharmacology. *Neuropsychopharmacology*, 5, 71–84.

Lehmann, H. (1993) Before they called it psychopharmacology, *Neuropsychopharmacology*, **8,** 291–303.

See also *Journal of Psychopharmacology* in general, but especially vol. 4 issue 4 and:

Beaumont, G. and Healy, D. (1993) The place of clomipramine in the history of psychopharmacology, *Journal of Psychopharmacology*, **7,** 378–88.

Sandler, M. and Healy, D. (1994) The place of chemical pathology in psychopharmacology, *Journal of Psychopharmacology*, **8,** 124–33.

Richter, D. and Healy, D. (1995) The origins of mental health related neuroscience in Britain, *Journal of Psychopharmacology*, **9,** pp. 392–9.

Rees, W.L. and Healy, D. The place of clinical trials in psychopharmacology (in press).

History of psychiatry

Claridge, G. and Healy, D. (1994) The place of individual differences in psychopharmacology, *Human Psychopharmacology*, **9,** 285–98.

There are a number of excellent histories of psychiatry which cover the emergence of the field and the shifting relations between biological, social and psychological camps and the differing views on nosology (the science of what constitutes a disease), and psychopathology (the science of what mechanisms are disturbed to produce the manifest features of mental disturbance). These include:

Berrios, G.E. and Porter, R. (1995) *A History of Clinical Psychiatry*, Athlone Press, London.

Pichot, P. (1983) *A History of Psychiatry*, Editions Roger Da Costa, Paris.

Shorter, E. (1996) *A History of Psychiatry from the Asylums to Prozac.* John Wiley & Sons. See also:

Healy, D. (1990) *The Suspended Revolution. Psychiatry and Psychotherapy Re-examined*, Faber & Faber, London.

Healy, D. (1993) *Images of Trauma. From Hysteria to Post-traumatic Stress Disorder.* Faber & Faber, London.

Masson, J. (1991) *Final Analysis. The Making and Unmaking of a Psychoanalyst*, Harper Collins, London.

In the field of therapeutics and the interface between science and therapeutics there are:

Gorman, J.M. (1990) *The Essential Guide to Psychiatric Drugs*, St Martin's Press, New York.

Healy, D. (1987) The structure of psychopharmacological revolutions. *Psychiatric Developments*, **5,** 349–76.

Healy, D. (1990) The psychopharmacological era: notes towards a history. *J. Psychopharmacology*, **4,** 152–67.

Healy, D. (1993) *Psychiatric Drugs Explained*, Mosby Yearbooks, London.

Healy, D. (1997) *The Antidepressant Era*, Harvard University Press, Cambridge, MA.

Kramer, P.D. (1993) *Listening to Prozac. A Psychiatrist Explores Antidepressant Drugs and the Remaking of the Self*, Viking, New York.

Pernick, M.S. (1985) *A Calculus of Suffering. Pain, Professionalism and Anesthesia in Nineteenth Century America*, Columbia University Press, New York.

Swazey, J. (1974) *Chlorpromazine*, MIT Press, Boston, MA.

Valenstein, E.S. (1986) *Great and Desperate Cures. The Rise and Decline of Psychosurgery and other Radical Treatments for Mental Illness*, Basic Books, New York.

Accounts from within the pharmaceutical industry are uncommon but the following contain some assessment of the issues facing the industry:

Baulieu, E.E. (1991) *The Abortion Pill*, Simon & Schuster, New York.

Breggin, P. (1991) *Toxic Psychiatry*, St Martin's Press, New York.

Healy, D. and Doogan, D.P. (eds) (1996) *Psychotropic Drug Development. Social, Economic and Pharmacological Aspects*, Chapman & Hall, London.

Lynn, M. (1991) *The Billion Dollar Battle. Merck versus Glaxo*, Heinemann, London.

Mann, C.C. and Plummer, M.L. (1991) *The Aspirin Wars. Money, Medicine and 100 Years of Rampant Competition*, Alfred A Knopf, New York.

Dramatis personae

Pierre Pichot (Paris)
Pierre Pichot was a psychiatric trainee with Jean Delay and Pierre Deniker when they discovered chlorpromazine. He was involved in early work on putative antidepressants and other biological treatments. He subsequently conducted important studies with haloperidol and clomipramine, championed clinical trial and statistical methodology in France and became Professor of Psychiatry in Paris. He is internationally known for his work on the History of Psychiatry, having through a series of books and articles introduced many mental health professionals to the intricacies of the field and to the differences in international traditions in diagnosis and treatment. He was a founder member of the Association for European Psychiatry.

Julius Axelrod (NIMH)
Julius Axelrod worked first at the famous laboratories in Goldwater Memorial Hospital in which he, Steve Brodie and others laid the foundations for modern pharmacokinetics and pharmacodynamics before moving to the National Institutes of Health during a 'Camelot' period, when Brodie and others were laying the basis for biological psychopharmacology. He was critically involved in the discovery of the microsomal enzyme system and later amine reuptake mechanisms for which he won the Nobel prize in 1970. This laid the basis for the development of drugs like fluoxetine. Although in his 80s, he continues to work – at present on cannabinoid receptors and their ligands.

Arvid Carlsson (Gothenburg)
Arvid Carlsson's career extends from early work with Steve Brodie at NIH to the present day. He was involved in the discovery of dopamine in the brain, in establishing the importance of chemical neurotransmission, in postulating that dopamine might be deficient in Parkinson's disease and that antipsychotics might act through the dopamine system. His work was seminal to the development of the 5-HT reuptake inhibitors (SSRIs) and the first SSRI – zimelidine. His is a unique perspective on the emergence of brain science and he is still producing novel hypotheses of great influence.

Frank Ayd (Baltimore)

Frank Ayd was involved in the founding of the first international psycho-pharmacology association, the Collegium Internationale Neuropsycho-pharmacologium (CINP) and subsequently the American College for Neuropsychopharmacology (ACNP) and the British Association for Psychopharmacology (BAP). He was the first to pick up the antidepressant effects of amitriptyline, the compound that 'made' the antidepressant market. He was also involved in early assessments of Kuhn's work on imipramine and the work of Cade and others on lithium. He put together the first meeting on the history of the discovery of current treatments. One of the first biological psychiatrists, the story of how he ended up in psychiatry is a dramatic one.

Alan Broadhurst (Cambridge)

After training in chemistry, Alan Broadhurst joined Geigy Pharmaceuticals in the United Kingdom, at a time when pharmaceuticals were a relatively small sideline for the company. Then imipramine was discovered. He participated in the developments that led to its discovery and in its subsequent launch, doing a great deal to make it the reference anti-depressant. Following this he retrained in psychiatry and entered clinical practice in time to see the transforming effect of the new drugs on that practice. He thus has had the unique advantage of being able to see the development of modern psychopharmacology from all sides.

Silvio Garattini (Milan)

Silvio Garattini was one of the first pharmacologists into the field with his work on the mechanisms of action of the new psychotropic compounds. Sensing the existence of a new frontier, he organized the first international psychopharmacology conference, a meeting that was an important first step in the creation of the institutional framework within which psychopharmacology has developed. He then founded the Mario Negri Institute, an institute that is independent of both the Italian university system and the pharmaceutical industry. From this vantage point he has been an influential commentator on developments in modern psychopharmacology in recent years.

Heinz Lehmann (Montreal)

Heinz Lehmann was born in Germany but emigrated to Montreal before the Second World War. He was the first in North America to publish studies of the effects of chlorpromazine and later imipramine and he played a considerable part in advocating their subsequent use. Far from being simply a biological psychiatrist, however, he has always spoken eloquently of the need to integrate drug treatment and psychological approaches to mental disorders. He became Professor of Psychiatry at McGill and Director of Psychopharmacology. He is a Past-President of the CINP as well as of ACNP and he is currently the Deputy Commisioner for Research at the New York State Office for Mental Health. He has received many awards for his work, including in 1957 a Lasker prize.

Hanns Hippius (Munich)

Hanns Hippius came into psychiatry in Germany in the 1950s, having first trained in chemistry, just in time to participate in birth of psychopharmacology. Along with colleagues he set up the Fünfer Group and AGNP, the German Society for Psychopharmacology, one of the first national psychopharmacology associations. From early on he believed that antipsychotic activity could be produced without extrapyramidal side effects and this belief led to the discovery of clozapine, the rediscovery of which in recent years has been one of the most exciting events in the field. He was also a founding member of the CINP and in recent years has served on its history committee with Tom Ban, researching the origins of the field.

Hannah Steinberg (London)

Having qualified in psychology, Hannah Steinberg, unusually for a psychologist in the 1950s, undertook postdoctoral research in pharmacology on the effects of nitrous oxide and other compounds with psychotropic effects. She then went on to study the effects of centrally acting compounds on animal behaviour, becoming one of the first to do so. Her work led to her being made a Reader in Psychopharmacology and later to a Chair in Psychopharmacology. She was possibly the first to hold an officially designated position in psychopharmacology. She continues to work on the effects of drugs on animal behaviour, as well as on non-pharmacological means of manipulating behavioural states.

Jonathan Cole (Harvard)

At the start of the psychopharmacological era, Jonathan Cole was recruited to the position of Director for the Psychopharmacology Research Centre, a branch of the National Institutes of Mental Health that had been established on the back of funding donated by Congress for the evaluation of the new psychotropic drugs. His brief was to inaugurate the first multicentre clinical trials and to support a wide range of research across all the disciplines relevant to psychopharmacology. He subsequently moved into mainstream psychiatry taking a Chair in Psychiatry at McLean and from this position has participated in the social psychiatry developments that psychopharmacology made possible.

Alec Coppen (Epsom)

Alec Coppen was one of the first of a new generation of biological psychiatrists in the United Kingdom. He did early research on electrolytes in mood disorders and followed this up with work in 5-HT in mood disorders, becoming the first to put forward a specific 5-HT hypothesis in depression. His subsequent research included studies on the role of plasma levels in the activity of antidepressant drugs, on the prophylactic effects of lithium in mood disorders and on the role of cortisol elevations in depression. He ran the definitive study of the dexamethasone suppression test. He has held a number of high offices including the Presidency of the CINP and of the British Association for Psychopharmacology.

Jules Angst (Zurich)

Jules Angst was born in Zurich, studied medicine there and subsequently psychiatry with Bleuler and Jung. He was involved in early trials on a number of antidepressants, lithium and clozapine, and played a significant role in developing methods to analyse the possible prophylactic effects of compounds like lithium. His subsequent work on the epidemiology of mental disorders has made Zurich a world leader in this field. This work has led to the recognition of recurrent brief affective disorders. In other work he has challenged many of the myths of the field – that antidepressants couldn't be used to treat mania and the notion that treatment should be aimed at target symptoms.

George Beaumont (Cheshire)

After training in medicine, Geroge Beaumont became the medical director of Geigy UK at a time when clomipramine was being developed. His strategies to ensure a market niche for this compound led to the virtual rediscovery of obsessive – compulsive disorders, which in 20 years have gone from being almost undiagnosed to being recognized as occurring very commonly and leading to significant disability. He also pulled together the first observations of the effects of psychotropic compounds on sexual functioning, laying the basis for an entirely new area of psychopharmacology but one which remains under-explored – some of the reasons for which are developed in this interview.

Donald Klein (New York)

Donald Klein underwent a conventional analytically-orientated training in psychiatry in the 1950s. In the early 1960s, along with Max Fink at Hillside Hospital in New York, he became identified with early pharmacotherapy and conducted a number of seminal studies on antidepressants and neuroleptics. In the course of this work he first noticed and described the phenomenon of panic attacks and proposed that these have a biochemical basis. Panic attacks have since become one of the most widely recognized psychiatric conditions. He has made significant contributions to thinking about depression and to clinical trial methodology and he was one of the key players in the framing of DSM-III.

Herman van Praag (Maastricht)
Herman van Praag qualified in psychiatry in Holland at the end of the 1950s. Impressed by the new psychotropic agents he began research in 'biological psychiatry' earning himself a reputation as a biological psychiatrist at a time when such a reputation was tantamount to being thought of as being in league with the devil. His lectures were picketed and he and his family received death threats. He later worked for a decade as Head of Department at Einstein University in New York during the 1980s before returning to Holland latterly. Throughout this period he has been one of the seminal thinkers within psychopharmacology putting forward and developing a range of theoretical positions, most notably proposals for a psychiatric physiology.

Merton Sandler (London)
After training in medicine, Merton Sandler specialized in chemical pathology but unusually for a pathologist he has been most interested in the origins and fate of those neurochemicals that have been implicated in the pathology of nervous disorders and in the mode of action of psychotropic compounds. Operating from a maternity hospital, he played a key part both by virtue of his work and also his organizational style in both the ante-partum and post-partum development of British psychopharmacology and in the monoamine-oxidase story.

Floyd Bloom (Scripps)
After studying medicine, Floyd Bloom went into psychophysiological research, first at NIMH and later at Yale and then NIMH again. He subsequently became a Director of Neuroscience Research at the Salk Institute and later at the Scripps Research Institute. His primary research interest has been in the psychopharmacology of the addictions. He has written or edited several key texts which have brought psychopharmacology to a mass audience as well as some of the benchmark reference volumes. He is currently the Editor of *Science*.

Alexandra Delini-Stula (Basle)
After qualifying in medicine, Alex Delini-Stula moved to Switzerland and a career in psychopharmacology within the pharmaceutical industry, first of all with Geigy, and then later with Ciba-Geigy and Roche. She has been associated with the development of maprotiline, the first SSRIs, the RIMAs and other psychotropic compounds. Her research has spanned the development of animal models, biochemical assays, and clinical trial methodology. She was a founder member of the European College of Neuropsychopharmacology.

Gordon Claridge (Oxford)

After graduating in psychology, Gordon Claridge began his research career with Hans Eysenck, at a time when Eysenck's theories of personality and predictions as to the likely effects of psychotropic drugs on personality made him one of the foremost pharmacopsychologists in the world. Claridge subsequently laid down many of the methodological principles which now guide work in this area. He also proposed a theory of schizophrenia as a nervous type – a forerunner of the modern schizotypy concept, which has had considerable influence.

Malcolm Lader (London)

After doing his PhD at the University of London, Malcolm Lader trained in psychiatry at the Institute of Psychiatry, where he became the first British clinician to hold the post of Professor of Clinical Psychopharmacology. His initial research was on the interface between psychophysiology and psychopharmacology. He became a leading authority on the nature and management of anxiety. His subsequent interests have also included the psychopharmacology of the addictions and his name has been prominent in debates on the use and abuses of the minor tranquillizers and more recently in debates on the possible abuse of major tranquillizers.

Herbert Meltzer (Ohio)

The initial part of Herb Meltzer's career was paradigmatic of the kind of career in biological research in psychiatry that developed following the introduction of the psychotropic drugs. His early work covered the field of biological markers in psychotic and mood disorders and clinical trial work on neuroleptics and antidepressants at NIMH and in Chicago with Daniel X Freedman. In the late 1980s, his career stepped out of the ordinary. With John Kane and others he was involved in the rediscovery of clozapine and developed from this a series of hypotheses about antipsychotic mechanisms of action which have been immensely influential in subsequent drug development.

Brian Leonard (Galway)

Trained in biochemistry and later pharmacology in Birmingham when it was one of the nerve centres of British neuropsychopharmacology, Brian Leonard later worked in variety of university and industry settings before moving to Galway as Professor of Pharmacology. He was involved in the development of mianserin and has been a strong advocate of the use of animal models in psychopharmacology. He has been the President of the British Association for Psychopharmacology and Treasurer of the CINP with particular responsibility for the CINP's educational programme.

John Hughes (Cambridge)

John Hughes is the Director of Parke-Davis Neuroscience Research Centre, Cambridge and Professor of Neuropharmacology at the University of Cambridge. After training in London with the Nobel-prize winner John Vane and subsequently at the NIMH, John Hughes went to work with Hans Kosterlitz in Aberdeen. There he played the key role in the discovery of the Enkephalins, in the brain, one of the seminal discoveries in modern neuropharmacology. This work led to the award of a Lasker Prize. He has since moved from a University base to working within the pharmaceutical industry.

Peter Waldmeier (Basle)

Peter Waldmeier was born in Switzerland and after studying chemistry joined Ciba-Geigy when it was the clear world leader in psychotropic drug development. He was associated with the development of the SSRIs, the RIMAs and other psychotropic compounds. For a variety of reasons, however, few of these Ciba compounds ever reached the market – the story of what went wrong is one of the most important in this volume. He has since become involved the development of agents designed to act on neurodegenerative processes, as Ciba have moved out of the area of psychotropic drug development.

Tom Ban (Toronto)

Born in Budapest, Tom Ban emigrated to Canada in 1956, where he completed his psychiatric training at the Verdun Hospital with Heinz Lehmann and the Allan Memorial Institute with Ewen Cameron. From there he became Director of Psychopharmacology at McGill University and later Professor of Psychiatry at Vanderbilt University in Tennessee and Chairman of the History Committee of the Collegium Internationale Neupsychopharmacologium. He has written, edited or translated 40 books and published over 650 articles in the scientific press and has been one of the leading theorists in field. He now works from Toronto where he has established a multinational psychiatric corporation.

Chronology of interviews

George Beaumont: February 1993 – London to Guildford train.
Merton Sandler: June 1993 – London.
Hannah Steinberg: June 1993 – London.
Silvio Garattini: November 1993 – London.
Alec Coppen: January 1994 – Epsom.
Gordon Claridge: January 1994 – Oxford.
Alan Broadhurst: February 1994 – Suffolk.
Malcolm Lader: March 1994 – North Wales.
Floyd Bloom: June 1994 – Washington DC.
Heinz Lehmann: June 1994 – Washington DC.
Herbert Meltzer: June 1994 – Washington DC.
Tom Ban: June 1994 – Washington DC.
Julius Axelrod: June 1994 – Washington DC.
Don Klein: July 1994 – Washington DC.
Hanns Hippius: July 1994 – Cork.
Herman van Praag: July 1994 – Cambridge.
John Hughes: July 1994 – Cambridge.
Brian Leonard: August 1994 – Galway.
Pierre Pichot: November 1994 – Paris.
Peter Waldmeier: November 1994 – Basle.
Alex Delini-Stula: November 1994 – Basle.
Jules Angst: November 1994 – Basle.
Arvid Carlsson: December 1994 – Puerto Rico.
Frank Ayd: December 1994 – Puerto Rico.
Jonathan Cole: December 1994 – Puerto Rico.

Also interviewed have been:
Philip Bradley: July 1993 – Birmingham.
Linford Rees: January 1994 – Taplow.
Derek Richter: January 1994 – London.
David Wheatley: January 1994 – London.
David Sheehan: November 1994 – Nice.
Michael Shepherd: June 1995 – London.
Gene Paykel: July 1995 – Cambridge.
Isaac Marks: January 1996 – London.

1 Pierre Pichot

Psychopharmacology and the history of psychiatry

Could we begin with your recollections of the 1955 Paris meeting, which was effectively the first world-wide meeting on chlorpromazine.

The meeting was organized in Paris by Jean Delay. It was supported by Specia, the pharmaceutical firm which had produced chlorpromazine, which was a branch of the Rhône-Poulenc Group. For the first time people engaged in what was called psychopharmacology came together. They came from many countries, including the United States. Both the efficacy of the drug and the mechanism of action were discussed. However, at that time the biochemistry of the brain, as it exists now, was unknown. It was only at the beginning of the 1960s, that we began to speak of the role of the neurotransmitters in the action of both neuroleptic drugs and antidepressants and of their potential abnormalities in the disease process. So in practice 1955 was only a meeting on therapy with chlorpromazine.

I have always been very much impressed by the fact that chlorpromazine, which had been introduced only three years before, was already used all over the world. Theoretical ideas take usually a very long time to travel from one country to another and sometimes they never make it. I quote always the case of Karl Jaspers' *General Psychopathology*, which is considered in the German-speaking world as one of the basic books of psychiatry. This was published in 1913 but appeared in English translation only in 1963, 50 years later and, even then, a paper published in the *American Journal of Psychiatry* wrote ingenuously that, until this publication, many psychiatrists in the United States had not realized that Jaspers was not only a philosopher, but also a psychiatrist. It takes a very long time for theoretical ideas to travel but in the case of new techniques of obvious practical value, the transmission is very fast. It was the case with ECT and it was even more striking with the neuroleptics because at the time psychoanalysis had an extremely strong influence, especially in the United States, and psychotherapy was considered the appropriate treatment for the mental illnesses.

There was some paradox in the fact that psychodynamically orientated psychiatrists, when confronted with psychotic patients in hospitals, could admit that, after all, drugs were useful. At the beginning of the 1960s I visited Yale University, an extremely well organized Department, in which a young British psychiatrist, psychodynamically orientated, specialized in the psychotherapy of schizophrenics. The programme combined intensive individual and group psychotherapy. At the end of the discussion, I asked my colleague 'But do you use any drug?' 'Of course', he said 'we give them chlorpromazine 200 mg a day but just for facilitating the psychotherapy'.

At the 1955 meeting was the issue of who had discovered chlorpromazine an issue?

No. The meeting had been organized by Professor Delay who had published on it. It was certainly not an issue. In the case of chlorpromazine, the problem is extremely complicated. At that time, there was already a great hope about the possibility of psychopharmacology. In order to put the events in perspective, I must return to the life and career of Professor Delay. His father was a well-known surgeon in the South of France and, as fathers are, he wanted his son to become a surgeon. Professor Delay came to Paris to study medicine and, by competitive examination, became a Resident of the Paris Hospitals. At that time, this was a necessary step if you wanted later to attain an academic position. Professor Delay went through the entrance examination brilliantly – he has always been considered as one of the most brilliant physicians of his generation. His father was convinced, by one of Delay's friends, to let him to give up surgery. So he became a resident in medicine and went to neurology which was – and still is – in France, and possibly in the UK, considered an 'aristocratic' speciality, being reserved for the best medical students. At the end of his residency he became 'Chef de Clinique', a position more or less similar to that of a Senior Registrar. It's the first step in an academic career, followed eventually by the assistant professorship, and then by the full professorship. Professor Delay was Chef de Clinique at the Neurology Department of the Salpêtrière, but, at the same time, he studied psychology at the Sorbonne. All his life he had both psychological/literary and biological/scientific medical leanings. During his stay at the Salpêtrière, he was co-author of a book on EEG, an expression of his keen interest in biology and during the same period of his life, he became a PhD with a thesis on memory and its pathology. He was to write other books on psychopathological themes, especially one on mood disturbances which was relevant to his later ideas in psychopharmacology.

After leaving the Salpêtrière, Professor Delay entered psychiatry. This was a tradition in Paris. For a long time, in fact since the creation of a University Department of Psychiatry at the end of the 19th century, the Professor has been originally a neurologist of the Salpêtrière who had later specialized in psychiatry. At Sainte-Anne Hospital, the seat of the Department, Delay became assistant Professor and then full Professor and

Head of the Department. Because of his dual background he was interested in both psychopathology and in biological psychiatry. His first interest in biological psychiatry was electroconvulsive therapy, ECT, at that time the only really active biological treatment in psychiatry.

In the UK they were also using insulin coma . . .

Yes, that was also used, but it was technically complicated – there was a special unit at the University Clinic. The efficacy was at best marginal, but at that time we had nothing better for schizophrenic patients. We used a technique which came from the United States and Great Britain during the War: psychotherapy with patients whose state of consciousness had been lowered by a slow intravenous injection of amobarbital. It was called narco-analysis and was considered as combining in some ways psychological and biological components in the treatment. As soon as he became Head of the Department, Delay encouraged his co-workers to develop research in biological psychiatry. At the end of the 1940s, I was personally involved in research on amphetamines. The drug was not known to be addictive and it had been used in England intravenously in combination with amobarbital to produce abreactions, considered to be powerful therapeutic tools. During Delay's period the general concept of 'shock' – an ill-defined term which implied that a rapid change in the state of consciousness could stimulate a recovery – was widespread. One spoke of insulin-shock, cardiazol-shock, electro-shock and of other now forgotten shock-techniques and, for that reason, Delay proposed the term amphetamine-shock.

In 1950 the first World Congress of Psychiatry was held in Paris, Professor Delay being President. As I have said, the main and practically only interest in biological therapy was in shock treatments: the inventors of the three best-known techniques – Sakel, Meduna and Cerletti – presented the main papers. The same year, Professor Delay had collected all his previous publications on biological psychiatry in a book called: 'Biological Methods in Clinical Psychiatry'. This gives a good idea of his interests and of the situation existing just before the birth of modern psychopharmacology. The book contains, among others, chapters on insulin therapy, electro-shock, narco-analysis, amphetamines and, interestingly, the first mention of drug therapy as we understand it today. Delay had published with Sizaret and Deniker the year before two papers on the action of a dinitrile preparation in depressive states. Dinitriles had been studied previously in Sweden by Caspersson and shown to have allegedly 'stimulating' actions in nerve cells. Delay had various types of dinitrile derivatives prepared, and made a clinical trial with one of them. I mention this fact to give a general idea about the atmosphere. The attitude at the Clinic was that, if we tried hard enough, we would find a drug with therapeutic properties.

At that time chlorpromazine appeared. It has been synthesized at the

Specia Laboratories. They had already created a series of antihistaminic drugs, some of which, like phenergan, had been used in psychiatry because of their obvious sedative effect. But chlorpromazine had different, and much more complex, properties. After it had been synthesized, its pharmacology was studied by Mrs Courvoisier at Specia Laboratories and it was then put at the disposal of Laborit. He was a navy physician, an anaesthesiologist. On the basis of a theory of the action of drugs in anaesthesiology, he proposed to use it in a combination he called a 'lytic cocktail'. During his work he discovered and published the fact that chlorpromazine, used alone, had a very specific action. The consciousness remained normal, but the patient showed a complete lack of interest about his surroundings. Laborit suggested that because of that type of action, the drug could play an important role in psychiatric treatment. Others had also received supplies of the drug: Hamon, Paraire and Velluz, the psychiatrists at the Central Military Hospital in Paris, the Val de Grâce, and Pierre Deniker who used it at the Clinic under the direction of Delay.

They also published in 1952 and this is one of the points of discussion. There were three groups involved. There was Laborit, who made the first clinical observations, who did of course not use the drug on mental patients, but who discovered its psychotropic action and suggested that it could have a special interest in psychiatry. There was the group at the Val de Grâce, which used it on mental patients and published the first psychiatric paper, and there was Delay and Deniker whose publication came immediately after. The debate has been very heated. The Lasker prize was given in 1957 to Laborit and Deniker. Delay and Deniker have always considered that they were the real discoverers of the clinical properties of the drug. Their argument is that Hamon, Paraire and Veluz, even if their paper was the first, had used chlorpromazine in conjunction with barbiturates in manic states to potentiate the sedative properties, whereas they had used the drug alone. The American author, Josephine Swazey, a supporter of Laborit, wrote a book on chlorpromazine in which she portrayed him as the real discoverer of the properties of the drug. I have heard – but did not see the documents – that the New York Academy of Sciences made a detailed enquiry in France and concluded that Delay and Deniker were the discoverers of the clinical properties. However, the representative of the Army medical services still claim that their role was decisive.

In September 1993, a ceremony took place for the 200th anniversary of the foundation of the Val de Grâce, an old abbey which became a military hospital in 1794, during the French Revolution. A large scientific meeting was held in the wonderfully restored building and, at the end, a marble plaque was unveiled on which was inscribed: Hommage à Laborit, Lasker prize 1957, and to J. Hamon, J. Paraire and J. Velluz for their discovery, in 1952, of the therapeutic effects of chlorpromazine in psychiatry.

From 1952 on, Delay and Deniker contributed enormously to the subject, whereas Hamon and colleagues did not pursue that direction, and Laborit, not being a psychiatrist, did not work directly in psychopharmacology. The momentum came from Delay and Deniker, who had realized the importance of the new field, and in this respect they were the real discoverers. This is my personal opinion but I believe the discussions about the precise role of the various persons and groups involved have had an unfortunate consequence. I have always thought that the Nobel prize was never given for chlorpromazine, when it should have been, because of this. Only two Nobel prizes have been given for psychiatric discoveries, namely for malaria therapy and lobotomy and chlorpromazine was just as important. My impression – but it is only a guess – is that our Swedish colleagues were afraid of being involved in an argument about the roles and the priorities – they had already had bad experiences in this respect – and preferred to abstain.

Is it possible to tease their respective contributions apart? Was Deniker simply acting under the direction of Delay?

It is very difficult, not to say impossible, to tease the respective contributions of Delay and Deniker apart. As I have said, Professor Delay was deeply interested in the potential possibilities of drug therapy in psychiatry well before chlorpromazine appeared, and he encouraged his assistants in that direction. Deniker was then assistant in charge of the men's wards, and had under him as resident Harl who is mentioned in the original paper. Of course Deniker was closer to the patients than Delay – and for that matter Harl was even closer – but, just as Harl discussed the results with Deniker, so Deniker discussed them with Delay. It was certainly not a one-man job.

At the 1955 meeting, Linford Rees reported on the evaluation of chlorpromazine using a randomized clinical trial method and he recalls you asking him about the English 'obsession' with clinical trials.

I probably meant – and it is still my opinion – that in cases where the changes produced by a treatment are of such a magnitude that they appear obvious to a naive observer, we do not need statistical proof. But it is fairly ironical that Linford Rees mentioned this episode, since I was already considered in France as a strong supporter of statistics. My training had been both in psychiatry at the medical school and in statistical psychology at the Institute of Psychology at the Sorbonne. I had published a book on mental testing and I had close connections with British psychologists and psychiatrists with the same interests. The British tradition in those matters was strong, and from the beginning, I had a leaning towards measurements in controlled trials. I am more or less considered in French psychiatry as the man who has been responsible for the introduction of quantitative assessment methods, both in psychopathology and in psychopharmacology. Indeed, I have been much attacked at that time by my colleagues for taking this position.

The French attitude was the result of a serious historical development. Statistical methods were born in France with Laplace and the mathematicians of the 'Ecole Polytechnique' such as Fourier, who developed the theoretic basis and the first great medical statistician was in the middle of the 19th century, a French physician, Louis. When the Royal College of Physicians started a section of statistical medicine, about 30 years ago, the first session was, significantly, an outline of Louis' work. However, statistics later lost any prestige in medicine, probably under the influence of Claude Bernard. Claude Bernard was, of course, a great scientist but in his field, experimental medicine, where a single well-planned experiment was sufficient for a discovery, statistics were of no use. Unfortunately, in some of his writings, he ridiculed statistics. The result was that, because of his considerable influence, the medical profession took a negative view on the method. It was seen as opposed to the traditional and allegedly typically French clinical approach, which rested on the accurate observation of a single case. Statistics were confined to psychology and, in medicine, were looked down on until the Second World War.

It came back mostly through the influence of the medical publications we were receiving after the end of the War from the United States, but its progress was very slow. A few years after the end of the War, Robert Debré, at that time the most influential medical man in France, organized a meeting on clinical trials and invited French colleagues and British statisticians. The lectures of the proceedings are very revealing. Debré's idea was to promote clinical trials in France but the reactions were, on the whole, not very positive: it was only conceded with some difficulty that statistics had some place in medicine. Debré managed, several years later, to have a mathematician, Daniel Schwartz, nominated in a newly created Chair of Statistics at the Medical School. Although Professor Schwartz was a brilliant statistician of engaging personality, who had a great talent for making complicated concepts understood by people without mathematical training, it took a long time to convince the traditional clinicians of the value of the methods. It was the same in psychiatry as in the rest of medicine: statistics and controlled trials were looked down as alien to the clinical spirit.

Hanns Hippius suggests that when the drugs were first introduced in Germany they weren't of any great interest to German psychiatrists because therapy was not considered to be part of science. The use of the drugs or the interest in the drugs would have been to see what they revealed about how the mind works rather than in terms of trying to get people well. To some extent, it was a little bit the same within the UK, in the centres of excellence like Oxford and Cambridge and the Maudsley. The idea that it might be a good idea to try to get people well has come from outside the big centres. Is that the same in France?

Not to the same extent, I would say. You must remember that in France, the Paris University Clinic was considered the centre of excellence, and that Head of Department, Professor Delay, had already shown a great interest in drug therapy, as I have mentioned earlier. On the other hand it is true that, in so far as you can speak of German, French or British schools of psychiatry, the German one had always been considered in France as mostly interested in theories. Since Madame de Stäel, Germany was seen, especially in the 19th century, as a country of philosophers and thinkers, producing beautiful but sometimes obscure theories. Two years ago I wrote a paper on the history of German psychiatry as seen by the French authors of the same period. The German school had always fascinated the French psychiatrists because of its theoretical points of view, so different from the French attitude prevailing since Pinel, which was basically clinical and descriptive. Of course, the atmosphere in those relations has been influenced by external events. During the First World War, German psychiatry, as represented then by Kraepelin, was attacked violently and considered as fundamentally aggressive, as aiming at imposing its ideas on the world, as the armies of the Kaiser were doing. But, even during this short episode, the main argument used against Kraepelin – of course, wrongly – was that his concepts were of a basically theoretical nature and had allegedly no connection with the clinical facts. Even if one leaves aside the role of national stereotypes which colour the judgements on another country, it can certainly be said, as Hanns Hippius mentioned, that German psychiatry has always shown a great interest in theoretical issues and in psychopathology, whereas the French had a more pragmatic, descriptive and clinical bent. This emphasis on the clinical approach probably favoured an interest in the therapeutic methods, but was at the same time responsible for the antagonism to the controlled trial. It was claimed that a clinician could realize, better than any statistical method, if a drug was active or not.

Well, this is what Roland Kuhn would still say to this day – that he didn't need clinical trials to discover imipramine and what have all the clinical trials, done ever since, shown.

In France such an extreme position is no longer supported. It was probably originally an idea dear to many 'classical' French clinicians, but nobody would defend it today.

When the antidepressants came in they looked very different to chlorpromazine?

Yes, but they were studied first in Switzerland. As soon as they were known, they were used in France too and found to be clinically very interesting. I shall mention in this respect a curious episode. Professor Delay had formerly developed a psychopathological model of disturbances of mood – it was the title of the book he wrote on the subject. He considered that mood could be altered by being pathologically either elevated or lowered. The lowering was the central element of hebephrenia which was in the French tradition seen as the core form of schizophrenia. This point of view had already been developed in France by Guiraud, who suggested the term 'athymie' – absence of mood. On the other hand, there were states with elevated mood, the hyperthymies. They could take two different forms according to the colouring of the mood: it could be a painful hyperthymie, typical of the psychopathology of melancholia, or it could be a euphoristic hyperthymie, typical of mania.

When the antidepressants came in, their therapeutic action could be logically interpreted as a lowering of an abnormally elevated mood. Possibly under the influence of Delay's model, the first documents published by the Swiss firm Geigy, which had introduced Tofranil, described the drug as having a 'thymoleptic' action – it lowered the mood. However, since the generally held view simply opposed the elevation of mood in manic excitement to its lowering in melancholic depression – as the term depression implied – the new word 'thymoanaleptic' – meaning elevating the mood was rapidly substituted, and was used by Delay himself in a paper on Tofranil, published in 1959.

There is a 1959 paper by Delay and colleagues on izoniazid and iproniazid in which was indicated that they had the impression that izoniazid might have antidepressant properties. It seems that this work was being done around 1953/ 54 which would have been very early. What was the basis for thinking that isoniazid was antidepressant?

At the beginning of the 1950s, there was a great interest in the new treatments of tuberculosis which were tried near Sainte-Anne at the Cochin Hospital, where the Chair of Pneumology was located. Professor Delay had discussions with our colleagues there and thought that, maybe, the general well-being experienced by the patients treated with isoniazid was partly related to a psychotropic factor. He used the drug at relatively low doses with depressive patients and concluded that, especially in the less severe cases, a positive result could be observed, and he published those results in 1952 with Laine, who was then Chef de Clinique, and a resident, Buisson. On the other hand, being interested in statistical assessments, I proposed to control the changes observed in tuberculosis patients and arranged for a group of them to answer the MMPI before and after treatment by isoniazid in Cochin. The results showed obvious changes in the psychological MMPI profile. I did not publish it but they were incorporated in a paper by Delay and Buisson published in 1956. After the discovery by Nate Kline of the antidepressant action of iproniazid, Professor Delay tried the drug, and the first results were published, together with the results on isoniazid, in a paper with Deniker and Buisson in 1959.

Did the idea of antidepressant activity mean anything like what Kuhn later claimed to have discovered – namely a compound effective for vital depression or did it mean something closer to a stimulant effect?

At the time concepts such as 'vital' or 'endogenous' depression essentially belonged to the German school of psychopathology. In the UK, if you look at a book which was a classic at the end of the 1940s, the *Textbook of Psychiatry* by Henderson and Gillespie, endogenous, neurotic and reactive depression are mentioned, but there is no emphasis on the sharp distinction which you find later in the book *Clinical Psychiatry* of Mayer-Gross, Slater and Roth (Mayer-Gross, Slater and Roth, 1954), and which was imported by Mayer-Gross from the Heidelberg school. We had, in France, an even clearer situation, the words 'endogenous' and 'vital' being never mentioned. As I said before, the prevailing psychopathological view was derived from Professor Delay's book on Mood Disorders in which no mention is made of endogenous – non endogenous distinction. The result was that the antidepressants, when they appeared, were seen as acting on depression generally and not, as Kuhn suggested, primarily on the endogenous – vital type. Delay presented his position in 1957 at the second World Congress of Psychiatry in Zurich. He suggested that psychotropic drugs could be classified according to their three possible actions on the psychological functions: depressing-sedative, stimulating and finally dissociating. The first class of drugs with depressing action – the psycholeptics – included the hypnotics, the neuroleptics and the tranquillizers. The second – the psychoanaleptics – included the drugs stimulating the awareness: the psychotonics like the amphetamines, and those stimulating the mood: the thymoanaleptics or antidepressants. The third – the psychodysleptics – included mescaline and other so-called hallucinogenic drugs. From this classification it is obvious that Delay's point of view was that antidepressants were stimulants of a specific psychological element, the mood.

Where the idea of calling the neuroleptics 'neuroleptics' come from?

It was Professor Delay's idea. It means that the drug is taking hold of the nervous system and depressing it. Delay's original model opposed shock therapy to chlorpromazine. In the book I have mentioned, and also in a later one which he published with Deniker on 'Chemical therapeutic methods in clinical psychiatry' (Delay and Deniker, 1961) he held a dichotomic view opposing shock therapies which tend generally to stimulate the nervous system, and chlorpromazine, which tends to act broadly in a sedative direction. Although the word neuroleptic is now widely used in Europe, its use has been strongly opposed, especially in the United States, where antipsychotic is usually preferred.

The French, I think more than any other nationality, tend to break the neuroleptics up into different groups of compounds. In the UK we see them as being all the same – a different profile of side effects maybe but essentially they are all the same.

There have been efforts, especially by Lambert and also by Delay and Deniker, to distinguish between sedative and stimulating or disinhibiting agents, some drugs having both types of action. Of course, such distinctions have also been taken over by pharmaceutical firms for marketing purposes – just as they stress today the difference of pharmacological activities on the neurotransmitters in antidepressants – but many French psychiatrists are convinced from clinical experience that some neuroleptics are more stimulating – or disinhibiting – and some more sedative. You can find such a distinction in all recent French textbooks.

What relationship, if any, did or does athymie bear to Janet's concept of psychaes-thenia. Was he still around in 1950?

There was no direct connection. Professor Delay was of course a pupil of Janet. His book on Memory was considerably influenced by Janet's ideas and Janet wrote the foreword. But the concept of athymie has another origin. It derived in part from ideas expressed in a book written by von Monakow and Mourgue which was very influential among French psychiatrists in the late 1920s. Athymie was really created as a concept by Guiraud who was a very respected clinician at the Sainte-Anne Hospital in Paris. It has certain connections with the ideas of Bergson about the élan vital. It was later used by Delay in his general model of mood disturbances but it had no direct connections with Janet except the fact that it uses analogies with physical notions such as power, level of energy and so on.

Janet died in 1947 at the age of 88. Until the end he was very well preserved physically and intellectually. He came every Sunday to Saint-Anne where Delay gave a public lecture which had a very large attendance of young and older psychiatrists. I was, at that time, already an assistant to Delay and I remember having met him there just before his death. I was, of course, very impressed. He was a very charming old man full of humour. Showing me a book which was on a table he said 'something extraordinary has happened. There is a book, which is a marvel'. At that time Jean-Paul Sartre had published his philosophical work, *L'Etre et le Néant*, which had become a bestseller. Very few had read it, of course, but everybody had to buy it to follow the fashion. Janet added 'it is wonderful. This young boy – that was what he called Jean-Paul Sartre – is a genius. He has managed to do something which no other philosopher has managed to do – to sell metaphysics as the Americans in Chicago are selling corned beef cans'. He was probably right in a way.

You raised the question of the needs of the marketing departments shaping the concepts that get used. One of the interesting things recently is that, with the introduction of the serotonin-specific reuptake inhibitors, the SSRIs, disorders like obsessive – compulsive disorder are being – not resurrected in that they never go away – but they are being recognized as being 100 times more common than we thought. There is also a revision in our ideas of how extensive these concepts might be − in the case of OCD it's not just people who wash their hands too much, it's a much broader concept − let's say the concepts have fallen on the fertile soil of marketing needs.

Nosological entities can become very popular for many reasons − some, of course, as you mentioned, because of therapeutic reasons. It's obvious that obsessive − compulsive neurosis, as it was called formerly, has become more interesting because it was discovered that a fair proportion of cases reacted well to clomipramine. Up till then it was really one of the most horribly incapacitating mental diseases. When it was severe, the only hope was that it would react to lobotomy − which it did in a very small proportion of cases. But even then one was afraid for various reasons to use the method.

So even the neuroleptics didn't work?

Everything has been tried. There have been claims of positive results with various methods, but nothing really worked. Then clomipramine − and later the SSRIs − was found to work and so automatically there has been an expansion of interest and, of course, an expansion of the limits, especially in the United States, where things tend to be pushed to the extremes. But there are other factors in the changes of interest for special categories of disorders. Right now there is an extremely interesting situation with the problem of multiple personality. Many psychiatrists in France have doubts even about its existence. Of course in the 1900s there was a huge and picturesque literature about the subject. I became acquainted with it when I was in High School. We learned then some psychology − including its pathological aspects as part of philosophy − and I remember vividly that my textbook included descriptions of multiple personalities. Claparede wrote a book *Des Indes à la Planète Mars* about a lady who claimed to be at some periods an Indian who wrote Sanscrit, at another a Martian, and so on. Her multiple personalities were extremely picturesque. Such cases belonged obviously to the same category as the parapsychological phenomenon of clairvoyance, so popular at that time, and have probably to be considered as the result of unconscious suggestions of the observer on a suggestible hysterical personality. But they have reappeared today: multiple personality disorder is now an official diagnosis of the DSM, and thousands of cases are described in the United States.

It is, however, interesting that the ICD-10, which because of its international character is more cautious, has accepted the diagnosis because of an agreement of compatibility with the DSM, but it clearly states that such a diagnosis is not accepted everywhere. Several interpretations have been proposed to explain this rebirth. It seems to be an indirect way of reintroducing hysteria, whose name has disappeared in the DSM. The claim which is now made − that such a disorder appears generally in patients who claim to have experienced sexual abuses as children – strongly recalls the stories told to Freud by his hysterical patients at the beginning of his career, stories which shocked him very much, but which he rapidly interpreted as being fantasies resulting from unconscious wishes, and not real facts. But if historical social factors can play a role in the rebirth or in the expansion of diagnostic categories, it is true then in other cases, as in OCD, drug therapy has played a role.

Panic disorder?

Panic disorder also. Panic disorder was created in its present sense by Donald Klein on the basis of differential responses to drug therapy. He has written down in detail how he came to the idea that there were two distinct disorders in the anxiety neuroses, one of them, the acute episode he named panic, reacting to the antidepressant therapy while the other component, basic permanent anxiety, did not. It is true that the importance of a new disorder was later increased by world-wide trials of drugs, the results of which tended to influence key people. At the beginning, many French psychiatrists considered it as an uncommon disorder. But of course one finds a condition if one searches for it.

Yes, absolutely.

You must remember that before panic disorder was isolated by Klein, the word 'panic' had been widely used in the American psychiatry. Homosexual panic, which was described first in 1920 had become an official diagnostic category which lasted until 1960. It was related to a psychoanalytic perspective of the pathology and it consisted of what we would call now an acute psychotic episode. Klein's concept has, of course, nothing to do with it. But I mentioned this now forgotten episode to suggest that the idea of describing a panic disorder existed already in American psychiatry.

The latest thing to be created in this way is social phobia. In some respects this seems to be a way to bring on stream some older ideas about what some antidepressants may do, particularly the MAOI antidepressants. There's always been an idea that these drugs are in some way personality strengthening, that is not caught by conventional rating scales.

The MAOIs have always been a mystery. It is perfectly obvious that clinically there are patients who react extremely well to them and to nothing else. But nobody has been able to pinpoint in advance which patient will react. There have been a number of studies, some impressionistic, some extremely sophisticated and well controlled, but, practically no convincing demonstration of a special target for the MAOIs.

More generally, the differential clinical efficacy of the antidepressants raises unsolved problems. If you survey the controlled trials of antidepressants, using the best possible methodology and the best clinicians, practically no single study shows in a statistically significant manner that one antidepressant is therapeutically more effective than another one whereas every experienced clinician is convinced that there are differences in efficacy. The controlled studies show, of course, very significant differences in side effects, but that is a different problem. The statistically naive clinicians and the pharmaceutical companies claim that, since you cannot find a statistically significant difference between the new and the old drug, both are equally effective. But that is a false statistical way of reasoning. The only thing you can say in such a case is that you cannot disprove the null hypothesis – which is that, with the method you are using, you cannot prove that the activity of one drug is different from the activity of the other. They may be different but you cannot prove it. Such results with trials of antidepressants are in sharp contrast to the results obtained with neuroleptics, which demonstrate often significant differences of activity between drugs.

But isn't this because the companies haven't been prepared to do the trials that would test these things out?

Maybe it's partly true, although I doubt it. After all the trials are the responsibility of the clinicians. The problem lies somewhere else, probably in the methodology. Years ago, the Japanese health authorities performed what is known as a meta-analysis, combining a number of studies done there, but restricted to depressions in bipolar disorders, the idea being that there would be as pure a clinical sample as possible. Even then the results show that you couldn't differentiate the level of activity of the different drugs, although you could differentiate on the level of the side effects.

Part of the problem, I suppose, is defining where the concept of depression begins and ends. In your article in the British Journal of Psychiatry *two years ago (Pichot, 1994), you said that one of the problems we are now faced with is that it turns out that most psychiatric disorders seem to be co-morbid with other disorders.*

My opinion is that right now we are going in the wrong direction and I am not the only one who says that. The DSM, which I acknowledge as an enormous effort, is in some aspects excellent. It has improved enormously, for example, the reliability of the diagnosis. But the trend now is to define smaller and smaller entities, with the background idea that the more homogenous the picture the greater the probability that the category so defined corresponds to a real species, which will have a typical reaction to a certain drug and so on. It is perfectly obvious that it does not really work. When chlorpromazine and the antidepressants came in, the famous Dutch psychopathologist, Rumke, who was an admirer of Kraepelin, said that their action proved the rightness of the Kraepelinian dichotomy, chlorpromazine being active in schizophrenia, the antidepressants in manic – depressive psychosis. But, he forgot to mention that chlorpromazine was also active in manic states. From the beginning the idea did not really hold up and we know now that there is only a very rough correlation between drug action and our present categories of mental disorders – except, maybe, to mention a category we have already discussed, the OCD, which seems to react specifically to a precise pharmacological type of antidepressant, but even there the correlation is not perfect.

The dream of the nosologists – to describe homogenous categories corresponding to natural species – is still far away and, maybe, will never be attained. You mentioned in this respect the now very fashionable problem of the so-called co-morbidity. When one uses the present nosological categories, the level of co-morbidity is high. In no other part of medicine can you have four diseases at the same time, unless you are a very old man and you have collected a few along the way. This means that there is something wrong with the trend which has begun with the DSM-III and has been accentuated by its successors.

Where will it go? What's going to happen?

I don't know. There must be some other direction which I foresee only vaguely. The DSM destroyed the concept of neurosis because it considered it, with good reason, to be controversial. But it didn't propose anything to replace it. An interesting example in this respect is hysteria. Hysteria does not exist any more. The DSM describes dissociative disorders, somatoform disorders, histrionic personality disorders and does not connect them. I am not personally a psychoanalyst and I do not claim that there is a special psychodynamic relation between them, but the existence of a statistical link in the form of co-morbidity seems to be present. My opinion is that there will be, in the future, a trend in the opposite direction – towards bringing the present categories together in some broader wholes.

In the early part of the psychopharmacological era it seems to me that the psychiatric profession, to some extent at least, was in the driving seat. The industry came and asked us our views, etc., etc. I get the impression in more recent years, in the last 10 years or so, that we are increasingly being marginalized.

In my opinion, if you look at the history of psychopharmacology, since, say, 1964–30 years now – nothing radically new has been introduced. Perhaps the only original idea was the discovery by Japanese colleagues that a drug such as carbemazepine, used as an anti-epileptic, could be protective in manic – depressive disease. The activity of clomipramine on OCD was also something new, but the drug had been introduced in 1962. There have only been new drugs in the old classes of drugs – new antidepressants, new neuroleptics, new anxiolytics. It is, for example, admitted by most clinicians that no antidepressant is more active say than clomipramine. The new drugs have fewer side effects, or different side effects, but more or less the same efficacy.

You have spoken with Hanns Hippius, who has probably told you about clozapine, which was in some ways a very original neuroleptic and even became at the beginning an object of a theoretical discussion. Professor Delay had originally made the hypothesis that there was a direct connection between the therapeutic activity of the neuroleptics and the extrapyramidal symptoms and, of course, clozapine did not fit the rule. It had a very good efficacy but little or no extrapyramidal side effects. But, as I said, on the whole, with relatively few exceptions, the differences between the older and the new drugs are small and there lies, in my opinion, the reason why the pharmaceutical firms have been compelled to increase their efforts towards marketing. For chlorpromazine there was very little marketing. I have still in my library some of the first commercial literature on chlorpromazine. It was matter of fact and somewhat drab. But since the efficacy was so obvious, and no other drug was available, no necessity existed for what one would call today aggressive marketing. The same is true with the first antidepressants.

Yes, sure, but it seems to me that as a group, the psychiatric profession could have taken the opportunity 20 years ago to say 'look, the drugs we've got all seem to be much the same. We should be doing the kind of trials and the kind of research that would pick out which is superior or under what conditions do people respond to one rather than another' but we didn't.

I wonder if the responsibility lies on the psychiatric profession. The public research organizations in Britain, France or elsewhere had relatively little interest in clinical therapeutic research. They preferred to leave the chemical and pharmacological research on the new drugs and also the organization of the clinical trials to the industry, since the industry was naturally interested in determining the clinical efficacy and the side effects of the drugs it had developed, in order to obtain eventually its registration. It was generally hopeless for a clinician to ask for a research grant in the domain; the public research organizations considered, possibly wrongly, that it was better to direct the money into other types of research, since the industry was taking care of this domain. There have been isolated efforts.

The German Ministry of Research funded a special programme endowed with a large amount of money to study the long-term efficacy of various types of treatments such as the comparison of long-term neuroleptic, social therapy, and a combination of both, in a population of schizophrenics. But such a programme has largely remained an exception. The public research organizations have always favoured basic research such as experimental work on brain chemistry and neglected clinical therapeutic research which was left to the industry: which was primarily interested in the type of clinical research which produced the results requested by the public health authorities for the registration of a new drug. Relatively short-term comparative trials were requested although, of course, the requirements are becoming more and more stringent.

It seems possible that the change in health care in the US could change all this. I wonder if the situation we've got doesn't depend to some extent on a socialized market-place in health care. In the US, with the move towards managed health care, there are indications that the purchasers of health care will be saying to companies 'Well, is there any evidence that your more expensive antidepressants are superior'.

There is now obviously much interest in the costs of health developments. This is a very complicated field, and the cost of the drugs is just one of its many elements. There are now a number of good studies on this issue. As far as the drugs are concerned, it must be kept in mind that already the basic conditions for the registration of a new drug – and eventually, as in France – for its acceptance by the social security system – are either a greater efficacy than the existing ones, or a lower cost. But because of the scarcity of really new developments in psychiatry, I believe one of our goals should be to improve the use of what we have already, to select the best strategies of treatment. The example I gave of the German research programme shows, in my opinion, a way we must follow in the future.

Are you hopeful that we'll go down this road?

Yes, it will come, and not only in psychiatry, for a quite simple reason that in all developed countries the cost of health increases at such a rate that Governments have to do something. One of the ways – but not the easiest – is to try to find the cost of the different strategies and to chose the best with the lowest possible cost.

We don't yet have a potent European psychiatric forum. Do you think we will have one?

I hope so. I was one of the founding fathers of the Association of European Psychiatrists just at the end of the World Congress of Psychiatry which took place in Vienna, in 1983. As President of this Congress I was impressed by the weight of the American psychiatry. I have a great respect for its scientific status and I have many American friends but I became convinced that such a disequilibrium was not sound – including for American psychiatry itself which was tempted to cut itself from other schools and, by doing so, to lose the benefits of interchanges of ideas. This is the reason why I supported warmly the idea of founding a European Association. It will certainly be a long and difficult process. There is no homogeneity in European psychiatry. Of course there is no more homogeneity in American psychiatry but our American colleagues are much more efficient when it comes to working together. We, Europeans, have only been able to build jointly the Airbus but fortunately there are many positive steps in that direction. If we could coordinate our efforts – I do not say homogenize, because I firmly believe in the virtues of a diversity of opinions – a European psychiatry programme, in a broad sense, could compare favourably with the American one. It would bring advantages both for the Americans and for us. The American psychiatrists are eager to have contacts with Europe and they show it repeatedly, but the interchanges would be much easier for them if we had some sort of coordination.

Who else was involved in founding the AEP?

As far as I remember, the idea also came from Peter Berner, who had prepared the Vienna meeting, and from Leonard Singer, who became the President of the AEP. He was the Professor of Psychiatry in Strasbourg. The original idea was to start from a German – French core, just as it had started in European politics, although we had no political model, and Strasbourg had, in this respect, a symbolic view. The others were Dufour from France, Hippius, Ackenheil, Dilling, Heimann and Rein from Germany, Bobon from Belgium and Pull from Luxemburg.

Was there a problem starting up a new organization at much the same time as the European College for Neuropsychopharmacology was starting up . . .

No. The European College was created a few years later. Maybe we indirectly suggested the idea of its creation since its basic purpose was, in their specialized field, probably very similar to our own in the larger field of psychiatry. It is true that its existence created problems for us because we had our meetings every two years and they also. We made a satisfactory arrangement in order that they did not clash.

Within groups like the American College for Neuropharmacology and the BAP there's a tremendous and increasing strain between the clinical people and the basic scientists, even though these associations were begun in order to bring these two groups together.

The story did not begin with psychopharmacology. More than a hundred years ago, a new Professor of Psychiatry had to be selected by the Medical School of the University of Vienna. One of the competitors was Meynert, a world-famous neuroscientist to use a modern word. The clinicians claimed that his basic research had absolutely no relevance to the real problems of psychiatry and opposed his nomination, the result being that the University had to take the diplomatic decision of having two Chairs of Psychiatry, one for the basic sciences and one for clinical psychiatry. The situation is the same now and is even probably more sensitive. The work done by the neuroscientists is extremely impressive. I don't dispute that, but until now very little comes out of it in psychiatry in terms of concrete clinical applications.

Indeed, and ironically we've gone down the scientifically rational route of producing purer and purer drugs and all of a sudden we find that it's an old dirty drug like clozapine which is more effective.

I have been struck recently by the commercial literature on a new anti-depressant, which stressed the fact that it worked simultaneously on three different neurotransmitters, that it was impure, to quote the bizarre word you were using. I thought that it was an original marketing idea. But in our present state of knowledge we have no conclusive proof that the disturbances of the neurotransmitters which have been observed – and eventually corrected by our drugs – constitute the central biological mechanisms, whose end results are the behavioural disorders. I do not deny that they exist nor that our drugs modify them but it is possible that they are only witnesses and consequences of underlying and more basic disturbances. The concepts of 'pure' and 'dirty' drugs are based on simplistic models which, as the case of clozapine among others demonstrate, are unable to predict reliably the therapeutic efficacy. The only proof of it is given by the clinical trials. At the present time a large gap exists between the scientifically impressive discoveries made on the neurotransmission mechanisms and the facts we observe at the clinical level. The same can be said about genetics. Thanks to molecular biology we have made tremendous progress in other fields of medicine, for example, in neurology, but in psychiatry, we are only able to entertain hopes and the results remain disappointing.

I have the impression that many neurobiologists realize now that their theories and the results of their research did not have the clinical relevance they expected. I, of course, hope that they will become relevant in the future. But for the time being it has, as you mentioned, created a tension in groups where there are both clinicians and neurobiologists. An additional factor is, of course, the technical aspects of neurobiological methods which have become so complex that clinicians like myself are usually unable to grasp their detail. They only try to understand the conclusion in so far as it has relevance to clinical problems.

When did you begin to become interested in the history of psychiatry?

I have always been interested in history. But, when you get older, you usually get more involved possibly because it allows you to put things in perspective, to discover that ideas you had thought were new had been defended before. It does not mean that nothing changes, as the French proverb 'plus ça change, plus c'est la même chose' implies. It would be a nonsense to say that psychiatry has not made any progress. Coming back to neuropsychopharmacology, it is fascinating to look from an historical point of view at its introduction. It is obvious now that it has been, in practice, responsible for an enormous improvement in the care of mental patients. I remember Sir Aubrey Lewis writing in the days of its birth, that if we had to choose between drugs and social therapy, the drugs would go. Nobody can contest the positive role of social psychiatric measures, but it seems historically clear that the primary role has been played by psychopharmacology and that many of the social measures have been made possible by it. What is fascinating in such interpretations is the discrepancy between the objective facts and the theoretical explanations which are obviously not satisfactory.

Not even satisfactory. There's no theoretical background. These things aren't actually derived from any theory at all.

It is also largely true in the discovery of new drugs. A Swiss pharmacologist said once that animal psychopharmacology was a retrospective science. Once you had discovered a drug which clinically worked in a certain way, say as a neuroleptic, the pharmacologists searched for other drugs which had the same profile on a battery of animal tests. With such a method you could not hope to find a new drug whose therapeutic action was based on a biological mechanism different from the original one. The search is based on empirically observed correlations, not on any theory.

As regards the antidepressants, you have had an overview of how they've been introduced. You've known all the key players, Kielholz and others.

Paul Kielholz was already a personal friend before the birth of psychopharmacology. He didn't have a role in the introduction of the antidepressants but mainly in promoting their use among the non psychiatrists, especially in general practice. Initially, there was a strong resistance of the general practitioners for two main causes. The first was that the teaching of psychiatry was a very small part of the medical training and consequently a general practitioner had practically no serious clinical knowledge about depression. It may be added that if they had some, it was usually about the most severe melancholic type and not about the minor forms, by far the most common among the patients they were seeing. The second cause was their fear of side effects. At that time the usual antidepressants were tricyclics and they had cardiovascular side effects, and, perhaps more importantly from the point of view of the practitioners, atropinic side effects such as dryness of the mouth, dilatation of the pupils or trembling, which can be very unpleasant. The result was that, even if by chance the correct diagnosis was made, the practitioner tended to prescribe anxiolytic drugs, usually benzodiazepines even if it was completely inappropriate. The main role of Kielholz has been in promoting a correct diagnosis and a correct treatment of depression in general practice.

Historically, another key player was Walter Poldinger. He was an assistant of Kielholz, became his successor at the Chair of Psychiatry in Basel, and has just retired. I discovered his role in a curious way. Some years ago a symposium was organized in Paris to commemorate the 20th Anniversary of the introduction of clomipramine and I was asked to preside at the meeting and to give the introductory lecture on the history of the drug. I did an extensive bibliographic search and discovered that the first clinical trial had been made by Poldinger who presented the results at the World Congress of Psychiatry in Madrid in 1966, but the paper was not published in the proceedings. I asked Poldinger about it, but he had no copy. Fortunately, there was, shortly afterwards, a symposium organized by Geigy-UK and the Chairman, George Beaumont, who was the medical director of the company, gave a detailed introduction in which he reported the contents of Poldinger's paper.

The story of clomipramine contains many curious episodes. For example, its synthesis was made by the biochemists of the Geigy Laboratories on the basis of an analogy of dubious scientific value. They reasoned that since chlorpromazine was more effective than promazine as a neuroleptic, clomipramine would be more effective as an antidepressant than imipramine. They were, at the same time, afraid that it would be more toxic but they took the risk and it worked.

If you asked the psychiatric profession generally which was the most potent antidepressant, they would probably pick clomipramine, even though there's no real evidence.

I absolutely agree. Any clinician who has worked with clomipramine is convinced of it but we are unable to present what is considered today a scientific proof. I still remember a patient taking part in our initial trial with clomipramine. She was resistant to imipramine and responded overnight to the new drug. There are many such anecdotes, but by our present standards, they prove nothing. A criticism one can make to the controlled trials is that they have been unable to demonstrate a statistically significant superiority of clomipramine.

Is it because we haven't done large enough trials, like the Isis trials in medicine? We haven't done this.

I don't agree. If you need a sample of say 10 000 patients to prove a difference, the difference, even if it is statistically significant, has no practical interest. If the present conviction of the clinicians on the greater activity of clomipramine rests on observed facts, then the difference must be large enough to be detected on a normal sized sample.

Is it because we've got heterogenous groups of depressives?

It is an obvious idea. But, as I have mentioned, the meta-analysis made in Japan using only bipolar disorders did not bring conclusive results. We believe that depressions in bipolar disorders constitute a homogenous group, but maybe we are wrong. My opinion is that we have not yet a satisfactory nosology of the depressive states and possibly also no good instrument for the measurement of the intensity of depression.

What about if we were to try and give up our ideas of trying to find the molecular biology of schizophrenia or depression and tried to look at the molecular biology of responsiveness to particular drug groups?

Some psychiatrists have hoped to base nosology on responses to drug.

Sometimes it seems to work. I have already mentioned the work of Donald Klein on panic disorders. At the present time there is a trend to re-group trichitillomania, nail biting, and similar illnesses with OCD on the basis of their response to SSRI treatment.

From a theoretical point of view it's very nihilistic isn't it? Recently, Herman van Praag, who's been very much associated with biological psychiatry, looking at dimensions of behaviour and trying to associate them with particular neurotransmitters, has taken a position that's rather like the position that Adolf Meyer took, over half a century ago, saying that what we've got in psychiatry is a series of reaction formations.

I am in agreement with most of the present ideas of van Praag on nosology as developed recently at the AEP meeting in Copenhagen. His evolution in this respect is striking because in his previous work on antidepressants he supported the notion that two categories of the disorder existed, each being associated with a specific anomaly of neurotransmission and therefore responding to a pharmacologically specific type of drug.

Who have been the key figures in the last 40 years? What we've been focusing on up till now has been the forces that shaped the period, but it's also interesting to speculate as to whether things would have gone the same way without certain key personalities.

It is an extremely difficult question. The importance of the role played by personality can only be judged after a sufficient period of time has elapsed and, even so, there can still be disagreements as every student of history knows. Everybody would agree that Freud has played an important role in the shaping of many modern ideas. But look at the conflicting opinions about the impact of psychoanalysis on our present psychiatric concepts. At the beginning of this century, Kraepelin had, in my opinion, a decisive influence on psychiatric thought. In France, in the generation before mine, it is clear that the two most influential people were Jean Delay and Henri Ey. The problem is more complicated in Germany because of the gap created by the War. Looking at the just retired personalities, Hanns Hippius and Hans Hafner, each in their own way, had a leading role. In the UK it is obvious that, since the end of the War, and for 20 years, Sir Aubrey Lewis has been a key figure. His role has been discussed but nobody can dispute the extent of the influence he had. I could also mention the contribution made by Willy Mayer-Gross who, through the textbook he wrote with Slater and Roth, introduced to British psychiatry ideas stemming from the Heidelberg school.

Max Hamilton?

Max was a very close friend. He used to point out with his well-known sense of humour that we had the same scientific training, both in psychiatry and in statistics, but he added: 'Look at the result. You are now the Professor in Paris, and I am at this dirty English town'. Max has certainly been influential, but not in the same way as Sir Aubrey or Mayer-Gross. His scale is now criticized on technical grounds but it was the right instrument when he created it. It is striking that, although we are now aware of its deficiencies, nobody dares to abandon it, even if, in modern trials, other scales are added. It has taken the value of a symbol, just as in another field in the BPRS (Brief Psychiatric Rating Scale) has.

I should have mentioned in the Scandinavian countries the name of Eric Stromgren, whose position was unanimously recognized. But he was not directly involved in psychopharmacology, mainly in psychopathology and in genetics. In Denmark I want to mention Schou because a comparison of his work with what Hanns Hippius has done illustrates the difficulty of comparative judgements. Schou's studies have concentrated on a single, but very important subject, lithium, whereas Hanns Hippius has acquired great merits in promoting, against strong resistances, psychopharmacology in the whole of Germany. And despite these differences, both are undoubtedly key historical figures in the history of drug treatments.

In the United States where, because of the number of people involved, a choice is more difficult than in the European countries. I would select Nate Kline. He had a decisive role at the beginning of the new therapeutic era by discovering the unexpected psychotropic action of new drugs. Thanks to his activity, to his optimism, and to the expansiveness of his personality, he became in his time the best internationally known American psychopharmacologist.

What about the larger questions of how the production of drugs that affect behaviour influences the culture – which brings us to the agenda of people like Julien Offray de La Mettrie, who put it that "once the physician can reliably influence behaviour, he will replace the philosopher'.

Since I am not a philosopher myself, I shall not discuss the opinion of La Mettrie, which has of course to be considered in the context of the period in which it was written. It was "l'ère des Lumières' and the word philosophy was used constantly. The title of Pinel's book on mental diseases was *Medico-philosophical Treatise on Mental Insanity*. The problems raised by today's drugs have always existed. I accept that we have more possibilities now and our drugs are more effective – and so the social consequences can be different, probably more complex – but fundamentally the situation is not new. Of course, we now have, for example, the case of the consumption of anxiolytic drugs. But basically it brings us back to the definition of the concept of a disease and of its limits. There is no really satisfactory definition. Take the case of the so-called sociological definition, so important for psychiatry. There is now a trend in the DSMs to consider as mental disorders – the modern nosologies are careful to use disorder instead of disease because its definition is even more vague – behaviours like pathological gambling. But gambling is a fairly common behaviour. The DSMs consider this behaviour as pathological if it interferes negatively with the social adjustment of the subject: a typically sociological definition of the limits between normality and pathology. The discussion on the socially defined disorders in psychiatry goes back to Esquirol when he described, more than 150 years ago, the monomanias. How can we prove that a behaviour recognized by society as negative, such as stealing, or provoking a forest fire, or for that matter ruining oneself gambling, belongs to medicine by being called kleptomania, pyromania or pathological gambling. The whole problem of the definitions of mental disease is a subject which has been dealt with in an excellent paper by Kendell (Kendell, 1975).

But all of that was worked out against the background of the psychotic disorders, the diseases that are found in hospitals. With the SSRIs do we need to rework these definitions for the population at large?

All the discussions about the limits of disease in psychiatry have started when psychiatrists began to treat patients outside the hospitals. There's a universal agreement also in the so-called primitive societies, that somebody who presents manifestations which would be called in modern terms an acute schizophrenic episode, is insane. Even the ethnologists who defend a relativistic position recognize that in all cultures some types of behaviours are considered pathological and it refers roughly to the psychotic states treated in hospitals. The problem of the limits is raised by the other and less severe deviations. Zarifian has recently written in France a controversial book on the subject. He analyses and condemns the trend to use drugs, according to him under pressure of the industry, for people who have only ordinary life problems and therefore are not 'ill' in the medical sense.

On the other hand someone like William Osler said 100 years ago 'human beings are the animals who self medicate'. The drive to take drugs comes from us. In a sense, we create the pharmaceutical industry to supply our needs rather than the other way around.

There is in my view a fundamental difference between people taking something spontaneously and doctors prescribing it. If we prescribe a drug, as physicians, we consider that the people to whom we give it are ill. We judge that they have some kind of pathology. If somebody drinks alcohol because he is sad, that is something completely different.

But let me give you the case of if they go into the health food shop and they buy vitamins or whatever; they do so because they've got a lay concept of disorder of some sort, a humoral model – Yin and Yang being the current fashion. Now with drugs, like the SSRIs, becoming safer and safer, they could be sold over the counter. You could remove the physician. This would seem to me to pose the possibility of a change in the concepts of mental illness completely. If the industry started to sell directly to the consumer would we revert to more humoral types of concepts?

It is true that in some cases drugs are becoming relatively safer, but there are obvious limits. It has been said that side effects are the price we must pay for efficacy. Without pushing this argument too far, it must be remembered that even the vitamins can be harmful when taken in the wrong way. We have seen it during the last War when mothers gave enormous doses of vitamin D to their children and provoked kidney troubles. We have always, in such discussions, come back to the concept of disease. To take spontaneously something to make you feel better if you are not ill in a medical sense is basically different from receiving from a doctor a prescription and taking a drug to improve your state of health. A doctor has no right to prescribe if he does not consider the state of his patient to be pathological.

I am perfectly aware of the difficulties involved, especially, but not only, in psychiatry. From its beginning and until now psychiatry has adopted the medical model: even if we call them now disorders, we consider the states we treat as diseases. There are, of course, people who consider that psychiatry does not belong to medicine, and that there are no psychiatric diseases. It was the position taken by some exponents of the anti-psychiatric movement. But, if we adopt the medical model as we do now, and as I believe we must do, we must look at the question of the use of drugs from the medical point of view – that is that the use of drugs is only appropriate to prevent or to treat a pathological condition. It is completely different from taking a product for your personal comfort or pleasure.

But in the UK you can get H-2 blockers for heartburn and ulcers over the counter, you don't need to go to a doctor.

Today the rules defending the drugs which can be sold over the counter are made by Governments and are, at least in part, related to the fact that in our countries the State supports the cost of medical treatment. Confronted with the increase of this cost, it authorizes the over-the-counter sale of drugs whose use is considered as not belonging to the treatment of 'real' diseases, and in such a case it is not financially involved. The health authorities have coined in France the word 'comfort drugs'. We are coming back again to the definition of the limits of pathology. The State, being financially involved, decides the limits. What we have here is to do with a typically social definition of the concept of disease. If you get older and need glasses to read, the cost in France will be reimbursed by the social security system to a very small extent, which is equivalent to saying that presbyopia is not a disease.

But this comes back to the social engineering element of it, in that it is clearly useful for society to give you a pair of glasses that improves your eyesight. The same arguments have been made about the SSRIs — without them people are myopic, on them life suddenly looks much much better and clearer.

Even if you are a perfectly normal person, you may feel better by taking a small quantity of alcohol.

But headaches and aspirin. This is presumably closer to an illness but the treatment is in my own hands. I can go to the pharmacist and . . .

Yes. But the sales over the counter depend on a combination of general factors. One, I have mentioned, is the link between disease and discomfort; another and very important one is safety. Aspirin has for a very long time been considered as a purely symptomatic analgesic drug — that is a comfort drug — without important side effects. But we now know that taken regularly at a low dose it has a protective effect against cardiovascular diseases We know also more about its side effects. It can provoke haemorrhages in the digestive tract and, at very high doses as it is sometimes taken for suicidal purposes, death by kidney failure. For that reason it is a common saying among the pharmacologists that, if aspirin had been discovered in our days, it would never pass the stringent tests requested by the FDA. This is, of course, a good story, but I doubt that it has any sense. Considering the extent of its consumption, aspirin is a remarkably safe drug and it is the reason why it is still sold over the counter.

Do we not have an issue of whether we are prepared to trust the populace with their own health care? One might argue that the situation is rather like the situation we had about trying to decide whether to give people the vote 100 years ago, with some people saying no you can't really trust people to make sensible decisions. In the same way we now say you've got to keep control in medical hands, but if you go to Asia, almost all the drugs short of the cancer therapies are sold over the counter. And people presumably learn how to manage the system.

But in the countries of Asia you mention the death rate is much higher than in ours. I would suggest, instead of your provocative comparison with the vote, to use a more relevant one. People, provided they have the money, can eat the food they want. It is clear that many do not make sensible decisions. Some statisticians claim even that in the western countries life expectancy could be increased by five years if people had a correct diet, if they had made the right choices of food. If the people need to be informed, as they are fortunately more and more now, by the specialists on the types and quantity of food, it is right to take steps to preserve their health, the same can be said about the drugs used to treat illness. There is, however, a difference. Whereas the choice of food is only related to the general purpose of maintaining health, the choice of drug is related to a specific situation, the existence of an illness. People without the special medical competence acquired by long training are, in most if not in all cases, unable to determine the nature of their illness and the right drug to treat it. If they are often unable to make the relatively simple choice of the food which is right for the maintenance of their health, how could they be able to make the much more difficult choice of a drug? The trend to self-medication is not new, but I consider that to support it is basically harmful. Social forces may favour its extension and some sociologists may claim that physicians are opposed to this in order to preserve control – but to approve of drugs to be sold without medical advice and control would be, for our part, a completely irresponsible attitude.

Can you account for the general hostility there is to psychotropic drug treatment? This was most clear in the States when these drugs were introduced but there is still a widespread popular prejudice that talking is the appropriate treatment for human beings in distress. I fancy that such attitudes are not without links to several of the big controversies in neurobiology such as the controversy at the turn of the century as to whether neurones were continuous or contiguous and the controversy during the late 1940s and early 1950s as to whether transmission in the nervous system was chemical or electrical. There's generally been a resistance to a particulate view of things and perhaps to the mechanical implications of such a view. Being particularly fanciful, one could suggest that there are connections all the way back to La Mettrie, when he proposed a radically material view of man and drew down the hostility of virtually everyone on his head and found himself consigned, more or less, to oblivion. Am I being too fanciful or are there other explanations?

There are, in my opinion, two distinct problems. One, very simply, was the initial hostility of the psychiatrists who were psychoanalytically trained, and who had a dominating position especially in the United States when psychopharmacology appeared. They claimed that the drugs had only a symptomatic action, and did not really cure the patients as they did by allegedly reorganizing the personality along normal lines. The same hostility and the same arguments existed when behaviour therapy appeared, especially in France among the clinical psychologists who were, contrary to the situation in the UK, usually psychoanalytically orientated. But it belongs now to the past. Another problem is the hostility of the general public which has, as shown by many researchers on the popular concept of disease, a model about the causes of the disease and about the method for preventing and curing them. In psychiatry, the basic idea is that mental disorders are of the same nature as normal psychological reactions, that they are the result of psychological or social causes, and consequently that they are best treated by psychological or social measures. The present fad for so-called natural food is possibly another expression of this popular model of disease. In this respect our drugs, which are the result of chemical syntheses, being non natural, must be harmful. It is probably one of the main ingredients of the resistance of many people to pharmacological treatments.

Many of those that I've interviewed, particularly people from Europe, when asked about the climate of hostility to drug therapy have cited the movement that led to the events of 1968. When I think of 1968 I think mainly of what happened in France and hence I wonder whether you might be interested to comment on the events of 1968 and the relationship to trust or distrust in the idea of scientific progress. In some respects maybe this question comes back to La Mettrie's L'Homme Machine *but whereas La Mettrie was all for scientific progress, since 1968 perhaps the idea of* L'Homme Machine *has not been received sympathetically.*

There is no good explanation of the origin of the 1968 events in France or, if you prefer, there are too many brilliant ones proposed, from the murder of the father suggested by the psychoanalysts, to André Malraux's crisis of civilization. But whatever the causes, one of its expressions has been obviously the dream of a golden age, where life would be free, without obligations and control, in a world allowing a supposedly natural life. Since you mention the 18th century author La Mettrie, I would suggest that some of those 1968 attitudes had more to do with a concept of the same period, the myth of the good savage, who was supposed to live a harmonious, natural life. I think that, if one wants to find a relation between the popular hostility to drug therapy and the 1968 events, one has to consider that in both cases a contrast is affirmed between the natural things which are intrinsically good, and the others, represented by the industrial civilization and its products, the drugs, which are bad.

Select bibliography

Delay, J. and Deniker, P. (1961) *Méthodes Chemothérapiques en Clinique des Médicaments Psychotropes*, Masson, Paris.

Kendell, R.E. (1975) *The Role of Diagnosis in Psychiatry*, Blackwell, Oxford.

Mayer-Gross, W., Slater, E. and Roth, M. (eds) (1954) *Clinical Psychiatry*, Ballière and Tindall, London.

Pichot, P. (1982) *A Century of Psychiatry*, Editions Roger Da Costa, Paris.

Pichot, P. (1982) The diagnosis and classification of mental disorders in French-speaking countries. *Psychological Medicine*, **12**, 475–92.

Pichot, P. (1994) Nosological models in psychiatry. *British Journal of Psychiatry*, **164**, 232–40.

2 Julius Axelrod

The discovery of reuptake

It may be of some interest to you that I actually began my research in psychopharma-cology working on 5-HT reuptake into platelets and so I came across your work very early on and so I'd love to hear about how it all came about – how you stumbled on the idea of amine reuptake. We probably should begin though with how you entered the field and we can move forward from there to what you've done since.

I was born in New York from immigrant parents. My mother's side came from Vienna and my father's side from Poland. I was raised on the Lower East Side of Manhattan. It was a Jewish ghetto at that time. There had been a tremendous influx of immigrants who arrived around the beginning of the century. I was born in 1912 and I was raised in an impoverished neighbourhood but it was colourful and lively, mostly of a Yiddish culture. My parents were poor. They were barely literate, well at least in English. They were fairly well cultured in Yiddish. I went to a public school where there was a spectrum of students. Some were almost illiterate, some literate, some wound up in jail, some became fairly distinguished. I then went to Seward Park High School on Lower East Side. I wanted to go to Stuyvesant High School where the bright kids went but I didn't make it.

Why not?

Oh I don't know. I just wasn't good enough. The High School I went to though was not too bad. It had a number of interesting graduates, mostly entertainers – Zero Mostel, Walter Matthau and Tony Curtis, who were actors and Sammy Cahn the composer – but no great scholars. I read a great deal when I was young. All kinds of books. The books that interested me most and gave me a feeling of what I'd like to be were two books, one by Sinclair Lewis, *Arrowsmith*, and the other was *The Microbe-Hunters* by Paul De Kruif, which was about the lives of the bacteriologists Pasteur, Ross and people like that and how they made their discoveries. My dream was to become a doctor, a research physician. I went to City College, a free college in New York City. If there hadn't been a City College, I don't think I could have afforded to go to College. It was a fairly selective school. You had to have high grades. I think it was an important influence on its students, mostly Jewish. It was highly intellectual and it graduated nine future Nobel laureates.

They were poor kids who were very bright. When I graduated from City College, I applied to several medical schools but couldn't get into any. At that time there were quotas for Jewish students; many of them were very bright and there were too many Jewish students applying for the limited number of places. I wasn't in the top echelon. My grades were good but they weren't extraordinarily good. I graduated from City College in 1933, during the depths of the Great Depression.

There were very few jobs and I decided to take an examination for a position with the Post Office, which I passed. At the same time, I was offered a position in a laboratory at New York University, which paid $25 a month, to help a fairly well-known biochemist, K.G. Falk. I got an offer for the position in the post office and I had to make a fateful decision. I decided to take the laboratory position. That decision was very crucial to me. I assisted Dr Falk in his research on enzymes in malignant tissues.

In 1935 I decided to get married and I needed to make more money. A position opened up for me in a non-profit laboratory to test vitamins in foods. Vitamins were a big thing in the 1930s. I remained there until 1945. The laboratory work was fairly interesting. I thought I was set for life testing for vitamins. I spent most of my time modifying methods which was important to my future career.

At that time very few people worked in research. To do research then you had to be wealthy and smart or a physician who did research in his spare time. I had no idea about doing research but in the laboratory we had periodicals like the *Journal of Biological Chemistry*, which I read, so I had a sense of what was going on in biochemical research. In 1946, the Head of the laboratory was a retired professor of pharmacology, George Wallace, who was also one of the editors of the *Journal of Pharmacology, Experimental Therapeutics*

That's about the most prestigious journal.

Yes, it was. And he came to me one day and said 'Julie I have an interesting proposition for you. A group of manufacturers of analgesic drugs are having problems. Some people taking the non-aspirin analgesics acetaniline or phenacetin have come down with methaemoglobinaemia. Would you like to work on this problem?' I said 'I'd love to but I have had no experience in research of this kind'. He told me that there was an associate of his, Bernard Brodie, working at Goldwater Memorial Hospital in New York and he advised me to go and see him and discuss the problem.

This was 1946. I remember the day – it was Lincoln's birthday February 12. I telephoned Dr Brodie and he invited me to visit him. He was working at Goldwater Memorial Hospital, in a unit associated with New York University. It had been set up during the war to test anti-malarial drugs. The Japanese had cut off the supply of quinine and the US had to develop new antimalarials. Goldwater was devoted to clinically testing new synthetic antimalarials. The head of antimalarial research at Goldwater was James Shannon. He was instrumental in later making the NIH what it is now. He was an MD working on secretory mechanisms in the kidney. During the War he was asked to set up a clinical laboratory testing the new antimalarials that were being synthesized. One of his great qualities was that he had a good nose for picking people. What he did was call up the professors of pharmacology throughout the country. 'Send me your best people', he told them. And they did – of course it was either that or going somewhere in the Pacific. So Shannon picked Brodie to do research on the physiological disposition and metabolism in man of the synthetic antimalarials.

Brodie was born in the UK, wasn't he?

He was born in Liverpool. He spent his youth in Canada. He was a graduate of McGill. He was an interesting and colourful person. Somebody told me he had been a boxer and also that at one point he had earned his living by playing poker.

He was 40 years old, when I first met him, 6 years older than me. But to me he was of a different generation. What he did was really revolutionary for that time. He measured plasma levels of drugs. And to do that he devised methods to measure the antimalarial drugs. There was a series of germinal papers that he published in the *Journal of Biological Chemistry*, with his close associate Sidney Udenfriend. To get back to my problem, I called Brodie up. Everyone called him Steve Brodie. There had been a Steve Brodie who lived in Brooklyn and one day he said to some people in a bar that he could jump off the Brooklyn bridge if anyone wanted to bet him. He did and survived. They called Bernard Brodie, 'Steve' because he was always prepared to take a chance.

You have to remember, when I visited him at that time, all I had was a masters degree in chemistry. While I worked in the food testing laboratory, I had taken a masters degree in the evenings after work at New York University. I came to Brodie with the problem of the toxicity of acetanilide. He told me that drugs or foreign compounds are transformed in the body. I vaguely knew this but this was an important piece of information for me. He suggested that it was possible that these analgesic drugs were transformed into toxic metabolites. I put the structure of acetanilide on the blackboard. We conjectured that it was possible that one of the metabolic transformation products would be deacetylation to form aniline. I looked up the literature and found that aniline could cause methaemoglobinaemia.

One of the most important things that I learnt that day was to ask the right questions and not only to ask the right question but know how to answer these questions – to have the right methods. Dr Brodie then invited me to spend some time at Goldwater to find out whether we could find aniline in the blood or the urine after acetanilide. We had to develop very sensitive methods to measure aniline. Brodie was one of the world's experts in developing methods because of the antimalarial research. We soon developed a method for measuring aniline (Brodie and Axelrod, 1948a) and sure enough when we took acetanilide – myself and others – we found traces of aniline in the urine (Brodie and Axelrod, 1948b).

We also developed a method for measuring it in the blood and we found it in the blood after taking acetanilide. We showed that there was a direct relationship between the amount of aniline in the blood and methaemoglobinaemia. Brodie and I solved that problem – it didn't take us very long. I just loved doing it; I'd never had experience of doing this kind of thing – particularly with a charismatic person like Steve Brodie.

There are mixed views about him.

He had charisma but he also had a lot of other problems but that is something else. He was very stimulating. He was almost magnetic. He fired you up. It wasn't just me, he did it to many people. So here I was really doing important work. We found that aniline only represented a few percent of the metabolic product; most of acetanilide was metabolized to something else. We looked for other metabolites of acetanilide and we found a compound which we identified as N-acetylparaminophenol. Brodie had this compound tested for analgesia and it was just a good an analgesic as acetanilide.

So you guys had a new drug then?

Yes, it is now called acetaminophen, commonly known as Tylenol. We recommended when we first wrote about it in the literature (Brodie and Axelrod, 1948b) that it should be used as an analgesic. Well, it took off. Anyway, I just loved doing research. I worked on the metabolism of antipyrine and phenacetin. I published many papers with Brodie but I got only one senior authorship, although I initiated and did most of our work. And I realized that I had very little chance getting any place in an academic institution with a masters degree. I needed a PhD. I was married with two children. Either I didn't want to or was afraid it would be too difficult to get a PhD. I didn't want to think about it.

I saw an item in the *New York Times* – Dr Shannon had been appointed the Director of the National Heart Institute in Bethesda. I wrote to him for a position and he offered me one. He also persuaded Brodie to come to Bethesda and when I went there I was assigned to Brodie's laboratory. I worked for a year or two and then I was offered a position in a drug company. When I told Brodie I would like to leave, Dr Brodie asked me what would make me stay. I told him that I wanted to do my own research. Brodie agreed and asked me to stay.

The first problem I worked on was the metabolism of caffeine. Nobody knew anything about what happened to caffeine in the body. I published the first report on its fate. I also became interested in a group of compounds called sympathomimetic amines, and I worked on the metabolism of ephedrine and amphetamine and published the first report on their metabolism.

At that time there was one problem that intrigued pharmacologists, which was how did the body know how to transform all of these synthetic compounds? There must be endogenous enzymes and I became very interested in this problem – this has been written up in a book called *Apprentice to Genius* by Robert Kanigel (see Glossary). It's about Brodie, me and Sol Synder. I also have a written prefatory chapter in the *Annual Reviews of Pharmacology and Therapeutics* in 1988 (Axelrod, 1988). Anything you miss now, you can find in these publications.

So I got interested in enzymes that metabolize drugs. I had a benchmate, a brilliant guy, Gordie Tomkins, who gave me a lot of good advice on enzyme research, which led to me finding a metabolite of amphetamine in a liver slice. I then found that ephedrine was also metabolized by a liver enzyme but in a different way. I wanted to find out more about this enzyme. I won't go into details but I found that there was a new class of enzyme that was present in the microsomes of the liver that required NADPH and oxygen. These enzymes metabolized both ephedrine by demethylation and amphetamines by deamination and I knew then that I was on to something very important (Axelrod, 1955a; Axelrod, 1955b).

I submitted two abstracts on the enzymatic metabolism of amphetamine and ephedrine for the usual meeting of the American Society of Pharmacology and Therapeutics. Brodie saw these later and was upset. He knew it was an important discovery and he set the whole laboratory to work on this problem. I hate to tell you this, I owe a great deal to Brodie, but this was something that upset me very much. Brodie wished to write a paper on this group of enzymes, the microsomal enzymes, as they are called now, with himself as the senior author.

I now thought I had to get my PhD and leave Brodie's lab. To get a PhD I took a year off and went to George Washington Medical School. I knew the professor very well and he said all the work on drug metabolizing enzymes would be very good for a thesis but that I would still have to take courses and pass exams – one of the courses, however, I would have to give myself, the one on drug metabolism. I did. By the time I got my PhD, Shannon had become the head of the entire NIH.

Tell me more about Shannon.

He had very good rapport with two important congressmen. One was Fogarty, the congressman from Rhode Island. And the other one was Lister Hill, a Senator from Alabama. Shannon convinced them that the best way to treat and cure diseases is not to invest large amounts of money on targeted research on diseases but to understand the fundamental process, the biology, etc. Congress were generous to the NIH while he was there. He also recruited some really top flight people to the NIH – Jim Wyngaarden, Don Fredrickson, future directors of the NIH, Christian

Anfinson, who became a Nobel laureate, and a whole lot of other excellent people.

There was considerable scepticism at the time that an arm of government, a bureaucratic institution, could possible be compatible with doing ground-breaking science; why did the NIH track-record turn out so well?

The reason why the intramural NIH and NIMH worked so well was due to Shannon's ability to convince Congress, during the period that he was director, between 1955 and 1968, that basic research was necessary to find treatments and cures for diseases. The generosity of funding meant that little grant writing was necessary and this gave the scientists and bright postdocs a free hand.

So you sent your application . . .

Yes. I sent applications out to both the National Cancer Institute and the National Institute of Mental Health and I received a call from Seymour Kety, who was at that time the Director of the intramural programme of the NIMH. He interviewed me for the position. I knew he was interested in me. He sent my application to several laboratories in the Institute. There was one laboratory I wanted to work in and that was Giulio Cantoni's, a well-known biochemist who discovered S-adenosylmethionine, but I didn't get to work with him. I was hired by Ed Evarts, a neurophysiologist and psychiatrist. I don't know if you know of him?

No, I haven't heard.

Evarts was a lovely man. He was the Head of a Laboratory of Clinical Science and he did a lot of fundamental work on the central control of motion. At that time Evarts was interested in biological psychiatry. He saw my papers on amphetamine and asked me to come and work in his laboratory. That was just as I was taking my PhD. He was working on LSD at that time. In my spare time, while going to class, I was working on the metabolism of LSD. We published a paper in *Nature* on the metabolism of LSD in 1955 (Axelrod, Brady, Witkop and Evarts, 1956). We developed a fluorescent method for measuring it and found that incredibly small amounts of LSD in the brain could cause behavioural effects.

The philosophy of Seymour Kety in the NIMH was to hire the best people you can and leave them alone because they are in the best position to know what problems are important, doable and possibly relevant to the Institution. That was a great philosophy for me. I knew nothing about neuroscience or the brain. I had worked in the Heart Institute and I felt almost intimidated by these bright physiologists and psychiatrists working on these electrical phenomena. They were all very good talkers – especially Kety.

Anyway, I started to work on the microsomal metabolism of morphine.

I had a theory of tolerance which I published in *Science* (Axelrod, 1956), which proposed a downregulation of morphine receptors – the term downregulation hadn't been coined then but in some of my experiments I showed a reduction in the number of receptors with tolerance and I proposed that this led to a need for more morphine. It was criticized at the time but I think the theory and also the experiments were not bad.

Well, anyway, I felt a little guilty because this was work on the liver – even though these were good and highly regarded papers. We used to have weekly seminars in the laboratory and at one of these Seymour Kety gave an account of the experiment by two Canadian psychiatrists, Hoffer and Osmond. Their work hadn't actually been published yet but he had heard from them that when they exposed adrenaline to the air, adrenochrome, an oxidative product of adrenaline, was formed and that when this was ingested it caused schizophrenic-like hallucinations. They proposed that schizophrenia could be caused by an abnormal metabolism of adrenaline to adrenochrome.

Anyway, I was intrigued by this. I searched the literature and there was nothing known about what happened to adrenaline in the body. I thought this would be a good problem for me because I had worked on amphetamine, which is related to adrenaline, one of the sympathomimetic amines – this fascinating group of compounds, worked on by Sir Henry Dale many years before.

First, I tried to look for the enzyme involved in forming adrenochrome. I spent three frustrating months looking for this enzyme and I couldn't find it. Then one day I came across an abstract in the *Proceedings of the Federated Society of Biology* by a biochemist, Marvin Armstrong. He found that patients with tumours of the adrenal gland excreted a large amount of what he called vanillylmandelic acid (VMA). It was a methylated compound and it struck me that this compound had to come from adrenaline. I knew about the deamination of adrenaline by the enzyme monoamine oxidase and VMA looked like it had been formed by the deamination and methylation of adrenaline. I found the methylating enzyme, catechol-ortho-methyl-transferase (COMT), that formed a compound which we called metanephrine – methylated adrenaline. It also methylated noradrenaline to a compound we called normetanephrine and we also found another metabolite called 3-methoxy-4-hydroxyphenylglycol (MHPG).

At that time, in 1955, there were two neurotransmitters known to be present in the central nervous system. One was acetylcholine and the other was noradrenaline. It was known that the mechanism for inactivation for acetylcholine was metabolism by acetylcholinesterase. But experiments showed that monoamine oxidase was not the means of inactivation of noradrenaline. I thought that COMT must, therefore, surely be the mechanism for inactivation for noradrenaline. However, just at that time we found an inhibitor for COMT. An inhibitor for monoamine oxidase, iproniazid, was also known but Dick Crout found that when both of these enzymes were inhibited, the action of noradrenaline was still rapidly terminated, even though neither of those enzymes were working. Therefore there had to be another mechanism for the inactivation of noradrenaline.

Just at that time Kety wanted to test Osmond and Hoffer's hypothesis that schizophrenia was due to an abnormal metabolism of adrenaline. To do this he commissioned New England Nuclear to synthesize tritium-labelled adrenaline. The idea was to inject it into humans to measure the amounts of radiolabelled adrenaline and its metabolites that resulted. We had identified all the metabolic products of adrenaline by this time. Briefly, no differences were found between the amounts of radiolabelled adrenaline or its metabolites between normal males and subjects with schizophrenia. When he had done this study, I asked him if I could have some of the radiolabelled adrenaline. Hans Weil-Malherbe and I had developed a method for measuring radioactive noradrenaline.

Where did Weil-Malherbe come from?

He was German and then he emigrated to Britain. He was well known at that time. He was one of the pioneers in the study of the biochemistry of mental illness in the 1930s and 1940s. He worked in the mental hospitals in Britain. It was actually Joel Elkes who arranged for him to come to my laboratory. Hans developed a fluorescent method for measuring adrenaline, which was very non-specific but I had radioactive adrenaline which made a difference to the specificity.

Seymour was prepared to give you the radioactive compound. Did he know though how critical it was going to be to your study.

No idea. He knew I worked on the metabolism of adrenaline and was very impressed but he didn't know where it was going to lead. We injected the radioactive adrenaline into cats and we measured it in their tissues afterwards and found that unchanged adrenaline remained in certain tissues for hours, long after its effects were gone. So we knew it was being sequestered someplace. Gordon Whitby came to the lab then from Cambridge. He was doing his PhD. We decided to study the tissue distribution of radioactive noradrenaline and we found the same thing – that it persisted in certain tissues – in those tissues that were very rich in sympathetic nerves. We suspected it was being taken up into sympathetic nerves but we had to prove it.

About this time, 1959, I was attracting postdocs and visiting scientists and one of these was George Hertting from Vienna. He was a classical pharmacologist and a very good one. Hertting and I had many discussions on how to prove that radiolabelled noradrenaline was taken up by the sympathetic nerves. One day we came up with the right experiment. We removed the superior ganglion from one side of the cat. After one week we had a unilateral denervated cat. When we injected radiolabelled noradrenaline very little was found on the denervated side, while a lot of radiolabelled noradrenaline was localized in tissues on the innervated side (Hertting, Axelrod, Kopin and Whitby, 1961a). This was the first crucial experiment to prove that noradrenaline was taken up into the nerves.

You made a marvellous comment some years later. You wrote an article in 1972 in Seminars of Psychiatry, *which said that because you were outside the field, that you were an enzymologist, you didn't come to this problem with the preconceptions that other people had.*

You have to have an open mind. One thing I tell my students when they are starting is don't read the literature too much, you might be influenced and you won't do experiments which you should do and would do if you have a naive approach.

I think that's almost the classic statement about science.

You have to be naive. You'll probably be frequently wrong but sometimes you will discover something new.

At that point there was no concept at all of a reuptake mechanism.

No. We knew we had it but we had to do further experiments. I did another experiment with George Hertting, where we perfused the spleen with labelled noradrenaline, and stimulated the splenic nerve. Every time we stimulated the nerve, there was an outflow of noradrenaline (Hertting and Axelrod, 1961b). We now knew it was taken up by nerves and released on stimulation. Then we did an experiment, where we gave phenoxybenzamine, and we found a much greater outflow – as Brown and Gillespie had also found. So we proposed that the mechanism of activation of phenoxybenzamine was to block reuptake into the neurone. We missed that one.

In the next experiment, we used radioautography with Keith Richardson, an anatomist, and David Wolfe who did radioautography. I was working on the pineal gland at that time and we knew that the pineal gland was rich in innervation from sympathetic nerves. What we did was to inject radiolabelled noradrenaline and after a few days we found that the sympathetic nerves of the pineal had a high concentration of radiolabelled noradrenaline – all of the radioactivity ended up in sympathetic nerves when we injected it and we knew we had it (Wolfe, *et al.*,1962). The concept of inactivation by reuptake which we proposed was accepted after some initial controversy. It was later confirmed by others.

We then examined the effect of drugs on the uptake of radiolabelled noradrenaline in peripheral tissues. We had to work on peripheral tissues because Weil-Malherbe and I had shown that there is a blood – brain barrier to radiolabelled noradrenaline. Whitby and I showed that cocaine blocked the uptake of noradrenaline in tissues that were heavily innervated with sympathetic nerves, such as the heart and the spleen (Whitby, Hertting and Axelrod, 1960). The reason we didn't work with dopamine was that there was no convincing evidence at that time that it was a neurotransmitter – it was just seen as a precursor for noradrenaline.

Brodie and co-workers reported a very important finding just around the same time. They gave reserpine to rabbits and showed that reserpine reduced the level of serotonin in the brain. He had a theory about serotonin at the time. A few months later Martha Vogt found that reserpine also depletes noradrenaline in the brain. It was also known that reserpine, if you give too much of it, causes suicidal depression. These experiments with reserpine indicated that noradrenaline and serotonin were involved with mental illness. The thinking was there but when you have the beginning of something, like this, there are all kinds of by-ways and sidetracks before you zero in on the real mechanism.

At that time, I had many bright young postdocs joining my laboratory – Sol Snyder, Dick Wurtman, Les Iversen and Jacques Glowinski. Snyder worked on circadian rhythms in the pineal. Wurtman on the role of glucocorticoids in the regulation of the enzymes that synthesize adrenaline from noradrenaline. Glowinski devised a procedure to introduce radiolabelled noradrenaline into the lateral ventricle of the brain. He also worked on the metabolism of catecholamines in the brain. Glowinski and I showed that imipramine and its chemically effective analogues blocked the reuptake of noradrenaline in the brain (Glowinski and Axelrod, 1964). We got a series of tricyclics, I think from Geigy, some of which were active as antidepressants and some inactive and we found that those that were clinically inactive had no effects on the levels of radioactive noradrenaline. So we knew there was some relationship between clinical effectiveness and an antidepressant's ability to block reuptake.

Later Iversen demonstrated that GABA was taken up in nerves. Joe Coyle, now Chairman of Psychiatry at Harvard, demonstrated that dopamine was taken up into nerve endings and Snyder found that serotonin was also taken up. Later in the 1970s, other labs showed that many amino acid neurotransmitters were similarly taken up by nerves. Recently the transporters that take up neurotransmitters have been cloned – two of them, the dopamine and serotonin transporters, were cloned in our laboratory.

Well, that was that. But I was mainly a biochemist. My interests were in enzymes so I worked on in that area. I found the enzyme that converted noradrenaline to adrenaline, called phenylethanol-N-methyl-transferase (PNMT) in 1962. I was particularly interested in methylating enzymes. Don Brown and I found the enzyme that inactivated histamine, histamine methyltransferase and hydroxyindole-O-methyltransferase, the enzyme that synthesizes the pineal hormone melatonin. I also found a curious enzyme which methylated tryptamine to dimethyltryptamine, which induces psychosis. I found this in both the lung and the brain. There were some very simplistic ideas around about dimethyltryptamine at the time – that it was responsible for psychosis – but I couldn't believe that. This was just a by-product of metabolism – the theory was too good to be true, too simple. I had learnt working in biology that things aren't as simple as they may appear. If something is too simple, you should distrust it but we published a lot of papers on the psychotomimetics that might be formed in the brain.

Now I was also interested in the enzymes that regulated noradrenaline metabolism. We found two regulatory mechanisms; we found a relationship between the adrenal cortex and the enzyme that makes adrenaline. Coupland, a British anatomist, found that in the dogfish, where the adrenal cortex is separated from the medulla, the principal catecholamine is noradrenaline – unmethylated adrenaline. However, in mammals where the adrenal cortex is contiguous with the medulla, the main catecholamine present is adrenaline. This suggested to Dick Wurtman, a postdoc, and I that the cortex had something to do with the methylation of noradrenaline to adrenaline. Remember I had found the enzyme that methylates noradrenaline to adrenaline (PNMT), so then we removed the pituitary gland from rats – this should deplete glucocorticoids from the adrenal cortex. After several weeks there was a profound drop in the medullary PNMT activity. Injecting glucocorticoids (dexamethasone) or ACTH (which induces the synthesis of glucocorticoids) brought about a restoration of PNMT activity. This was the first demonstration that a substance from the cortex could regulate the medulla (Thoenen, *et al.*, 1969).

The other regulatory mechanism we discovered was with Hans Thoenen, who is now a Director of Neurochemistry, at the Max Planck Institute, in Munich. He's a very distinguished cell biologist, who discovered the ciliary nerve factor and other nerve factors. When he came to me, we found that when we gave reserpine there was an increase in tyrosine hydroxylase in the adrenal gland. We thought about it – what's happening? We realized that what reserpine did was to increase the firing of the nerves and this firing caused an increase in tyrosine hydroxylase. When we denervated the adrenal gland, there was no increase. We called this the trans-synaptic induction of tyrosine hydroxylase (Snyder, *et al.*,1965).

These were the kind of experiments I liked to do. I didn't try to develop drugs – my students, Sol Snyder and Leslie Iversen, did that.

Tell me more about Sol Snyder and Leslie Iversen.

When Whitby went back to Cambridge, Les Iversen was his graduate student. Les did a lot of important work exploring further the details of the reuptake mechanism – how it is regulated, the effects of competition; he showed that sodium was involved in the uptake. He was very good and I think he became a fellow of Trinity when he graduated.

Les came to me with all these credentials and we worked on the metabolism of noradrenaline in the brain. He wanted to do more detailed neurochemistry and fortunately Glowinski, a neurochemist, was there at the same time. They developed a method for dissecting various parts of the rat brain. Their paper on the Glowinski/Iversen dissection technique is still highly cited. That's how Leslie learnt neurochemistry. He stayed a year and in that year he wrote his book called *The Uptake of Noradrenaline by Sympathetic Nerves.*

That was in 1967

No, in 1965. He was a Rockefeller fellow and they gave him an automobile, so he could travel with his wife Susan across the US. I don't know how he did it. He then went to Harvard for a year to work with Kravitz, where he did the GABA work, and Susan worked with Peter Dews, a psychiatrist in Harvard, on operant conditioning.

Sol Synder, also, wanted to become a psychiatrist. He worked as a graduate student across the hall from my lab with Don Brown, who is now a distinguished molecular biologist. Sol was interested in schizophrenia and he talked to me a lot about my work. I was working on the pineal at that time. After getting his MD, Sol came to my lab as a postdoc. I put him on a project on pineal gland. I won't go into the detail, it's too complicated, but he first worked on histamine metabolism. He says he's a klutz in the lab but he wasn't when he worked with me. He was very good. Sol had a sharp mind; he knew how to do the right experiments.

We developed a very sensitive method for measuring serotonin, the precursor of melatonin. We could measure the serotonin level in a single pineal gland and we found that it was highest during the daytime and lowest at night. When the rats were kept in constant darkness, there was free-running rhythm in serotonin levels which we abolised after denervation of the pineal. These experiments told us that there is a circadian rhythm in pineal serotonin which was controlled by the brain. We knew that there was some internal clock. Well anyway that's what he found. A very fundamental discovery. The assay for serotonin was very important for this; methods are very important.

On the question of methods, how important was Sidney Udenfriend?

Oh, he was very important. Sid was involved in the development of a new type of spectrofluorimeter. He worked with Brodie when they were measuring quinine in the blood in the 1940s. They developed an instrument, with the help of some engineers, that could measure fluorescence – the instrument had two filters, one that measures incoming light at one wavelength and another to measure outgoing light at a different wavelength. They developed this instrument and Sid wrote a book on fluorimetry. They used fluorimetry for their antimalarial work.

Who was the crucial person there, would you say?

Udenfriend and Brodie together. I owe Brodie a great deal despite everything else I've mentioned. Udenfriend and Brodie developed a fluorimeter
using filters on the antimalarial project, during the War in 1943–1945.
This enabled them to measure blood levels of atrabine and other antimalarials. It was very important that they got this right because the Japanese
had cut off the supply of quinine used to treat malaria. So atrabine was
used instead but the troops found atrabine unpalatable and they didn't
want to take it because of side effects. Using the fluorimeter to measure
blood levels, Udenfriend and Brodie developed a dosage regime for atrabine that was more palatable.

The spectrophotofluorimeter was the next development; this was
developed by Bob Bowman, also at NIH. He also came from Goldwater.
In 1955, Bowman improved on the original fluorimeter by using prisms
instead of filters. They named the new fluorimeter after him – the
Aminco-Bowman fluorimeter. It was more sensitive and easier to use and
its introduction made it possible to measure blood and tissue levels of
serotonin, noradrenaline and dopamine and this revolutionized catecholamine research. I used it in 1955, when I was measuring LSD. Bowman
allowed me to use it when it was still in development. I was lucky to
have it because I could then measure very tiny amounts of LSD in the
brain.

Where did he come from, Bowman?

Bowman was a physician. He came from Goldwater and worked on the
antimalarial project. He loved tinkering with instruments. He also
developed an instrument called the flame photometer to measure sodium
levels in plasma. People forget this – how important instruments are.

*I agree completely. The instruments are absolutely critical. So much so that you
wonder about the theories. You have people who say that science is all about
theories, having the right kind of theories, trying to suss the theory out.*

It's all about the right methods and asking the right questions. The
introduction of radioactive noradrenaline and other radioactive neurotransmitters also had a great impact on neuropharmacology and on neurochemistry research. This was how fluoxetine was developed. They used
labelled serotonin and tried out thousands of drugs to see what blocked
the uptake. People often don't realize how critical technical developments
like these are.

I agree completely with you.

Some of these young people have no idea where some of these developments come from and how important they are. Anyway, talking about Sol
Synder, he took a residency in psychiatry but he was hooked on research.
His early work demonstrated the importance of dopamine in schizophrenia, showing the relationship between binding to dopamine receptors

and clinical effectiveness of drugs in the treatment of schizophrenia. These were important experiments. Seeman also did a lot of work in this area.

Sol Synder, I think, did more for receptorology than anybody. He revolutionized the field by using radioactive ligands of high specific activity to measure the binding constants of ligands to receptors. The grind and bind approach. He showed, for example, that there are two serotonin receptors – these were important experiments – and also the existence of an opiate receptor. They sound very crude experiments now but they were germinal at the time. The whole field of receptorology exploded.

He seems to keep on coming up with things – for instance, the work on nitric oxide recently.

With all kinds of things, yes. He did and still does a lot of very good experiments. He's a brilliant guy. He has a skill at picking the right things at the right time. One thing I am very pleased about are the people who worked with me – almost all of them became distinguished in different fields – pharmacology, physiology, psychiatry. I have a very small laboratory. I never have more than two or three post-docs at any one time. I feel a great sense of pride in the type of people who work with me and in getting them involved in research. I don't know what it was but I tried to make it as pleasurable an experience as I could. Most of them came out of the grind of studying medicine and I said 'Relax, no more exams, just enjoy yourself, let your mind explore things'. With my help and their intelligence and enthusiasm, it worked out very well.

One thing about psychopharmacology is that these drugs are such powerful tools biochemically as well as pharmacologically. Drugs like reserpine, the monoamine oxidase inhibitors and the uptake inhibitors, they were really important tools. Well let's see, from 1970 I became . . .

Before you go onto 1970, let me ask you about a few people whose careers began during the 1960s and you might like to comment on. There's Arvid Carlsson.

Arvid was trained as a pharmacologist. He came to Brodie's lab just around the time I left – 1956. Brodie had a tremendous influence on Arvid, as well as on Pletscher who was working there in the lab at the time. Brodie had many brilliant people working with him. Costa was there. There was a real ferment about that time. Soon after Carlsson left Brodie's lab, he got into the dopamine field. He showed that dopamine was present in the brain and he did the preliminary experiments showing that rats can develop a Parkinson-like syndrome by giving reserpine which reduced brain dopamine. This influenced the thinking of Hornykiewicz who examined dopamine levels in patients who had died of Parkinson's and found that it was decreased in the striatum.

I have nominated Arvid for a Nobel prize many times. It's a pity he didn't get it. I think he deserves it. He has done so much important work. Not only the work I've just mentioned but work showing that dopamine might be involved in schizophrenia. He was the one who started to make dopamine what it finally became. He tells me he owes a great deal to Brodie.

There really are very many people who would say that he was extremely important. Silvio Garattini, for instance, would say he had the pharmacological 'attitude'.

Well, Brodie wasn't a pharmacologist at first. He was a biochemist. He was very imaginative. What a fund of ideas he had and he really swept you up with his ideas and . . .

Are you saying that even when he was wrong he was convincing?

Very convincing. He had a theory of the inhibitory action of serotonin in the brain which had considerable influence even though it was incorrect. But you know, in order to be a productive scientist you have to have lots of ideas which you can try out. Even if only one or two of them work out, it will have been worth it. If you have no novel ideas, nothing happens – you can do incremental work – that's just improving on something already known. But to do something original you have to have really bold ideas which Brodie had and he was also convincing. He was very stimulating and you wanted to rush to the lab to try out his ideas.

The other thing you hear about though was that he used to work by night, sleep by day.

Well, yes, he used to come to the lab about noon. He would then talk a lot to the people in the lab and sometimes he wouldn't get home until late. Sometimes he would call me at two in the morning if he had an idea.

He also seemed, in the mid 1960s, to vanish from the scene.

He always complained about his health when I worked with him. He led a life which wasn't very healthy. He ate hamburgers and stayed up late. It finally caught up with him in the 1960s. He had all kinds of medical problems in the 1960s and he just faded away because of that.

I think he had a great influence on all the people who worked under him. He was one of the father figures in psychopharmacology. His fame could rest just on the reserpine experiments. I shall tell you how that started. Sid Udenfriend and Herb Weissbach described the metabolism of serotonin to 5-hydroxy–indole–acetic acid (5-HIAA). Park Shore, then, discovered that if you gave reserpine to rats there was an elevation in 5-HIAA levels in the brain. Pletscher and Brodie started to theorize about that and came up with the idea that maybe reserpine was doing something to serotonin in the brain. So it was Park Shore who made the initial observation but it was Brodie . . .

Who really picked it up and ran with it.

Yes, that's how it started. You needed the imaginative bold thinking by someone like Brodie to really drive something like that forward. Sometimes it may not work out but sometimes it does and it happened to work in this case. But then his idea about the function of serotonin in the brain was wrong. He was very disappointed when Vogt and Carlsson found that reserpine also did the same thing to catecholamines. His theory was shattered. But anyway, it didn't matter. You forget the things that don't work but you remember the things that do.

If we move on to the 1970s. When did you get conferred with the Nobel prize?

In 1970. I knew I was nominated by Seymour Kety and Irv Kopin but it was a surprise.

What role did Irv Kopin play?

Irv Kopin came to the NIMH as a clinical associate but he had a nose for laboratory research. He happened to be in my laboratory when we were doing the crucial experiments on denervation with Hertting. Every time we did an experiment Irv Kopin showed up to help so we made him a co-author on some of the papers. Kopin and I discovered MHPG. He shifted from clinical research and wound up working in my lab most of the time. It was a very crucial period with the uptake experiments and in metabolism of catecholamines. He was a co-author on many of the papers. He remained in the catecholamine field longer than I did and he still is in the field. He's now the Director of the Neurological Disease Institute.

And after the Nobel prize?

In the 1970s, I mainly worked on the pineal gland, on methylation reactions, and started work on signal transduction. We discovered a new transduction pathway, in which arachidonic acid was a second messenger. I continued with this during the 1980s with the G-proteins which are heterotrimers – with alpha, beta and gamma units. When a receptor is occupied by a ligand, the G-proteins dissociate to alpha and beta-gamma subunits. The thinking at that time was that it was the alpha subunit that activates adenylate cyclase and phospholipases. But Carol Jelsema and I found that the beta-gamma subunits of the G-proteins can activate phospholipase A2 in the retina. We sent the paper to *Nature* in 1986 and it was rejected.

But they don't reject things from a Nobel prize winner.

They sure do. Our manuscript was published in the *Proceedings of the National Academy of Sciences* in 1987. About that time a paper appeared in *Nature* showing that the beta-gamma subunit can activate a potassium ion channel. A few years later more than a dozen papers were published in *Nature* showing that the beta-gamma subunits of G-proteins can activate adenylate cyclase, phospholipase C, kinases, etc. Evidently, by then, even the reviewers for *Nature* had started to believe it. But I have to say that almost all of our papers (about 30) that we submitted to *Nature* were accepted.

Why do you think they'd turn down a paper like that?

Well, they did it because it was too revolutionary. Any time a dogma is challenged, it meets with scepticism. The criticisms were just lousy and nit-picking. They just didn't believe it. They questioned lots of things but it was true and it was confirmed later on.

You said that you were surprised to get the Nobel prize.

Most scientists dream about getting a Nobel prize. In the 1960s, catecholamines and neurotransmitters were hot – they still are. There were several people working in the area at that time that were likely candidates for the prize – von Euler, Carlsson, Bernard Katz, Hillarp, who was working on mapping catecholamine nerve pathways; Vogt and Blaschko. Von Euler, Katz and I got it. They decided to give it on neurotransmitters. So they gave it to Bernard Katz for his work on release of acetylcholine. They gave it to von Euler because he discovered noradrenaline as a neurotransmitter and they gave it me for inactivation. So I just happened to be doing the right thing at the right time.

Has it changed your life?

Not much. You become a minor celebrity. You get called up by news reporters. You get many honorary degrees and a lot of important lectureships. People recognize you – it makes me feel uncomfortable. But it hasn't changed my life very much. Of course, I'm delighted to have it. It's a great honour. I think I deserve it, but a lot of other people do too and don't get it.

What about your more recent work?

To continue with the rest of my work, in the 1980s I was beginning to wind down. I still loved to do research. Most of my work in the 1980s was on signal transduction, mainly phospholipase A2.

In 1984, I officially retired from government and became a unpaid guest worker in the laboratory of my former postdoc Mike Brownstein. I am still active and I am presently working on anandamide, the endogenous ligand for the cannabinoid receptor. The cannabinoid receptor was cloned by Mike Brownstein and Lisa Matsuda, a postdoc in Mike's laboratory. This meant that there must be an endogenous ligand for the receptor and Bill Devane and Raphael Mechoulen found it and called it anandamide. Bill and I described the enzyme that synthesizes anandamide. We have preliminary evidence that it is a neurotransmitter. Anandamide has a bright future I think – it has a receptor, it has an enzyme that synthesizes it in nerves and we know a few of the things that it does. That's a very exciting project and I have really got caught up with it.

Let me pick up two things — radiolabelled antidepressant binding and of course the whoe SSRI story with fluoxetine and all that. Now that Steven Paul, who worked with you, has moved to Lilly, you have close links in a sense with both of these developments

Yes, Steven Paul was a postdoc in my lab. He was a very bright guy and he's done a lot of work on antidepressant mechanisms.

But was the radiolabelling of the antidepressant binding site, which he played a part in making fashionable with his early reports that there was decreased binding in people who were depressed, a mistake? It seems to me that the earlier work looking at altered uptake in people who were depressed was more promising in a sense but the field was seduced by the glamour of this new hi-tech approach and a great number of groups became bogged down in trying to sort out what has not been methodologically sorted out.

No, I don't think it was a mistake. It led to the next great development which was the cloning of the noradrenaline, dopamine, serotonin, GABA and glutamate transporters. It now appears that labelled antidepressant drugs do bind to these transporters.

I agree with what you say from the point of view of the basic sciences but do you not think that clinical research went down the wrong path, when they radiolabelled the antidepressants? So many groups got involved with this assay expecting it to be a diagnostic marker and it has led nowhere.

You have to try. If you do nothing, nothing will happen. As long as you're able to recognize you are on the wrong path. Some people become a prisoner of their ideas. They put so much work in it, that it must be true and they can't stop. You have to know when to stop and cut your losses. I've made a lot of mistakes but I found out fairly soon and I didn't waste my time. Things don't always work out the way you hoped they would but you have to try out your ideas. The binding of antidepressants indicated that there must be something there. It didn't pick up the transporter but it showed that there must be something there. It was the revolution in molecular biology that made the cloning of transporters possible.

Costa was someone who was into this area as well as GABA and other things.

Yes, he was mainly into GABA. He and his co-workers discovered a natural compound that inhibits benzodiazepine binding. Costa is very bright. He's done a lot of work on GABA and benzodiazepines, a lot of important work. Nothing germinal but very influential I think. He was greatly influenced by Brodie. Brodie was his hero. At the very end, when Brodie died, he took care of his wife. He's a warm-hearted person and he has trained a lot of good people, particularly Italians. He is the guru of Italian neuropharmacology.

How do the 5-HT reuptake inhibiting drugs look from your perspective?

I think they were an important development but there has been a lot of hype about what these drugs can do.

As I understand it when they were introduced first, there were at least two groups, and maybe more, which appear to have been involved. One was the group with Arvid Carlsson who thought it would be a good idea to make the 5-HT reuptake inhibitor as an antidepressant . . .

I didn't know that. I thought there were several but I thought it was the Lilly group who were first. I don't know the history other than what I read in the book by Kramer (see Glossary). But you know the old saying: there are a lot of fathers to success and a lot of orphans to failure. You can never pin these things down. Take the discovery of dopamine; Carlsson had an important role and so did Seeman and so did Snyder. All of these things build up – it isn't any one individual that does it. There are several people contributing and it becomes compelling after a while. I'm sure Brodie and Carlsson had a lot of ideas that didn't turn out, but when they do, they're remembered. You have to have a lot of ideas and Carlsson had many.

What role do you think Seymour Kety had in everything?

Seymour Kety was a germinal figure in neuroscience. A statesman of neuroscience. He was the one who set up the NIMH in a way to do solid science. There had been some psychoanalysis research at the NIMH but he wanted basic science included as well. And he also had a nose in hiring good people.

He also had the ability to enthuse people.

Well, no, not in the way Brodie did. Kety had an analytical mind and he wrote an influential review in *Science* critical of the sloppy research in biological psychiatry – the pink spot and the Akerfelt test, for example. Kety believed that without sufficient basic knowledge doing targeted research on mental illness would be a waste of time and money. He did pioneering research on cerebral blood flow. His work and that of Lou Sokoloff provided the underpinning for PET scan imaging today.

What was the Akerfelt test?

Akerfelt reported that he had a blood test for schizophrenia. It was later shown that the Akerfelt test was a test for vitamin C deficiency. It so happened that schizophrenics in mental institutions were lacking in vitamin C. At the time there were many psychiatrists and others who were looking for abnormal metabolites in the urine of schizophrenics using paper chromatography. Some did find abnormal metabolites but they were later shown to be artefacts. This was the kind of thing Kety was very critical about. This was very different from Brodie who was very enthusiastic.

Pink Spots were a big industry at one time.

Yes, you have these fashions which peter out after a while. We found that in a group of schizophrenics and controls, schizophrenics always had two spots and the controls never did. So we couldn't believe that. It was too good to be true. So we analysed the diet of our subjects and found that our controls were Mennonites – they didn't drink coffee. That was Kety, that type of thinking. A great analytical mind. He was a very nice person. And the thing was he never took advantage of you. He left you alone. But if you did something important he really pushed you, recognized it.

I've had two or three people who've talked about you at length – particularly Merton Sandler.

I always found Merton stimulating and amusing. It's interesting, in his interview he talked about a meeting in 1958 where he met me; actually I was never at that meeting. It was at a meeting in 1961 that I met him.

Well, this says something about history in a sense – maybe the way we remember things is in one sense more important than the way they actually were.

Select bibliography

Axelrod, J. (1955a) The enzymatic deamination of amphetamine (Benzedrine). *Journal of Biological Chemistry*, **214**, 753–63.

Axelrod, J. (1955b) The enzymatic deamination of ephedrine. *Journal of Pharmacology and Experimental Therapeutics*, **114**, 430–38.

Axelrod, J., Brady, R.O., Witkop, B. and Evarts, E.V. (1956) Metabolism of lysergic acid diethylamide. *Nature*, **178**, 143–44.

Axelrod, J. (1956) Possible mechanism of tolerance to narcotic drugs. *Science*, **124**, 263–64.

Axelrod, J. (1972) Biogenic amines and their impact on psychiatry, *Seminars of Psychiatry*, **4**, 199–210.

Axelrod, J. (1988) An unexpected life in research. *Annual Review of Pharmacology and Toxicology*, **28**, 1–23.

Brodie, B.B. and Axelrod, J. (1948a) The estimation of acetanilide and its metabolic products, aniline, N-acetyl-p-aminophenol and p-aminophenol (free and total conjugated) in biological fluids and tissues. *Journal of Pharmacology and Experimental Therapeutics*, **94**, 22–28.

Brodie, B.B. and Axelrod, J. (1948b) The fate of acetanilide in man. *Journal of Pharmacology and Experimental Therapeutics*, **94**, 29–38.

Glowinski, J. and Axelrod, J. (1964) Inhibition of uptake of tritiated noradrenaline in the intact rat brain by imipramine and structurally related compounds. *Nature*, **204**, 1318–19.

Hertting, G., Axelrod, J., Kopin, I.J. and Whitby, L.G. (1961a) Lack of uptake of catecholamines after chronic denervation of sympathetic nerves. *Nature*, **189**, 66.

Hertting, G. and Axelrod, J. (1961b) The fate of tritiated noradrenaline at the sympathetic nerve endings. *Nature*, **192**, 172–73.

Snyder, S.H., Zweig, M., Axelrod, J. and Fischer, J.E. (1965) Control of the circadian rhythm in serotonin content of the rat pineal gland. *Proc. Natl. Acad. Sciences* (USA) **53**, 301–6.

Thoenen, H., Mueller, R.A. and Axelrod, J. (1969) Increased tyrosine hydroxylase activity after drug induced alteration of sympathetic transmission. *Nature*, **221**, 1264.

Whitby, L.G., Hertting, G. and Axelrod, J. (1960) Effect of cocaine on the disposition of noradrenaline labelled with tritium. *Nature*, **187**, 604–5.

Wolfe, D., Potter, L.T., Richardson, K.C. and Axelrod, J. (1962) Localising tritiated norepinephrine in sympathetic axons by electron microscopic autoradiography. *Science*, **138**, 440–42.

3 Arvid Carlsson

The rise of neuropsychopharmacology: impact on basic and clinical neuroscience

How did you come to go to NIH?

In Sweden, I had been working mainly in the area of calcium metabolism. I went for a position and the expert committee who gave the position to my only competitor let me understand that the area of calcium metabolism is not really a central field in pharmacology – this is something that has changed lately but that was how it was. Since I wanted to remain in pharmacology, I decided to switch into a different area, so I went to a friend of mine, Dr Sune Bergstrom, who was in the same building – he was Professor of Physiological Chemistry, in Lund, and he was often very helpful. He later received a Nobel prize for his work on prostaglandins. I told him I would like to switch fields; I knew he had lots of good contacts in the US, so I asked him to find a lab in the US, where they were doing biochemical pharmacology, which at that time was something I felt very strongly for.

He wrote to his friend, Bernard Witkop, a very clever chemist – he was originally from Austria – who had done lots of synthetic chemistry that others have profited from enormously. He was behind very important successes in organic chemistry and biochemistry. Witkop transferred the letter to Sidney Udenfriend. Udenfriend was not independant at that time so he had to give it to his boss, Bernard Brodie. Brodie wrote to me and said 'we would be more than happy to have you but we have no money'. I managed to get a modest sum of money in Sweden so I could go. When I came there, in late August 1955, the first thing they did was to invite me to the cafeteria for lunch. Brodie and Udenfriend were there and I figured out that that was the time when Brodie finally made up his mind whether he would accept me or whether he would give me to Udenfriend. He accepted me.

Coming from outside the area, there can't have been much that you could have actually impressed them with in terms of the knowledge of the area.

No, I didn't know anything about this actually. My first pieces of work in pharmacology dealt with central nervous system drugs but from there I had switched to calcium metabolism. I had worked a little bit on convulsants and on what was called, at that time, central analeptics, metrazol – a drug that could wake up barbiturate-sedated animals, and humans for that matter. But that was the only research I had done in CNS pharmacology.

What was NIH like at that time?

Brodie's lab belonged to the National Heart Institute, funnily, which really shows that the labels don't mean that much. It was called the Laboratory of Chemical Pharmacology and the building, where I worked, was building 10, which is the biggest one. At that time, it was said to be the building in the world that had the largest number of bricks. I don't know if that's true, but it was a huge building and, of course it has expanded a little bit, but it isn't that much different actually from how it used to be. At that time, it was new and in the lab of chemical pharmacology they were still buying equipment and there were still big boxes of equipment that hadn't been unpacked yet. It was really at the beginning of that period, which was to be so significant a period in the development of neuropsychopharmacology.

There was a stream of visitors. Almost every day people would come from all over the world to interview Brodie and find out the latest news. Why did it attract that much attention? I think there were three things. One was that Brodie was the real pioneer in the area of measuring drug levels. Pharmacokinetics more or less sprang out of the work that Brodie started originally in New York and then at the NIH. So they were doing a lot of work on that and it was a really fashionable thing at that time and of course it was very important.

Another thing was that they were in the process of developing the spectrophotofluorometer, which is not used so much any more, but which was of such a tremendous importance over two or three decades. The only instrument in the world, when I came there, was the model that Bowman had built. It was the prototype but still not really packed into anything. It was composed of loose parts all over the room, more or less. You had to put out the light in order to work it. So that was a very important development. Then finally there was the discovery that they had just made that if you give reserpine to animals serotonin disappears from tissues, including the brain. I think it was mainly this last finding that attracted so much attention.

This was really the first hard-core neurochemical finding wasn't it?

I think so, yes. This really bridged the gap between biochemistry and psychiatry – and neurology as it later on turned out. So I think it was a very important discovery. Of course, before that you had a few pointers.

You had the discovery by Gaddum that LSD can block the effect of serotonin in the uterus, on which he built his statement that serotonin is needed to keep us sane. And, there was at the same time two Americans, Woolley and Shaw, who had said the same thing. Actually, they corresponded a little bit about the issue of who was first to come up with this statement. I think they were independent. Before that, of course, was the discovery of serotonin in the brain and also Marthe Vogt's study of sympathin as she called it, in the brain, which was also important in the early 1950s.

But this was the first change in anything in the brain that had been shown to correlate with a change in behaviour wasn't it?

Absolutely, yes, because LSD was rather a loose connection, but to give a drug with a very powerful psychotropic action and discover a very striking biochemical change in the brain, that was absolutely the first breakthrough.

You were working on platelet 5-HT. How did all of that go? Because harvesting platelets is quite tricky isn't it?

Well, there was something tricky in it and I must tell you that I still don't know what it was. When I arrived there in late August I was put on this immediately. They had the equipment ready for me, very good equipment, so they told me exactly how to do it. And I did it. I isolated these platelets. It's not difficult at all.

But if you use the wrong anticoagulant and the wrong G-force . . .

Yes, it doesn't work. That's true but in this case, with EDTA, there was no problem. For some funny reason, they told me I had to use siliconized glassware, which we found out was not at all necessary. I worked, I think, for more than one month on this – I isolated the platelets, put in the reserpine and measured serotonin in the supernatant and in the platelets – and found no effect. That was frustrating because as you already indicated I was entirely new in the field, so they thought probably I was just a joke. But then what happened was that I ran out of the sample of reserpine and they gave me a new one and, as soon as I got that, it worked beautifully. I think there was something wrong with the first batch of reserpine.

Having cutting your teeth on 5-HT, despite Brodie's great enthusiasm for it, you were quite keen to look at catecholamines and not just 5-HT. This was heresy.

Yes, it was, and the reason why I wanted to do that was that I did a little bit of work on my own on these platelets. For some reason, probably because Hillarp back in Lund had discovered that there is a lot of ATP in the adrenomedullary granules and I wondered if there was any ATP in the platelets. I did some analyses on that. I don't think they were very good qualitatively but at least they convinced me that there is ATP in the platelets and in fairly large amounts. Since this was the case, I felt it was a reasonable hypothesis that the storage mechanism for serotonin and catecholamines could be basically the same and therefore if you gave reserpine something might happen to the catecholamines as well.

So I told Brodie, shouldn't we do that and he said 'no, that would be a waste of time because it's serotonin that's important'. He insisted on serotonin for an unreasonably long time – why did he do that? Well, partly perhaps because of his particular character but perhaps also he had started out with an hypothesis and this experiment with reserpine and serotonin confirmed the hypothesis in his mind. The hypothesis was based on Gaddum's ideas. They had done sleeping time, which at that time was very fashionable – you give either ethanol or a barbiturate to a mouse and you measure the time the mouse is in anaesthesia. Then you put in LSD and you could shorten the time or put in serotonin and you could lengthen the time. Reserpine lengthened the time. So LSD and reserpine were antagonists and serotonin acted like reserpine.

So then they said well suppose that reserpine releases serotonin. That's why they did the experiment and it came out exactly the way they thought. Now that's what they felt on the basis of these rather simple experiments but, of course, they were not really interpreted correctly because serotonin doesn't get into the brain. The interpretation was basically wrong. Nevertheless, they thought that, when you give reserpine, there will be more free serotonin and it is this free serotonin that sedates the animals. That was the story and they were firm on that.

But on the other hand, I must say that Brodie was very generous to me. When I was considered for a position, a Chair in Lund, and the Faculty demanded references, Brodie wrote very generously that I had astounded the world by showing that catecholamines are also depleted by reserpine. On the other hand, of course, we also had some debates, which got a little bit harsh every once in a while. Not so much with Brodie himself, as with some of his younger colleagues.

Such as?

The most memorable debate was with Mimo Costa. There was a meeting in Stockholm, in 1961. It was actually the first international congress of pharmacology. Costa reported on continuing studies that proved that reserpine acted on serotonin and that catecholamines were not important. I discussed his paper and demonstrated that they had misinterpreted their data. While we were debating, it became very lively I must say. Brodie came into the room – he hadn't been there in the beginning – and he said later 'lucky Carlsson that Costa didn't have a knife', because he really was so furious. Actually, it was in the Swedish newspapers the following day. Twenty-five years later, there was an International Symposium on Clinical Pharmacology, that Sjoqvist chaired in Stockholm, and he had been at this debate and thought it was so memorable, that it must be repeated–25 years later. So he invited me and Costa . . . but it was rather friendly at that time.

How do you rate Brodie?

Brodie I think was really the top. You cannot measure him by conventional academic standards because he might not do very well. Part of his science was very solid but he went out speculating into areas where he was ignorant. He was not a traditional scholar – I think one can say that for sure – but as I indicated before, in a way, that was his strength. It may be that the most important people, the most creative people, do not fulfil conventional standards. But that is also the reason why some people think he was nuts, because if you look at him from a certain point of view, he was. It's enough for one individual if he's got one or two great ideas, that they can elaborate on and bring to a certain level of truth. Then they have contributed haven't they – even if they are crazy in every other respect.

Should he have got the Nobel prize with Axelrod?

In my opinion he would deserve a Nobel prize. But it depends on how you read what Alfred Nobel put in his testament. Certainly, in terms of contributing to neuroscience or pharmacology for that matter, Brodie is far above anyone else. The problem was that he was an organic chemist and his knowledge of physiology and medicine was really not a heavy burden on him. He didn't know much about it and I think that was one of his strengths – his ignorance, yes. He didn't have any idea how complex the brain is for one thing, so he could come up with some very simple concepts. There are several things to be said about Brodie but one of them was his ignorance in physiology in combination with this ability to formulate simple concepts that were testable, which was very surprising. Many times he could sit at the meeting and listen to very complex presentations and then come up with some very simple question at the end that made a lot of sense even though people probably wouldn't accept it. But he would go home and do something about it. So that was the strength, together with his ability to develop methods and to collect people around him who were clever, such as Udenfriend and Bowman and Axelrod.

So he was a terrific guy but when it came to interpret his data – when it came to a stage where knowledge was needed in order to bring it further, that was where he failed. It was his strength and his weakness. By means of this way, he could make a breakthrough but he couldn't develop the concept any further because he didn't know that much. He was an organic chemist and you couldn't demand from him that he should have an understanding of the function of the brain.

So you went back to Sweden and did the catecholamine work with Hillarp. Tell me about him.

He was a very interesting personality. He was a genius, I think one can say. He started out in histology but he was very much focused on function, so that he became just as much a physiologist as histologist. He was very clever and had very fine experimental skills. He had acquired a range of techniques at that time, that were so important, such as homogenization, differential centrifugation to isolate the different organelles in the cells, and so forth. He had set up methods for analysing catecholamines and ATP – he was also a very good biochemist, as a matter of fact. So, when I thought of this in Bethesda I thought I must ask Hillarp if he would like to work on this with me and, luckily, he said yes. So we did some work actually on the binding between catecholamines and ATP but then also we gave reserpine and we analysed the adrenal medulla for catecholamines.

Now I had been very much impressed by the spectrophotofluorometer, which I had started to work on in Brodie's lab. At that time, they had just started to manufacture and sell this Aminco-Bowman spectrophotofluorometer. The first thing I did after coming back home to Lund was to order an instrument. It was very expensive. I didn't have the money. So I applied for money to the Swedish Medical Research Council and got it, but when we were doing these first experiments I didn't have the instrument. However, Hillarp had set up a colorimetric method and it worked beautifully – you add an oxidant, which converts adrenaline into a red-coloured compound, adrenochrome, which you can measure colorimetrically. Of course, when we did this experiment, we found we didn't need any colorimeter because, after we had given reserpine, there was no colour at all. You could see it with a naked eye. It was very dramatic.

At the time, was there any feeling that changing the world from Lund was unusual and people weren't going to pay any heed to you? You weren't operating out of the NIH or Oxford or Cambridge.

Sure, and that came out fairly strongly a couple of years later when Hillarp and I went to a meeting in London on adrenergic mechanisms and there was this . . .

Yes, I was going to ask you about . . . I've read the volume from that meeting. Tell me about that because there are two or three of your articles where, you still to this day, express surprise that the people in the UK at least didn't realize the implications.

Yes, disappointment in a way. But at the same time it aroused opposition and perhaps even aggression to some extent that these people couldn't understand that this was very important.

The really surprising thing is that the participants at the meeting were the very people, who had campaigned for so long on the importance of chemical neurotransmission.

They were the pioneers, they were all there. Dale, Gaddum, Marthe Vogt, Feldberg, Blaschko, everybody was there. Burns, Zaimis, Bulbring, everybody in the field was there. An interesting thing is that the discussion was actually printed, so you can really see what was said. There were very few things that were omitted but one thing that was omitted was that at one point, when they expressed their scepticism against the idea that these amines could be so important in the brain, Blaschko, who had actually replicated some of our most salient experiments, became annoyed and said I think you should recognise that Carlsson has made a great discovery here. What he alluded to then was the effect of the L–dopa on the reserpine treated animal . . .

I'll pick that up in a moment but can I ask you what were Dale and the others like?

I may have seen him a couple of times in other situations but in this symposium we saw each other every day. He was a magnificent personality and it was funny to see how he behaved with the younger guys. The younger guys, of course, were in their 50s or 60s but they behaved as school children more or less to this man. Sir Henry! He was terrific but, also, it was clear that you should be careful not to come up with any statement that was not well taken by Sir Henry Dale. So, for example, coming back to when Blaschko said that they should really recognize that Carlsson has made an important discovery here – he came to me later privately and said that he was sorry that he was so irritated that he said this. In fact, his remark was omitted in the proceedings. That, I think, is a sign of how the people around Dale felt they should be careful. If a statement was not approved by him it should be deleted and he was obviously very doubtful about the whole idea of this L–dopa story, dopamine and so forth. One of his comments at the meeting was, isn't it strange that here we have an amino acid, dopa, that is toxic?

Toxic, why toxic?

Well, the reason why he said toxic was that Weil–Malherbe had done some experiments with L–dopa. He gave large doses of dopa in combination with MAO inhibitors and the animals looked terrible and died. Because he was one of the guys in Britain, what he had seen was more important than what we had seen and for that matter Blaschko or the Polish fellow Crusciel, who was working with Blaschko and had done the experiments, had seen. Weil–Malherbe belonged to the 'real people' and somebody coming from Lund or Poland or whatever, coming to

Britain and telling you stories, that would not be immediately accepted, that's for sure.

From there yourself and Hillarp went on to develop the histofluorescent methods and the mapping of the brain pathways, which was so important.

Actually this was related to this meeting in London because we were both very disappointed. We travelled back together. One of the things that was said at that Adrenergic Mechanisms meeting was that maybe these amines after all were only in the glial cells – it was mentioned in the proceedings there. So we said it would be terribly important if one could demonstrate the presence of these amines in neurones. So Hillarp and I decided we should try it. I had just been appointed to the Chair in Pharmacology in Gothenburg, he had an Associate Professorship in Lund, and we decided we should apply to the Swedish Medical Research Council to enable him to be set free from his teaching position, to come with me to the new department and work on this. We got the money and started on the work.

In the first stage we tried to apply the same fluorimetic procedure we had used for catecholamines before, adapted for a histological preparation, and it worked but it worked only for the adrenal medulla. Nevertheless, Hillarp was very excited by this and he said we must do this in some different way. What he started out from then was another analytical method developed by Udenfriend, where he had added formaldehyde to serotonin and converted serotonin into a fluorescent compound that could be measured. So, Hillarp started then on formaldehyde gas added onto films. Thieme was his technician and Thieme came with him to Gothenburg and what they did was to have a solution with serotonin, for example, and a protein and they put it on the slide, allowed it to dry, so they had a film, and they put the slide into formaldehyde gas and looked at it in the fluorescent microscope. They had to change the various conditions but finally it worked beautifully.

One day in August 1961, when Hillarp went down to Lund, he and Bengt Falck, who was his former pupil, decided they should try a preparation that Hillarp had used in his thesis – stretched preparations of omentum or iris. You just take omentum from a rat, put it on the slide, allow it to dry in the air, or you take the iris and do the same thing, stretch it on the glass and then you put it into formaldehyde gas. That was when Hillarp was just down for a weekend in Lund. And it worked. They put it into the fluorescent microscope and all of a sudden they could see the same reticulum that Hillarp had described in his thesis, using methylene blue. So the adrenergic nerves were there. It took another two or three months for them to repeat it. They couldn't repeat it, so they had to work on all these various conditions – to change the humidity or whatever and so forth – and they got it working again and then they could apply it to histological preparations. So that was how it was done but the model experiments were done by Thieme and Hillarp in Gothenburg actually.

When did they get to the stage of mapping the various pathways?

Well, that was rather soon. Hillarp liked to do a lot of work and then to publish the work in very extensive publications that were not accepted usually by the journals themselves. They had to be a supplement. So there was a couple of important supplements in *Acta Physiologica Scandinavica* from 1962 and 1963 that nobody knows about.

He wasn't too concerned to get his name in lights.

No. I don't think he really understood that. He was a fairly shy man. In his whole life, he had been only to one international meeting. That was the meeting in London. So he didn't know much about the world. He had also been to one meeting in Helsinki. So this idea of how to distribute information, he didn't understand so well. Also he had the idea, adopted by *Acta Physiologica Scandinavica* that authors should always be in alphabetical order. You can see that in all his publications. I didn't mind, because my name C is before H. So the first publication demonstrating the neurocellular localization of monoamines in the brain was by Carlsson, Falck and Hillarp.

What was the impact of the maps when they came out?

Oh, it was enormous. I think that probably there were two things that led to a general acceptance of the monoamines as neurotransmitters. One of them was the histochemistry and all the work that we did on pharmacological manipulations, with reserpine and precursors and seeing how monoamine levels changed. The other thing, I think, was the discovery by Hornykiewicz that you have a depletion of dopamine in Parkinson's disease. We had, of course, proposed that on the basis of animal data but it was Hornykiewicz, who really demonstrated the low levels of dopamine in post mortem analyses.

The other big debate in this area at the time was whether vesicles were of functional importance, with Axelrod on one side saying 'no, it's not, it's the neurotransmitters in the cytoplasm that count' .

I connect different issues with different meetings. This was at the 1965 meeting in Stockholm where von Euler, Rosell and Uvnäs were editors of the book called *Mechanisms of Release of Biogenic Amines*. At that, von Euler and Axelrod and Udenfriend said it's the cytoplasmic pool that is the important thing and they quoted especially Udenfriend, who said that the vesicles are garbage cans. We fought this very strongly. At the time, we had just collected pharmacological data by means of the histochemical fluorescense technique and we could actually demonstrate a condition, where you had an excess of amine in the cytoplasm and yet when you stimulated the nerves, they did not respond, because there was none taken up by the granules. The 1965 proceedings are nice because there was a discussion where people really stated what they thought. We reported on our monoaminergic synapse model that we had proposed a couple of years earlier.

The effects of L-dopa in reversing reserpine-induced behaviour was the point that proved it was the catecholamines rather than 5-HT. 5-HTP didn't make any difference, how did Brodie take that?

Well, he had his own interpretation. In 1957, he actually visited Lund and we did the experiment there so he could see it, so he didn't doubt the finding but he came back then to an idea that goes back to the Swiss physiologist, Hess, who talked about the trophotrophic and ergotrophic systems. The trophotrophic system was serotonin, according to Brodie, and the ergotrophic system was the catecholamines. So he said, okay, what you see here is exactly what I'm saying – if you elevate the function of the ergotrophic system it will counteract the effect of the trophotrophic system that is now over-stimulated by the continuous release of serotonin. So he could easily handle that.

Did that idea come back 10 years later, when you put forward the proposal which led to the 5-HT reuptake inhibitors, that maybe the catecholamines were involved in motor activation and 5-HT was more involved in mood.

Well, no, not really. The reason I proposed this, which may not be true after all, was based on the data by Kielholz, who had this beautiful picture with all the tricyclics and on one side he had a spectrum of mood elevating effects and on the other side he has a spectrum of restoration of drive. And you could see from Kielholz's scheme, which was based on his clinical impression, that it was the secondary amines that were on the activating side and the tertiary amines that were mood elevating. Then we found that serotonin uptake was also inhibited by antidepressants and that it was more so by the tertiary than by the secondary amines and we just put that together and said look it's noradrenaline that is activating and it's serotonin that is mood elevating. That was in 1969, I think.

And this was the idea that led to the 5-HT reuptake inhibitors . . .

Oh, yes, and especially after our data on the effects of clomipramine on 5-HT reuptake. Actually I went down to Basel, to Geigy, it hadn't fused yet with Ciba, and talked to Theobald and the pharmacologists there. I showed them the data that clomipramine was acting preferentially on serotonin reuptake but they were not terribly interested. They had another alternative to develop as a follow-up to imipramine, but apparently the other drug had some problem in the toxicity studies, so they picked up clomipramine finally. And then, of course, clomipramine turned out in the clinic to have a profile that was not the same as imipramine.

It was clomipramine that made us so excited and also we felt that, on the basis of Kielholz's scheme, imipramine and amitriptyline, the tertiary amines, were perhaps more mood elevating than the secondary amines. We were also impressed by the fact that the tertiary amines were the ones that were used more; the secondary amines never came into any broad use, except perhaps for nortriptyline.

Except in the States. Desipramine sold extremely well in the States.

That's right and the reason for that was Brodie. He did a nice experiment. He simply gave desipramine followed by reserpine and he could see then that reserpine, under those conditions, had a stimulant action. Therefore, he said that imipramine acts via its metabolite, desipramine, and it's desipramine that's the antidepressant. It makes a lot of sense and, of course, Brodie was at that time a major figure. So that's true but in Europe desipramine never sold very much. Nortriptyline did a little better but actually it acts relatively more strongly on serotonin. Nevertheless all the careful, well controlled, clinical studies always show the same thing – if you compare any two of these tricyclics in depression you see no difference. Therefore, it was concluded they are the same. Kielholz had a different view he based it on his clinical impression, while all the so-called solid data showed no difference. I think it's partly because the instrument that is used is so crude – so you cannot pick out any subtle differences.

Anyway, we felt that since the tertiary amines are so much more popular it may be due to their serotonergic activity. Then we found that certain anti-histamines also had serotonin uptake inhibitory properties, even though they were not terribly selective. They acted on noradrenaline as well. But, on that basis, we picked up brompheniramine and chlorpheniramine. These were the most potent serotonin uptake inhibitors, among the antihistamines. On that basis, Hans Corrodi, a very clever Swiss organic chemist employed by the Astra subsidiary Hässle, with whom I had close collaboration for several years, came to zimelidine, which is actually very close to brompheniramine in terms of chemical structures.

Now, I know zimelidine was the first 5-HT reuptake inhibitor on the market but was it the first 5-HT reuptake inhibitor? There's some controversy about this. Ciba had one from fairly early on and Lundbeck with citalopram.

I know because I came down to Lundbeck and gave them a seminar and I told them the whole story as we had it and also I told them that if you add a halogen or similar things on the molecule of a noradrenaline reuptake inhibitor, you will switch it and it will become more serotonin uptake inhibiting. So the chemist there, Bögesö, had lots of noradrenaline uptake inhibitors, and he went back to the lab and modified his molecules, so as to make them serotonergic and that is how they got citalopram, which I'm sure was not before zimelidine.

What about fluoxetine?

Clearly, fluoxetine came after zimelidine. The first preclinical lab test of fluoxetine for 5-HT uptake inhibition at Lilly was performed in May 1972, two months after publication of the first patent demonstrating the selectivity of zimelidine as a 5-HT reuptake inhibitor.

Alec Coppen mentions that even after fluoxetine was developed the company weren't particularly thinking of it in terms of depression.

Yes, well . . . zimelidine came first both preclinically and clinically. I suppose that the demonstration of the antidepressant efficacy of zimelidine had an impact on the other drug companies. I'm not sure they would have even developed fluoxetine if it weren't zimelidine hadn't been shown to be clinically active.

We've gone down the road of producing drugs which are more selective to the 5-HT reuptake site. And this has been a major step forward but there's a hint from the literature, it's hard to put it stronger than a hint, that while these are good antidepressants, if anything they aren't as potent as some of the older tertiary amines were. Should we be going back from the route of trying to produce purer drugs to producing dirty drugs?

Well, if we do that, they will not be dirty in the same sense as in the beginning. because then they just happened to be dirty. This is a kind of rational dirtiness, isn't it?

Is there really such a thing as rational dirtiness? . . .

I think so. I think that is how ideal drug development should be. Number one usually is serendipity. You come across something. You have rather a dirty drug that's doing something. The next step is you try to find out how it works and in some cases you find one major site of action and in other cases you find a couple of candidate sites, so to speak. What you do then is you develop clean compounds and they had to be taken to the clinic to see whether they work. Then, for example, we can say serotonin uptake inhibition is an antidepressant principle but I think we can also say that noradrenaline reuptake inhibition is an antidepressant principle. So you've got two at least. The next step then would be to make molecules that are doing exactly these things but built into one and the same molecule. That would not be the same thing as just going back to the tricyclics because they have lots of other problems.

It's going to be very hard to actually persuade people that it isn't the same thing.

Not really. Because if you can develop a drug that is a serotonin uptake inhibitor and a noradrenaline uptake inhibitor and it does not have the cardiac problems, it will be a winner. However, I'm not sure about the anticholinergic action, whether that could also contribute. This is, of course, generally asumed to be just a side effect. I'm not so sure. The main argument is that an anticholinergic agent does not have anti-depressant activity and I think that is true. But that is not the same thing as saying that if you add an anticholinergic component, to a serotonergic or noradrenergic component, that then it won't do something. We have lots of experimental data showing that a drug, that in itself does nothing, can do a lot if it is combined with another drug that has a different site of action. So I don't think we can disregard this possibility . . .

Can you give me an example?

We have lots. This is an area we're working very much in now. Take clonidine, which is a rather striking example. If you have a monoamine-depleted animal and you give clonidine, you see practically nothing in terms of psychomotor activation. Now it was discovered by Anden, in our lab, many years ago that if you give apomorphine in a moderate dose to reserpine-treated animals, you get a stimulant effect and then if you add clonidine you get a lot more. So clonidine, which in itself does nothing, in the presence of a dopamine receptor agonist becomes a very powerful psychomotor stimulant.

You've just reminded me of Hannah Steinberg's work showing that if you co-prescribe amphetamines and barbiturates you get a much greater degree of excitation than you would expect to get from the amphetamines on their own, which seems remarkable. The whole area of the use of two different groups of drugs together is completely unexplored really.

Yes, it is. Actually my daughter, Maria, is very much involved in this field now. There are tremendous interactions at the post-synaptic side. Anden's experiments showed this but now we have so many examples. Another one is with atropine. If you give atropine to a monoamine-depleted animal you see very little. But if you give atropine combined with clonidine or with a sub-threshold dose of a NMDA receptor antagonist, which does nothing in this dosage, you will have a lot of psychomotor excitation. There are so many examples of these interactions. I think this is a very important area actually. The whole field of schizophrenia, I think, is now moving in the direction of trying to look for interactions and trying to look for patterns of aberrations that involve more than one neuro-transmitter.

It's very hard to see how treatments which will involve two or more drugs being co-prescribed will get through the FDA because the FDA is geared to handling one compound at a time.

That's true. I think they will have to re-educate and maybe we will have to wait for another generation of FDA people. But I think this concept of powerful interactions between neurotransmitters will have its day. I'm sure of that but not perhaps for the next few years.

One of the curious things to come out of the 5-HT reuptake inhibitors was the idea that the purer the compounds you get, the more specifically you can actually influence very discrete behaviours very quickly. The obvious example is that you can give a low dose of one of the 5-HT reuptake inhibitors and influence sexual performance within hours of having had it. This runs counter to the old idea that it takes a while for the drugs to get in the brain and they work terribly slowly on the receptors, etc., etc. and this explains why antidepressants take so long to work. But the effects of 5-HT drugs on sex prove that this can't be the case. How can we now explain the two or three or four week delay in response of depression to antidepressants?

Some of the therapeutic actions are also rapid. One example is premenstrual tension. That actually was pioneered by a fellow in our department, Elias Eriksson. What he did was to treat PMS patients with 5-HT reuptake inhibitors and the effect was dramatic. There is a very high percentage response and it's a dramatic response. Not only are the patients very grateful but their husbands are too. Now the point is this – they started treating people for the whole of their cycle but then they found out you can actually do it for a very short period of time. Just start a few days before the symptoms usually show up and it will work. So here we have another case of almost immediate response and, therefore, we are left with the problem how come that the antidepressant response shows such a sluggish onset. Maybe there is no true latency but certainly there is a slow development, of response over several weeks.

I have no explanation for it. But the way I try to envisage what happens is that presumably when a patient goes into depression, it takes a long time. Whatever is the first mechanism that becomes deficient, a series of secondary events happen and bring the patient into the final stage of depression. If this is so, it makes a lot of sense that if you manage to rectify some of the aberrations, that were at an early stage of the chain of events, you will have to wait for all these things to normalize and that takes time because it may involve protein synthesis, trophic effects in complex chains and complex circuitries to start to operate again. You get more or less the same lag, if you give serotonin inhibitors, MAO inhibitors or ECT. So it rather suggests that it is the disease that is the cause of this slow onset and now that we see that other symptoms that are not depression can show improvement very quickly, that also brings the focus onto the disorder as such. If this is true, it could have some important implications, namely that maybe there will never be a drug that will act immediately on the depression because it's impossible. Even though, one cannot be sure – one day maybe somebody will find something.

Coming back to dopamine and Hornykiewicz. The story goes back before Hornykiewicz to the idea that dopamine might be a neurotransmitter. Can you tell me how that came about?

Well, that goes back to the original experiment where we gave reserpine and found that catecholamines are also depleted. At that time dopamine was not in focus at all. Actually it had not yet been demonstrated to occur in the brain. After seeing this depletion, we stimulated the adrenergic nerves and found that they didn't respond any more so that argued against Brodie's idea of an excess release and in favour of a depletion. Therefore, we wanted to see if we could refill the stores in the brain. We couldn't give the amines themselves because we knew they didn't get into the brain but the precursors were known to get in. Actually, Udenfriend had given 5-hydroxytryptophan to reserpine-treated animals and I think he had also given L-dopa but probably in insufficient doses, I don't know. He hadn't seen much and he never published on it. But we did it and we were luckier. We could see a very dramatic effect of L-dopa on reserpine-treated animals–10 minutes after L-dopa they were up and running. We published it in *Nature* in 1957 but at the time when we submitted the paper, we hadn't yet analysed the brains. When we did we were really very disappointed because there was no noradrenaline in the brains of these animals.

It must have been very puzzling.

It was indeed. We were forced to look for dopamine because we had evidence that it was an amine that we had to look for. When we gave an MAO inhibitor it strongly potentiated L-dopa actions. So we had to develop a method for dopamine and we found dopamine tied up beautifully; it can be correlated in time and so forth with the arousal. Then we looked for dopamine normally in the brain and found it is there in amounts that are more than noradrenaline, so it couldn't be just the precursor.

Then, of course, there have been some statements that we were not first in the discovery of dopamine in the brain. This is partly true because there was a paper by Montagu, where she showed on a paper chromatogram a compound she called X. She said X has the same migration rate on paper as dopamine but she didn't say it was dopamine and she didn't say anything about the amounts it was present in or anything else for that matter. There was nothing in her publication that suggested that she thought this had any particular significance. You see everybody, of course, believed dopamine is in the brain from the work of Blaschko and others on the synthetic chain of catecholamines – dopamine had to be in the brain because there is noradrenaline in the brain. What we did was to demonstrate specifically that dopamine is in the brain, that it is depleted by reserpine, and that it comes back when we give L-dopa and we proposed that dopamine is an agonist in its own right in a paper to *Science* in 1958.

Shortly after that two of my students, Bertler and Rosengren, came to me asking if they could pursue this a little bit. I said, 'okay, you can look at the distribution' and they did and they found that the distribution is so different from noradrenaline. You have most of it in the basal ganglia and on the basis of that, we proposed that dopamine was involved in extrapyramidal functions because the basal ganglia had been recognized for a long time as being somehow involved in the control of motor functions. And, of course, it was known that reserpine can produce the picture of Parkinson's disease, so we proposed that the depletion of dopamine leads to Parkinson's syndrome.

All too often the only findings that get quoted are those of Hornykiewicz.

That's true but it was very clearly stated both in the volume from the First International Catecholamines Symposium in Bethesda in 1959, and also in the original paper by Bertler and Rosengren (Bertler and Rosengren, 1959), but it was elaborated on in a paper in *Pharmacological Reviews*.

So did Hornykiewicz come to this idea totally separately?

No, he knew about our work. There was a time lag in between. He knew about it even though he doesn't emphasize this a lot, I think one can say. What he rather emphasizes is that after spending a year with Blaschko, apparently the last thing Blaschko told him when he was departing was 'please remember dopamine'. So that was his story.

And when did that lead to people treating Parkinson's disease?

Well, you have two stories – Birkmayer's story and Hornykiewicz's story. Birkmayer said 'I came back to Hornykiewicz and told him that we must get started with giving L-dopa to Parkinson's patients' and if you ask Hornykiewicz he says 'I came to Birkmayer and told him when are you going to start to do this L-dopa in Parkinson's patients'. I don't know. Apparently they remember this in different ways but any way these were the two guys who did it. Birkmayer was a clinician in a neurogeriatric setting and he had lots of Parkinson patients and they gave it by injection.

Of course, they had problems. They saw something but not everybody who tried to replicate these injections could see it but there were some that saw it. I am convinced that they saw something and actually Birkmayer went on with it for a long time. In 1966 Hornykiewicz expressed doubts about the therapeutic usefulness of L-dopa. But Birkmayer insisted and one thing that really shows that Birkmayer was on the right track was his story about the decarboxylase inhibitor that Roche had, benserazide. Actually Roche supplied the drug to Birkmayer, rather reluctantly. They didn't seem to believe much in Birkmayer's L-dopa trials. I don't know who was the initiator of this, again I hear different stories, but in any event, he started to use it. The Roche people said that what you are going to see now is that you will block the effect of L-dopa because this is a decarboxylase inhibitor but he gave the two together and found it was the opposite. It potentiated the action of L-dopa.

Then, of course, Roche had to do what Birkmayer called retrograde pharmacology and they found that this drug didn't get into the brain and the Roche people had missed that. So that's how the first peripheral decarboxylase inhibitor came about and I think that really proves that Birkmayer saw something very significant and I am sure that if Cotzias had not come at about the same time as Birkmayer had made this discovery of the interaction with benserazide, then it would have developed further in Vienna, I'm sure.

But then Cotzias came in and what he saw was so dramatic. He was a Greek fellow, who as a rather young person had come to the US and got an MD degree there. He had access to Parkinson patients. He had some ideas about neuromelanin, that I never understood really, but of course neuromelanin disappears in Parkinson's – there's no doubt about that – and he thought that was important. So, he reasoned that one should give dopa orally in escalating doses and he did that, using the racemate, and discovered a much more dramatic effect on the symptomatology than Birkmayer had seen, at least before he was using the decarboxylase inhibitor. Then, he switched to L-dopa. The doses were rather shockingly high – up to 6, 7 or 8g per day of L-dopa and Birkmayer says that what Cotzias discovered was the side effects. And of course that's true – he discovered the side effects. But that's not the whole thing of course. Birkmayer hadn't seen the dyskinesias.

I heard about this for the first time at a meeting in Canada in 1967. Cotzias had a movie to show that his Parkinson patients responded very dramatically. I remember Duvoisin was there. He is a neurologist who specialized in Parkinson's disease. So I asked him 'what do you think, do you think this is a real thing?'. He said 'yes, I think so because of the dyskinesias. That could not be faked in any way'. I went home and I told the neurologists in Gothenburg and they got started. Of course it spread out world-wide very quickly – in a few years there were lots of observations of this effect.

So you think it was the combination of that and the Falck/Hillarp mapping that led to the change in attitude.

Yes, at the Adrenergic Mechanisms meeting it was argued that the issue as to whether these amines are doing anything in the brain was a matter of how you manipulate brain amines, what kind of doses of drugs you use – it was put down as a kind of manipulation of the system that had no physiological meaning. In addition there was the argument that the amine might be located in the glia.

This is so remarkable seeing that that very same group had been at war with Eccles and others saying that chemical neurotransmission was important.

Yes, and it may be that Eccles had an impact on it in a negative sense – although, of course, you know that Eccles is the one who later claimed that he was the one who first argued that you had chemical transmission in the brain. After fighting with Dale for so many years, all of a sudden he did an experiment that I don't think was terribly conclusive but he said, now look what I have found, there is chemical transmission in the brain. But I think his attack on Dale had made Dale very cautious. He didn't want to spoil the solid story he and his colleagues had as regards the peripheral system by any claim about the CNS. Of course there were also some good arguments – the synaptic delay in the brain was really very short in contrast to what you had in the periphery. The electron microscope pictures came at about the same time, showing how densely packed everything is in the brain, suggesting there was a lot more possibility for an electric impulse just to cross directly without any chemical intervention. As late as 1963, there was a nice book on synaptic transmission by a Canadian fellow – McLennan – in which he stated there was really no evidence even for acetylcholine as a neurotransmitter.

Talking about dopamine and Parkinson's disease leads on to dopamine and schizophrenia and the neuroleptics. Can you tell me how you got into working on the mechanism of action of chlorpromazine.

We were puzzled by the fact that the pharmacological profile of reserpine and chlorpromazine are very similar in animals and also in the clinic and yet one of them is a depletor of monoamines and the other one is not. We felt that maybe chlorpromazine was doing something to the metabolism of catecholamines. Axelrod had discovered catechol-O-methyl-transferase and we were interested in that. We were looking for the metabolite of dopamine, which is 3-methoxytyramine, and we found it normally in the brain. In order to measure the formation of 3-methoxytyramine we felt we should block monoamine oxidase because then we would have a closed system as it were. We thought that would be a nice way of looking at release because we had some data, which suggested to us, that 3-methoxy-tyramine formation is related to release. Actually this was one of the things that I brought up at the meeting on Adrenergic Mechanisms but Gaddum didn't believe in it at all. We had found that in order to be O-methylated, the amine has to be released first and therefore formation of 3-methoxytyramine would be an indicator of release. This is now generally accepted, but at that time, it was not at all accepted.

Anyway, what we did was to give an MAO inhibitor, chlorpromazine, haloperidol and a number of other compounds and looked at the rate of accumulation of 3-methoxytyramine and we looked at normetanephrine at the same time, the corresponding noradrenaline metabolite, and showed that there is an acceleration of the formation of these metabolites, while there is no change in the level of either dopamine or noradrenaline. So, if you have no change in the neurotransmitters but you have an elevation of metabolite, on that basis we said what is happening here is a stimulation of synthesis and release. In order to make this fit with what was known otherwise, especially the background knowledge that chlorpromazine and reserpine have the same profile and also some other data showing that the behavioural effects of L–dopa can be antagonized by chlorpromazine, it wasn't really far-fetched at all to say that here we must have a blockade of a receptor.

Receptors at this stage though were still theoretical entities. No one had actually labelled them and we didn't really know, for sure, that they existed.

That's true, but receptor theory in pharmacology goes back decades. It was well accepted in pharmacology long before any biochemist ever started to think of it. So it was not a problem to postulate the existence of a receptor that was blocked here, even though, of course, we couldn't say what kind of receptor it was. But we did experiments with phenoxybenzamine and it didn't do anything to 3-methoxytyramine, so there was some slight hint that maybe there are different receptors but we didn't postulate that – we left it at catecholamine receptors. Actually, in that paper we didn't even exclude an effect on serotonin receptors. So, as perhaps one does often with patent claims, you try to widen the claim as much as possible so we included serotonin – and serotonin receptors are, of course, now very much being discussed in connection with antipsychotic activity.

The way it was interpreted by others was that we claimed dopamine. I do not argue against it; certainly dopamine was in it. Shortly afterwards Anden and his colleagues in my lab and Nybäck and Sedvall in Stockholm studied a fairly large number of antipsychotic agents and found that the effect on dopamine is the common denominator, so that narrowed the whole thing on to dopamine.

Every so often when people write articles on the dopamine hypothesis, you see the name van Rossum mentioned. Where did he come in?

Actually in our 1963 paper, we didn't say anything about the pathogenesis of schizophrenia. This paper deals with the mode of action of antipsychotic agents and van Rossum said 'look, schizophrenia involves dopamine'. That's what he said and of course he may be right, he may be wrong, we still don't know. But what we do know is that neuroleptic drugs have an impact on dopamine and that is important for the effect.

Van Rossum was one of the pupils of Ariens, who has contributed a lot, I think. Ariens was the one who introduced the concept of intrinsic activity, which was very important. This is an example of how far pharmacology had gone before any receptor had even been isolated. There was a whole doctrine about receptors, affinity versus intrinsic activity and so forth. So he was his teacher and van Rossum did a lot of work together with Ariens but this is what is especially known about him.

The next thing was that Randrup and Munkvad found, together with a number of others, that amphetamine depends on the synthesis of catecholamines for its stimulant action. That led to the suggestion that amphetamine acts by releasing catecholamines and especially perhaps dopamine. They became very interested in the stereotyped behaviour that all dopamine receptor agonists induce, and they proposed that this stereotyped, disorganized behaviour was a model of schizophrenia. This is probably not true, in the strict sense, because we now know that in Parkinson patients, L-dopa can induce severe dyskinesia without inducing any psychotic symptoms – even though L-dopa can of course induce psychotic symptoms. Still, it could be true in a somewhat different sense – if the same type of disorganized output that you have in the motor system that leads to dyskinesia were to happen in those parts of the system that are involved in the mental functions, that could lead to psychosis. It's a perfectly sound idea.

Merton Sandler, however, would say that one problem with that is that during the 1950s and 1960s, in the UK at least, probably the US as well, thousands of housewives were having amphetamine to treat mood disorders and they weren't becoming psychotic from it, so much so that when the idea that these drugs can induce a psychosis came out, it wasn't widely believed.

I don't think that argues against the whole thing. It's trivial that we have different vulnerabilities among people. I think that one of the things that really had an impact in this area was the observations in Japan after the War when apparently the American troops had left stores of metamphetamine that came out on the black market. There was a widespread abuse of metamphetamine in Japan and a large number of cases of paranoid schizophrenia. The picture mimicked it so faithfully, that it took a while to find out about it.

That's the first I've heard about that.

Is that right? Oh, there must be a literature on it, I'm sure, it was so striking. It was a thing that happened during such a short period of time and there was so clear a relationship between these stores and the disorder – maybe the Americans don't like to write about it. But, of course, there were also lots of publications from other parts of the world, with a lower number of cases showing that the picture of paranoid schizophrenia was mimicked very faithfully by the amphetamines and of course later on with L-dopa and the directly acting dopamine agonists you can see similar things. Moreover, experiments on healthy and psychotic volunteers confirm this action.

Let me push you on this. Do you think it's the picture of paranoid schizophrenia or paranoid psychosis? Because now these days, of course, a different picture comes out from using drugs like ketamine which act on the glutamate system. Giles Harborne who works with me has been looking at this and it is very different to the effects of amphetamine.

Yes, I think you are right. Observations with PCP, phencyclidine, are also compelling. Adrienne Lahti and Carol Tamminga gave ketamine to schizophrenics and found that the patients say when they inject it 'now I feel exactly what I felt when I became ill'. So perhaps it's more like the natural symptomatology of schizophrenia than what you can produce by means of metamphetamine. However, some people claim that neuroleptics are not at all efficacious against this symptomatology, whereas in schizophrenia, the neuroleptics are efficacious in a fairly large number of cases. So that would argue a little bit against glutamate deficiency as being important.

Well, the interesting thing about these reactions when ketamine is used for surgery is that the minor tranquillizers are used to control the post-op reactions.

Yes, the benzodiazepines are the drugs of choice. So that's another thing that is hard to reconcile – there is no ideal model.

It's fairly complex. Do you think we made a mistake when people moved from saying that the neuroleptics work on the dopamine system to the idea of a dopamine hypothesis of schizophrenia?

Yes, maybe we should have called it the dopamine hypothesis of psychosis. That might have been closer to reality, but even that may not be quite adequate in view of the fact that neuroleptics act on a number of conditions, all of which probably involve hyperarousal. Maybe it's hyperarousal that these various conditions have in common – maybe we should have a dopamine hypothesis of arousal perhaps.

You seem to have moved from thinking in terms of neurotransmitters to thinking in terms of complex circuits lately?

Actually we started out with a very simplistic concept, aiming to explain why neuroleptic drugs can have such an impact on the cerebral cortex even though their main target is probably dopamine D-2 receptors, which are very scarce in the cerebral cortex. Now, the few D-2 receptors that you have, could still be the ones that explain everything but, to me, it seems more likely that the main action of the antipsychotic drugs is in those areas where the D-2 receptors are abundant. If this is so, we must explain how a change in the basal ganglia have such an impact on the cerebral cortex.

In the striatum, in the broadest sense, including the ventral striatum, there are two major inputs – glutamate from the cortex and dopamine from the brainstem. The striatum then has as its main target the thalamus. We postulated that if you had an inhibitory effect of the striatum on the thalamus, it should have an impact on the amount of sensory information being relayed further on to the cortex and if you open this 'filter' too much you may overload the cortex with sensory information and that would lead to delirium, confusion, hyperarousal and psychosis maybe.

If dopamine is assumed to have an inhibitory effect on the striatum it will be inhibiting an inhibitory mechanism and, therefore, dopamine will open the filter and that will lead to hyperarousal. On the other hand, if glutamate is an opponent to dopamine, a deficiency of the glutamatergic cortical input to the striatum would lead to the same thing. PCP would induce psychosis by weakening the glutamatergic input on the striatum.

Looking at psychomotor activity taken broadly, if you remove dopamine from the brain, you get virtually complete immobility. This immobility, according to this simple model, is due to an active predominance of the glutamatergic input to the striatum. Therefore, the simple experiment one can do is to deplete the brain of dopamine, with reserpine and an inhibitor of the synthesis of catecholamines, and you have a virtual complete immobility and then you give an antagonist to glutamate and they should move. And we found that they do. So that was how we started. Of course, it was a simplistic model and sure enough we are not simply dealing with one negative feedback loop, there is also a positive feedback. So going into it, the thing becomes very complicated but still I think the most powerful mechanism in this complex system is actually this negative feedback loop, where dopamine and glutamate control each other in the striatum.

So that is what I have been working on together with Maria Carlsson and collaborators and this is different from what was done before in this area in one important respect, which is that people, who had earlier been working on NMDA receptor antagonists such as MK801, and had found that it is a psychomotor stimulant, had postulated that it is so by means of elevating the release of dopamine. Everything has been assumed to be mediated via dopamine. But this model says that you can control psychomotor activity independently of dopamine by controlling the glutamatergic tone from the cortex to the basal ganglia. Now, we have evidence that this is true not only for glutamate but you can bring in acetylcholine, noradrenaline and serotonin – especially by 5-HT-2 receptors. They can also operate independently of dopamine. So you have a lot of different pathways that go into the striatum and they can operate in opposite directions. Some of them will, in this way, elevate arousal and others will have the opposite effect.

There is, therefore, a very complex interaction between a large number of neurotransmitters and one shouldn't have any predjuice about which neurotransmitter is most important. There may not be just one. It may be a complex imbalance that we are dealing with.

This prompts me to ask you, how frustrated do you get by clinicians. Clinically, there's a range of psychoses. You really need to get one or two of them to match up against the model you've got, rather than say this is a model for all of schizophrenia.

That's exactly the way of thinking that we are pursuing now and we have actually a little bit of evidence that we find quite encouraging. Let me tell you a little bit about this. This is a rather strange story and I would like to see the thing confirmed before I really believe in it. We have done postmortem studies on schizophrenics and controls and measured monoamine levels, precursors and metabolites in different brain regions. In each individual, we use 60 variables. In order to handle this you must use multivariate analysis and we have a very clever guy in our group who can do this, Dr Lars Hansson. Before he came we couldn't get anything out of this material. We tried the usual statistics and couldn't see anything really striking. And then he came and showed that these schizophrenics form two different clusters that are actually located on either side of the controls. The most amazing part of it was that when we looked at the cases that were on one side, they were the paranoid schizophrenics and the other ones were the non-paranoid schizophrenics.

This makes sense. If you look at the genetic inheritance of schizotypy versus paranoia, they don't go together.

We also found something with family history there, and that was that the non-paranoids had a much greater family history than the paranoids. Another very interesting part of it was that there were 10 out of the original 30 schizophrenic patients, who were discarded by the psychiatrist who made the diagnosis, Dr C.G.Gottfries. He said applying strict Bleulerian criteria. So we put those 10 back to see where they ended up and some of them ended up among the controls, some of them among the non-paranoids and some of them among the paranoids. Then when we looked at the family history of those that ended up among the controls, none of them had family history. Those that ended up among the non-paranoids had the heaviest family history and in between you have the paranoids.

Now, coming back to your question, could we come up with a model that will deal with only one of these groups and not with all of it? After having done all this, we went back and did the conventional statistics on the paranoids versus controls and non-paranoids versus controls, and there were statistical differences. We hadn't discovered that because, actually, I hadn't paid much attention to the distinction between paranoids and hebephrenics and catatonics. I stupidly thought this is rubbish; this is psychiatry – I don't want that. But now we found that the paranoids, for example, have higher levels of serotonergic metabolites, such as 5-HIAA, whereas these are reduced in the non-paranoids. So there is a pattern of changes involving dopamine, noradrenaline and serotonin that distinguishes these groups.

What we then did was we gave rats, MK801, and we analysed the brains in the same way as we had analysed the brains of schizophrenics and we did multivariate analysis and we found that the pattern of deviations involving dopamine, serotonin and noradrenaline, was similar to the paranoid schizophrenics. We think that this may be a strategy that can be used – you could try to replicate a pattern of deviations by means of a drug with a known site of action. If you can do that, you could formulate a hypothesis that this is a site that is out of order in the disorder in question. I think it's a fascinating approach.

Now, we were a bit surprised by some of our findings. We would have predicted, if anything, that the paranoids would have been the ones where dopamine would be primarily involved because neuroleptics are much better for the paranoids but it was not the case. Actually, there is a trend for dopamine to be low in the paranoid schizophrenics and we think this could be a compensatory phenomenon. Suppose that the primary deficiency is in the glutamatergic system, if the brain is smart it will reduce dopamine in order to try to restore the balance and if it cannot do it sufficiently, adding neuroleptics may help.

That's exactly the opposite to the conventional dopamine hypothesis. How does this fit in with the pure D-2 story? Under the influence of the dopamine hypothesis of schizophrenia, the companies went down the route of producing purer and purer compounds and we possibly got to the purest with Astra's compound, remoxipride, which may not have been the most potent but it seems to have been a good agent that was reasonably free of side effects. Now with all the fuss about clozapine, we've gone back to the old idea that we want dirty drugs, acting on D-1, D-2, D-3 D-5, plus 5-HT-2, etc., etc.

Well, you can use two arguments. Take remoxipride – you could say that look here we have a very clean compound and it seems to be very useful; it has a profile that's very acceptable and that would argue in favour of getting drugs that are very clean. On the other hand if you compare it with haloperidol, which is reasonably clean too, it has a different profile and we don't understand why the pharmacological profile and the clinical profile of haloperidol is so very different from remoxipride. There are a number of possible explanations but we don't know – and, as for clozapine, I don't think we have the answer to your question.

The dopamine hypothesis seemed to fit in with an older idea, which may date back to Jean Delay and Paul Janssen, that you've got to produce extrapyramidal symptoms in order to have a neuroleptic. Hanns Hippius and clozapine seemed to be arguing the opposite case but no one paid any heed to it, until of course clozapine came on the market again, then all of a sudden we hear people now saying 'well you don't have to produce extrapyramidal symptoms to have an anti-psychotic drug'.

That is true and that's a most important contribution from the clozapine story. You can be sure of this now. Of course, earlier one could have said that, I think, because in many cases you could find a dose of other neuroleptics, where you had an antipsychotic action that was satisfactory without extrapyramidal side effects. So that would also argue in favour of what is now accepted. But the most puzzling thing for me is remoxipride versus haloperidol. I think the pharmacology of remoxipride should be studied more carefully. We have some data that indicates that it has some preference for autoreceptors.

The remoxipride story also contains the twist about how one company can be struck by lightning twice. Astra, if anything, seem to have been the company that has been most guided by rational principles in drug development, but after having the misfortune they had with zimelidine, it seemed a cruel twist of fate that remoxipride should also have had problems. God doesn't want us to be rational!

That's right. That is the moral of the story and I was involved in both to some extent. So maybe it's me. I was closely involved in the zimelidine story and I was consulted by them for remoxipride. The idea was to distinguish between locomotion and stereotypy. They were using apomorphine and were looking for drugs that would antagonize its effect on locomotion rather than stereotypies and, therefore, would not have extrapyramidal side effects. It was a very simple concept.

So they haven't consulted you since!

That is only partly true. Actually, shortly after zimelidine, serotonin was a word that you shouldn't mention at Astra. It was a bad word. Even after zimelidine, they were in an extremely fortunate situation. They had all the know-how. They knew exactly how to make another SSRI in a short time and they could still have been the leaders in the SSRI field but they dropped it altogether. Actually the boss of the company was inclined to stop doing research and to switch Astra into a generic company.

That would have been terrible.

Yes, a disaster of course but he died from cancer shortly afterwards. And remoxipride, yes, that was really very sad. Anyway, it may be that remoxipride has relatively low EPS problems because it is a preferential autoreceptor antagonist. We have such compounds and they don't cause EPS. They have a very interesting pharmacology because they are what we call stabilizers. This means that if you have a high baseline activity they will inhibit behaviour and if you have a low baseline activity they are stimulants. So, they are very interesting drugs.

Why has Scandinavia has produced so many neuroscientists and psychiatrists? On the psychiatric side you've got Langfeldt, Stromgren, Gottfries and then Hillarp, yourself, Hokfelt and others – there is an endless list of people who've made major contributions, I'm sure out of all proportion to the number of people who are actually in Scandinavia. And you had one of the first psychopharmacological associations.

Yes, it came early. I was among the founders of this Scandinavian Society for Psychopharmacology – that was in 1959. I think it's a chance phenomenon because one cannot link it to any particular school or individual. For example, von Euler, who was early in this field, was not linked to any of the rest. He had some very successful pupils. Then you have Hillarp and actually his school was very strong because he was really very good in gathering skilful people around him. And it was in a way fortunate that he started out in Lund, then he moved to Gothenburg and then from Gothenburg he went to the Chair of Histology in Stockholm. Since he started out in Lund and Falck was still there, on the basis of the histochemical fluorescent technique, a group could be formed there and then in Stockholm so there was another one.

In the case of the Society, the originator of this Society was the Danish Lundbeck Company to some extent. Because Lundbeck had been very successful with both antipsychotic and antidepressant drugs thanks to a clever medicinal chemist, P.V. Petersen. There was also a clinician – Jörgen Ravn, who came to Lund to visit David Ingvar. It was the three of us who started the Society in 1959. Lundbeck served as generous sponsors from the outset.

But the neuroscience interest isn't just in Denmark and Sweden. There are people in Norway and Finland, like Linggaerde and Toumisto – and Scandinavian work always seems methodical and systematic.

Thank you. Maybe we have more crazy people up there so we have a greater need for this kind of research I don't know. I have no statistics to support that, but there are some very interesting families in the North of Sweden with genetic disturbances, porphyria and various schizophrenic disorders. That has attracted a lot of attention.

As regards the methodicalness, to be philosophical about that, perhaps one could say the further out you get in terms of climate you have to be careful. In warm weather down around the equator, you can almost sell your bed in the morning, can't you? But in the far North, you have to plan in order to survive, because the winter is quite severe. So it's possible that there has been some kind of selection of people who are planners, I don't know if there is anything to it.

Some years ago, in Human Psychopharmacology, *you wrote an article saying that we're really on the brink of an era where we won't just be treating mental illness, we will be engineering personalities and human abilities. This was before all the fuss about cosmetic psychopharmacology. Do you still think that, or . . .*

Yes, I think this is something that will come. I am sure there will be a lot of debate and a lot of emotions will be stirred up because of this trend but it will come. I am sure that when we have a drug that will improve the memory of old people without causing that much side effects – it's going to be used. Even if the doctor says 'never mind getting a little bit forgetful when you're old, that's normal'. People will take it regardless of that. They are not so impressed by clinical diagnostics. If they feel better when they take a drug and even if they are aware of the possibility of long-term use causing severe problems, they may consider, nevertheless, that they are taking a good chance by using it because they gain so much.

I think that is true now with fluoxetine and all these drugs. There are people who feel so much better, who didn't have any diagnosis really. For example, if you are shy among people, so-called social phobia, which is more or less normal isn't it, and if you get rid of that it must be a tremendous, a dramatic change for a person, mustn't it? Someone who has been shy and deprived of so much and all of a sudden you can do it, of course you will take it. I remember from the zimelidine period, that there were people whose income went up when they started to take the drug. If there are such very striking results as this, people will say all right, I will take the risk. I feel reasonably okay and the side effects are not that much.

As this field develops we will have more and more drugs that will do this and people will be taking more and more drugs. It will become a natural part of life – well it is already – we tend to forget that we use caffeine as coffee and tea all the time and we do it as a drug of course. We need to get a little bit more stimulation in order to work a couple of more hours – this is pharmacology isn't it? We have done this for a long time – take alcohol. Alcohol has done more good than bad to mankind. I am convinced of that. There is so much that has come out of the increased interaction between individuals because of alcohol. Some individuals have had to pay very much for this but mankind has done very well I think. And this will go on I am sure. Prozac is perhaps the most striking example but before that we had things such as the beta-blockers for stage fright. Those violinists, who started to perform a lot better while on the beta-blockers, you cannot say that they were sick. They just performed better.

The companies have begun to move away from trying to give drugs which act on the classical neurotransmitters to look at the neurodegenerative disorders, which seems to me to offer scope for some more radical engineering.

Oh, yes. I think molecular biology will come in very strongly. It has done a lot already even though it has not had too much of an impact on the clinic yet. But you also mentioned neurodegeneration and it could be that things that we don't think about so much in terms of neurodegeneration will turn out, I would guess, to have a component of neurodegenerative mechanism. For example, take the kindling phenomenon that comes up in many different contexts. If you have changes like that, isn't it very likely that it involves neurodegeneration? What I think here, of course, it's again very simplistic, is that in many cases, you have two glutamatergic inputs, one directly onto the neurone and the other indirectly via an interneurone that's GABAergic – now if these operate at a moderate level, you will have a kind of a balance and your output will be at a modest level. Suppose the GABAergic neurone is especially sensitive to cytotoxicity: if it goes, all of a sudden you would only have the gas; the brake has gone and you will have a tremendous elevation of the output that will remain forever because the GABAergic neurone has gone. And I wouldn't be surprised if this kind of mechanism is involved in kindling and it could also be in some aspects of memory and learning. When we learn, do we kill neurones, in order to get a more efficacious message through, what do you think? When we talk about addiction, which lasts forever – once an alcoholic, you will never be the same. And also if you think about tardive dyskinesia and kindling.

Does any of this link in with the issue of redundancy in nature?

This is extremely interesting. I think it has a lot of support from molecular biology. Various random phenomena such as gene duplication and sub-sequent mutations can sometimes lead to the production of proteins without any function.

Another thing that was brought up by C.W. Bowers in a recent article in TINS (1994) entitled 'Superfluous Neurotransmitters?' deals with gene regulation. There are mechanisms that determine whether or not a gene is going to be expressed in a given cell and these mechanisms are not always very precise. That means that you could very well have expressions of proteins in cells, where they are not functioning. The genome is the same in all cells so, in principle, all cells can produce all the different proteins that other cells can but the expression is restricted in different cells. The regulation of this expression is not precise – this means that you can have protein in places where they have no function. You should be particularly careful if you see the occurrence of a certain protein, maybe an enzyme or a receptor, in a site where you don't have it in the same region or organ in a related species. For example, if you have it in a rat and you don't have it in a mouse or in a guinea pig, you must start to wonder. Is it really likely that this protein is going to be an essential thing in the rat, while it's not needed in the mouse or the guinea pig. So that brought in the idea of superfluous neurotransmitters, and a number of neuropeptides were given as examples in Bowers' article.

In 1988 I published some rather similar speculations. I called my paper 'Peptide Neurotransmitters – Redundant Vestiges?' (Carlsson, 1988b) I came to a similar conclusion from a pharmacological point of view, starting out, for example, with naltrexone or naloxone, where you have so little functional loss even if you have blocked the receptor as indicated by a blockade of the action of morphine. There are other examples where antagonists of peptide neurotransmitters aren't doing anything.

My reasoning was based on evolutionary considerations. The peptides are enormously powerful as signalling molecules because they have an identity that is terrific. By means of changing just one amino acid you have a different identity. And they are tremendously powerful because you can have very high affinities. And they are easily made by the cell because after all the cell is a peptide manufacturing machine. So all this makes the peptides so convenient as hormones or neurohormones. But, once upon a time, one of these endocrine cells started to make a process to become a neurone. At that point, there is a drawback, because the production has to be around the nucleus and you had to transport the transmitter to the nerve ending. If the thing has to operate very quickly, it may become awkward to have a peptide as a neurotransmitter.

In evolution these things can be solved. What nature does is to produce enzymes and a machinery and so on that is transported down the nerve and they will manufacture the neurotransmitter – a small molecule – at the nerve ending. That is how the small molecule neurotransmitters evolved. So how about the neuropeptides? They are made in very small amounts. The negative selection pressure on such small amounts is virtually nil, so they can go on forever being there because they don't make any harm and that's why we have such a tremendous assortment of them. Now, if that is how they evolved, it's not surprising to find that there are enormous species differences because if a mutation happens and this peptide is no longer functional in a certain species it doesn't make any difference. That was my way of looking at it.

This idea would open up a whole new way of looking at chemical neurotransmission because, at the moment, the fashion is for people like Sol Snyder to write articles talking about the neurotransmitter orchestra – that there are hundreds of them. This is quite a different idea.

Yes. One thing that has to be added to it, which I think is important, is that we have now reached a sensitivity of analytical methods down to the levels of the background noise. We can pick up practically everything. So it means that while in the 1950s, when I started in this field, we could detect a compound by means of the techniques that were available at that time, it had a much higher likelihood of being functionally relevant than today.

Another fascinating possibility is this. Suppose it's not true when we say that different genes are expressed in different cells. Suppose all genes are expressed in all cells. What would happen then is that the expression is suppressed but nature doesn't take the trouble to suppress it all the way down to zero. Why should it – I mean it's down to a level where it doesn't matter. If so, when our methods become sensitive enough we will find that all cells produce all the proteins that the genome can produce. What made me think of that was when I went to see a colleague in Gothenburg, who demonstrated this enormously sensitive capillary electrophoresis. What they could do was to take one white cell, put it in a little funnel at the end of this tube and then extract this single cell and do electrophoresis. They found dopamine, tyrosine–hydroxylase and monoamine oxidase in this white cell.

One might feel that dopamine is an important compound in immunology but suppose what they see is just background values. It's just that nature doesn't take the effort to suppress the genome 100%. There is a little bit left. If that is true, people should be aware of it because otherwise we will waste a lot of resources on things that we should perhaps use on something else.

Select bibliography

Bertler, Å. and Rosengren, E. (1959) Occurrence of distribution of dopamine in brain and other tissues. *Experientia*, **15**, 10.

Carlsson, A. (1959) The occurrence, distribution and physiological role of catecholamines in the nervous system. *Pharmacol. Rev.*, **11**, 490–93.

Carlsson, A. (1966) Physiological and pharmacological release of monoamines in the central nervous system, in *Mechanisms of Release of Biogenic Amines* (eds U.S. von Euler, S. Rosell and B. Uvnäs), Pergamon Press, Oxford, pp. 331 – 46.

Carlsson, A. (1982) Recent observations on new potential and established antidepressant drugs. *Pharmakopsychiat.* **15**, 116–20.

Carlsson, A. (1987) Perspectives on the discovery of central monoaminergic neurotransmission. *Ann. Rev. Neurosci.*, **10**, 19–40. Also published in: *The Excitement and Fascination of Science: Reflexions by Eminent Scientists*, Volume 3, Part 2 (ed. J. Lederberg). Annual Reviews Inc, Palo Alto, California, pp. 1335–58.

Carlsson, A. (1998a) The current status of the dopamine hypothesis of schizophrenia. *Neuropsychopharmacology*, **1**, 179–80.

Carlsson, A. (1988b) Peptide neurotransmitters – redundant vestiges? *Pharmacology and Toxicology*, **62**, 241–42.

Carlsson, A. and Lindqvist, M. (1963) Effect of chlorpromazine or haloperidol on the formation of 3-methoxytyramine and normetanephrine in mouse brain. *Acta Pharmacol* (Kbh), **20**, 140–44.

Carlsson, A., Lindqvist, M. and Magnusson, T. (1957) 3,4-Dihydroxyphenylalanine and 5-hydroxytyramine in brain. *Science*, **127**, 471.

Carlsson, M. and Carlsson, A. (1990) Interactions between glutamatergic and monoaminergic systems within the basal ganglia – implications for schizophrenia and Parkinson's disease. Trends in Neurosci., **13**, 272–76.

Dahlström, A. and Carlsson, A. (1986) Making visible the invisible. (Recollections of the first experiences with the histochemical fluorescence method for visualization of tissue monoamines), in *Discoveries in Pharmacology*. Volume 3. Pharmacological Methods, Receptors and Chemotherapy (eds M.J. Parnham and J. Bruinvels). Elsevier, Amsterdam, New York and Oxford, pp. 97–128.

Hansson, L.O., Waters, N., Winblad, B. *et al.* (1994) Evidence for biochemical heterogeneity and schizophrenia: a multivariate study of monoaminergic indicies in human post-mortem brain tissue. *J. Neural Transm.* (GenSect) **98**, 217–35.

von Euler, U.S., Rosell, S. Uvnäs, B. (eds) (1966) *Mechanisms of Release of Biogenic Amines*, Pergamon Press, Oxford.

4 Frank Ayd

The discovery of antidepressants

Let's begin with the CINP. If you look at the history the way it's been written these days, people talk about the importance of a meeting that was organized in 1957 by Silvio Garattini, but you and Hanns Hippius have drawn my attention to the fact that there was another meeting in 1957 that was organized by Ciba. Do you want to tell me about that meeting?

To my knowledge, Silvio Garattini's was a scientific meeting at his place. It was not intended to be an organizational meeting. The meeting that Hanns Hippius and I refer to was convened for the express purpose of discussing the formation of an international scientific organization devoted to psychopharmacology. The meeting was held in Milan. It was attended by people from various European countries, North America and Australia. England, for example, definitely had some representatives. Among those from England, Frank Fish stands out in my mind. He was an impressive fellow to meet. Richard Boardman I believe was there. Most of the people that were there actually had done a lot of the early work in psychopharmacology. From the United States there were Sid Cohen, Herman Denber, myself and Nathan Kline . . . I think Fritz Freyhan was there but I'm not really sure. From Austria, there was Hans Hoff and Dr Arnold, who was Hoff's assistant. From Switzerland there were Paul Kielhotz, Jules Angst, Walter Poldinger, from Germany was Hanns Hippius and . . . from France, Pierre Deniker, Jean Delay and Pierre Lambert were there.

Ernest Rothlin?

Yes. He was definitely there. I can't recall who came from the Scandinavian countries. The idea was to assemble a group to discuss formation of an international organization to enhance communication between researchers.

So this was almost completely clinical.

Yes, definitely. We met in Milan for about four days and at the end, there was a decision to organize. The Swiss were given most of the organizational duties because they were right there and could deal with the people at WHO and also deal with Ciba, although Ciba did not try to control the organization in any way. Ciba's major function was to contribute the money to fund the travel expenses for the people who participated.

The decision was made that not only would we organize but we would start right off with an international meeting that was to be held in Rome. Since it was to be held in Rome the decision was made to extend an invitation to Pope Pius XII to address the meeting and indeed he did. The meeting was held in the fall of 1958 and that was the beginning of the CINP.

How did the Pope end up being at CINP?

Well, the invitation was extended to him and he accepted it. He was provided with copies and reprints of a number of articles because he wrote his own speeches. He was particularly interested in medicine which was one of the reasons why he agreed to do this. After his death, all his addresses – about 200 different talks to medical organizations – were published, and there were several hundred pages. The Pope was supplied with information and he wrote his own speech. It was a remarkable speech for a Pontiff and particularly for a layman, in that he appreciated immediately the potential of the psychoactive drugs – he spoke primarily on chlorpromazine, some on reserpine but not a great deal and of course by then we were in the early days of the anxiolytics. So he had some idea of what the potential was.

The importance of that meeting was that, for the first time, we assembled, not only psychiatrists but pharmacologists, psychologists, and a number of basic science people. The idea was to have an exchange of information between the clinicians and the basic scientists and so this was a revolutionary meeting. It attracted a large number of people and really provided a basic membership for the CINP. It, to me, was perhaps the most important meeting in the early days of psychopharmacology.

It also gave people a chance to meet each other. I was one of the fortunate ones. I had already travelled. I had been to England, Ireland, Germany, France, Italy, Switzerland, Spain and Portugal. So I had covered Europe pretty well and I knew many of the pioneers in psychopharmacology, but very few Americans knew them outside of Will Sargent, who frequently came to the United States. This meeting started an interchange and so now Hanns Hippius was no longer a name, he was a person that you could relate to and that was true for Angst and for Poldinger and for other colleagues.

It makes a big difference doesn't it? Its curious how often you can be hostile to a person's ideas, when you see them put on paper, but when you meet the person you get a completely different perspective.

Sure, for example, Mike Shepherd was there. Now my initial reaction to

Mike reading his papers was that he's negative. At that meeting, the first day we sat next to each other on the bus from the hotel to the meeting centre, so we had a half hour to talk and my impression of him changed completely. Also Pichot was there and my initial reaction to him was also negative – until I met him and then it changed. And I think that probably happened to others, when they met me. The meeting led to a lot of useful exchange of ideas, as well as a formation of mutual respect for people. In my judgement, it was most important thing that happened to psychopharmacology in the 1950s from the standpoint of really having a dissemination of respected material.

In the early days the CINP hit problems. When the meeting was held to found the ACNP you hinted at some of these problems, some of the clashes of personality, you mentioned I think that you had been left off the membership list and . . .

Yes, but whether that was deliberate or accidental who knows. There were some power struggles. Some of the early men in psychopharmacology were somewaht vain and looking for promotions and prestige. You would expect there would be some conflicts and a power struggle, but that was true also within the ACNP.

Well, can I ask you about ACNP? It appears that one of the reasons to organize the ACNP was because CINP was seen as being too European – and very much linked to the major European companies.

Well, we were thousands of miles away. That made a big difference and you have to look at it from the perspective of the people who wanted to participate actively in things. They had to get funded, which in those days was not yet an accepted thing. They either had to persuade the institution where they worked to pick up the tab or pay for it themselves. Consider one like myself. I'm in private practice. I have to get a locum while I'm away. I've got to pay him, the plane fare, the hotel bill and other costs. It was not inexpensive to do. And I think it is better to have a national group and that the national become very active in the international. The ACNP now has become a powerful force within the CINP, very much so.

Who were the key people behind getting ACNP going?

Ted Rothman. Ted was an unusual fellow and a very personable gentleman. He was an analyst in Los Angeles, who had an interest in what the drugs were doing to his patients. He felt that there ought to be an organization of people interested in psychopharmacology. He talked to Leo Hollister, to me, and some others about his idea. Then he talked to friends at Ciba in the pharmaceutical industry. The decision was made to get a group together. We met in New York at the Barbizon Plaza Hotel for a weekend. It was a good mixture of people. There were people from academia, State Hospitals, private hospitals, people from different geographic parts of the United States and Canada, and people who were just starting in psychopharmacology.

There were some very forceful personalities as well.

Some very strong personalities. Ted put together a list. I don't know exactly how he did that. I know he called a few people and asked if you were going to do this who would you want to have at the meeting? When you look at this list, I was in private practice, Henry Brill, of course was working in the Commissioner's office in the State of New York, Bernie Brodie was at the NIMH, Eugene Caffey was with the Veterans' Administration, Jonathan Cole had been at NIMH, Bill Dorfman was a board certified internist with an interest in psychosomatic medicine. He was one of the founders of the Academy of Psychosomatic Medicine and editor of its Journal. Ed Dunlop was connected with a private psychiatric hospital in Vermont. Paul Feldman was from Kansas, Paul Hoch was from New York State Psychiatric Institute, Doug Goldman from the State Hospital in Cincinnati, Bernie Glueck, the Institute of Living. Some were primarily interested in basic science; others had no real interest in basic science.

Heinz Lehmann put it to me that one of the reasons that either Ted or others were keen to have you there was because of your awareness of the legal angles.

Yes. That would be, in part, because when I was at Rome, I taught a course called Modern Medical Moral Problems. My students were ordained priests studying for their Doctorate in Canon Law. Part of the course covered informed consent, making a valid contract, the autonomy of the individual, and human experimentation. I had some pretty strong feelings about doctors giving medicines to patients without telling them anything at all about the risks and benefits. I didn't think that was right or ethical. Anything that could damage psychopharmacology bothered me because I saw this as a really great blessing for mankind.

Think what it was like to be connected with a psychiatric hospital prior to 1952. There were hundreds or thousands of patients for whom you could do very little. You had hydrotherapy, insulin coma, and ECT, a lot of bromides, paraldehyde for controlling some symptoms. You had patients who were in the hospital for 25, 30 or 40 years and they weren't 60 yet. Abandon hope all ye who enter here – you're not going to leave except in a pine box. Then consider the dramatic change that took place when chlorpromazine and other antipsychotics, and the monoamine oxidase inhibitors, were used properly. Although limited to a certain number of patients, MAOIs offered an alternative to ECT. Then came the tricylics. It is difficult to accurately described the remarkable changes that took place in psychiatric hospitals in the 1950s.

One real value of these drugs in the early days to me was they stimulated inquisitiveness. When you swallowed that pill, what happened – where did it go, what did it do? When I gave ECT, I wondered when the current passed between the temples and crosses through the mid-brain, what did it do? I was so glad Bernie Brodie was there because he had similar interests. Already we were thinking in terms of, what is now the pharmacokinetics and pharmacodynamics of drugs.

Yes, well that comes through quite clearly. I think it's actually probably yourself and Brodie, who actually contributed the most towards the ACNP organizational meeting. If you look at a word count, I'm sure the two of you will come out as . . .

Yes, we were active participants. Bernie was very interested in trying to explain why and how drugs worked. It was very dramatic. Take ECT – a psychotically depressed patient is given 10–12 treatments at most and he's normal. Then you give this very psychotic individual chlorpromazine and the first thing you saw, of course, was sedation and then gradually, particularly if he was acute with what we call today the positive symptoms, these would disappear. Even some patients who had predominantly negative symptoms, did respond. So this revolution was going on, which I saw as being important, not only to the current patients but to the patients of the future, and I gave a lot of time to this – that is one thing my wife will tell you. Sometimes she used to say 'you're like John the Baptist – you're out preaching what's coming'. That's true: I lectured all over the place.

What about side effects. You were one of the first to report some of the side effects of these drugs. The whole issue has to have been tricky in terms of you guys weren't really sure what was going to happen. Some people got well, okay, but . . .

We weren't sure. There was minimal animal and human data. Basically it took a lot of courage because we really didn't know what was going to happen. Yes, I had a fatal agranulocytosis and that will wake you up, if you've been kind of cavalier. I will never forget within the first 6 weeks of chlorpromazine, I had 2 patients who got jaundiced. The first one had only gotten 2 doses. He had just been hospitalized – it turned out in fact that he had a viral hepatitis – whether chlorpromazine brought it to the surface I don't know – but it kind of rocks your boat if you've admitted someone to the hospital and he has 2 doses of this medicine you're giving and the nurse calls you up and says 'hey, this fella's turning yellow on us' and you go see him and he's got a full blown jaundice. The second patient who got jaundice, I didn't tell her this was a risk because I wasn't sure in the first patient whether chlorpromazine had any role in the jaundice. This was a woman who had been chronically agitated and so forth and really was more of an agitated depressive than anything else. I gave her chlorpromazine and when she returned for her next appointment she was jaundiced. I said to her 'Mary, how long have you been like this?' and she said 'doctor you've tried so hard to help me and I do feel better, even though I'm yellow'. So I said 'well I hope you've stopped the medicine' and she said 'oh no, it's helping me'. So I learned that chlorpromazine can cause jaundice but if you keep it up the jaundice doesn't necessarily get any worse. In fact, if you can keep it up, which I did with her, it went away. So it was a transient hepatic reaction to chlorpromazine. But you also get a hint as to how valuable these drugs were to patients.

I also reported the first case of severe dystonia with chlorpromazine. In fact, I filmed this patient and I took it to SmithKline and French and showed it to them. They had never seen or heard of this and they arranged for me to show the film at the annual meeting of the American Neurological Association in Atlantic City. I showed it there and I got everything from hysteria to 'I don't know what this is'. There were a couple who said 'well it looks like torsion dystonia' but there were some differences, in their judgement. Anyway, I realized that I couldn't go around and just extol the benefits of the medication; I had a moral obligation to keep track of the side effects and to try and present a balance; not frighten people away but fulfil my duty to give them as much information as they need and can handle to make an informed decision about their treatment.

I soon realized that if you stop neuroleptics, relapse occurred pretty quickly. So it was obvious that neuroleptic therapy is equivalent to treating an epileptic or a diabetic: long term treatment is going to be important. I got into that very early. I lectured about one year's experience with chlorpromazine, and at the CINP meeting in Munich I reported on 10 years' experience with chlorpromazine. I gave a paper at the World Psychiatric Congress in Montreal on one year's treatment with imipramine patients and then wrote a paper on long-term perphenazine therapy, which the *New England Journal of Medicine* published. This helped psychiatry. Psychiatrists were not publishing in regular medical journals. My paper on drug-induced extrapyramidal symptoms was a lead article in JAMA in 1961, and I'm proud to tell you that when the 100th anniversay of JAMA was celebrated they listed the 100 most frequently quoted articles published in JAMA in 100 years. My paper on EPS was No. 20 (Ayd, 1961). There were only two by psychiatrists among the authors of these 100 publications.

I had an article on chlorpromazine in JAMA showing photographs of patients who were quite severely anorectic, who looked like they were from concentration camps and who after chlorpromazine gained weight. I reported neuroleptic-induced galactorrhoea. I even had the local heath department analyse the breast milk, collected from women who were lactating on chlorpromazine, and it was absolutely the same as normal breast milk in terms of fat content and other constituents. I was one of the first to report false pregnancy tests on phenothiazines. This was all new. We had to really know what were we doing. It really was a puzzle. Here's a drug that can twist a man like a pretzel, can make him stiff as a board, produce jaundice, cause agranulocytosis, sedate people and people could take a huge amount without dying. It caused all kinds of endocrine changes, some people had total amennorhea, others had galactorrhea. It was very interesting – what's this drug doing in the body and how is it doing it? This led to endocrinologists getting interested in it.

I got letters from all kinds of specialists based on the articles I had in JAMA and the New England Journal. It changed attitudes towards psychiatry and that was a very important thing. I can tell you the pioneers in psychopharmacology were looked upon as quacks and frauds. I was accused of being no different than the guys who sold snake oil in the wild west days. I gave a lecture in New York on my experiences with chlorpromazine and one of the discussants was the Past President of the American Psychiatric Association, Nolan Lewis. Dr Lewis was very gracious and complementary but at the end he said 'I have one word of advice to the audience, hurry up and prescribe this drug while it still works'. There was such scepticism in the early days.

There was more than just that though. There was hostility in certain quarters that the proper treatment is psychotherapy and this is a quick fix that is going to be harmful to both you and the patient.

That's right. You're not really getting to the problem. You're masking the problem. Oh yes that was certainly true. The analysts dominated, and here you're giving a pill and not talking about the Id, the Ego and the SuperEgo. And you're not even considering the psyche and that was just anathema. They missed the point. The point was sure we were enthused, look what was happening, but we weren't forgetting that this was happening in a human being and just as you don't treat a diabetic with insulin and diet alone, there's a whole lot else that's involved in psychopharmacologic therapy. We were doing psychotherapy but not dynamic psychotherapy. You had to explain to patients what this medicine was, what it could do, why they should take it, how we thought it worked and you had to encourage them to be patient because it wasn't miracle medicine. If you give chlorpromazine and the family would say 'oh yes he's quieter but he's still hearing voices and he's talking about the crazy ideas he has' because you don't get an antipsychotic effect early. You had to educate the family as well as the patient.

I personally was convinced of the value of proper pharmacotherapy. Sure I had a bias – you couldn't experience this and not get a bias – but I tried to be balanced about it. But then I attracted a lot of attention, there's no question about that. Here I am, relatively young, out of medical school not even 10 years and I'm testifying before Congress about these drugs and I'm on different programmes. Ciba had a weekly television programme, prime time Sunday afternoon in the US, called 'Medical Horizons'. It originated almost exclusively from hospitals and it covered surgery and obstetrics, internal medicine and so forth. They asked me if

I would do the first one on psychiatry and I did. I did an electric shock treatment on national television and I learned how ill-informed my colleagues were. Some physicians wrote me saying I faked ECT because they didn't see a convulsion. They didn't know what succinylcholine could do, they had no idea what giving brevital sodium meant or what the new equipment was doing in terms of controlling milli-amperage and all the other things that would influence ECT.

I had a neurosurgeon on the programme with me who had done some lobotomies and we had some patients who had had lobotomies. These were not transorbital, they weren't the original pre-frontal, these were stereotactic psychosurgery and these people made quite an impression.

It also provoked a lot of envy and hostility. That didn't just happen to me. Heinz Lehmann was defending psychopharmacology, in the early days, at a public meeting and a guy walked up to him and smashed a pie in his face. Heinz just wiped it away and continued. I could have never done that. I would have been so angry. But this was the kind of hostility that you encountered. There were people who risked their jobs. Henry Brill risked his job.

Henry Brill's move to introduce chlorpromazine to Pilgrim State Hospital was one of the big breakthroughs. Why did he take the risk?

As you know, initially, psychopharmacotherapy was not embraced by the psychoanalysts who dominated American psychiatry. Some viewed psychopharmacology as a threat to be opposed. Their hostility was not verbal. If the introduction of CPZ by Brill resulted in serious adverse effects, the opponents would have gone for his head. Henry knew he was taking a risk but he believed that patient welfare justified the risk.

In the US, 1956 was a big year for psychopharmacology. The annual meeting of the American Psychiatric Association was in Atlantic City. I gave a paper on chlorpromazine and reserpine. The first papers on meprobamate were presented. Now in part, because of some of the promotional efforts, there was a 'whispering' campaign – have you heard about this drug, meprobamate. It's just as good as thorazine but without the side effects – the press got more interested than usual.

Meprobamate is a drug that has vanished at least in the UK but it had a big impact during the 1950s. When the history gets written of this period, it gets written in terms of the antidepressants and in terms of the neuroleptics. Meprobamate is written out. What role did it play?

Oh I thought it played a very important role. Actually first of all it was an effective anxiolytic and it didn't have some of the disadvantages of the barbiturates. It is a barbiturate-like product but it was a little bit different. When it was used initially in lower doses and people were put on it and left on it for long periods, it proved to be a fairly safe drug and there weren't problems with dependance and withdrawal per se. As time went on that became a problem and it became, in the eyes of many doctors another barbiturate, but the important thing it showed that you can have a non-barbiturate, which can do many of the things that a barbiturate can. So, it actually was responsible for Roche coming up with the benzodiazepines.

So why did Librium replace meprobamate?

Well, there were two reasons. First of all a very small company had meprobamate and when sales began increasing, they had no sales force. They had cross-licenced with Wyeth, who produced it as Serax. The company was in a sense a one-doctor company – Frank Berger. He was a good man, a very fine man but he was doing more administration than research. Eventually, combination products with meprobamate replaced meprobamate.

Getting back to the APA meeting.

Yes, the most important thing was, attending that meeting was Mike Gorman. Mike Gorman was an experienced press man who was national executive director for the National Association of Mental Health. He was a very astute man. He heard the message and he then approached Nathan Kline, Henry Brill and myself and said 'if you doctors will come to Washington I'll arrange for you to appear before Senator Lister Hill's Committee and you can tell your story. Maybe we can get these people to put up some money' because at this point there was little being done in Washington at all in any way to help psychiatric patients. They were considered hopeless, incurable.

We agreed, and Nathan, Henry and I went to Washington. We appeared before the Congressional Committee. We told our story and we asked for funding and for the establishment within the National Institute of Mental Health of a psychopharmacology branch. Senator Hill was impressed. I was not sure when we left how much of a persuasion we had exerted on any of the other Committee members but if you get the powerful Chairman convinced, he can move the rest of his Committee and so money was made available.

There was an organizational meeting held in Washington. That was an interesting meeting because it brought together pharmacologists, statisticians, psychologists, and a good number of psychiatrists. There was a good mix of elderly and young people. Ralph Gerard, from Michigan, who is famous for his statement 'behind every twisted thought is a twisted molecule', chaired the meeting. Ralph had trained Jonathan Cole and so he played a role in the appointment of Jon Cole to head the psychopharmacology branch at NIMH. That was an excellent choice.

Tell me why. Because he was actually pretty young at the time.

He was. Jonathan had a good, open mind. He is energetic. He got involved in the ACNP and became very active. He, Bernie Brodie, and I formed a committee to discuss issues that we were all interested in. As a matter of fact, we had all been in a meeting in New Jersey that was sponsored by Warner Lambert, which was interested in MAO inhibitors. On a train back to Baltimore and Washington, we talked about some of these issues and expressed concern at the lack of real work going on in this area. We were giving drugs without knowing what we're giving really and why it's working.

There's a feeling now that ACNP may not be going down quite the right route that it may be becoming too neuroscientific. It's led Don Klein to form ASCP, what do you think?

Well, I'm not surprised. Don approached me several years ago. We were the young turks when this started and the initial idea was to have an exchange of information between clinicians and basic science people and for a while that was certainly true. But now what's happened is coming from the basic sciences to the clinician with no input from the clinician back to the basic science people. You only have so much time to give to things and if you come to a meeting like this and 80% of it has no real meaning for you in a pragmatic way, as a clinician, you have to ask yourself 'am I investing my time, my money, my energy in the wrong way?' And this is what basically Don was asking and Max Finx was asking. Oakley Ray will tell you that he's heard from me more than once about what I saw coming. It came a little faster than I thought it would and that's both good and it's bad. Don Klein is a very intelligent man and a good man. He has the power to make this new College a very viable and meaningful organization for a lot of young people who will never get in the ACNP. You know we have a restricted membership.

Has that been a bad idea – the idea of a closed membership?

Well, it's one that is been debated off and on for years. In the beginning I thought it was good because if you're going to have a really viable organization people have to know each other and respect each other and have some admiration for each other and be willing to contribute. So the idea was to have a small number of people – almost like old boy club meetings, where everybody got to know each other. There was enough time for the papers and to go out on the beach for an hour or two for nothing more than serendipity. Then we got accused of being exclusionists, so it was decided to enlarge membership, but everytime you increase the membership you had less time for any exchange of ideas. That to me has been the worst thing that has happened. This is a very big meeting now. It's 700 or 800 people.

There are still people who are very upset that ACNP is not taking in any more members. Last year I think we took in four new members; that's because someone has to die or retire. We may have a suggestion from within the membership and I'm not saying this facetiously 'hey you're getting old, please resign and let somebody else come in' . I've thought about it, I really have. I'll be 75 soon. I miss, what to me was the greatest teaching force of this College, the individuals whom you could challenge and they could challenge you and make you do some thinking.

You were also involved in helping get BAP off the ground.

Well, the first person I really talked seriously to about it was Max Hamilton. Max and I became friends when he came too work at St Elizabeth's in Washington. He would come over to Baltimore with Tony Hordern and visit me at home and have dinner with my wife and I. When we were in Rome Max visited us for a couple of days. Max was very interested as to what was going on in the USA. He knew of my role in the ACNP and CINP and he lamented to a certain extent that nothing like this was really happening in England. But he never said that he was going to do something about it.

Then David Wheatley, who I got to know at NCDEU meetings started coming to some of the ACNP meetings; he asked me if I would share my experiences with the founding of the ACNP with him and with Tony and I agreed to do that. I went over to London and met with them and then we did some by correspondence. I encouraged him to go ahead because I felt that it would be important to British psychiatry. I have attended some BAP meetings.

Let me take you back then to the founding of the ACNP again. You say Ted Rothman was one of the key people. Any other key people?

Joel Elkes was important. He was the first President. Joel, of course, was working in Washington at the time. He was at St Elizabeth's Hospital and he had established a fairly good reputation before he came here because of his work in England. He was doing controlled studies and this was something that was new. Joel is a very personable fellow and a very articulate and diplomatic man. We needed someone who, in a sense had all of those qualities because we were hoping we were going to have to do a lot of dealing with the public and with the government, a lot of dealing with the industry and even a lot of dealing within the profession. Joel was highly respected and he was going on to become the Professor and Chairman at Hopkins, one of the most prestigious medical schools in this country, so he was really ideal. He fitted the bill and he was enthusiastic but he wasn't overly-enthused; he was a very prudent man and he was a good leader. He was a very good choice.

Talking about the psychopharmacology service centre brings up Gerry Klerman – where did he fit in?

Gerry was a man with a tremendous mind. I envied the clarity of his thinking and his logic and his courage. Gerry didn't hesitate to speak out, regardless of how unpopular it might be. Gerry initially was not so much interested in the drugs but applying the drug to the right diagnosis. He was very interested in nosology, in establishing good criteria for diagnoses, but he was also very impressed with what he was witnessing. He went from the Carolina's to Washington for a short stay before going from Harvard to Yale. Then came the opportunity for him to be an administrator at NIMH and, American politics being what they are, you had to have a broad based support, I campaigned for Gerry because I felt he was an extremely ethical man, with an awful lot to offer and he got the appointment to ADAMA.

Gerry was very interested in comparing non-drug treatment with drug treatments. He became a champion of the drugs but not to the exclusion of psychotherapy – he was very interested in extracting the best out of both psychotherapy and pharmacotherapy and he devised interpersonal psychotherapy.

And the use of the two together. Whereas it had always been the case of either drugs or therapy one or the other, he introduced the idea that maybe they could help each other.

Absolutely. And that was very important and he funded some very important studies. He took a very strong position – it wasn't a very popular one but it was a strong position – about the shortcomings of psychoanalysis, not because he was anti but he asked where's the proof of its efficacy. He urged and urged that studies be done and he tried to get funding for that but that was rather difficult to do. First of all even designing a controlled study of psychoanalysis is very difficult.

Just from reading the literature in that period, there was a feeling among the analysts in particular that the rating scales that were beginning to be used in drug trials were a travesty of evaluation – they argued that you could not evaluate people's responses in this way . . . and it actually took time to change the whole climate of opinion on this one.

Absolutely and Gerry played a major role in that. Methodology was something in which he was very interested. He was very interested in seeking the truth, even though he was not a well man. His diabetes was giving him some trouble but he was tireless. He worked very hard for the good of the psychiatric patient and for the good of psychiatry. He had a capacity to fuse people – to get them to work together. He was a great organizer. You couldn't help but like Gerry. Those who knew him would work hard for him.

What about the role of Nate Kline in all this because he was one of the group who went to Congress and changed their mind to come up with the money.

He came up with a lot of money. He had a lot of influential patients and he travelled in an influential circle in the New York area. Nathan in my mind contributed very much to the advancement of psychiatry. It's very hard to quantify it. He was a very flamboyant fellow. He tended to be a little hypomanic on occasions and he tended to get carried away. He would embellish things, not greatly but, at times, he would rub people the wrong way – not intentionally, it was just his style. He knew how to persuade people and he knew how to use the press . . . and he used it.

In your article in Neuropsychopharmacology *(Ayd, 1991) you quote the phrase 'that it's not always the person who makes the discovery first, it's the person who persuades the world of the importance of the discovery, who gets credited with a discovery'. In terms of who actually discovered the antidepressant use for iproniazid, did Nate snatch this out from under other people's noses? There are these two articles, which sit side by side in the same journal, one by Nate and the other one by George Crane. Who was really the first?*

Well that's very hard to say. Nate didn't keep the best records in the world. He had a big operation going. He had a very busy private practice and he was working part-time at Rockland State, primarily seeing chronically ill people, and not seeing a lot of true affective disorders – manics maybe or psychotically depressed patients. Be that as it may, he at least recognized that there was more to this than first meets the eye. Now, whether George Crane ever realized that or not – I have my doubts, I don't think he did.

I knew George well. He and I became friends when George left NIH and came to Baltimore. He was an intelligent man there's no question about that and a fairly astute observer. If you read some of his early observations on tardive dyskinesia, you will appreciate how astute he was but he didn't really appreciate the significance of what he saw with iproniazid – Nate did. And Nate grabbed that ball and ran with it. And he deserves a lot of credit because even though there was some initial hepatotoxicity and some fatalities with it and Marsilid was pushed off the market pretty promptly, that didn't deter Nate from still saying MAOIs are good drugs. Otherwise, I think we would have had the death of the MAOIs, in this country at least. It's to Nate's credit that that group of drugs was saved in this country.

Nate got two Lasker awards for his work with reserpine and his work with the MAOIs. That was most unusual and that made a few people envious to say the least. When he was working with reserpine he was dealing with Ciba and with Jack Saunders, who was employed by Ciba. Nate persuaded Saunders to leave Ciba and join him at Rockland State. Jack was very bright. He liked Nate and they worked very hard together. Jack felt he should have received more credit than he did for his work on the MAOIs. Jack sued Nate. That was the beginning of a series of court battles over who really made this discovery.

As you know, in 1970 Barry Blackwell and I organized *Discoveries in Biological Psychiatry*, to which I invited all the people who had made the major discoveries in biological psychiatry up until that time. Now here I was faced with George Crane and Nate Kline – and how do you decide what is the truth? Frankly, I talked to the Roche people and it was their impression that it really was Nate. I did that because I didn't want to offend George Crane and deny him an honour if it really was his. I was quite convinced that it was not George who had made the important observations here. No doubt he saw the effects and he may have contributed some input but on his own he would have never taken it to where it was taken by Nate. That was my impression; it's still my impression. So I decided to go ahead and we had Nate on the programme.

I had a similar problem, also at that same meeting, and that was who really was the fellow who made the true clinical observations and really could be considered responsible for chlordiazepoxide – Librium – being known as more than just another barbiturate. There were two people who had done early work. Joe Tobin out in Eau Claire, Wisconsin – a friend of mine, a very nice fellow, and Irv Cohen. At that time Irv had moved to Houston but when he did the chlordiazepoxide work he was at Galveston, Texas. Again, it was Irv who really capitalized on what he observed. His paper was published in JAMA – it went to a peer reviewed prestigious journal and it got accepted. In those days, it was unusual for a psychiatric report to be published in a leading non-psychiatric medical journal. Maybe to ourselves we were coming a long way but to the rest of the medical world we were still suspect. Joe Tobin's article was in a non-peer reviewed journal. I approached Roche for their view and they used Cohen's data. Irv was the first, who presented the data in a persuasive way. So, we finally decided on Irv Cohen and thank God that decision was accepted by Joe.

Before Nate and George set to, the idea that the MAOIs might be euphoriant was around, wasn't it? You have an early publication on these 'side effects'.

That's right, Dr Serra who was Chief of Medicine at Franklin Square Hospital where I was Chief of Psychiatry was interested in tuberculosis. He worked part-time at a hospital which had a large TB Unit. He said to me one day, 'Frank', have you ever looked at this drug isoniazid'. I said 'no', he said 'well, that's a pretty good drug for tuberculosis but there's another one called iproniazid, which I'm not convinced is very good for tuberculosis, but it sure peps up patients, you might want to try that for some of your depressed patients'. So, he told me how it had been widely used and that it seemed to be reasonably safe.

And this was before Nate had come out with his paper.

Oh, yes. In those days you could accumulate drug naive patients who had not been exposed to anything pretty quickly, because there wasn't a whole lot being done yet. I frequently would call general practitioners who referred patients to me and say 'if you've got someone who's depressed, who would be willing to be a participant in a study, I can take care of them and it won't cost them anything' – that's how you got patients. I submitted this one-page report to the *American Journal of Psychiatry* which published it (Ayd, 1957) and Nate Kline blew his cork. He wrote me a letter; he felt that I was stealing some of his thunder. And I wrote back and said 'Nate, the truth of the matter is I didn't know you were working with iproniazid. This was an idea that came from the Chief of Medicine who works with TB patients and I just tried it'. And it was more of an energizer than really a true antidepressant. If it had been a really good antidepressant, I don't think Roche would have capitulated as quickly as they did, when the few cases of hepatitis came along.

To change from one group of antidepressants to the other, you were at the talk that Kuhn gave in 1957 on imipramine – one of the few people still around I'd imagine because there were about 12 people there, as I understand it.

You're right there were very very few people there. Now, I have to tell you one of the reasons I was interested. I had a relative who was manic – depressive and who had his first depressive episode at college. Within a year he had a spontaneous remission and went back to school. He graduated and was very successful. In 1929 he had another severe depression and was ill for three years. He had to be tube fed to keep him alive and he had to be kept from killing himself. The next serious episode occurred when I graduated from medical school. I was determined he wasn't going to go back to a hospital if I could prevent it because of what I had seen of psychiatric hospitals as a medical student.

You had absolutely no interest at this stage in doing psychiatry.

None whatsoever. There was a psychiatrist in Baltimore who was doing ECT. I called him. He came and saw my relative and said 'yes, he's got to have ECT'. David, the first ECT treatment I ever saw was on one of my own relatives. I was at St Joseph's Hospital in Baltimore then, and the ECT was done in the radiology department with sandbags under his back. There was no ECT machine as we have now, no succinylcholine, no Brevital sodium, nothing. You saw what a real grand mal seizure was and the scream, not really a scream of pain, but as the air was inspired. Quite an experience. It was a horrible one for me.

Your relative was prepared to have the treatment, was he?

If I had to say we got informed consent, no. I made the decision to go ahead. He was in no condition to at all. ECT worked. Eight treatments and he was out of it. He had mild memory impairment for a while. You know if you're a classical unipolar or bipolar, episodes get closer and closer together, as you get older, and tend to be a little bit more severe and so forth. Two and a half years later, my relative had another episode and again he received ECT. This time it was started earlier and the psychiatrist who was doing it had the latest machine. We had succinylcholine and brevital sodium. He recovered very nicely, some memory impairment but within six months he was back at work. So that's why I was interested in antidepressant treatments.

Tell me about Kuhn's talk at the World Congress first.

Well, it was dramatic. There were very few people in the room. Kuhn is a rather tall man, slender, very soft spoken, very cultured, very dignified and very erudite. He gave a very, very nice description of the clinical manifestations of the illness he was treating. He didn't say, 'this is a good antidepressant'. He said 'this is a good drug for depressed patients who have *these* symptoms'. That was basically his message. He was very impressive. He mentioned the more common side effects, primarily the anticholinergic and some of the sedative effects of imipramine. He gave a very convincing talk.

I'm not sure how many people in that room really appreciated that we were hearing the first announcement of a drug that was going to revolutionize the treatment of affective disorders – and do more than that. If one thinks of what imipramine can do. It's not just an antidepressant, it's an anxiolytic, it's an anti-panic. We would have never had all these things if Kuhn hadn't given a very lucid and convincing paper. I'll tell you David you want to read the English translation of his first paper – it's as good as the Gettysburg address.

Why did it take Geigy so long to market this compound. They did the studies in 1956, in 1959 they marketed it – which was a long time compared to chlorpromazine.

The important thing about Kuhn's paper was not that he said that imipramine is an antidepressant, although that was very important, but he said in what kind of depression it is most likely to work. Kuhn was not well known then. I didn't know who he was. No one I asked prior to the meeting knew anything about him at all. And I think in part that would have been one of the reasons why there were not a whole lot of people there to hear this history-making paper. I subsequently came to know him. He is a man who's basically a philosophical psychodynamic psychiatrist who is a very ethical physician who has devoted his life to working with the mentally ill in a public hospital in a little out of the way location in Switzerland. He had not done any drug studies before imipramine, but had been carefully observing patients and keeping meticulous notes on them.

If you look at the structure of imipramine it looks very much like a phenothiazine. The early neuroleptics were selling like hot cakes then. Geigy's animal data suggested that imipramine had phenothiazine-like properties and therefore they felt it possibly could be another phenothiazine anti-schizophrenic drug. They looked for investigators, who had access to a fair number of schizophrenic patients. They borrowed, I think from Rhône-Poulenc's experience, that the best way to get this done is to go to the guys who work in the large public hospitals – Pierre Deniker and Jean Delay in France and certainly in the United States chlorpromazine got on the map when the work was done in the large state hospitals.

Kuhn was working at this mental hospital with a fair number of patients, who were not exposed to any medications yet, and I presumed that played a role in the decision to ask him to test imipramine. Kuhn did that. He was a very careful observer and he noticed that some improved and some didn't and to him the question was, what was the difference between them. He found that the difference between them was that those who had depression did reasonably well compared to those who were without any depressive symptoms. Then he asked himself, what kind of depressive symptoms and he looked at the vegetative symptoms and concluded that if they had predominantly vegetative symptoms and particularly the basic biologic things – disturbances in sleep, appetite, sexual drive, etc. that these were the people who were more likely to respond.

Kuhn clearly also realized this was not the only thing: that dose played a role and that low doses were ineffective – you had to give a minimum of 75–150 mg and in some patients even a little bit more. He made these observations and he reported them to Geigy.

Was the idea there that you couldn't have an antidepressant because analytic theories suggested there was an object loss and drugs can't replace objects?

Well, that certainly played a role in some of the people's thinking because there were analytically orientated people in Switzerland, as everywhere else, and Kuhn himself was analytically inclined. Now the other question that immediately came up was 'well, what do we have for depression now'. And the answer was simple. We had ECT and the only drugs that had any possible antidepressant effects were the psychostimulants, mainly amphetamines at that time. Ciba had already had a bit of work done on methylphenidate. The question was with what would imipramine be competing? Are we going to have a pill that will do what ECT does? Nobody thought that. Is it going to do anything more or less than the amphetamines? Is it a drug that could become addictive? For the business people, the central issue was, okay, let's say that this an antidepressant in a pill, how many people get depression, how widespread is the illness depression? No one had any answers for that. These business people were sharp enough to realize that. You might say 'oh, it's very common', but how common, how many cases are there per year.

In a sense, at the time depression was quite rare because the only people who had depression were the ones who were so bad that they ended up in hospital. No one else was prepared to admit to it. At least in Europe there wasn't the outpatient psychiatry that you had in private practice in the US.

Well, let me tell you how I got involved in this. I published in 1961 a book called *Recognising the Depressed Patient*, and this was based on 500 patients who I saw in a general hospital, not in a psychiatric hospital. I became well known for that – it got very good reviews and as a matter of fact, Merck Sharp and Dohme bought 50 000 copies of it and distributed it, not just to psychiatrists, but to family doctors and internists and so forth. It was translated by Jean Delay into French and then subsequently into a German edition and it did very well. That brought attention to me in this area. Now no one really knew the answer to the question of how common depression was. There were no epidemiological studies worth a tinker's damn. In fact, epidemiology as we know it today in psychiatry didn't exist then. So here you have men whose livelihood depended on making the right decision for the company because if the company succeeded, they succeeded and if they made the wrong decisions they were fairly certain that their days were going to be limited in a highly competitive industry, as it was becoming then. So they asked some very pointed questions.

The advent of imipramine sparked many studies, including some done by WHO, which culminated in Sartorius' very well-known paper, in which he said on any one day there are at least a 100 million people in the world with clinically recognizable and possibly treatable depression. Well 100 million people, that's a big market. That's a very big market but in 1957, that was a way off. Unless there was a motive for doing these kind of things, which had never been done, are we going to market a drug that's only going to be good for a few hundred, or possibly millions?

Let me move on and ask you, since you were also involved here. As is often the case, the first drug in the field helps to make the field but the second drug becomes the best-selling one, and you were involved with amitriptyline, do you want to tell me about that?

Well, amitriptyline's animal's data suggested it too had phenothiazine-like effects. Merck approached me, along with Doug Goldman and Fritz Freyhan and Nate Kline, and asked us to look at this. It could have been 1957/58, I don't remember the exact date. I made the observation that it had some antidepressant effects. In part, I was stimulated to look for that because this is what Kuhn said and here's a drug, structurally almost identical to imipramine except for a slight change in the nucleus. So I reported my observations to Merck and that stimulated Merck to investigate further.

Hoffman La-Roche also had amitriptyline. In fact, they had synthesized amitriptyline in Europe as a possible antipsychotic. When Merck applied for the patent, they applied for the patent as an antidepressant, not as an antipsychotic. So they got the patent in the United States – and once you get it here it's world-wide basically. My understanding of what transpired then was that there was a gentleman's agreement between Merck and

Roche that they would, literally split the world market. Merck got the United States and Canada and they got Australia and I think the other countries were areas that both companies could compete and essentially that's what happened. That was a very satisfactory arrangement for both companies apparently, until Schering and Merck entered into an agreement with the combination of perphenazine and amitriptyline, which Schering marketed as Etrafon in the United States and Merck marketed as Triavil. Well that product turned out to be a huge commercial success. Family doctors loved it because it was sedative, it had some definite antianxiety as well as antidepressant properties and the amitriptyline protected against perphenazine's potential of causing extrapyramidal symptoms.

It wasn't long after that when Roche filed a patent suit in the Federal Courts in the United States. I was deposed in it, mainly because I said it was an antidepressant. The decision favoured Merck. I have never seen the court decision.

As I was saying to you, I think Linford Rees even found in a trial that he did that it wasn't superior to placebo which caused him quite a surprise because he clearly believed that it was an antidepressant.

Oh yes, I know Linford did because I gave lectures in the UK under Merck's sponsorship and he was the man who introduced me at many of these dinner meetings that were held around England, except in Max Hamilton's territory, where Max did the introductions. And there was Tony Hordern, who did a huge study with amitriptyline and showed that it was an antidepressant drug. But there again even though you said to the company, look this is an antidepressant, the pragmatic questions were 'how common is this illness? – we don't want to market an orphan drug so to speak'. Nobody really had any idea. That's one of the reasons why Merck picked up on my book. Here at least was something that showed that this is not something that's unknown in the non-psychiatric hospital world. It's a very common thing and, in fact, these people are numerous in medical and surgical clinics. So now you've got something that you could advertise.

I did another thing. I made a film on the depressed patient, which was very well received. Not only was it done in English but we got people at the United Nations to do a simultaneous translation and it was sent around the world in 12 languages. It also won an award at a film festival in Tokyo. This was an unusual film in that it showed patients in a doctor's office. What we did was the patients agreed that they would be filmed but they didn't know when. A hole was put through the wall, over my shoulder and back but the camera was between books and unless you were really looking for it you wouldn't see it. The filming was done on a random basis. The patients may have come in three times and the setting was always the same but sometimes no film was made. And then the relatives sat with them and described what these people were like at home. It was a quite successful film as a teaching instrument.

Is there a sense in which drug therapies are always going to have the advantage on things like cognitive or behavioural therapy because there's not going to be an industry doing that kind of thing. Could you see a video which shows what the cognitive therapist does being sold in blocks of 50 000? Is there a sense in which the dice is loaded toward drug therapy because there's money to be made out of it in the way that there isn't for other therapies.

Probably. After all, if you're a business man and you've been funded by investors, you've got to produce a return for them. And it's the old story, success breeds success too. If products do well, you get more investors, you get more money to do things. That's why it took lithium a little while to get on the market – there was no one fighting for it. No drug company could get a patent on it. There was a big question of medico-legal issues associated with its use.

So you picked amitriptyline out and when you looked back and it was the people who were depressed that were the ones that seemed to pick up . . . but did you actually test it out on people who were depressed before the patent?

Initially no. Initially these were all presumed schizophrenic patients or schizo-affective, and once I became convinced that this drug did have some antidepressant properties, I switched over and looked at it now in people who were specifically diagnosed as having an endogenous depression. I did not give it to people with neurotic depression.

What did the others think – Kline, Goldman and all.

Well, initially they hadn't made the same observations. Later they did. They didn't attack my findings at all. I think there was some scepticism and probably if I were in the room and somebody else was saying this I might be sceptical as well. But I think that the people who needed the most convincing at that time were first, the medical people and then secondly the management people who had to make that important decision – how much money do you invest in this new product?

There are so many complexities to what's behind a drug getting on a market and for what indication and so forth. Temaril, for example, is a phenothiazine drug – I looked at it for SmithKline French and it turned out to be predominantly an antipruritic type product and not an antipsychotic. Fritz Freyhan did a fairly large study in schizophrenics at Delaware State Hospital and got negative results basically except for the sedative effects, but I found the antipruritic effects and how did I find them? Well, I had a patient to whom I had given this drug who had had an allergic condition with a lot of itching before starting Temaril, and suddenly the itching stopped. The historical truth is, at that same time three of my children came down with chickenpox and they were driving my wife and me crazy. So I gave it to them. And they stopped itching.

Remarkable.

I reported this to SmithKline – in fact I wrote a paper on it – because I then gave it to a number of patients who had various pruritic conditions and it worked. Here was a drug that was originally looked at for a psychiatric use and it ends up being used by the dermatologist. Just simple clinical observations.

You've also met one of the other key people – John Cade. Can you tell me about John and about the problems trying to get lithium into the US because it's been quite a saga.

Well, John Cade was a host for me in Melbourne when I was on a lecture tour. John met me at the airport and we hit it off. We had a mutual interest. We were both Catholic, both Jesuit-trained. I happened to be interested in beautiful scenery and nature and John was very much interested in that and he took me to see some lovely gardens. We went out to some State parks together. He was very very good to me.

What were the problems he had using lithium then – because they didn't have the brand name forms that we had.

Well, first of all it's a naturally occurring product that couldn't be patented. The real problems were that he hadn't done much in the way of human studies. His work had been with his guinea pigs. He gave the lithium to some chronically manic patients – not really full blown mania, thank God, because if he had it wouldn't have worked. We know that severe mania is not responsive to lithium but hypomania or low grade mania is responsive. That took a lot of courage because there was no way to measure blood levels. It was just careful observation; he was fortunate in that he guessed, so to speak, the right doses. He was very prudent. He started with a very low dose and depending on response he gradually escalated. He carefully observed and kept good notes on those patients. I've seen all his notes. They were meticulous. Then he wrote his famous paper which was published in the *Medical Journal of Australia* (John Cade, 1949). Up to this point John Cade was unknown outside of Melbourne.

In this country, as you know, we had had the problem of lithium being marketed as a salt substitute for cardiac patients resulting in a lot of lithium retention, lithium intoxiciation and a number of fatalities. So much so that lithium was banned.

Mogen Schou deserves a lot of credit because he picked up the ball and ran with it. He did the very important controlled studies and the good observational studies. John was not interested in becoming a great research man. He was a very happy administrator of a public hospital. A very devoted family man. Limelight did not appeal to John Cade. He was a very humble person and as a matter of fact he was somewhat reluctant to be on the programme for *Discoveries in Biological Psychiatry* (Ayd and Blackwell, 1970). When I first wrote and asked him to come, his reply was 'it's not on the market. Why do you want me to come over and talk about the discovery of a drug you can't even get in the United States'.

But at that point I knew there was a good possibility that it could get on the market. A fellow by the name of Paul Blatchley had picked it up. He was a fine psychiatrist, very much dedicated to alleviating suffering in his patients. He was a pioneer in multi-monitored ECT. He worked primarily with affective disorders, therefore the antipsychotics did not particularly appeal to him. Antidepressant drugs did but his real interest was lithium. He was convinced from what he had read and from what he had done on his own with a local pharmacist making it up for him and by careful clinical observation, he became quite convinced that lithium was an extremely important drug. I was doing the same thing in Baltimore but not on the scale he was doing it.

Paul wrote letters to Congress but got nowhere. He decided to take the next step and that was to turn to the media. He called me and asked me to join him. We did a series of interviews with some media people and that really generated some real interest in lithium because actually when you stop and think about it, you had two choices for a severe manic. One was ECT, but the number of treatments you would have to give almost invariably is going to cause some memory impairment. The other one was to use the neuroleptics, which meant that if you use the high potency ones you're going to get some extra pyramidal symptoms and if you use the low potency ones like chlorpromazine you're going to get a lot of sedation and a lot of postural hypotension. So we really didn't have a good treatment. That's why I willingly joined Paul Blatchley.

He picked some magazine with a national circulation and that really got to families who were faced with the problem of what do you do for a relative who's manic and you don't want any more ECT and you don't want to make zombies out of them as you would with fairly heavy doses of neuroleptics. So there was pressure brought to bear and in the meantime, fortunately, Schou was doing what he was doing in Aarhus and also ways of measuring lithium were developed, so the stage was set and people began writing to their congressmen. Actually SmithKline was the first to market lithium in this country. In part, because they felt they had a duty to it. They wanted to maintain their image as a leader in psychopharmacology. They were making money on all their other products, so this was a chance to make available what could be called an orphan drug to people. That's how we got lithium.

There were two or three other people who played a part in helping raise awareness, one was Nate Kline.

Oh, yes. Very much so. And there again it's another testimony to Nate really fundamentally wanting to advance the science of psychiatry and to provide alleviation of suffering to people. Admittedly he could be quite dramatic and so forth but in actual fact he was highly ethical and a highly motivated person, so again Nate picked up the ball. I never published on lithium. I had no reason to. My interest was being able to help a few of my patients.

In the early days the person who prescribed the drug would be seen as the 'druggist' and often in quite a few of the hospitals the medical people would try to make sure they were uncontaminated by prescribing. I seem to remember something about you being the only person prepared to prescribe when you were in the Navy.

Yes, at Perry Point. I was in the Navy and was assigned to the VA Hospital at Perry Point. I was giving ECT. And that gave me an idea of what could be expected before we got the drugs. Syphilis was around and we had Pick's disease and Alzheimer's and a lot of organic patients and you really got a pretty good idea of what uncontrolled mania is like, what a severe depression is like and the people who get very negativistic and almost catatonic. There was a certain feeling of frustration that there were so few things you could do.

Isn't it curious though that in a sense although the neuroleptics don't cure schizophrenia, they go very close to curing some forms of it. You don't see classic schizophrenia anymore – you don't see the same hebephrenias or catatonic pictures any more, that I still saw when I entered medical training, in the early 1970s.

That's right. I now go down to Eastern State Hospital in Virginia, as a consultant. There I see psychopathology that I will never see in my office. I saw a first case of acute neurosyphillis with a delirium recently, the first since I left Perry Point. I've seen Pick's disease there. I have seen some very bizarre forms of excessive reactivity, over-activity. One patient there that we've checked now for three months has never slept more than two hours a night. He has a pervasive developmental disorder. He has been in that hospital since age 6 and he's now 60 but he's never had a physical illness and suddenly he developed this very peculiar syndrome, which has been totally refractory to all interventions. Now I am sure he has some organic lesion but the CAT Scan and MRI were negative.

Do we need an asylum yet? The answer is yes we do. There are patients who will never be able to live in the community regardless of what kind of medications are developed. There are people who are refractory to antipsychotics and there are those who can't tolerate or don't respond to Clozaril or Risperdal. The number has whittled down a little bit more with each new entity but we've got a long way to go. I think one of the things that the ACNP is going to have to do is to now champion hospitals – you can't care for all patients in the community. We are going to have a renaissance of the hospital. They will be different from the old days; we're not going to warehouse large numbers of people but we are going to have to provide humane care for people who just cannot care for themselves in the community. I think the future is bright. I may be too sanguine but I think there are going to be technological breakthroughs. I think we are getting closer to treating the true psychopathology or a pathophysiology of schizophrenia.

I wonder; I have my doubts. The industry needs to make money.

Well, the hope lies in the industry's needs to make money. The hope also lies in that there are non-industry people, who are motivated by what has been accomplished, to carry on to improve on what we have. And there is a better educated public, so Congress is not going to be able to cut off all funds. They may prudently want to withhold certain funding and the people at the NIMH are going to have to say we've put our funds in those areas which are most likely to produce some concrete results. The public expects that. But the one thing that I think psychopharmacology has done is that it has made the public realize that psychiatric patients are sick people and that they are entitled to treatment.

There are now powerful national organizations that are influential advocates for the mentally ill. They are collaborating with psychiatrists to ensure government support for psychiatric patients and to ensure government approval for new psychoactive drugs. But drugs must be prescribed prudently. Doctors who are pill dispensers shouldn't prescribe psychoactive drugs. To be a good psychopharmacotherapist, one has to be a good physician who does a good diagnostic work-up, takes a good personal and family drug history, who knows the physical status of the patient, and who carefully observes the patient's response to drug therapy.

How did you get into psychiatry Frank?

Well, I graduated from medical school in 1945, when the War was on. I did a rotating internship and started a residency in paediatrics at the University of Maryland Hospital in Baltimore. After six months into the residency I got called for active duty by the Navy. I was assigned to the Bethesda Naval Hospital for surgery. I have no manual dexterity. The only exposure to surgery I had was during my internship. When I learned my assignment, I said 'my God I'll kill more people than the War will'. I didn't have any hesitancy to ask for another assignment. At that time the Army and Navy were staffing VA hospitals. Hence I was assigned on loan to the Veterans' Hospital at Perry Point, Maryland, a large psychiatric hospital.

David, to be honest, to me that sounded like a fate worse than death. My memory of psychiatry was a few lectures from people who talked about the unconscious and things of this sort and then we would visit the State Hospital and be taken on a tour like through a zoo. You really got no feel for it. Well there was another doctor at Bethesda who had been a friend of my father. I went to talk to him because I was really down. I thought I should have kept my big mouth shut and he said 'Frank, go up there, you only have to be there for two years and why don't you just decide that you will take care of all the physical problems of the patients. You be a physician and you won't lose the touch'. So he gave me a very good pep talk and I went to Perry Point with an open mind. There were a couple of thousand patients at that hospital and only eight doctors and that's why the Army and the Navy were pouring extra doctors in. After a very quick indoctrination, you were sort of turned loose, like during the internship during the War.

I was there only a short time working on the admision service when I was transferred to, what was called, the continuous treatment service. There were 800 patients in that service, who had been in that hospital on average anywhere from 20–40 years and none of them were yet 65. So these were really chronic patients. What did we have? Paraldehyde, bromides, barbiturates, cold packs, tubs, all kinds of hydrotherapy, some insulin coma therapy and ECT and that was it. I quickly learned that schizophrenics are really different people. Their pain and temperature senses are different.

I remember one fellow vividly who stuffed himself with newspapers and set himself on fire. When I got there they had put that out and here he is sitting, burned pretty badly, still hallucinating and responding to the voices, but we didn't have to give any narcotics at all. It was just amazing to me. There was a fellow who escaped from the shower. It was about 4 a.m. that night and the old attendant who was in charge of that ward called me, as I was the Officer of the Day, and told me this fellow had escaped. In my naivety I said 'he won't be gone long, it's so damn cold out there, he's going to come back in'. I'll never forget it but he said 'Doc, you don't know schizophrenics, we've got to find that fellow, if we don't he's going to freeze to death'. So we started a search party and we found him. He was hypothermic but we saved him and that made me do some real thinking.

What's wrong with these people? And I'll be honest, the people who were training us were basically psychoanalysts and I could never get a satisfactory answer to questions such as 'You can explain to me why this fellow thinks he's George Washington instead of Abraham Lincoln but why does he have this delusion in the first place?'. Well, they didn't have the answers for that. And I felt that sure you could give what seemed to be plausible explanations but that doesn't really explain anything. So my perennial desire to ask a question why and look for a answer got me interested in psychiatry. I willingly got involved with ECT because I could see what it could do for some people, even people who were called schizophrenic, who probably were schizoaffective or bipolar patients, who were misdiagnosed as schizophrenic.

By the time I had resolved that I was going to be a psychiatrist and had taken my boards and passed them, my time at Perry Point was up. I had stayed on longer than I was required to stay on because I wanted to get the extra training. That hospital was a museum of psychopathology. You could see everything – all kinds of organic brain diseases.

One of the things that I know David Wheatley was very concerned to get right at the start of BAP, which he says he picked up from looking at ACNP, were the links between the organization and the industry. Now, let me just broaden this out to ask you generally about the industry. You've mentioned issues to do with the editors of various journals having to be, not so much industry friendly, but the next best thing.

Well, to a certain extent that's true. This is not a new one. I was subpoenaed to testify before the Blacknick Committee in Congress at the House of Representatives. It was an official congressional investigation into pharmaceutical advertising. How did I get involved? Well, Congress has a lot of power and they can hire people to investigate things and one of their investigators went through some journals that were suspect and made the interesting observations that the summary and conclusions from a paper I had written were not published, but they were in a reprint. So I got subpoenaed to come over there and explain this thing. What came out of that hearing, not just from me but from others that they subpoenaed, was that when you submitted an article to certain journals, before they send it out for any peer review, if they did send it out for peer review, they sent it to the manufacturer and said 'look, we're thinking of publishing this article on your drug, do you want to buy advertising space in the same issue?'

This was when?

In the late 1950s, early 1960s. Now, what came out was if the company said no don't publish that or we'll stop advertising, that article was rejected. Or in the case of mine it turned out that it was sent to the company and the company deleted the summary and conclusion, which is what most people look at. That's still happening. Some of our prestigious journals have by inference, without proof, lately been considered guilty in this area – that they don't want to publish anything that's not going to please their advertisers. Senator Kennedy has raised this issue a couple of times.

All of this is grist to mill of someone like Peter Breggin – look at Toxic Psychiatry (see Glossary).

You're right. He picks this stuff up and there's a certain element of truth to it and you know money is a poweful motivator. I think anybody who does what I do or who does research has to be very, very careful about having a distant relationship from the company because they can increase your bias, there's no question about that and I've sat in on enough meetings to see that actually happen. The industry has changed. When I first started, and you ask anybody, what it was like 35–40 years ago, you dealt with physicians. They ran the pharmaceutical industry. Today they aren't running the industry, they have some input but not a major input. Decisions are made by the business people who think in terms of the bottom line and that's their prime interest, there's no question about that. Some companies are a little bit more aggressive than others and I think all Colleges have to be very careful.

There have been some publications recently about, for example, journal supplements and certain journals have been identified now as taking huge sums of money from the industry and publishing supplements. How peer reviewed these are is a big question and how much are they really used for promotion rather than scientific purposes is another concern. And if a company wants to get a speaker on a programme they can do it. You've seen this in England and it happens almost everywhere.

It's a very fine line, because Peter Breggin won't be taken seriously other than by people who are on the fringes.

Yes, it is. We're all human and it's very difficult not to become biased. You really have to say consciously in advance I am going to do my best to avoid that, which means that you say no to certain invitations however nice they might be. I'm well aware of the other problems that have been going on and the gifts that have been given to influence reviewers and teachers here and in England.

Now, in 1970 you organized the 'Discoveries in Biological Psychiatry' meeting, why? We work in a profession that's not terribly interested in history.

I had worked at the Vatican from 1962 to 1965 and you cannot work in that environment without becoming very conscious of history. You're living in a city where everything is older than the country where you were born and raised. I have been very fortunate. I have met a lot of the people who were pioneers in psychiatry and it was a pleasure to meet them. As I say, you put a face to an article and so on. I had been instrumental in getting Barry Blackwell to come to the United States because I was a consultant for Merrell Dow Pharmaceuticals and they were looking for a psychiatrist so I suggested Barry. He was famous for the cheese reaction observations. I met him at a CINP meeting in Washington, where he gave a paper on the MAOIs and I was very impressed with him and we corresponded. So I suggested Barry and they asked me if I would call him and ask if he'd come over for an interview. I called Barry and he was interested. He was interviewed and, as I expected, they were very favourably impressed with him and they offered him a job.

Barry came and we are good friends, although I don't see him as much now because he's interested in the homeless and does a lot of work in the area of the homeless and their psychiatric needs in Wisconsin. Anyway we were both at an APA meeting and we had been to dinner and met with Mogen Schou. Barry and I sat around and talked for a while and concluded it would be a good idea if we got together all the men who made these discoveries in biological psychiatry, while they are still alive so they could tell the story in their own words. And we kicked it around and that to me was the end of it for a while.

Then I got thinking about this idea and this was another example of picking up the ball and running with it. I called Barry. I then proposed this to Taylor Manor and they agreed to fund it. Barry and I discussed things by phone – primarily who we ought to invite and so on. What he really did was he helped greatly with the editing of the book. One of the things we wanted was early publication. Two weeks after that meeting was over the first copy was out. The man from Lippincott stayed over the weekend, attended the meeting, and then came round to my house and had dinner with me and left with the galleys to take on Monday morning to the printer. We had page proofs within five or six days and within a few weeks the book was published.

Let me ask you – it seems almost that the era of drug discovery is over. There are some drugs coming through but at nothing like the same rate. The golden era was 1954 through to 1974 or thereabouts. In last 20 years, there have been great advances in neuroscience but not clinical advances to anything like the same extent: why is this?

Well, for a long time of course there was a search for me-too drugs, which is understandable. You've got to have money from something to do research on another area and me-too research is relatively inexpensive. One thing about chemists is that they are molecule manipulators and they can produce an awful lot for you but as you know you've got to screen a whole lot before you get one that looks like it's worth doing work beyond an animal stage. So the end result was we got a lot of tricylics, got a lot of phenothiazines, a lot of thioxanthenes and so on. The real change came with clozapine and now risperidone in the antipsychotic field. The serotonin uptake inhibitors are an advance to a certain extent. Whether venlafaxine is going to be another breakthrough in the sense that it may have all the assests and none of the liabilities of amitiptyline, we'll have to wait and see, but that's a possibility. Wellbutrin still has some promise and nefazadone is about to be approved.

There has been a real change in the industry. I have already said to you that 30 years ago, the industry was run by the scientists and that's no longer true, it's the business man who runs the industry. I've seen large companies take and put all their eggs in one basket – gambling because their hope is that this product is going to be a megabuck product and therefore other things fall by the wayside. Look what's happened. Squibb at one time was very active in the CNS field: they decided to go into cardiology because it's a much bigger market. That didn't materialize. They had to merge with Bristol-Myers. Now Bristol-Myers gets into cancer drugs and later the AIDS market, which was a big market at that time. So money that was being used for CNS research and development was diverted and we had drugs like nefazadone, which was approved almost two years now and in England it's still not on the market.

This is the change. Management looks at that bottom line first. This is why there are all these mergers, in my judgement. I can understand that. They do have to make some return on their investment for their stockholders. Merck and SmithKline have bought into the pharmacy business and they're all getting into managed care one way or another. It's a very interesting time to see what's going on. It's got to be of interest to this College because there are fewer and fewer companies looking at the psychiatric field as a field where there's going to be a big return. In part because it is true that for many people, the tricyclics are still very good drugs and I can treat many patients with them as safely as I can treat them with the serotonin uptake inhibitors, with no greater risk of unpleasant side effects really and there's a big difference in price. The industry are going to have to come up with some very good products if they are going to produce a lot of money from them.

The cost of doing research for the industry has just escalated. I think I did the first 100 patients on chlorpromazine for $1000. Of course everything was cheap then. But the requirements of the baseline data you've got to get, the EEGs, ECGs, the ophthalmological and all these other things. There's no way someone like me can do this kind of research now.

You've been an independent practitioner through this period, which hits me as a drawback in this respect in that the way politics works within any scientific community, you've got to be part of one of the powerblocks and you're not. If you read reviews of things the reviewer cites 'our' guys and doesn't cite the other guys. But being in the middle, the way you've been, you're not going to get that recognition.

That doesn't bother me. As a matter of fact I've been fortunate. I've got five honorary degrees, four Doctor of Laws and one of Science. I've been honoured twice by the ACNP and I've received other awards and honours. So I've gotten my recognition but my most important thing is I go to bed every night with a clear conscience and with a sense of satisfaction that, thank God, today I did the best I could to help some people, somehow. I have lectured extensively and that took a lot of time, lot of effort, sacrifice and you're away from your family, fighting all the vicissitudes of travel. And why do it? What I do it for is, if I can lecture to 50 physicians and convince 10% of them to do a little better, I've helped more patients that day than I would staying in Baltimore in my office and if it weren't for people who were kind to me and shared their knowledge with me I would not have been able to do what I did. Knowledge gives you strength. It really does. It gives you the courage of your convictions and it makes you willing to roll up your sleeves and take legitimate risks for the benefit of your fellow man. That's been my motive.

Select bibliography
Ayd, F.J. (1957) A preliminary report on marsilid. *Am. J. Psychiatry,* **114,** 459.
Ayd, F. J. (1960) Amitriptyline (Elavil) therapy for depressive reactions. *Psychosomatics,* 320–25.
Ayd, F.J. (1961) A survey of drug-induced extra-pyramidal reactions. *J. Am. Med. Assoc.,* **175,** 1054–60.
Ayd, F.J. (1961) *Recognising the Depressed Patient.* Grune and Stratton, New York.
Ayd, F.J., Blackwell, B. (1970) *Discoveries in Biological Psychiatry,* Lippincott, Philadelphia, PA.
Ayd, F.J. (1991) The early history of modern psychopharmacology. *Neuropsychopharmacology* **5,** 71–84.
Cade, J. (1949) Lithium salts in the treatment of psychotic excitement. *Med. J. Aust.,* **36,** 349–52.

5 Alan Broadhurst

Before and After Imipramine

Can we go back to the start?

My first contact with Geigy was in England, in 1949. Before going into the Services, I had acquired a modest knowledge of pharmacology and, on demob, I looked for a job in this field. The advert sounded interesting. It said 'If you would like to join a small pharmaceutical operation in the UK . . .'. I went to an interview in Manchester, in a luxurious office suite in a large building just off Piccadilly. In my naivety I spent the first half of the interview believing that this was where I might be working. Eventually I was sadly disillusioned to learn that it was not. Leslie Robinson, who was on the other side of the desk, said 'this is, of course, not where the job is. If we decide to accept you, you'll be based outside Manchester in a little mill town called Rhodes'.

Well, to cut a long story short, I was accepted for the post and I found my way to this rather curious place, 729 Manchester Old Road, Rhodes. It was a small house, detached, but at the end of a terrace of mill workers' cottages. I was surprised to find the pharmaceutical set-up at such an early stage of development. The house was quiet and virtually empty. One room was devoted to small-scale packaging of products brought across from our parent company in Switzerland. There was an order office, a secretarial office and a few spare rooms. In charge of it all, was Leslie Robinson – a delightful and extremely competent scientist. He had started the Geigy pharmaceutical operation in Britain and this was the whole of what was then known as Pharmaceutical Laboratories Geigy Limited.

When had it actually begun?

He had begun it in 1948, a year before I arrived. There had not been a pharmaceutical division of Geigy in the UK, before that. You might ask why it was started in such an out of the way spot as Rhodes? The real reason was that right opposite this place there was a Geigy Dyestuffs Warehouse. The dyeing industry, of course, centred on Lancashire because of the cotton and woollen industries close by and this Geigy warehouse had been there a very long time. The management of that warehouse had been asked if they could find somewhere local to set up the pharmaceutical operation and this was the little house that they found.

What was your role in this enterprise?

In broad terms, my job was to act as an assistant to Leslie Robinson and, in particular, to be concerned with the scientific side of the operation. He was an interesting man, originally a pharmacist, with strong research interests. He had been trying to encourage out-of-house projects but he was very heavily involved with the administration of the firm.

I must add that when I was first accepted for the job at Geigy, I felt – and was – extremely junior and was uncomfortably aware of the depth of my scientific ignorance. I wondered how I was going to fit into this important pharmaceutical set-up. Within 48 hours of my arrival, I was alarmed to find that I was, in fact, one of the senior members of the British company. This was, of course, simply due to the fact that there was such a small staff! Indeed, apart from our packers, order clerks and secretaries, there were only two of us actually in the HQ at Rhodes. Outside we had two reps calling on doctors. At the most senior level there were a couple of directors of a holding company; they were mainly concerned with DDT and dyestuffs and had only a minimal input into the pharmaceutical business.

Despite my discomfiture, my somewhat paradoxical situation made it easier for me. There were very few guidelines and I was able to use and develop my rather limited abilities without dampening interference. At first all went well but then, sadly, within a year of my arrival, Leslie died and I found myself overloaded with all aspects of the business. Suddenly I had to learn a whole lot of new things, such as how to cope with the importation of drugs from abroad. How to apply for an Import Licence and how to deal with Key Industry Duty. I was, incidentally, so hopeless at these things that HM Customs took pity on me and sent a Customs Officer each week to help me fill out the forms. But it wasn't all admin. and I was keen to push forward with other work.

Other work meaning?

Well research. Not necessarily out-of-house research. There was a thought that we ought to try and do something within Geigy UK itself, to develop some sort of scientific base. My remit was a fairly broad-based one and we were able to pursue a number of different lines. Our parent company in Basle had, of course, a lot of drugs already on the market. Some of these needed looking at again. Other drugs, not yet marketed, were in the process of investigation and we tried, so far as possible with our very limited resources, to get some work going on parallel lines. This in quite a small way, of course.

What kind of things were you developing?

My very first major task was to work within the field of anticoagulation. In particular, I was looking at one of the early coumarin derivatives called Tromexan. For me, this was a fascinating area of study because I had very little knowledge of it and I needed to learn a great deal before I could start work. I was indebted to one of the Geigy scientists in Basle, Dr C. Montigel, for his skill and enormous kindness in teaching me what I needed to know. This was the start of a period of my life when I was practically commuting between Rhodes and Basle.

At about the same time, I was working also in the antirheumatic field. We were devising laboratory tests which would detect the anti-inflammatory effect of drugs. Geigy had already produced a compound known as Irgapyrin. This was an early antirheumatic, only available for injection – which may have reflected the Continental trend for parenteral therapy. It consisted of amidopyrine in a solvent. Amidopyrine was a troublesome drug which could produce agranulocytosis. Curiously, the incidence of this blood disorder seemed higher in Anglo-Saxon populations and we were worried about the use of Irgapyrin in the UK.

These days that kind of compound . . .

Almost certainly could not have been marketed. It would not have got through our CSM. So, we looked at possible ways of reducing this potentially dangerous side effect. The solvent used in the injection bore some chemical similarites to amidopyrine itself and we investigated it for possible anti-inflammatory properties. The solvent was phenylbutazone and it emerged that it did have a powerful anti-inflammatory effect. We wondered if it could be used as an antirheumatic. Clinical trials were set up in Britain by a colleague and it soon became clear that phenylbutazone represented a major advance in rheumatology. It was orally active and became widely used as a non-steroidal anti-inflammatory agent.

When you say clinical trial, what did they involve at this stage?

Oh, this was way back in 1951. There was almost no question of doing double-blind studies – strictly controlled trials at this time. These were 'suck it and see trials'. And yet, even without controlled trials, phenylbutazone was a great success and, until a few years ago, was used extensively.

Where did the work go from there?

I should tell you that this was a time of particular change in my life. Working with Geigy had brought it home to me how restricted one was in this type of field, without a medical qualification. Research could be taken so far, but then there was a barrier. At times I felt rather like the poor child looking into the party window. I was not happy with the situation and it was not good for Geigy, who, in the UK, had no medical staff. So I decided to go to medical school, this in parallel with my work for the firm.

That must have been quite a load?

It probably sounds a bit hectic but it was a challenge and I enjoyed every minute of it. I was still travelling frequently between Manchester and Basle. There in Switzerland I had a corner of an office shared with Dr Paul Schmidlin and a bench in Dr Montigel's lab, working from there with Dr Wilhelmi and Dr Pulver.

What were you working on at this time?

Well, it was a time of great excitement. The infant science of psychopharmacology was only just emerging. The phenothiazine antihistamine, promethazine, had been used by Henri Laborit to reduce surgical stress and he noted that it seemed to have some central anxiolytic effect. Subsequent further investigation by Charpentier had produced chlorpromazine, which, apart from its antipsychotic action, also possessed a thermolytic effect and this seemed fascinating.

Why did thermolysis look interesting?

Mainly because this action could inhibit the response of a warm-blooded animal to maintain a constant body temperature. This was the time, of course, when open-heart surgery was starting and chlorpromazine was to revolutionize the technique by allowing body cooling and thus permit brief interruptions of the blood circulation.

At Geigy, we also were involved with antihistamines. At first, I found myself working with halopyromine. But our chief of pharmacology, Professor R. Domenjoz, a brilliant man possessed of an energetic, questing mind, pointed out that other routes to antihistaminic – and perhaps other related activity – seemed entirely possible. So, with mounting interest in the phenothiazines, we wondered if we already had any compounds of similar molecular shape available, so that they might be tested for similar properties.

How do you mean available? How did you think you might find them?

Well, in the basement of the Geigy building, opposite the German Railway Station, the Badische Bahnhof, in Basle, there was and probably still is, a kind of museum of long-forgotten, mainly useless compounds, gathering the dust of half a century of more. There was a search for likely substances amongst this collection of chemical curios. Attention eventually focused on a substance called iminodibenzyl. This had been synthesized in 1898 by Thiele and Holzinger who had described its chemical characteristics (Thiele and Holzinger, 1899) . It had been of no interest and had not been investigated further. It was a tricyclic compound, which apart from its central ring structure, closely resembled the tricyclic nucleus of phenothiazine. It looked interesting and a decision was made to examine it closely. We spent a lot of time talking about structure and activity relationships, which was a big thing in those days. We thought it would probably not be very active in the parent compound form.

Why not?

Because it didn't have a side chain and wasn't likely, therefore, to be absorbed adequately. And so our chemist colleagues, Drs Schindler and Haeflinger, produced a series of basic alkylated derivatives of iminodibenzyl, by adding side chains at the H- position on the central ring (Schindler and Haefliger, 1954). I should add that when chemists are asked to produce a series they do not do things by halves. In fact, they produced 42 different compounds.

Did you test all of these?

Yes, but in a pretty basic way. After the routine chemical tests, animal tests were used to look for evidence of sedative activity and thermolysis. We also tested for spasmolytic and antihistaminic activity in the isolated rabbit and guinea-pig gut and for analgesic effect. Interestingly, a quaternary C-atom in the side chain increases analgesic activity but none of the substances possessed major pain-relieving properties. As far as I remember toxicity testing at this stage required no more than LD-50s in a single species. All of the compounds showed some antihistaminic and anticholinergic activity; some of them had moderate sedative effect and some did produce thermolysis.

What about human pharmacology?

Based on the animal results a few were tried out in human volunteers. Doses were tiny at first and then were increased progressively to look for sedative or hypnotic effect. Otto Kym and Paul Schmidlin went out to see Dr Roland Kuhn at the Münsterlingen Hospital on Lake Constance to ask him if he would be prepared to try out one of the compounds as a hypnotic, a substance given the Geigy nomenclature G22150. In fact, the hypnotic effect of this drug, at least at the dosage then being used, was unsatisfactory.

Soon after this, in 1952, Delay and Deniker in Paris reported on the remarkable effect of chlorpromazine in schizophrenia. Our chemists had already produced the analogous iminodibenzyl derivative designated G22355. Further pharmacological testing of this compound was carried out, including some human pharmacokinetic and general observational studies in human volunteers.

Were you a volunteer?

Yes, I think I was one of the first people to try G22355. Volunteering came with the job. At the time, we hadn't quite worked out the human dose equivalent and the net result was my first and, happily, only OD. Anyway, the results were not particularly promising. It seemed to have similar properties to chlorpromazine in the laboratory but it was less potent and, moreover, its effects were less predictable. Nevertheless, we thought it would be worth trying to arrange a clinical trial and we had another meeting with Dr Kuhn.

What kind of a person was Kuhn?

He was a man who had been brought up in the old, strictly non-biological school of psychiatry, with a strong psychodynamic and psychotherapeutic component. I thought he might well have been difficult to persuade but, in the event, he wasn't. The success of chlorpromazine in schizophrenia provided a strong stimulant to interest. He was keen to try out G22355 and he was asked if he could assess its action, particularly in a group of chronic schizophrenic patients to see if it was as effective as chlorpromazine. Some of his patients were on chlorpromazine and others were on nothing except for hypnotics at night, if necessary.

What were the hypnotics being used at the time?

I can't be sure so long after but they were probably barbiturates. Administration of chlorpromazine was discontinued in those individuals being treated with it and G22355 was started and in others not being treated with it the new experimental drug was given directly. It should be added that, as we were saying earlier on, that in those far off days, sophisticated clinical trials employing double-blind techniques were virtually unknown. So any effect produced by G22355 would have to be quite obvious for it to be regarded as significant.

In fact such was the case. The whole team of workers, both staff at Münsterlingen Hospital and scientists from Geigy, waited with bated breath. Within a period ranging from three days to three weeks, certain results began to appear and, in truth, the results were not only fascinating, they were, in some patients, quite disastrous! Many quiet, formerly well controlled schizophrenic patients began to deteriorate with increasing agitation.

What kind of dose were you using?

We were using the sort of dose that we would be thinking about now, as an antidepressant dose, about 150 mg a day, in the beginning by the parenteral route. Some patients began to deteriorate with increasing agitation and a few went into frank hypomania. One gentleman, in such a state, managed to obtain a bicycle and rode in his nightshirt to a nearby village, singing merrily, much to the alarm of the inhabitants. This was not very good PR either for the hospital or for Geigy. Of course not all schizophrenic patients deteriorated in this way. Some even improved, especially if there was a major depressive component in their illness.

When we talk about patients who have schizophrenia, as you know in the late

1960s and afterwards many patients who had been diagnosed as schizophrenic were redesignated as manic – depressive rather than schizophrenic, how many of these patients do you suppose had schizophrenia proper?

I think it would be very difficult to exclude that possibility in retrospect. But certainly many of those patients being treated were the same group of people who are labelled schizophrenic these days. They were experiencing auditory hallucinations, they had paranoid ideas, there was thought disorder. I think, in fact, a very significant proportion of them were true schizophrenics by modern diagnostic criteria.

Would you expect these days if we gave a group of schizophrenic patients antidepressants that they would produce that kind of reaction?

Well, we were rather surprised at this, I must confess. It seemed to be an extraordinary reaction. Of course, it could be argued that those patients who went high were probably suffering from manic – depressive psychosis and they had just been pushed into it. But I think there is evidence that some people with schizophrenia who are given tricyclics alone, without the benefit of simultaneous neuroleptics, may deteriorate in this way. The Geigy team viewed the situation with dismay and, as gracefully as possible, retired from the scene for the time being.

Can I ask you about the mood at the time – obviously it must have been a fairly remarkable time – the first drugs . . .

Absolutely incredible. So exciting. That a drug should produce mood changes like this. We were simply at a loss to explain it. A series of discussions with Dr Kuhn took place over the next few months. We all asked ourselves what could have happened to precipitate such a reaction in certain patients. I remember sitting on the harbour wall at Gottlieben, overlooking the Bodensee with Roland Kuhn and Paul Schmidlin, trying to work out what imipramine was doing in these patients. Clearly the reaction we had seen in some patients was not the effect of a simple withdrawal of chlorpromazine, for similar hypomanic agitated episodes had occurred in a few patients who hadn't been having chlorpromazine.

It seemed as though G22355 could in certain patients actually precipitate some kind of hypomanic reaction. We stumbled around considering a variety of unlikely hypotheses and possible mechanisms. Then, basing our thoughts on the most naive scientific reasoning, something I now look back on with horror such was the lack of logic, we began to wonder if the flattened affect of schizophrenia were somehow elevated by the drug to hypomania, might a similar elevation of mood be possible in patients with depression.

And so in 1955, G22355 was tried in a number of patients with endogenous depression. By the time three patients had been treated it was clear that the drug was having a dramatic effect. By the time the whole series of 40 patients had been treated, we became certain that G22355 represented a major advance in the treatment of depressive illness.

On the 4th of February 1956, Roland Kuhn sent a detailed report on his findings to the Pharmacology Department at Geigy and on 31 August 1957, he published a paper in the *Swiss Medical Journal* (Kuhn, 1957) describing the research results (Kuhn, 1957). At the Second International Congress of Psychiatry in Zurich on 6 September 1957, he gave a paper on the results to an audience of 12. In the spring of 1958, G22355 was given the generic name imipramine. After a slightly hesitant start, I think while doctors accustomed themselves to the idea that many cases of depressive illness could be treated with medication, it began to be prescribed.

Can I take you back to the Zurich meeting. You said there were 12 people in the audience; what was it like, were you there?

Yes, I was. It was a very small meeting in any case. It was divided into sections and in one of these Dr Kuhn gave his paper. One had the feeling almost that those doctors who were in the audience had come reluctantly. There was a considerable lack of enthusiasm amongst those present.

Had Kline actually come out with his work on iproniazid at this stage?

It was running in parallel. I can't remember exactly where the two were at this particular time but I think that I'm right in saying that the first published results of an antidepressant study were with imipramine rather than iproniazid. That followed but not very long afterwards. As far as I remember Kline did not speak at that meeting, nor did he mention his work with iproniazid.

Tell me more about Kuhn's presentation, was it 5 minutes, 10 minutes, half an hour or what?

He spoke for about half an hour. The presentation was an interesting one – really rather along the lines of what I would have expected, knowing Roland Kuhn and his particular fields of interest. He spoke for rather a long time about the psychodynamics of depression and, at some point in this discussion, brought up the question of his research and the results. But there was a great deal more in the paper than just the description of a clinical trial.

So, how did he actually account for the effects of imipramine, given the background he came from?

Well, I think this was very difficult. He was clearly baffled. I know he was very surprised. But of course he was not the only person with a particular interest in psychodynamics who had become involved in research work with imipramine. I'm thinking of a trial carried out in England by Hilda Abraham, who was the grand-daughter of Abraham the psychoanalyst, who herself was a psychoanalyst. She got in touch with me and said, 'this compound sounds remarkable and although I haven't ever really thought about using medication in the treatment of depression, could we talk about it?' and she carried out a very important trial, which strongly reaffirmed the antidepressant effect of imipramine.

There was a very lengthy period from 4 February 1956 to when you said his report was published on 31 August 1957. It seems remarkable given that everything else happened so fast, that it took so long for the publication to come out and for the data to be presented

Yes, I don't know why that was so long. I don't think there were any queries. I think it was simply the case that in those days there was often a tremendous delay between submission and publication.

You weren't aware of any sort of comments that were made. Could it have been held up by referees saying you know this isn't possible.

I'm not aware of that and I think I would have heard.

The other odd thing about the compound that must have caused people some surprise was the fact that here was a drug that was being reported as an antidepressant that was sedative. Everybody expected that an anti-depressant when it came would be a stimulant of some sort. It was counter-intuitive in a sense . . .

I think that's right but I think also that that was one of the most attractive features about it, because obviously amphetamines had been used and they had been seen to be highly undesirable in treating depression. In a sense, it was helpful to be able to say to people with whom one was discussing this new drug that it did not have a stimulant effect. People felt it was something entirely different and would probably be without the hazards of the amphetamines.

Yes, but people like Brodie, who were working on these drugs, were left with the problem that the MAOIs were rather more what they actually expected − a drug that was somewhat stimulant − and now they had this problem of trying to work out what common action there could be for class of drugs, some of which were stimulant but others of which were sedative.

But, of course, we must remember that we had discovered this drug by serendipity and not by logical development of a pharmacological principle and, as is often the case with such a discovery, we hadn't the remotest idea how it worked. This was a great stimulus to further research.

If the effects of G22355 were as obvious as you say to all concerned with the development programme, can we really say that Kuhn was the person who actually discovered imipramine? In a sense, surely the whole ward of the hospital must have discovered it and he was the figurehead who promoted it rather than the one person who saw something that no one else was seeing.

I suppose you are right in some measure. He was inevitably working, not on his own, but as the head of a team at the hospital and he was also working closely with scientists from Geigy. One certainly would not want to detract from his observations and discovery, but there clearly was a team element, as I am sure he would agree. And don't forget, that even if the antidepressant effect were obvious when it occurred, he was the man who saw it first in his patients.

Did you personally see any of the trial group of 40 people? Did you call in at the hospital?

Yes, I was frequently at the hospital – whenever I was over in Switzerland – and I did see many of the patients being treated with imipramine. I was very impressed with their response to treatment but you must not forget that, at that time, I had no higher psychiatric training and I was fairly ignorant of the natural history of untreated depression. And it didn't strike me as being all that unusual that if one gave patients an effective form of medication it would cure the illness from which they were suffering. If I had known more, I think I would have been even more excited.

What about the odd fact that it took two or three weeks to work ?

Again, this was a very difficult thing for us to understand. We, of course, had some vague ideas about mechanisms. We knew about Woolley and Shaw's work, who in 1954 had suggested that 5-HT had some effect upon mood and even at this time we were wondering whether in some way we were seeing an elevation of 5-HT due to the imipramine and we assumed that if there were an elevation of 5-HT that it was something that couldn't happen instantly. That there was a gradual build up. In a sense, we rather quaintly explained away the latent period before the therapeutic effect became apparent, in this way.

You say Woolley and Shaw rather than Gaddum?

Gaddum's work with 5-HT was also germinal. He and Woolley and Shaw separately, but simultaneously, had advanced the notion that schizophrenia could be a result of disturbed 5-HT metabolism. I think Woolley and Shaw had suggested that depression also might be associated with a 5-HT abnormality.

On the 5-HT front I must ask you about Archie Todrick, who was of course the first to report biochemical changes with antidepressant therapy in humans. He blames you for getting him involved in this work. Do you want to tell me about that.

Well, it was a time when a lot of people were trying to discover the mode of action of imipramine – and not having much success. I had the responsibility not only of setting up all the clinical trials of it in Britain but also of trying to organize basic research. The latter was slow to get off the ground, so I was delighted when Archie Todrick got in touch with me from the Crichton Royal to say that he and his colleagues were interested in undertaking some biochemical research with imipramine. I had never been to the Crichton Royal before and I thoroughly enjoyed my first visit there. This must have been in 1959. Archie was working with a delightfully friendly team, Allan Tait who was Director of Clinical Research and Elizabeth Marshall, a charming and very bright biochemist. We spent the best part of a day discussing their plans and we firmed up an experimental method. The idea was to estimate platelet 5–HT in patients who were to be treated with imipramine, both before they had received the drug and at various points during their treatment. We celebrated the completion of the plan for the project by going out to dinner in Dumfries that night and then they put me on the night–sleeper back to Manchester. Within a few days, Archie was in touch to tell me that they had exciting results (Todrick, et al.,1960). I dashed back to Scotland to discover that the platelet 5HT levels had fallen dramatically following administration of imipramine. I remember that we were all terribly excited.

One of the curious things about this of course was that the findings were the opposite to the effects on 5-HT Pletscher had reported with the MAOIs.

Yes. These findings were difficult to explain, but they pointed the way to the later discovery of the effect on reuptake mechanisms. In retrospect, it all looks so simple but we mustn't forget that it wasn't until 1958 that Zeller discovered iproniazid to be an inhibitor of monoamine oxidase.

What other basic work was around at the time?

It is difficult to recall all the details now but I do remember helping to set up some basic studies in Birmingham in the Department of Experimental Psychiatry – it was an outstanding department with a main base in psychopharmacology. They were doing important research on LSD, neuroleptics and then on antidepressants. I persuaded Brian Keay to look at the effect of imipramine on the process of habituation to external stimuli in rabbits.

Was your own in-house research programme still running?

It gradually faded, so far as the Manchester end was concerned. I think its heyday was when we were doing the anticoagulant work. Subsequently, we found that we were carrying out very similar, if not identical, studies to those being performed in Basle. Our facilities were very simple and sparse compared with theirs, so apart from the waste of time arising from duplication, we could not deal adequately with the later, more sophisticated programmes. One of my later Manchester investigations with imipramine was to look for any evidence of local anaesthetic activity. In fact, it emerged that the tricyclics are quite powerful compounds in this respect.

We also went through that phase, beloved of pharmacologists, of examining the metabolites of compounds – in this case, imipramine – in the belief that a metabolite could be less toxic, have fewer side effects, would act more quickly and, indeed, perhaps be the true active substance. The simplest way of examining the metabolites was for a few of us to take imipramine and collect our urine. This entailed collecting all one's output over a week or two. Hence the famous enquiry of one's hostess when arriving at a party – 'where can I leave my Winchester?' The outcome of the study was, of course, desipramine, which was something of a disappointment.

What about basic research with imipramine in Switzerland?

That was continuing apace. We still had no animal model for depression but a variety of behavioural techniques were in use and further pharmacokinetic testing was carried out. But don't forget that we were, at that time, limited in what we could do. We had no real knowledge about the mode of action of imipramine – Arvid Carlsson's paper did not appear until 1969.

You were also responsible for setting up the clinical trial work with imipramine – you mentioned Hilda Abraham.

Yes, I was responsible for setting up virtually all of the early British clinical trials. This was an interesting task, for within the sphere of clinical psychiatry in those days, there was much scepticism that depressive illness could be treated by means of drugs. Indeed, our only therapeutic tool in those days, apart from psychotherapy, was ECT. But gradually people became interested, excited even, by the possibilities. I visited Newcastle and met Kiloh and Ball who conducted the first British trial (Kiloh and Ball 1961). This must have been in 1958.

Why did you go to Newcastle, why not to Linford Rees or someone like . . .

Well, Leslie Kiloh was then a young and keen research psychiatrist, eager to get his teeth into something interesting. He had read Kuhn's paper and he got in touch with me to say that he would, in company with John Ball, like to run a clinical trial. This was before the marketing of imipramine and, apart from a small quantity of the active ingredient in my office, there was none in this country. The first small clinical supply of imipramine and placebo in Britain arrived here in a slightly devious manner, wrapped in my laundry after a trip to Basle – to avoid the horrendously long and complicated exercise in obtaining documents and so allowing these enthusiastic researchers to get started.

Did Martin Roth participate in all this?

He was there when I went to Newcastle and I met him on that first occasion. He was interested and wanted to hear about it. We were sitting in what was probably his office in the medical school. But it was Kiloh and Ball who did the work on that first trial. Then, of course, Martin really organized the MRC trial.

This was in 1965.

It was published in the *BMJ* in 1965 but work started on the trial long before that. Altogether some 35 important British studies were carried out. One of the earliest of these was by Jan Leyberg and John Denmark working in Bolton, which was published in the *Journal of Mental Science* in 1959 and served to stimulate other potential researchers.

Another important contact I made at that time was with the MRC Brain Metabolism Unit in Edinburgh. This was based at Craig House, a hospital with real style. The doctors' dining room was a large oak panelled hall complete with stags' and boars' heads and various heraldic devices. The MRC people were a cheerful group and very hospitable. George Ashcroft, Donald Eccleston, Philip Barker and John Binns were all there at that time, together with the legendary Elizabeth Robertson. George Ashcroft became a close friend and we shared a hospital flat in Cambridge later. Their paper on imipramine in depression was published in 1960.

In London, I went to see Silvio Benaim and later Linford Rees and Alexander Brown. They carried out a beautifully designed trial, as you can imagine.

I also went over to Ireland. My remit was to stimulate research in the UK but Eire seemed like a good place for an extension of the limits. So I found myself in Dublin. I met John Dunne, a wonderful character and he introduced me to Mary Martin, who knew a lot about imipramine; she conducted a first-class trial comparing it with phenelzine. I also met Norman Moore, who was the superintendent of St Patrick's Hospital and had dinner with him in his beautiful home on the banks of the Liffey, just outside the City. He was a delightful man and he too carried out an excellent trial with imipramine.

I'm intrigued by Hilda Abraham's request to do a trial.

Yes, I was fairly staggered by the request. She was determined to be scientific in her approach to the work. She joined forces with three colleagues and between them and with some gentle prodding from me, they came up with a well-designed double-blind trial. One of them, Ismond Rosen, who played a major part in the trial design, remains a distinguished psychoanalyst to this day.

This was still the stage, though, when the trials didn't necessarily have to be placebo double blind

This was the time when things were beginning to change, certainly in Britain. At some point in about 1959 or 1960, most trials became fully controlled. Only a few of the early trials here with imipramine were non-controlled.

In a sense, the discovery of clinical trials was as important as the discoveries of the new compounds.

Absolutely, but of course the other thing, too, is that double-blind studies were regarded as much more important in psychiatry and psychopharmacology than they were in the investigation of other drugs at that time. I think the reason for this was that we were dealing with rather small changes in many people. We were not looking at the effect of streptomycin in tuberculous meningitis, where virtually 100% died unless they were given an antibiotic, in which case there was a high survival rate. We were dealing with patients showing, in some cases, marginal improvement in their depression and there it was much more difficult to make a clinical judgement unless, of course, you did actually control very, very carefully. This was, of course, also the era of the introduction of rating scales.

Max Hamilton.

Yes, indeed. I got to know him very well from the first moments that I became involved with the imipramine trials in the UK. I got in touch and asked him if I could visit him in Leeds. I remember his dismal office in what I suppose was part of the Medical School. He sat there completely surrounded by piles of books and papers. He explained all about his Depression Rating Scale to me and I could see that it would vastly improve the imipramine research, if only I could persuade people to apply it. As you know, he had had some mathematical training and was extremely precise and logical in his thinking. One could not discuss something with him in even a vaguely slipshod manner. In a sense, he was quite schoolmasterish. But he was a delight to know and eventually we became good friends. We often went to the same meetings around the world and sometimes we travelled together. Its amazing how well you get to know somebody when you have eaten breakfast together in Paris, lunch in Quebec City and dinner in Tokyo – not all in the same day of course! His death was an incalculable loss to world psychiatry. When I met him first the HAM-D was ready for take-off and it was marvellous to see how rapidly it was universally accepted.

What did you make of the MRC trial? It did for the the MAOIs.

I thought that was an extremely unfortunate outcome. I was surprised because it seemed to contradict the work of Sargent and Dally, who had demonstrated fairly conclusively the great efficacy of the MAOIs. By then, I was certainly using MAOIs myself with considerable effect. I was very surprised at the outcome of that study and looking back on it now I find that part of it very difficult to believe.

You said that being a chemist in the industry was a little bit like the poor child looking in the window, but talking to George Beaumont he would say that being a medic in the industry, in those days, was not the best of positions in that in medical terms the idea of working within the industry wasn't awfully highly thought of. In that sense do you think things were very different in Europe and in particular in Switzerland?

Yes, I think that's right. There were certain negative feelings about doctors working in the industry at that time. Only a few of us were there because of its being our primary choice. Many people went into the industry because they couldn't get a Senior Registrar, or Consultant job they wanted in hospital medicine. In a sense, therefore, a number of doctors in the industry were disappointed men and, in some cases, this showed. The other thing, which was difficult and caused envy, was that disproportionately high salaries were paid to medics in the industry to attract them there and keep them.

Is there any reason though why you think that the pharmaceutical industry within Britain has taken time to become respectable in a way that it hasn't say in parts of Europe or parts of the US. To work in the pharmaceutical industry in Germany was a very respectable position from the last century but it's taken much longer in the UK.

Partly for those reasons I've just mentioned, there was some tarnishing of the industry. In Europe those slightly negative feelings were not there and, not infrequently, medical students planned to go into pharmaceutical medicine long before they qualified. In this country, it is, of course, very pleasant to work within academia but, because of underfunding and short tenures especially among the more junior people, the industry has distinct attractions. I think there have been progressive changes in attitudes towards doctors in the industry in the last 25 years. There's been a gradual recognition that pharmaceutical medicine is a speciality in its own right and it is beginning to control its own fortunes and produce its own examinations. Now there is a high quality of doctor going into the industry and these doctors must inevitably command respect. But this is a big change.

You eventually left the pharmaceutical industry and went on to become a psychiatrist

During my time at Geigy and following the development of imipramine, I had become fascinated not only by the capacity of drugs to affect mental illness but also by the practice of psychiatry itself. I had enjoyed my time at Geigy immensely and had found the work there fulfilling, but now I wanted to explore this branch of medicine further and I wanted to be closer to patients. It would be a very big step, but after discussing matters with many colleagues and with particular encouragement from my friend Edward Beresford Davies, I came to Cambridge in 1960 to begin a formal training in psychiatry – a decision I have never regretted.

Going on to do psychiatry means that you have had a unique perspective – seeing both how the drugs came about and then being involved clinically at a time when the impact of these compounds was changing everything.

Yes, when I first went to Fulbourn, I found wards full of people with chronic psychiatric illness. Many of them had schizophrenia but a considerable number also had depression. I think there were nearly 1000 beds full when I arrived. I remember David Clark had a big chart in his office, showing a gradual decline in in-patient numbers over the years. I'm not sure what the capacity is now, probably about 400 beds.

In the early 1960s we had become accustomed to the idea that persons with chronic schizophrenia would suffer institutionalization but it is easy to forget that the same thing happened to large numbers of patients with depressive illness, who could stay in hospital for very long periods of time, hoping for a natural remission. Others came in and went out but then had another acute exacerbation of depression and came back again a month or two later. It was quite remarkable to see the impact of imipramine in Fulbourn. It had, of course, only just begun to be commercially available when I arrived in Cambridge and was able to use it. We were able to discharge people who had been in hospital for very long periods of time. I realized that we would not see such large numbers of chronically depressed patients again.

It was interesting, too, to sit in the outpatient department and realize that general practitioners, in those days, despite the availability of the new drugs, wouldn't use them. I suppose they felt that they were insufficiently trained in psychiatry. Most of us, of course, in those days had received only very scanty undergraduate training in psychiatry. It meant that even quite uncomplicated cases of depression were being sent to the clinic. Often all one had to do was put them onto imipramine and many such patients recovered without difficulty.

On that point, I suppose one of the really big changes was the disappearance of involutional melancholia. Concepts like this just went out of use.

Just disappeared, yes. Involutional melancholia was an odd disease. I suspect that if there is such an entity, cases are now recognized early as affective illnesses and treated so that the fully developed state never appears. I haven't seen a patient for years whom I would regard as suffering from involutional melancholia.

So, looking back on things over the last 30 years or so, you're one of the few people whose careers has actually spanned the psychopharmacological era, what has it all meant?

I think one of the most important things that I see is that in those early days people came to see a psychiatrist only because they were very seriously ill indeed. They would usually be very profoundly depressed or psychotic. Being referred to the psychiatric outpatient clinic was somehow thought to be highly undesirable and even to go to a general practitioner complaining of depression, for example, in the early 1960s was something which most people found very difficult. Gradually the threshold at which psychological symptoms have become acceptable and psychiatric treatment has been applied has been lowered until now we see people with really trivial psychiatric complaints. And I think this is the major change. There's been a huge escalation of the number of patients passing through the doors of psychiatric clinics.

What do you say to people who say that there are far too many people passing through our doors and we give drug treatment to far too many − I guess the minor tranquillizers in particular were a case in point where we seemed to be over-medicating.

Yes. I would certainly agree with that. I think we do use pharmacological treatments too readily, especially for stress reactions and anxiety but, of course, there is an all too ready demand as well, which makes it extremely difficult for the doctor to refuse. Having said this, I think we need to be very careful not to miss cases of depression, perhaps appearing under the guise of other symptoms. Unless there are very clear reactive features requiring just the healing effect of time or a psychotherapeutic approach, then almost every case of depression should be treated as early as possible with appropriate medication.

One of the unfortunate accidents in the whole period is the Thalidomide story. How did that affect the field .. it led of course to the creation of the Dunlop Committee here and the CSM later. It set in train a sequence of events that has led to the major complications we have now with any drug coming on the market, if there is any side effect of any sort, we now have a threshold for removing them that may even be too low and perhaps because of thalidomide we are now losing many useful drugs too soon?

Well, that's probably true. But I believe we cannot be too careful and I'm totally in favour of the much tighter controls we have now. These controls have, of course, had enormous financial consequences for the industry because the screening of drugs now is such an expensive exercise. But you are quite right, also, when you imply that we may be throwing the baby out with the bathwater.

And it takes a long time now to get a drug to the market compared with what you were faced with in the case of imipramine.

Yes, we did it very quickly indeed. I can't quite remember the precise dates but it was within a matter of four years. Of course, the pre-clinical pharmacology was pretty basic stuff. By today's standards, we didn't do much in the way of toxicological studies. We did some animal and some human studies, including pharmacokinetics, but not much beyond that. I wouldn't like to suggest that the tests were never done but there were not too many relevant tests available in those early days.

Behavioural work with animals?

We were not in a position, at the time, to do much because we didn't have the relevant animal models. It was only after Brodie's work with reserpinised rats, that we carried out such studies with imipramine and other tests as they became available. Studies of the effects of imipramine on normal behaviour had been done – tests such as the ones which had been used for chlorpromazine, including the usual maze and swimming tests. But the results were not specific and were far from uniform. Modest doses increased exploratory activity and vigilance; at larger doses sedation and ataxia were seen.

Can I take you back to some early meetings. You mentioned the 1957 one in Zurich; there were a group of very important meetings to happen around then, including the first CINP meeting in Rome in 1958. Were you at many of them?

I went to Rome for the CINP meeting. It was wonderful. I remember, at the time, thinking what a lot of people there are interested in the same kind of things that I'm interested in. I have no real knowledge of how many people were there but maybe there would have been 400–500 people altogether. If I go to the CINP meeting nowadays, there are thousands of people there and I think one of the most extraordinary things is the enormous escalation of people working in psychopharmacology.

There are people who say, yes there's an enormous escalation of people working in psychopharmacology but with no enormous output as a consequence.

That's right. There is a vast increase in numbers mainly for drug-testing purposes, partly for safety reasons, and what happens is that individuals work within quite limited boundaries on specific tests – but there is no broad vision. In our day, we worked much more as generalists. Because of this we could see the way a drug or group of drugs was moving towards pharmacological fruition. There were no such people as clinical research associates, no pharmacologists working just in toxicology or in preclinical work. Within limits, one had to do a bit of everything. People have become much more highly specialized now because there is so much to do in terms of screening and safety studies.

Are you saying that because of this that it is possible that we won't ever actually discover much more that is new? We have gone 30 years without really discovering much.

No, I'm not saying that. But perhaps our relatively low rate of success is due to our looking in the wrong directions. Nowadays we have several groups of drugs which affect 5-HT, many of them of widely disparate molecular shape. Because of the particular way in which some of them modify 5-HT, we have learned to say that they are likely to exert an antidepressant effect. But one wonders sometimes if the effect on 5-HT is really responsible for the antidepressant action or whether it is just a concomitant effect, simply a marker of something more important going on. Maybe we are getting a bit blinkered by 5-HT and a consequent rigid mental set prevents us seeing and exploring other issues. The psychopharmacological world runs in phases of fashion and we may be on the brink of exhausting the serotonin fashion.

At this stage were Geigy as big as the other Swiss companies?

I suppose so. I don't know the precise relative sizes but Geigy, Roche, Sandoz and Ciba were about comparable in Basle and although there was nominal rivalry between them, in fact there was a great deal of mutual respect and support. At the scientific level, many of the researchers were friends. The firms themselves shared some facilities. Although it is not well-known, behind the scenes, they shared at least one intermediates manufacturing plant at one stage.

Geigy UK remained at 729 Manchester Old Road for about five or six years, and then moved to Wythenshaw, which is on the southern outskirts of Manchester. The new home was a smart, brand new building with much larger and vastly improved facilities. It was splendid but I felt nostalgic about our little place in Rhodes, where so many exciting things had happened.

By this time, we had a large administrative staff. We had started to manufacture our own pharmaceuticals rather than import everything from Basle. We had some outside contracts for tableting and ampouling and we were just starting with some in-house manufacture. There were a couple of pharmacists to oversee this work and, of course, some materials were still coming in from Switzerland.

On the breadth of vision issue, these days it seems to me that with clinical trials being multicentred no-one has an overall feel for what a trial really demonstrates anymore

That's quite right and of course that's something that one did not see in the early days. I suppose this is something inherent in multicentre work, but clearly there is a need for it, especially when large numbers of patients must be recruited. In psychopharmacology, I think the MRC trial of antidepressants was the first work of this kind.

Mentioning the MRC trial raises the Newcastle connection again and I have one further question here which is that the notions of endogenous and reactive depression which people like Roth and Kiloh pioneered fitted like hand in glove with what you brought to them. I've often wondered if the Newcastle formulations didn't become so influential because the early clinical trial work with imipramine internationalized their formulations.

I suppose it could have played a part in putting that kind of classification of depression more firmly on the map. Certainly it appeared that imipramine was far more effective in what was called endogenous depression and, interestingly enough, that the MAOIs were superior in what were called the neurotic or atypical depressions. The Newcastle classification and the differential effects of the two kinds of antidepressants all seemed to fit together very well.

The same point could be make about the Hamilton Rating Scale; imipramine helped make it as well known as it became because you could argue that the Hamilton rating scale was geared towards picking up a tricyclic kind of compound, something that was going to be somewhat anxiolytic and somewhat sedative in effect. It isn't going to pick out another kind of antidepressant as quickly.

That's true. Max Hamilton was very excited about the introduction of imipramine and it certainly did fit in beautifully with his rating scale. Years later he still referred to it as a happy coincidence.

Since moving into clinical work, you've continued to do clinical research on tryptophan, biochemical aspects of cognitive function, hyperventilation and other things: can I pick up on a few of these. What about tryptophan?

I became very interested in tryptophan a long time ago. Reports of early clinical research with it, in the 1940s and 1950s (Rose, *et al.*,1954) had fascinated me. These stemmed from work with the early synthetic diets given to prisoners and students in America, which gave rise to our knowledge about essential amino acids. Diets of this kind, but with the omission of one ingredient at a time, were given to volunteers. When tryptophan was not present, subjects became listless, suffered general malaise, anorexia, nervous instability and were depressed. Addition of tryptophan to the diet rapidly restored health. So based on this and our newer knowledge of 5-HT and the bioamine hypothesis, it seemed reasonable to try to treat depression with tryptophan.

You went ahead with this?

Yes, but before we got under way, I went down to see Alec Coppen at the MRC Unit in Carshalton. Alec was extremely kind and helpful and eventually he in Carshalton and I in Cambridge carried out separate but parallel double-blind studies comparing imipramine with tryptophan. Both Alec and I found that they were of nearly equal efficacy as antidepressants. But tryptophan never really became popular as an antidepressant. It found its main use as a constituent of various cocktails used for the treatment of severe or resistant depressions.

I am still interested in tryptophan which, in fact, seems to turn up everywhere in medicine. Some of the areas of tryptophan activity are so widely different from each other, that workers in the general field might have no idea what is going on in other areas. Therefore, to disseminate information about tryptophan more widely and to minimize the risk of duplicating research, the International Study Group for Tryptophan Research, ISTRY for short, was founded in 1974. This is still going strong.

Another of my interests was the relationship between drug dose and clinical response. The work with nortriptyline, and what seemed a reversal of effect at higher plasma levels, had already been published and seemed fascinating. For our own rather obscure technical reasons, we were keen to use a molecule with a halogen atom in it and I decided to look at clomipramine in the same kind of context. Initially, there seemed to be no relationship between plasma level and response, but when we looked at the major metabolite, desmethylclomipramine (DMCl), we discovered an inverted-U relationship – shades of nortriptyline. This rather suggested that DMCl is the active antidepressant substance and not the parent compound.

What about the psychomotor studies?

These arose out of an interest I had always had in aviation medicine. There had been concern about aircrew using the more obvious sedative drugs since flying began. But as new drugs became available, I was, as a former pilot, concerned at our general lack of knowledge of the possible effects of these on flight safety. With a non-medical colleague, Paul Richens, we decided to design and build a machine by means of which we could detect even very small changes in psychomotor function. This was about the same time as Ian Hindmarch was becoming active in the field.

We made a random complex reaction timer. It's different from Ian's Leeds machine. The presentation is variable and is in the form of a line of lights, with or without an auditory signal. The lights in the first, second and fifth row might be illuminated, for instance, with an associated tone and the subject is told to respond to this pattern when it appears again. The machine is then set in random mode, producing an ever-changing display until, at some indeterminate point, the initial pattern reappears. By increasing the complexity of the stimulus we can slow down the response, thereby making it much easier to pick up very small changes induced by drugs.

What drugs were you testing?

We were testing a whole range of commonly used medicines. I was particularly interested in the beta–blockers. Some drugs of this type do impair psychological function but their effect varies according to their degree of lipophilicity. The strongly lipophilic compounds such as propranolol produce the greatest slowing of psychomotor response, whereas the hydrophilic atenolol has barely any effect upon functional capacity.

One of the things we discovered was that propranolol has a significant effect on psychomotor function and eventually the CAA forbade civil airline pilots to use propranolol for the treatment of hypertension.

You can't have been very popular with industry for that.

I don't think there were any hard feelings. Besides, if there had been a tragic outcome, which were later ascribed to propranolol, there could have been serious consequences for ICI.

People like David Shaw and Alec Coppen were critically important in getting biological psychiatry going – in bringing enthusiasm to the field. Somehow bridging that gap between what were very simplistic hypotheses and clinical reality.

The bioamine hypothesis was the most marvellous thing to hang our work on and it gave us some kind of basis for what we were doing. It may be that we shall one day discover that it was wholly flawed but it doesn't matter. It enabled us to have a framework when we needed it and allowed us to move forward.

In psychiatry, during the 1960s, people from all areas seem to have been quite happy to work together but during the 1970s there was a change. Was it a reaction to Laing and the antipsychiatry movement?

I think you're right. In the decade starting in the mid-60s, there was a movement into psychiatry of people with excellent clinical and scientific skills, which the earlier psychiatrists may not have possessed. Why those people came into the speciality is not entirely certain, but, at first, there were people who were frustrated by the long wait for senior registrar vacancies in other disciplines. They simply made a career move to where there were jobs. Of course, there was the hurdle of retraining to negotiate but many galloped through that process. The new scientific developments in psychiatry were particularly attractive to these new recruits and so there was a snowball effect. The new knowledge changed the balance in psychiatry, especially in respect of treatment techniques. Treatment was much more clearly in the hands of the scientifically trained doctors. Inevitably, this caused resentments in other workers in the field, heavily fuelled by Laing and this translated and developed into a more general antipsychiatry lobby.

In a sense then, the drugs created biological psychiatry. When you think of people before doing ECT, they weren't biological psychiatrists in the same sense. One of the areas that seems to have suffered though is the area of psychosomatic medicine, in which you've had interests. This has never really properly found its feet.

Yes, that's right and I suppose the reason for this is that there are not too many psychiatrists working in the general medical field and, therefore, it's been very difficult to put heads together and come up with answers. I was fascinated by the inter-relationship between psychological and general medicine, especially with the respiratory disorders such as bronchial asthma and hyperventilation syndrome, which is more common than many professionals realize. After getting my DPM, I went to work at Papworth as a medical registrar for a couple of years and later I became a Consultant in the Department of Chest Medicine in Addenbrooke's Hospital as well as being a psychiatrist.

Ten years ago we would have said that most people we now diagnose as having panic attacks were hyperventilating. Panic disorder is a relatively new concept − derived ironically from observations of the effects of imipramine on anxiety − is it valid?

Almost certainly: most people having a panic attack do hyperventilate and most people who are hyperventilating do experience feelings of panic. There is a bit of a chicken and egg situation here − we have to ask which comes first. And, of course, the two conditions are not identical, despite what some people think. There is no doubt that some people hyperventilate without experiencing panic.

Hyperventilation may be triggered by all sorts of physical and psychological states. Of the latter, most cases seem to fall into one of two classes. Either they are a response to a sudden anxiety-laden situation or current pattern of thinking, which might or might not have a phobic element to it, or they may arise spontaneously out of the blue. This second type occurs in people who over-breathe for much of the time and consequently have a persistently low level of carbon dioxide. Although it has been criticized, I use the reduplication method to make an initial assessment. Voluntary over-breathing in a person who is already low in carbon dioxide rapidly produces intolerable symptoms, whereas a normal individual can cheerfully continue for a couple of minutes or more. I think it is amongst this group of patients with persistently low carbon dioxide that panic attacks may occur. But to complicate the issue we have carried out respiratory studies in many anxious patients who complain of a sensation that they cannot take a deep enough breath, only to find that their blood and respiratory carbon dioxide levels are normal.

Now, this is interesting, because this relates to current debate. Where panic disorders are concerned people who take a cognitive approach talk about a pathological cognitive style. They would say that panic disorder is not a physiological disorder because it can be provoked by a wide range of physical stimuli, therefore it can't be actually related to any one of those stimuli − the common interpretative style is what is important. But you're arguing that hyperventilators really are physiologically different − that certain mechanisms are set at a different threshold.

We are getting into very complicated matters here. Interpretation of the meaning of physical symptoms is all-important. But going back to a point before the physical symptoms are experienced, I do believe that anxiety alters inspiratory and expiratory trigger thresholds in the respiratory centre. Once this alteration is present the individual concerned is, in a sense, physically different from other people and exhibits shallow and rapid breathing.

Can I put one final thing to you. The replacement of the hyperventilation syndrome by panic disorder is a good example of the ability of the pharmaceutical industry to shape the language we use. Hyperventilation disorder suggests a condition in which people can do a lot to help themselves, whereas panic disorder suggests something that arises for biochemical reasons which must be treated with drug therapies. Now if we ask why the concept of panic has replaced that of hyperventilation, one has to say that Upjohn at the very least had some part to play in the change in culture as it were. Any comments?

There are many such examples. Staying with the benzodiazepines and going right back to the start, the various manufacturers of drugs of this type were fairly successful in persuading doctors that benzodiazepines were the definitive and only reasonable treatments for anxiety and insomnia. Enormous sales followed. Now in the light of some of the problems associated with those drugs these early views have been modified. There is no doubt that the pharmaceutical industry is a significant factor in influencing prescribing through both high quality educational programmes and sometimes, sadly, less sound material. The industry may occasionally exploit results from a small number of clinical trials, in which a new indication has been explored, and in this way, as you say, they can change the culture. This is not necessarily for the worst, of course. But on the whole the pharmaceutical world is a highly ethical one and is fairly strictly governed by widely accepted codes of conduct.

Select bibliography

Kiloh, L.G., Ball, J.R. (1961) Depression treated with imipramine: a follow-up study. *British Medical Journal*, **I**, 881–86.

Kuhn, R. (1957) Ueber die Behandlung depressiver Zustaende mit einem I minodibenzylderivat (G22355). *Schweiz Med. Wschr.*, **87**, 1135–40.

Rose, W.C., Haines, W.J. and Warner, D.T. (1954) The amino acid requirements of man. The role of lysine, arginine and tryptophan. *J. Biol. Chem.* **206**, 421–30.

Schindler, W. and Haefliger, F. (1954) Derivatives of iminodibenzyl. *Helv. Chim. Acta*, **37**, 472.

Thiele, J. and Holzinger, O. (1899) Ueber O-Diamidobenzyl. *Ann. Chem. Liebegs*, **305**, 96–102.

Todrick, A., Tait, A.C. and Marshall, E.F. (1960) Blood platelet 5-hydroxytryptamine levels in psychiatric patients. *J. Mental Science*, **106**, 884–90.

6 Silvio Garattini

The role of independent science in psychopharmacology

Your book Psychotropic Drugs *(Garattini and Ghetti, 1957) was pretty well the first modern book on psychopharmacology and the meeting, on which it was based must have been close to the very first psychopharmacology meeting.*

The meeting was in 1957, before the first CINP meeting. I think the only thing that was before that was a small meeting at the New York Academy of Science on meprobamate in October 1956, published in the *Annals of the New York Academy of Sciences* in 1957. Our meeting was in May 9–11 1957 and we published during May 1957.

That was a fast job. There has been some debate about who was responsible for this meeting and the subsequent development of the CINP, with Dr Radouco-Thomas seeing Emilio Trabucchi as the key figure (Ban and Hippius, 1994 – see Glossary) but others I have interviewed, such as Philip Bradley see you as the prime mover. How do remember it?

Well, I was in the department of pharmacology of Milan University at that time and I felt that what was happening was really a new branch of pharmacology. Professor Emilio Trabucchi was the head of the department at that time and he supported the idea. You must remember that in 1956, when the idea arose and the initial organization took place, I was only 28 years old. Therefore many contacts with authoritative scientists were made directly by Professor Trabucchi, although the activities necessary for the meeting, including the list of speakers, came from me. My official profile therefore was only marginal, although the action of Professor Trabucchi was the result of my input. I have the impression that too many people are claiming an essential role in the steps towards CINP. I can only say that the organization of the 'Psychotropic Drugs' Symposium and the preparation of the following meetings have required a lot of effort and energy from me. My role in the 1957 symposium is clearly shown by the fact that I was the Editor or the proceedings, with Dr Vittorio Ghetti, representing Ciba, one of the major sponsors of the meeting.

We had support from other companies but Ciba was the most interested because they had reserpine. At the time of meeting reserpine was, of course, available and there was the knowledge that reserpine had a mixture of sedative and hypotensive effects, which one could perhaps separate and get something that could be more specific for the vascular system and something more specific for the brain. Then there was also chlorpromazine and the first very positive results in psychotic patients and there was the first tranquillizer, meprobamate, for which the term tranquillizer was established. It was Dr Frank Berger, working in Wallace Laboratories, the discoverer of meprobamate, who utilized the term tranquillization because it wasn't really a type of sedation in the classic sense and proposed that this was related to effects on the central nervous system but also to some relaxant activity on the skeletal musculature. There was another drug, hydroxyzine, which was also a centrally acting drug but with less clear effects compared to the others. Then we had the monoamine oxidase inhibitors and later on the tricyclic antidepressant compounds.

We at the Mario Negri Institute were very interested in serotonin, which at that time was known mostly because of its presence in the platelets of certain animal species and in the gastrointestinal tract. In the brain there were very small concentrations and many people believed that these traces – you'll find this, for instance, in one of the articles of Erspamer, who was one of the discoverers of serotonin – were really only something that remained from the presence of serotonin in blood in the brain. The amounts were so small that nobody believed that serotonin had a function. It was only later that the neurochemical mediation induced by serotonin became apparent. We were interested to investigate this issue at that time with methods which were rudimentary in a way, hoping to establish how drugs could change the level of serotonin in the brain. I remember around this time we had got a spectrofluorimeter which gave us the methodology to measure serotonin in a more specific and quantitative way than with the spectrophotometer. At the meeting Dr Luigi Valzelli and I reported the effect of electric shock on levels of brain serotonin. He was a very close colleague of mine and he was in the Mario Negri Institute from the beginning until he passed away. He did a lot of work during the years on serotonin, and in particular on aggressive behaviour.

The meeting was actually a mixture of experimental and clinical data and we mixed up, as much as possible, the two things. I remember there was enthusiasm because there was something new – an enthusiasm I experienced some years before working on isoniazid, the antitubercular drug which changed the treatment of tuberculosis, from which iproniazid was derived as well as the monoamine oxidase inhibitors.

It was also during that meeting that we had received from Dr Rothlin from Switzerland, the idea that it would be useful to have a branch of pharmacology called psychopharmacology and the basis was laid for establishing the Collegium Internationale Neuropsychopharmacologium (the CINP). The idea first came up during this meeting, after which it was of course implemented, and from then they have had regular meetings of the CINP. I was involved with the organization of the first meeting of the CINP in 1958 because Professor Trabucchi was involved and therefore I was drafted in to help him with various duties. Dr Radouco-Thomas was another key person.

What do you recall from the 1957 meeting? Are there any talks or any people in particular whose work interested you that you recall clearly now.

Well, there were several people who were quite outstanding in the field. You can get some feel by looking at who was at the 1957 meeting. On the question of metabolism of neurotransmitters, there was Dr Blaschko who gave a very good paper on the enzymes metabolizing monoamines. Dr Hoffer, he was the one, who believed that adrenochrome was exerting effects on the central nervous system to cause psychosis.

There was the group of Dr Himwich and Dr Emilio Costa. Dr Costa was a young man at that time. We had been colleagues at the Institute of Pharmacology because he came from the Cagliari Institute of Pharmacology, where he worked with a pupil of Professor Trabucchi, by the name of William Ferrari and he spent some time in Milan with us as well. Then he went to the United States and worked with Himwich on amino acids in the central nervous system and later, as you know, he became a member of Dr Brodie's staff before going on to his own career.

Could you give me your thoughts on what role Brodie has played in the field because he was also the editor of Neuropharmacology *wasn't he and he's had a very big influence.*

Yes. This came a little bit later but certainly *Neuropharmacology* was a very important journal as was *Psychopharmacologia*, another journal devoted to psychotropic drugs. *Neuropharmacology*, in fact, was born in St Tropez, during a meeting between Dr Brodie, Dr Costa and myself. Dr Costa contributed a lot in basic fields for the understanding of brain function. Actually, in 1959, I visited him at the Galesbury State Hospital, where he was working with Dr Himwich and we did some work together. It was immediately after Dr Kuhn had discovered the antidepressant effect of imipramine. There was a lot of scepticism about the reality of this discovery because imipramine was so close to chlorpromazine in terms of chemical structure that nobody really believed it in the beginning. But it generated a lot of activity in trying to establish some way to show antidepressant activity.

I was working with reserpine and I got an idea which was refined by Dr Costa. Since reserpine was an agent considered to have depressant activity, we thought that an antidepressant agent might inhibit its action. In fact, we established and we published that imipramine and its metabolite, desipramine are inhibitors of some effects of reserpine, including sedation, hypothermia, ptosis and diarrhoea. We published a paper in 1960 on this in *Experientia* (Costa, et al.,1960). Unfortunately *Experientia* is not a journal that is read by pharmacologists, so that paper, although it was the first one to show the effect of imipramine as an antidepressant agent in a test, was never quoted by anybody. They quoted subsequent papers.

You will remember at that time there was a lot of work on reserpine and there was also a lot of work on the mechanism of action of anti-depressants – it was about that time it was discovered that these agents blocked the uptake of noradrenaline in the brain and affected noradrenaline transmission. This was Dr Axelrod's work.

In terms of the people who were involved – Costa, Himwich, Axelrod, Brodie – who for you were the key people?

I think the most influential man for me was Brodie. I don't want to diminish the fundamental contributions of Julius Axelrod and Sidney Udenfriend, but Dr Brodie had more of a pharmacological attitude. As you know, he was the man who established the basis for pharmacokinetics, drug metabolism and the importance of measuring blood levels and so on. He represented a great impetus because Costa worked with him and really became known working with him. Dr Pletscher, who was respons-ible for monoamine oxidase inhibitor work, spent a lot of time with him. Arvid Carlsson, who was extremely important for his work in the area of catecholamines, worked with him. Dr Bowman developed the spectro-fluorimeter in his labs. So there was really a large number of people that have exerted a lot of influence in psychopharmacology that originated or at least made contributions in psychopharmacology while working in his labs. Obviously many key investigators in psychopharmacology passed through the labs of Dr Axelrod: Dr Glowinsky, for example, and Dr Udenfriend also.

What type of a person was Brodie?

He was a very interesting character. I had the privilege to spend a lot of time with him on various occasions in Bethesda or Milan – because he came from time to time to visit us particularly when I established the Mario Negri Institute in 1963. Steve was a man that was always working. One couldn't find him doing nothing; he was always working, thinking and enquiring. He had the capacity to discuss problems with people putting the right questions, insisting on getting answers, insisting on getting opinions. He was really what you might call, I don't know if there is an English word for it, a maieutic, which is a Greek word to say he could extract ideas from people by asking questions. He was quite good in this respect.

I remember that he used to work a lot during the night. With him, it was difficult to go to bed before 2 or 3 o'clock in the morning. There were all these sessions he was asking questions and he alternated discussions with correction of papers. I learned from him a lot about the logic of writing scientific papers. He was never completely happy with a scientific paper. He was always thinking about the possibility to improve it. For me it was really a very important schooling and I remember him always with great affection and gratitude. I think that he has really helped a lot in the development of psychopharmacology.

Who else was important . . .?

Well, Denber. He was working on a system to categorize psychotic reactions to the various drugs available at that time. Rothlin was the man who really helped made LSD available and undertook a lot of studies on the action of LSD.

What kind of a person was Rothlin? There has been some ambiguity about his role in the establishment of the CINP. Philip Bradley remembers him as being a key figure canvassing support for the idea, while Hans Hippius remembers him as being initially against the idea of a CINP but later emerging surprisingly as its first President.

Rothlin was a very good scientist, a very methodical person. He was a nice person although he had very clear ideas about what he wanted to obtain. We in Milan organized the 1957 meeting with the idea that a subsequent international association was desirable. I put a pressure on Professor Trabucchi to lead this organization but he did not want to become President because of his poor knowledge of English at that time. Clearly, many people had the same idea but I think without the 1957 meeting, in all probability the birth of CINP would have been postponed.

Did Hoffmann play much part in any of this or did he just accidentally find LSD and then fade out?

Well, without him there would have been no LSD but he was more on the chemical side. The man who developed knowledge on LSD from a biological point of view was Rothlin. Weiskrantz was important for studies on reserpine. Stata Norton was also important in the beginning because she was the one that tried to establish the action of various psychotropic actions on behaviour because at that time behaviour in pharmacology was certainly not very developed.

Observations of behaviour were already happening but all the tests this time were still simple tests. Obviously there were already people involved in behaviour but these were not known to pharmacologists. Neal Miller was one. Dr Leonard from the Roche Institute was involved very much in the effects of drugs on behaviour. Looking retrospectively I think we got a very good selection of names. I'm surprised. At that time I was a young investigator and although I asked advice from many people, to be able to put together a programme of this kind surprises me.

Erik Jacobsen was another one. He was studying benactazine but he didn't have much luck. And there was Dr Gatti from the Istituto Superiore di Sanita in Rome. He didn't get enough credit at this time. He was working with Bovet at the time and he really did some fine work on behaviour and in fact he was using conditioning tests in rats at that time. Actually some of these tests would be useful even now seeing that looking at the effect of neuroleptics on operant behaviour is now a relatively modern way to look at drugs.

Now, of some historical interest on the programme, we had Thuillier, a psychopharmacologist who played a role in the early days of the CINP. Nakajima who is now Director of WHO was working with him then. He was a pharmacologist and I think at that time he had a fellowship in France with Dr Thuillier to work on what they called the turning mice. They were giving dinitropropyl and they were testing what the various drugs were doing on this turning behaviour. At that time there was very little known but I don't know if we have any better screening tests today. They reported at our meeting an extensive series of drugs that they studied on these systems.

Moruzzi and Bovet were present. They gave basic papers on electrophysiology and the function of the reticular formation. Dr Bovet and Dr Longo were interested in the effect of psychotropic drugs on electrophysiology. Philip Bradley was there and he was already using microelectrodes to study effects of drugs on the reticular formation. Another neurophysiologist was Monnier. And Killam was also an important person because of course he started the techniques of self-stimulation in the brain and studying the effects of drugs on self-stimulation.

Gastaut was at the meeting but he was actually more interested in the effects of neuroleptics on behaviour and then there was Unna. From a cholinergic point of view there was Feldberg from the MRC. He was mostly interested in behaviour with particular reference to the control of body temperature, which was affected by some of these psychotropic drugs. Dr Bein gave one of the direct papers on psychopharmacology, in which he discussed in great detail all the actions of reserpine. Dr Plummer was also important. He was also from Ciba but from the American branch. He did a lot of studies on the behavioural effect of reserpine and then a lot of studies on a large number of derivatives and these studies led to more chemically simplified compounds, such as tetrabenazine. Roche were working on derivatives of this while Ciba was working on analogues of reserpine.

Arvid Carlsson, who was the first to establish that reserpine was affecting catecholamines, was there. I remember at that time the puzzle as to why there should be an increase of catecholamines without changing the synthesis of catecholamines. This created the basis for the concepts of release, reuptake and storage. Arvid was very important in this respect. He was able to put together biochemical findings with physiological techniques. He is still in fact very active in the field.

We also had Courvoisier, who was the person who discovered chlorpromazine and the person who did all the early work on structure–activity relationships in the area of the phenothiazines. She was working at Rhône-Poulenc.

There's some dispute among the French as to who was the most important person clinically in the discovery of chlorpromazine – was it Henri Laborit or Jean Delay?

Yes, I think they had different roles. Laborit was using it mostly to produce deep hypothermia to make possible certain surgical operations but I believe Deniker was really the person who established the antipsychotic effect.

Erspamer was there and gave a talk on the relationship between the gastrointestinal enteramine (which was his name for serotonin) and cerebral serotonin. Shore and Brodie reported on the depletion of brain serotonin by reserpine, which they followed up by looking at its effect on noradrenaline. There were a great deal of interesting discussions as to why animals treated with reserpine took so much time to recover from depletion of monoamines. It was quite unusual for drugs to have such a long biochemical effect. There was not a complete correspondence with the pharmacological effect and this gave rise to the concept of 'hit and run' drugs, which do something and then the drug is no longer present but the effect is there.

We had Tripod there; he tried to characterize agents on the basis of their effects on the chemical transmitters that were then available. He was working on the action of the various drugs on acetylcholine, adrenaline, histamine and trying to make up patterns for the various categories of drugs. We know now how difficult this is considering that what we see may be the effect of a result of an action on multiple subtypes of receptors.

We also had Alfred Pletscher, who gave the first observations of the antagonism between iproniazid and reserpine. This was a marked antagonism which was quite different from the one that is observed between imipramine and reserpine. At this meeting he reported on some of the biochemical effects of this interaction looking at the levels of serotonin that were antagonized by the action of iproniazid.

Clinically, then, there was Delay and Deniker. There were a number of psychiatrists commenting on the use of hydroxyzine and there was Frank Ayd.

You don't hear much about meprobamate these days but it seems as though at the time there was almost as much interest in it as there was in chlorpromazine.

Yes, meprobamate actually was a drug that enjoyed quite a good market and it could have been done even better if in the States it hadn't been marketed by a relatively small company, Wallace, which actually became quite large because of the sales of meprobamate. Dr Berger was the man who had an essential role in developing and sustaining the knowledge of meprobamate. But then with the advent of the benzodiazepines, there was a decrease in its market. I don't know if it was good or bad because certainly we didn't have any knowledge at least at that time of any dependence to meprobamate.

Why do you think things took off as quickly as they did? Chlorpromazine was really only produced clinically in 1954 and by 1957, three years later, you have such a meeting. It's pretty remarkable, isn't it.

I think that this happens at the beginning of a new field. Things are ripe, so when something starts there is a flourishing. I think we have had the same type of experience with the cytokines. The various interleukins came about in a relatively short time. And now I guess it will take some time before they will discover other cytokines. It seems to be a pattern, at least in pharmacology, that you have a burst and then improvements and then a sort of plateau, where you try to understand the mechanisms of action. But actually if you look at the situation, in practical terms the progress was not so fantastic. We already had a tranquillizer, meprobamate – now we have benzodiazepines, many of them, but they are all more or less the same. In terms of antipsychotics the only thing that was new was haloperidol and all its derivatives. Haloperidol, well it's different from chlorpromazine, maybe it's an improvement over chlorpromazine because it's more specific. We had the monoamine oxidase inhibitors and in 1959 we have the first tricyclic antidepressant. There has been no important progress after 1959. Some differences in the mechanisms of action but equivalence in potency. Maybe smaller differences in side effects which have not really been exploited in clinical practice. Clozapine may represent a progress in the treatment of the psychoses but that's all.

So why then did so much happen during 10 years and nothing very much since despite huge research enterprises?

Perhaps one of the reasons is that we depend for new drugs very much on the industry and the industry rather than wanting to find out more about various areas, aims at finding a better drug than the previous ones but always keeping a large spectrum of activity. Now this can't be. We have already got something for anxiety, for depression, for psychosis. The only thing which is new is the effect on compulsive behaviours. Whether or not the SSRIs are superior or not is open to discussion but it's a new area where something can be done. In this situation it's basically difficult to have new things – unless you start to think that within anxiety you have different components and you try to find out agents that are useful for that particular component. But this doesn't really appeal to the industry because probably the market is too small and they don't want to have a large investment just to get a part of the market. But in reality at least retrospectively most of the companies that have developed one of the hundred antidepressants available didn't have a big piece of the market anyway. So they tried to have a large market but in essence most of them got a relatively small market, so there was no real advantage.

Now all the potential research available is addressed to the area of cognitive function but for the moment there is very little happening. But that's probably the next area. There will be something available in the future which means being able to do something for senile dementia. It looks like we may not be far away from that particular development.

The Mario Negri Institute is now extremely famous. Why did you want to go independent when you did?

Actually the reason for which I sought to develop an independent institution was my first visit to the United States in 1957. I had two big impressions. One was the fact that at that time in the United States research was considered a professional activity. In Italy, in the University, research was considered a way to make a career in the University it was not considered a value in itself. It was instrumental to do something. The second thing that I was impressed by was the variety of institutions. There were universities. There were private and public universities. There were the big company research laboratories and there were these foundations.

I was interested in the concept of a foundation because it had, at least in my simple way to look at it, at that time, the advantage that foundations were not submitted to the bureaucratic laws that govern the public institutions, including the universities. A second advantage was that you don't have to make profit. You can devote yourself to the public interest so that in the way I understood the situation it could be a sort of simple statement of private initiative in the service of the public interest that appealed to me very much.

So in 1957, actually after this symposium, I visited the main institutions in the United States for a period of three months. Coming back, I got my group together. I said, well, if we are serious about doing research, we have an alternative: either we all go over to work in the United States where there was a request for us as scientists at the time or we try to do something different if we want to stay in Italy. In the end the idea was why don't we try to establish something different in Italy.

Who was Mario Negri?

Mario Negri was a self-made man, an industrialist in the field of jewellery, who came to me because he invested some money in a company called Farmacosmici, which represented Burroughs Wellcome in Italy. He and his director, Dr N. Damiani, wanted some advice about new drugs. I had a chance to talk to him about this on a number of occasions and after a while he was persuaded to establish a foundation. He wanted to when he was alive but unfortunately he got cancer of the liver. About two weeks before he died he called me in the clinic and told me to make sure I did what we had discussed. He died in April 1960 and when the Will was opened there were all the indications to establish the Institute with all the general policy that we had worked out together. In the Will, he named me as the Director of the Institute. At that time, what he left was a fair amount of money.

We started on the legal and financial aspects. We first got recognition by the US Government and then from the Italian one and at the end of 1961, we started to build the Institute and on 1 February 1963 the whole group of 22 people moved into this new building with a lot of anxiety but also with an interest to start the new adventure.

The Institute should have three aims – the first was to perform research, not so much in trying to discover new drugs but in understanding the mechanism of action of drugs, thinking that if you understand how a drug is acting you are in a good position to have a better use of the drug. The second thing was to train young people to do research. This is now something very common but in 1963 the idea of having trained people in Italy to do research as a profession was something relatively new. The third thing was to disseminate information that was collected from the research phase. By dissemination of information we mean not only in scientific journals but also to inform in various ways physicians about the results of research and even the public. Again, in 1963, this was rather revolutionary, when at least in Italy for an academician to talk to the public was considered something that was likely to lead to a loss of prestige.

In the beginning we had a lot of interest because this was the first example of a foundation in Italy that was doing research. We had quite a lot of hostility from academia. I left the University with the whole group and since I was very close to get a Chair this was considered by the academicians as a sort of insult. So we had a hard time for the period.

We established a few simple rules for our practice – the first one was not to spend the money that was not available. The second one was to establish as much as possible a situation where there was autodiscipline so in the Institute we never had a union but equally we never checked the time of anybody. This is based on the idea that everybody has to do as much as possible. The third rule was not to accept grants or contracts for more than 10% of our total budget. This was to keep independence of judgement. The fourth rule was not to take out any patent – again, in order to be free. So the Institute doesn't take out any patent even if we have something to patent: the results are either given to the ones with whom we have collaborated or they are published. So, these were the simple rules that we put at the beginning. Because of the experience we had in the University we wanted to be free from political, industrial and academic influence and be able to say at any time our opinion about things which...

You think the Universities aren't free?

They are not entirely free because they depend very much on the Ministry of Education or the Ministry of Health for their support and if you depend entirely on a single entity it is not easy to criticize what the supporting entity is doing. But if you get just a fraction of your total income from any one source, then it's easier because you can afford to lose something if it is necessary to speak out about certain things.

So the first six or seven years were really difficult in Italy but fortunately we had a lot connections at the international level and this is what really was very helpful to us. At the beginning we had grants from the Wellcome Trust to buy equipment. We had quite a lot of support from the National Institute of Health at Bethesda and also from some American foundations, such as the Gustavus and Louise Pfeiffer Foundation in New York. And after that the Institute was gradually accepted by academia here and supported also by the Italian sources. In the beginning almost 50% of our budget came from abroad and now it's much less.

The training of young people is an important goal for us. We now have about 850 people divided between the Institute in Milan, the Institute in the South of Italy, one in Bergamo and the other one that is being completed. We have tried to separate the field of interest of various groups. In Milan it is mostly cancer, psychotropic drugs and some aspects of cardiovascular pharmacology. In the South, it is mostly thrombosis, coagulation and neuroendocrine problems. In Bergamo, it is mostly renal diseases.

With time we have integrated our activity. We started purely on an experimental basis in the laboratory and then little by little we moved into the clinical area. The first one was to add clinical collaboration to protocols and then to arrange multicentric studies that were directed by the Institute of which the best known are the GISSI studies. These were studies on myocardial infarction. They were large-scale studies. We had three studies. The first one was a demonstration of the efficacy of streptokinase after heart attacks; we had a 12 000 patients. The second one was a combination of streptokinase and aspirin in comparison with tPA; there were 20 000 patients in that. The third, which has just finished, was the combination of ACE inhibitor with nitrates.

This was really world-wide, wasn't it?

Oh, yes, as I say, in order to collect 20 000 patients we needed 200 centres in all of Italy, 200 coronary units and about 600 cardiologists – it was a very big organization, only possible because of the collaboration of the Associazione Nazionale Medici Cardiologi Ospedalieri, but now it's established as a network and the mortality of myocardial infarction has been almost halved in these 10 years of studies.

So, we integrated the laboratory with clinical work with epidemiology and then Bergamo was established because we wanted more direct access to patients. In Bergamo, we have joint appointments at the Institute and in the Department of Nephrology at the Hospital so that we can have a movement from the lab to the clinic to the lab. The Negri South is our institute to help young people in the South of Italy to enter biomedical research.

The last location of the Institute is at Villa Camozzi. This is a place where we want to establish a unique clinical research centre which will be devoted to rare diseases – why rare diseases? Because patients with rare diseases are doubly unlucky; they have a disease and nobody can help because there is no competence, no financial support, no knowledge. This will be a big place actually, with 350 rooms and a beautiful park. There'll be three main activities there. One is to function as a centre of information for rare diseases where everybody can come and present their case and network with specialists. We'll keep an update of information about their disease and also an indication of the best Italian or foreign places where they can get assistance – if they want we will help them to establish a connection. This is work that is done free.

Then we will have a day hospital with 10 beds and there will be by the end of September 30 beds for chronic patients with all the necessary diagnostic facilities – a small hospital. The idea here is not to get the patients as they want to come in but to organize research on patients where they will be for one week. One week we will collect patients with a given rare disease and this we hope will trigger a number of specialists from all over the world to come because they will have such an opportunity. We will give hospitality in the same building and for one week there will be intensive work with a given group of patients with a particular diagnostic label – collecting biological samples, establishing therapeutic protocols, etc. And then there will be another disease. Of course we will have our own projects in our own field of interest but the place will be available to foreign groups to use the facilities in order to study certain problems that they are interested in. Most of the work to remodel this building has been done with private money and by the end of September, as I said, it will be running.

What about the questions of not being prepared to spend money that wasn't available and the autodisciplinary issues?

Yes, well, the first one means that we have been always working with our own money. In other words we never borrowed any money even for a very short period of time and this was vital because in the history of every Institute you find years in which it is easier to get support and years in which it is less easy to get support and then years of difficulty such as the one that we are having in Italy today. If you have your own resources you can survive. If you don't have them you are in trouble because you start to need to get loans and you have to pay interest.

Autodiscipline is the idea that you don't make too many controls that are meaningless. People can be there at a given time and if they don't do things they don't. The idea is that if you give freedom then of course people become more responsible. In previous periods of Italian history in which the unions had been extremely powerful in all the organizations, we never had any union inside the Institute and we never had strikes or whatever because people felt that the future of the Institute depended very much on them and not just other people. This I think was a very important part of the Institute.

You've been extremely careful about maintaining your independance – has it paid off?

Oh, yes. I think so. Of course, independence means so many times that you have less resources. It means that you have more difficulties because you don't have any 'padrino' (godfather) that is taking care of your needs, but in a period of scandals in Italy, it was very important that we didn't have anything to do with the politicians. So this has paid off because the public gets a clear understanding of these problems and I think that the Institute has been looked at by the public as an independant and reliable organization, a scientific organization that was close to people. This was shown up also by the support that we have received. Donations represent right now every year over 20% of our total budget – from private people, from banks or other organizations.

I think that there have been some important periods. One certainly was in 1972 when I was part of the committee to select the drugs for what was at that time our National Health Service. There were pressures to put in drugs, you know there was a lot of industrial pressure and so on, I resigned and I explained why I resigned. I think the public understood the fact that I wasn't willing, actually not me but the Institute wasn't willing to support things that were against scientific knowledge. Another important moment was in 1976 when we had the Seveso disaster, where the Roche factory blew up.

At that time through television and the media, the Institute said clearly what they thought about things, while industrial and political interests were trying to cover up or to minimize the importance of these events. We did a lot of work at this time. This happened on the 10 July and more or less half of the Institute announced that they would not take a summer vacation in order to work on this problem and I think that the public understood that to have a scientific institution is not just to have people who are working on their problems but to have people that care about what affects society.

The Institute was also well known because we took a public position against the presence of useless drugs in the Italian market. This was also unusual because in a way we have always been working very closely with industrial research and we think it is absolutely necessary and useful to collaborate with industry but I have always thought that we should not confuse the roles that cooperation with research is one thing but this doesn't mean that you are forced to help industry in public relations. This was also very difficult but I think we managed to keep the two things quite separate.

I have been involved many times in public discussions about problems of the use of useless drugs. Recently, for the first time, I should say under the pressure of the public, I have been asked to take part in a committee for approval of new drugs, but this is happening for the first time after 40 years of work in pharmacology.

From a neuropharmacological point of view, what have been the achievements of scientists within the Institute: Samanin, Mennini these are names I am familiar with.

Dr L. Valzelli has been involved very much in work related to aggressive behaviour. Dr E. Mussini has been very active on benzodiazepine kinetics and metabolism and actually we have been the first to show that many of the drugs that were put on the market as new drugs in fact were metabolites of other drugs such as temazepam or oxazepam or desmethyldiazepam. We have done a lot of work in that area. Dr R. Samanin has been very active in antidepressant agents as well and has made a lot of contributions to the mechanism of action of anorectic drugs and to the role of serotonin in drug activity. He has done pioneer work to show that serotonin was important for the control of food intake.

The group of Dr Mennini has been quite active in the area of receptors. Dr Consolo is well known for her work on acetylcholine and all the various drugs that effect the cholinergic system. I think she is one of the few that has developed methods to measure acetylcholine with a microdialysis technique which allows you to determine what is the extracellular level of acetylcholine. More recently Dr G.L. Forloni and Dr M. Salmona have been working on those peptides that are neurotoxic and part of the amyloid structure; one of the papers was recently published in *Nature*. Dr S. Caccia has contributed to the relationship between brain levels of drugs and their metabolites and pharmacological activity.

Then we have the clinical part where Dr A. Spagnoli is mostly interested in Alzheimer's disease at the clinical level and he has done multicentric studies. Dr E. Beghi is working on epilepsy. Dr B. Saraceno is in psychiatry and he is mostly interested in epidemiology of mental diseases and the quality of the mental health service – psychotropic drug utilization by hospitals as well as by practitioners. So these are some of the things that we have been doing. I think we have probably close to 1000 papers published in neuropharmacology and related fields.

The Mario Negri South has more recently contributed to outlining the mechanism of second messengers, the mechanism of secretion of chemical mediators, both of these areas are covered by Dr A. Luini and Dr D. Corda who have both worked for a long time with Dr Axelrod at NIH. They came back when we established Negri South. Work on molecular biology is led by Dr A. De Blasi. Dr G. De Gaetano, the director, Dr M.B. Donati, Dr C. Cerletti and Dr A. Poggi have contributed to knowledge of drugs acting on platelets, which may be considered a model for nerve terminals.

You've had 30 years to look at the interaction between neuropsychopharmacology and culture generally. Obviously the whole field has influenced popular culture when you get articles in the popular press and on TV and radio about fluoxetine for instance. Do you want to comment on how the field has influenced culture or how the larger culture has influenced the field?

Sure. Well, you go through phases and there was a phase in which everything was wonderful – wonder drugs or magic bullets that were able to change psychiatry. This was part true particularly for the psychotic patients because it was possible to dismantle somewhat the psychiatric hospital due to the fact that we have these drugs available. And then there was obviously the phase where criticism occurred and after all you had a lot of non-responders and you had a lot of problems caused by the drugs, side effects and so on. Now, I think we are in a phase where the drugs have established a pattern for determining whether a treatment is with or without efficacy. We have recently raised the problem of the legitimacy of psychotherapy and the various forms of psychotherapy, how it's justified and how they can justify whatever they do – as you know there are now up to 250 different methods of psychotherapy.

I had, as a result of this, a debate with a group of psychotherapists, where they invited me to express my view and where I strongly suggested that they are professionals and they have to justify what they do. Up till now there were only a few studies available and very little was done in Italy. Of course, it is much more difficult to prove the efficacy of psychotherapy than prove the efficacy of drugs but this is not a reason not to try. As a result of that I think there has been a lot of people, particularly young people, who want to collaborate on research in Italy to try to evaluate psychotherapy. This is certainly not an easy job.

The other way around our culture influences psychiatry or the use of drugs. That in my opinion is less obvious. At least if you look at the Italian scene, we don't have the problems that were typical of the triazolam story or the fluoxetine story. There were newspapers who reported some of the discussion but there has never been a real dramatization of the situation, so I don't really see much influence from the culture.

I could be wrong on this but it seems to me looking at what's happened over the last 30–40 years, not all Europeans have actually contributed equally to psychopharmacology. France was very crucially involved in the start. For some reason perhaps Italians have always been involved the whole way from the start. Is there any reason why psychopharmacology has taken root in Italy?

Probably the reason is that Italy participated since the beginning and I think this is always important in any new field. For instance, we are having difficulties in molecular biology because it came at a later time and we didn't participate in the development. In the area of psychotropic drugs, we were there perhaps by chance but we were there since the beginning. There have been some good groups – Dr Gessa in Cagliari, Dr Bovet, Dr Moruzzi, the department of pharmacology in Milan, Dr Racagni, Dr Cuomo, Dr Clementi, Dr Costa and others. There has been not only a presence from Italy in the beginning but also there has been a lot of cross-fertilization with foreign groups.

One can argue that there is a certain cultural imperialism about psychopharmacology. It supports a very US/UK view of what the mental illnesses are – that has become prevalent in DSM-III? How does that go down in Italy?

Well, I think that Italy has been very weak in psychiatry. There was little science, a lot of talks, a lot of comments, a lot of theories, but psychiatry has never been as strong and therefore either they follow psychoanalysis or they have to follow whatever has developed in the Anglo-Saxon countries – there is no other way. There is not enough strength to develop something autonomous.

Can I pick up a point you raised earlier which is the question of drug specificity. It seems that for 10–20 years after the 1950s we went down the route of trying to get more specific drugs and that seemed to be a good thing to do but in the last 5–10 years there's been something of a crisis of confidence. It seems almost as though the purer the drug the less effective it's going to be.

Well, for the moment this is the impression but there is no scientific basis to say that but I think that we should distinguish two areas in psychopharmacology. There's an area that I would say is the area of knowledge, where we have a lot of interest in having extremely specific agents because it is by having a specific agent that you can pinpoint the importance of a given chemical mediator or a given receptor or a given enzyme in general brain functioning.

But this has to be distinguished in a way from the practical applications and perhaps the strategy to develop new psychotropic drugs is not necessarily the same as that which improves your knowledge. So, there must be some distinction, although it is not known where you have to draw the line. Certainly you shouldn't use the first approach as the best approach in order to fulfil the second aim.

Well, then, is the idea of trying to develop a rational psychopharmacology something of a myth?

It is a myth for all science in a way because the complexity of a living organism is such that if the aim is to cure something it is difficult to proceed only on a very rational basis. I think we will probably come back to the idea that you need models of given psychiatric disorders, which you have to try to correct and then work out what has happened.

Obviously its an osmotic process because on the other hand you develop agents, which affect given chemical mediators or whatever and if you achieve this you try to see if they are doing something in the models of mental diseases. But while there is at present a lot of interest in establishing tools for research, there is an imbalance in terms of looking at models and investing in models.

What do you mean by investing in models?

I mean anything that you develop in order to mimic the whole or an aspect of a given disease. Such as, for instance, you can see that schizophrenia is a disease with many symptoms; you have positive and negative symptoms and you should be able to develop models on which to test if you. can modify any of these symptoms. It is obviously very difficult to modify these symptoms reliably in real life but if you have the model, in which it is simple to modify these symptoms by proper drugs, you can then go to man and see if the extrapolation is possible. This is neglected at the moment.

Certainly for schizophrenia but there are a lot of animal models of depression.

There are animal models for depression. Yes, there are many, but of course each one covers only a small aspect of depression. One should try to modify them by drugs but I think one should try to modify it by a primary approach because obviously if you test these models with only drugs that have given effects on chemical mediators you pre–establish what you are going to test. And that will not give you a new type of drug. In other words I think that you should apply new tests if you want to find new drugs. If you are using old tests for a known mechanism you are going to reproduce the same drugs.

Why is the industry so conservative then?

Well, the industry in this area is probably not convinced that you can make a lot of progress. Therefore they try to get a slice of the market. I think that the concept of me-too drugs depends always on the fact that you don't believe that we can develop something new. In Alzheimer's, where there is nothing, the industry is investing with determination. There is also another aspect, which is that there is a great discrepancy in the sophistication with which we look at the mechanism of action of the various antidepressant agents and establish whatever can differentiate one drug from the other and then when we arrive at the clinical level, there is extreme uniformity in testing them, as though you would not be interested to see differences (Garattini, 1996).

We use the same two or three rating scales and force all drugs to conform with them . . .?

Yes, the type of protocol that is used is used not to show difference but to show equivalence: industry makes a bet. They say if they can get an antidepressant agent through the FDA they may have a chance to have a big slice of the market. And since they know how to do this in terms of development, it is an easy way to go. Industry establishes pre-clinical differences for different drugs that it doesn't use in its clinical trials but it does use to exploit the market. Marketing is not based on the fact that my drug is superior to the other. It is based on the fact that my drug is affecting dopamine more than serotonin or more than noradrenaline with respect to another drug.

Coming back to the question of purity, on the question of testing for the toxicology of new drugs, I've heard you say that we cannot always rely on cell lines, that sometimes we have to go back to the whole animal. Do you want to comment on that because it's very politically correct these days to praise the virtues of cell lines?

Yes, I've just come from a meeting in Baltimore which was the world meeting on alternative techniques and there was a session called Point/ Counterpoint where a man from OECD was defending the alternative method and I was supposed to defend the animal methodology. I presented practical cases to show that a certain effect could not possibly be seen in tissue culture. The organism is so complex that the idea that we can mimic this complexity in a tube, it's really absolutely irrational. The approach taken by many of these groups that are interested in alternative tests is that essentially they are saying that since the mouse or the dog or the monkey is not man, therefore it may be misleading to extrapolate to man. I take the same approach and say if you go down to a level which is even further away and hope that by simplifying things you can solve a very complex problem, you are unlikely to succeed. Politically it pays because again there is money available to study alternative testing. There is little money to do animal research because it is not popular anymore.

This again is something that our Institute has been very strong in Italy in trying to tell people why we need to use the animals. I have had a lot of debates in public and on television to indicate that this is what we have to do if you want to make sure that you have better drugs, chemicals that are not damaging man, you have to rely on animals. That's the best thing that you can do now and the fact that in the future you may have alternative techniques, doesn't mean that you have to put obstacles in the way of the present line of research. Philosophically I'm convinced that it will never be possible to do without animal work in toxicology because I would like to know how a cell could tell you about convulsion, tremors, anorexia, cachexia, hypothermia. These are things that cannot possibly be seen in any cell, whatever you do, whatever type of methodology you may have available. But it is very unpopular to say this.

Well, now can I ask you why 40 years into the psychopharmacological era, the more rational we become about how we develop drugs, the more irrational people on the street have become. They prefer to go out and buy health foods thinking that they are safer even though the compounds in health foods haven't been tested and sometimes even are old drugs that have been rejected by orthodox medicine as unsafe. Why is this happening?

Well, first of all there have been all these Green movements and they have popularized a concept that seems logical – that nature is good and what man does is bad and so we should follow nature. I always try to say that this is tragic; it is stupid to think that nature is good and man is bad because nature may be good or may be bad. Viruses and bacteria are not all that good. Most of the poisons are present in nature. The rational way to look at the problem is not to generalize about nature or man but to look at the various compounds one by one and try to evaluate them one by one and one may discover in some cases that nature is good and in other cases it is bad. In the same way man as part of nature: sometimes he makes good things and sometimes bad things and you have to evaluate each one on its own. This applies to everything. The idea that herbs or health extracts are good because they are made by nature is stupid. It is irrational; it is a kind of subculture.

Why are we so influenced by this kind of thinking?

Well, because the environment is becoming an important issue, Having lost a lot of meaning in our life, religious and moral, then you must have some value and the environment appears to be something good for many people. Not for all. The Greens are still, after all, a very small minority, a very vocal minority, who may seem to be more than in reality they are but because it is fashionable nobody opposes these views because if you oppose you become unpopular. But I think that the role of science and the role of scientific institutes is sometimes to be unpopular because we are interested in what appears to be the truth and it's our duty not to follow fashion but to follow what we think is rational. Unfortunately I should say that the scientific community is not outstanding in this respect and most people prefer the quiet life rather than to expose themselves and to discuss these issues.

It's easier to get on a TV chat show as well if you're going to take the popular point of view.

Sure. If you defend the animals you are immediately popular and a good man. If you say look, if you want to have safe drugs I don't know of any better way at the moment than to use animals and then you become somebody that is cynical or questionable.

As we have lost cultural, moral and religious values in recent years, have the larger pharmaceutical companies become centres of culture in their own right?

Yes, this I see as dangerous for science because now there is relatively little freedom in science. If you look at most of the meetings, they have sponsorship and nobody sponsors anything unless at the end it gets some interest. Most of the journals that physicians are receiving are paid for by advertising; this creates a sort of distorted information that is very difficult to compensate by free information, independent information. I always say that in Italy the industry is spending about 3,000 billion lire every year to advertise their products in various forms and probably we are spending a few millions to have independent information. This is very bad.

In the long run it is not in the interest of the industry because the industry in order to improve must be stimulated. The industry must have a relatively difficult life in order to become productive. If you give it an easy life, obviously you are not going to make a big improvement. So in the end it is also in the interest of the industry to develop criticism, to increase the level of critics. But it doesn't at the moment I think. And this at the end influences all our knowledge and also the evaluation of efficacy. It is not by chance that we don't have any comparative studies among drugs. Because it is not in the interest of the industry. The state apparently doesn't seem to be interested in these problems and at the end what is done is only what . . .

When you say the state is not interested, is it that they don't want to lose their pharmaceutical companies?

I don't think so. I think it's a lack of culture. There is no culture, at least in the Italian National Health Service. They should be interested because if they take drugs and they establish that there is no difference or that one is better than the other there is a lot of consequence in terms of what they would do and also how much they will spend so they should be interested but at the moment there is not this type of culture.

When I raised the question about the industry being a centre of culture, I was thinking actually about something slightly different which is that they will sell antidepressant drugs to treat people who are depressed, they will sell antipsychotic drugs to people who are psychotic; but at the moment they've got a great number of drugs that will enhance sexual peformance for men and women, drugs that will delay orgasms for men who have a premature ejaculation problem, and bring it forward for women, but they don't market these. The smart drugs are another example. Companies are happy to get involved with drugs to treat Alzheimer's but social engineering . . .

Makes them very wary. Well, they may fear public disapproval. It's the same reason for which Roussel doesn't want certain countries to use their abortive drug − in countries where there are strong religious groups who would object and say to their members 'don't buy drugs from that company'. They may feel that it would be counterproductive.

Pursuing the issue of culture. The range of psychopharmacological cultures around

Europe is interesting. You get antidepressants that are best selling antidepressants in France, like maprotiline, which don't sell in the UK and then dothiepin which sells well in the UK but nowhere else in Europe . . .

I made an analysis of the 50 most sold drugs by value for the 4 biggest European countries: Italy, France, Germany and England and it's amazing to find out that there are only 7 drugs in common to the 4 countries (Garattini and Garattini, 1993). The differences are amazing. In Italy there are 3 preparations containing interferon, which is not present in the 50 most sold drugs in any other country. In Germany it's ginseng which brings to the rational use of drugs an alternative medicine – that is really crazy. The success homoeopathic medicine is having in Italy is unexplainable. People buy nothing. Homoeopathy contains nothing. And how nothing can do something it's really astonishing. But apparently people are interested.

Despite the improvement in scientific culture there is still a lot of interest in magic. Perhaps it's a reaction against science. People are afraid of science and they take refuge in magic. It's very strange in a way because people take advantage of all the scientific developments but they are afraid and that's probably because the growth of science has not been accompanied by a growth of the scientific culture in the public. You can see that the schools are not teaching elementary things belonging to science. If you talk with normal people about basic problems such as what is a risk, what is a probability, what is a risk factor people don't know. They have, for instance, a perception of a risk which is many times inversely proportional to the real risk.

Well, in a sense, clinical trials and all that have highlighted that there is a small risk of things happening that we wouldn't have known about if we hadn't done the trials, but the trouble is once people become aware of any risk, panic sets in.

Yes, and for other aspects when they travel in a car they have a much bigger risk but that risk has become part of culture. Other risks have not. And that's where the school should have a lot of influence but they don't teach these things at school.

Can those kind of things actually be taught?

Yes, I think so. If you start with children to tell them what the meaning of probability and of risk is and if you give them examples of effects, for instance, if you smoke you have a much higher risk than anything else you can do, that should be illuminating and something that will then remain in a culture but if you are teaching them . . .

In a sense we are talking about trying to teach people to do things that are very unnatural, aren't we. The calculation of risk up till the late part of the 20th century are things you do spontaneously. You don't work out with a pen and a piece of paper. Now we are saying we are in an era where we can put weights on all of these risks. It's very . . .

Yes, but what I find is that people may have a relatively good perception of the acute risk but they don't have a perception of the chronic risk because they don't see the relation between cause and effect. It is so far away from the effect that they don't ever see it. For instance, if you talk with people about the risk that could be intrinsic when we eat a given food, a given vegetable and so on, their reaction is well people learn what is good and what is bad. Yes, they have learned but nobody knows if a given vegetable contains a carcinogenic agent and after years of eating it you may get a cancer. This is out of the imagination of people to think in this way. Again it's a question of teaching.

When the adverse effects of drugs reach public consciousness through the media and newpaper reports, they do so as 'acute' risks in a sense . . .

And they don't have the knowledge to distinguish one case per one hundred from one case per one hundred thousand. They don't see the difference; they see them as all the same. And the public doesn't appreciate the fact that you cannot find out the toxic effects of drugs before they go to market. You can find out the very evident and very frequent effects but not problems that occur one in ten thousand and when you withdraw a drug from the market they are extremely surprised. They don't think that this is a good outcome because you have been able to localize a toxic effect. They think that this should be possible in the beginning. But it is not possible and it's necessary to explain these things to people.

I've heard this put quite well recently in terms of for some reason now we seem to feel that we are born with a warranty in a way that we didn't really feel 30 years ago. When people began taking the first psychotropic agents 30 years ago they felt life was a thing in which there were risks and if things went wrong tough luck. Now we've got this feeling if things go wrong there's someone to blame, a pharmaceutical company or some researcher somewhere and we want to be able to sue them.

Yes, this is partly what we have taught people. Because for a long time the pharmaceutical industry and whatever was connected with it denied any possible toxic effect of drugs which were depicted as magic bullets and then if you give something that is wrong you pay for that. Now we are paying for the extreme degree of confidence that we tried to instil into people about drug efficacy and safety. We haven't mentioned toxic effects and we haven't told them that a drug is after all what comes out from the ratio of benefit to risk and that benefits have to be there in order to justify the risk. The culture has always been safety first which is wrong in terms of drugs. It is simply meaningless; there is no benefit if there is no risk. And we are paying for some of the distortion in things that we have been inserting into the public whether in a conscious or unconscious way I don't know but that's what we have told them and now they react because we have told the wrong things.

I should like to explain. I have recently been involved in a sort of scandal because of a report showing that in Italy there were killer drugs in circulation. I had a role in looking at this data and then in explaining to the television and to the people what was the problem. What I said was that you shouldn't be surprised that there are toxic drugs – all drugs are toxic. What is important is the use that you put the drug to and I gave the example that if you take a drug which is an anticancer agent which everybody knows is extremely toxic and if you give it to a patient who has cancer you expect that the benefits are much more than the risk and even if you have a risk of a second cancer nobody cares because it means that you can survive for 15 years or so in order to get the second cancer. But suppose you give the drug to a patient for whom the wrong diagnosis has been made. He has no cancer. It will be devastating because you have no benefit since he has no cancer. He has all the risks. See how the ratio of benefit to risk is something that applies to given indications. It shows that toxicity is not a problem if you have enough benefits.

But this way of reasoning is not the way in which the effects of drugs are presented. Industry wants to show safe compounds. They wrongly think that whatever will raise attention on toxicity will decrease sales and they are against it. In the long run it pays to tell people how things are in reality because if you don't it will boomerang.

Select bibliography

Costa, E., Garattini, S. and Valzelli, L. (1960) Interactions between reserpine, chlorpromazine and imipramine. *Experientia*, **15,** 461–63.

Garattini, S. and Ghetti, V. (1957) *Psychotropic Drugs*. Elsevier, Amsterdam.

Garattini, S. and Garattini, L. (1993) Pharmaceutical prescriptions in four European countries. *Lancet*, **342,** 1191–2.

Garattini, S. (1996) Experimental and clinical activity of antidepressant drugs, in *P sychotropic Drug Development. Social, Economic and Pharmacological Aspects* (D. Healy and D.P. Doogan, eds), Chapman & Hall, London, pp. 1–12.

7 Heinz Lehmann

Psychopharmacotherapy

I guess the easiest thing to begin with is you were the first person in this part of the world to use chlorpromazine. Do you want to tell me how this came about?

I don't know whether I was the first one to use it but certainly the first one to publish on it and to do a systematic study on it in North America (Lehmann and Hanrahan, 1954). It all happened because of a drug salesman. You know they make the rounds. I worked in a mental hospital in Montreal and they would come around and leave their literature. I was extremely busy at the time and didn't have much time to see the detail man, the Rhône-Poulenc salesman that was, so my secretary couldn't give him an appointment. So he said 'I'll leave this literature – two or three reprints – with him and it will be so good it will sell itself, I don't have to see him'.

She gave me these reprints and she reported what he had said to me, which I thought was pretty arrogant and ridiculous and because of this I read it. I read it the following Sunday in the bathtub, where I do a lot of my reading, and it was very intriguing. It was in French. Now, we were in French Canada, in the province of Quebec; my wife is French Canadian and we speak French at home. So it was not very difficult for me to read it. Nowadays, of course, there isn't any difficulty, even the Anglophones learn French, but at that time Anglophones just wouldn't speak French. Anyway, I read it.

It was very strange, they made statements such as this is a sedative that produces something like a 'chemical lobotomy' – somehow it was different from other sedatives. I really didn't believe this. In those days we had the barbiturates, of course; they were the reigning sedatives. But we also had morphine and scopolamine injections for extreme agitation. We also had paraldehyde which was the cheapest and the most frequently used sedative. It smells awful; you could smell it when you got into a mental hospital. So I said, well it's just another sedative and they are kind of dramatizing it.

But it sounded somewhat different. The authors were Deniker and Delay. I didn't know anything about them but from their language and from the way the articles were written I realized they knew what they were talking about. So the next morning, which was a Monday, the first resident I met was Dr Hanrahan and I asked him 'do you want to start some research with me on a new drug?' and he said 'yes'. So we did it.

Now, at the time, all we knew was this would be some sort of a new sedative. There was nothing specific about an antipsychotic or antischizophrenic action or anything like that. We decided we would try it out on about 70 or 75 patients. Nowadays, of course, this would take years but in those days it didn't take very long. We just chose 70, and we did them all, practically simultaneously, within one or two months. Also, I didn't have to ask permission from the Director of the Hospital. I didn't have to get permission from the FDA or the Government. There were no ethical committees at the time, no guidelines, laws or regimentations. The only thing I had to ask myself was, was the thing reasonable, was it worthwhile and was it responsible? I don't remember – this was in 1953 – whether I even asked the patients. Certainly there was no such thing as informed consent at that time. I might have, but I don't think so. I just ordered it. I might have told the families if they visited. They were always very happy about anything being done because in those days you couldn't do anything for patients that would help them really.

So we did this and in the first two weeks there were two or three very peculiar events in some patients who were acutely psychotic with schizophrenia. We included schizophrenics, depressed patients and we also had some organic dementias; we didn't know who to give it to. We gave it for agitation, not for any nosological entity. And two or three of the acute schizophrenics became symptom free. Now I had never seen that before. I thought it was a fluke – something that would never happen again but anyway there they were. At the end of four or five weeks, there were a lot of symptom-free patients. By this I mean that a lot of hallucinations, delusions and thought disorder had disappeared. In 1953 there just wasn't anything that ever produced something like this – a remission from schizophrenia in weeks.

Well, then, okay, so Hanrahan and I decided when we had about 75 patients treated for 4–6 weeks to write a paper. Something which is not often mentioned nowadays, but quite a few other investigators had found the same: there were quite a few depressed patients who got better too, quicker than they would ordinarily have done.

I should have said that before we gave chlorpromazine to ill human subjects, the 70 plus patients, I wanted to see first of all whether it really was another kind of a sedative. So I asked for volunteers among our nurses for a research project. Nowadays it's difficult to get research subjects – it's almost a bad word, research, but in those days, Sputnik days, everybody wanted to be in on research, so quite a few nurses volunteered. What I did was give them chlorpromazine one day, enough to make them quite sleepy.

Roughly how much did you give them?

I think I gave them 50–75 mg orally which was quite a bit. And then a week later, they were given secobarbital, enough to make them sleepy to the same extent. Of course, we didn't expect it, but several of the nurses fainted from orthostatic hypotension. We were scared, Hanrahan and I. We didn't know what it was, but since they very soon came to, we realized what it was. Anyway, what we then did, before and after giving them chlorpromazine, we gave them a series of tests, such as reaction time, and digit symbol substitution tests – now they would be called neuropsychological tests. What we saw was that all subjects would get equally sleepy on both drugs and sometimes fall asleep. The ones on the secobarbital were dopey; they didn't do very well on the tests, they could hardly understand what they were supposed to do. But the ones on the Chlorpromazine, once they were awake, they did as well and sometimes even better than they had done before on the tests. That was, of course, unheard of, unthinkable at the time.

There were therefore some indications that this was really an entirely different kind of sedative. So then we started on our patients. We started in May and by August we had written the paper and then we sent it to the publishers of one of the larger psychiatric journals.

Which journal did you send it to?

The Archives of Neurology and Psychiatry. We were quite ambitious. We didn't hear a thing from August until January. Nowadays a six-month wait wouldn't be so unusual but in those days it was, because there wasn't so much to be published. I finally thought there was something a little bit fishy, so I wrote to them and asked them to send me my paper back and I would send it to someone else. They didn't; they published it in the March issue. What happened, or what I now deduce was probably the reason for this, was that the Americans wanted to have the scoop. Two months later somebody called Winkelman published on chlorpromazine – but actually as an anti-anxiety agent. And then five or six months later Kinross-Wright in Texas published on its antipsychotic effects. I think it was only because I pushed them asking them to send the manuscript back to me that they published it in March of 1954.

The first important papers in France had been published in 1952 by Deniker and Delay. Between August 1953 and March 1954, Rhône-Poulenc the company had sent my manuscript around to quite a few people in the States. One of them was a friend of mine Henry Brill; he was the Director of a large hospital in New York State.

Pilgrim's?

At Pilgrim's, yes. I think it was the biggest in the world at the time – some 10 000 patients or something. He knew me and trusted me and trusted the paper. On the basis of that alone I think he was the first one to use this new drug officially in the States. At that time, he also had an official position in the New York State Office of Mental Health, where I am now Deputy Commissioner of Research. He arranged on the basis of this paper to give the drug to a lot of patients at Pilgrim's and based on the results he published papers on the reduction of restraint and seclusion and on how the admission rate remained the same but the discharge rate went up, and so on.

When the article was published in 1954, I think it was the first English-language paper on chlorpromazine. Then there was another one, I wrote in German, which was published in Germany. So that is how it all started; it came about really because I married a French Canadian and we spoke French at home.

Interestingly, while this was happening a Professor of psychiatry from Scotland visited the hospital and was introduced to me. I told him about the research I was doing. I was very enthusiastic because I had never heard of hallucinations disappearing in a few weeks with a pill and so I told him about it. He gave me a little pat and a patronizing smile. I said 'well you are close to it in Scotland, you should fly over to Paris and really look at it first hand' and he said 'you know the French!'.

Let me go back and just ask you why you ended up over here. You actually come from Germany?

I come from Berlin. I actually am one of these rare people who decided to go into psychiatry before they went into medicine. When I hear about that now, or meet such people, I am very suspicious. Usually they are a little weird. They may be very good but there aren't many of those. My father was a surgeon. He was, of course, aghast when I said I would go into psychiatry and he said 'you don't know what you are doing but as you are going into medicine, there will be lots of time to change your mind'. But I didn't.

Psychiatry interested me because I had had a depression as an adolescent and rather than leave school as my parents were advised for me to do, because I would never make it, they hired a tutor for me, a student, and he was very interested in psychoanalysis. He gave me Freud's books and I had read all of what Freud had published at that time, when I was 14 or 15. This bibliotherapy might have helped. Anyway, for a year or two, I was not able to work at all and he had to do my homework for me. That was when I decided psychiatry was a very fascinating kind of thing. I had always wanted to become like my father, a physician, but I decided then to become a psychiatrist and stayed that way all the way through medical school.

You did your training in Germany before you came over.

Yes. In Germany the system was different; there were no medical schools like in the States, for instance. You went to University rather than into philosophy or jurisprudence or medicine. You just registered and in those days you would go from one University to another as often as your parents could afford to let you go. So I went to Freiburg to start with, because my father had studied there, and then I went to Marburg because Kretschmer was there. In those days Kretschmer and Schneider were the big stars in psychiatry.

What was he like?

I don't remember very much. I mean Kretschmer was just one Professor and I did all kinds of other things as well. I learned Russian. I did a lot of philosophy. I remember more of Heidegger in the seminars discussing existentialism than I remember of my medical lectures. After Marburg, I went back to Freiburg and then to Vienna and I met Wagner-Jauregg there, the only psychiatrist who ever won the Nobel prize.

Then, finally, I graduated in Berlin. On the way I had always taken extra lectures in psychiatry, which you could do because what you have to take wasn't prescribed like it is in a medical school today. There was a certain minimum that you had to have but then you could take extra lectures in whatever you wanted. So I did a lot of philosophy and psychiatry at the time as well.

So, coming from that background, how did you interpret the effects of the drugs? People like Roland Kuhn who were psychotherapists at heart had tremendous problems it seems to me from what I have heard him say, just trying to work out how a drug could be helping a psychological disorder.

That was not difficult for me. While I had a philosophical and existentialist background, I never had many problems with the mind – body problem. Now, of course, you have a biopsychosocial model but I think this is just an *aide memoire*. I don't believe that anyone really can integrate things into one biopsychosocial concept. If people claim to do it they are either deluded or they are lying. I don't think they can do it. I think what you do is, anyway what I do, is to oscillate, and you have to learn to do that very quickly. I look at somebody completely biologically and a fraction of a second later completely psychologically and a fraction of a second later I look at his social environment, and so on. And that keeps going like in a film, until it seems to become a continuum – but it isn't really a continuum, at least I don't think of it as such.

So how did you explain the effects?

Well, before 1953, I had always thought of psychoses as something essentially different from anything else in psychiatry, because of the loss of contact with reality. I always thought that there must be a 'centre' for hallucinations and delusions and I still think so. Seriously. Something that specifically keeps you in contact with reality and if that centre, or whatever function, in the brain, is disturbed and the physiology connected with it, you then begin to lose your contact with reality. Because contact with reality is such a solidly anchored function, no matter how sick you are with depression or with agoraphobia or obsessive – compulsive or whatever, you may be extremely sick, you may be paralysed in your home for 10 years, you still are not psychotic. On the other hand, overnight you can suddenly become psychotic, that is, lose contact with reality and become hallucinated or delusional or develop a formal thought disorder – the three hallmarks of psychosis.

Because of this I always thought that there must be something physical about the psychoses. I thought of the neuroses and personality disorders as different – they were intrapsychic but there was something extrapsychic in the psychoses. So I did all kinds of things to see if I could make a difference. I gave huge doses of caffeine. At one time I remember being intrigued by the polarity of the manic – depressives. I tried to change their metabolism by giving them ammonium chloride in large doses to make it more acid and at other times more alkaline and so on. None of this worked, of course. But I was always looking and hoping for some physical intervention that might make a difference and at the same time I did a lot of psychobehavioural tests, such as reaction times and so on.

Why did you do those?

Well, for one thing I was working in a mental hospital, during the war, when most of the staff had gone to war. I was an immigrant, a refugee from Germany, and I had my own difficulties with that. I had up to 600 patients alone; there were no residents or interns at the time and only one registered nurse to help me – otherwise untrained personnel. In order to keep up my morale I had to do some research and so I always went around with a little scratch pad and had patients draw on it or did association tests or something or other. I also felt that by doing things like after-image experiments or reaction times I might find some physical, neurophysiological function that was disturbed and would be correlated with hallucinations, for instance. Because an after-image – you know if you look at something bright red and you look at a white ceiling afterwards you see a green image – that's actually like a hallucination. It's a perception without an external stimulus. I did a lot of work with after-images and with critical flicker fusion thresholds.

I was always hoping and looking systematically for psychophysiological and neurophysiological correlates of psychotic disorders and doing all kinds of other things. In those days it was all trial and error. You produced huge skin blisters in order to do something to the reticulo-endothelial system and the immunological system. I injected oil of turpentine into the abdominal fascia – that produced a big sterile abscess, which you then had to open in the operating room. It also produced a great deal of leucocytosis and fever which you wanted. Patients, for a day or two, would show improvement – enough to keep on doing all this sort of thing.

There was a lot of trial and error going on in those days. The only one who had been somewhat successful was Klasi in Switzerland, with his continuous sleep therapy in the 1920s. I did that too but that was both expensive, because you needed a lot of nursing, and risky because quite often the patients would develop pneumonia and we didn't have penicillin yet. So that was a risky thing. But anyway I did all this constantly in order to keep my morale up while looking after 600 patients. So when finally a pill did work, you can imagine how I felt.

About a year before that or even just a few months before that – we used to take students in the hospital on their clerkships – and one student asked me one day, when he looked at the patients who were looking at the ceiling talking to their hallucinations, 'will there ever be any kind of pill that could help these people?'. I thought the question was rather ridiculous, but I was quite benign and patronizingly said 'well, there would never be a pill but somehow eventually we might be able to help them'. But a few months later we had a pill.

Even so I didn't quite believe it and it took almost two years until I really would talk fairly freely about 'anti-psychotics'. I had correspondence with colleagues in the United States, who worked with these drugs and none of us were really talking about antipsychotics – we couldn't believe that there would be something specifically antipsychotic. Some even said antischizophrenic, which I have never believed of course – antipsychotic, yes, but antischizophrenic, no. I said in a talk to the Canadian Medical Association in the early days, I said it is almost like the antibiotics, one could almost call it antipsychotic. I was very apologetic about it and made it clear I was talking only metaphorically. Although in our correspondence, we would say that chlorpromazine really did remove delusions and hallucinations, it took two years really until we were comfortable with this idea.

How did I explain what it was doing? Well, we didn't know anything about dopamine at the time. Dopamine, in fact, was not something that we considered to be important. It wasn't even a neurotransmitter. We knew about noradrenaline, and I still remember talking to a pharmacologist once who said 'mark my words, dopamine eventually will become very important'. I thought that wasn't very likely because at the time it just seemed to be a precursor of noradrenaline.

So how did I explain the mechanism of action to myself? I have published on this once or twice. I thought it was kind of a new sedative; that was something I had established experimentally. It was a new sedative, which did not destructively interfere with wakefulness or arousal. Patients might doze off, but once you had aroused them, you could immediately awaken them and they would be quite normal, not doped any more. I thought that, clearly, psychotic patients have a lot of trouble. They are terrified by their delusions, hallucinations, experiences; their psychotic anxiety which is different from neurotic anxiety. And if they could be given a sedative which would not interfere with their cognitive functioning, as this obviously didn't as I had established experimentally, they would not have their disturbing agitation and panicky anxiety. So their self-help potential, which is always there, their own healing power, would have a chance to get through – if it was not held back by the anxiety and the emotional disturbance. So it was because it was a sedative that did not interfere with cognitive performance; it therefore allowed patients to cure themselves.

I still think there may be a good deal to this even now. I don't think it is just all neurotransmitters and receptors. In the same way I think that depression is a learned illness, and that maybe one of the reasons why antidepressants, which physiologically or pharmacologically should work very quickly don't – this may be because it takes two or three weeks before you unlearn what you have learnt in your feelings and your perspective of the world. Anyway so that's how I explained it to myself at the time – patients use their own recovery potential because they are sedated without being doped.

How did you view the side-effects that happened? This again must have been virgin territory seeing some of these side-effects for the first time. You can't have known what they meant.

No. At first I remembered the hospital having been visited in the late 1930's by Sakel, the inventor of insulin coma therapy. We were one of the first hospitals to use it. I slept in the same room with him once and he told me that when he developed this treatment a few years before in Vienna, he always had his passport under his pillow at night, because he didn't know what would happen, he might have to leave the country very fast because of a toxic fatality in one of his patients.

What was Sakel like?

I was just starting out as a very junior psychiatrist when I met him – in 1938 or 1939. I had the impression then that he was a bit flaky. He got his idea when he was treating heroin addicts with insulin in Berlin to help them over their withdrawal symptoms. I don't remember what his rationale was but it calmed them down. Once one of his addicts who was also schizophrenic, accidentally slipped into a hypoglycaemic coma. Sakel was scared but brought him out of the coma quickly with an injection of glucose. To his amazement, the patient showed a considerable improvement of his schizophrenic symptoms. Sakel then wanted to use hypoglycaemic coma as a treatment for schizophrenia. But they would not let him do it in Berlin, so he went to Vienna where they let him set up a clinical trial and he had some success.

When Hitler came, he accepted an invitation to the US. He lived in a hotel – I forget its name and it does not exist anymore – in New York

City. I thought that he liked the good life and to feel important. He died fairly young – I think in New York City.

Where you surprised when insulin coma was shown not to work?

No. It was an utterly nonspecific therapy. A shock to the brain and to the whole organism – like banging a watch on the table to make it go again when it stopped. I never thought of it as a cure. It was a very risky, cumbersome and messy method of treatment. But it was the first and only game in town then.

So you felt a bit the same way as Sakel in terms of possible problems.

Yes. Particularly since we didn't know how to dose chlorpromazine. The French had gone up to as much as 300 mg or something like this but not much higher. I decided that we had to get some sort of a guideline. So we agreed that we would aim at making patients sleepy. But some people didn't get sleepy even though they got 600 or 700 mg. It was hard to know how high to go because I was never quite sure that the drug wasn't possibly quite toxic in a way that might take several months to become apparent.

This was at the time of Moruzzi and Magoun, so beside my psychological self-healing potential theory, I had the explanation that the drugs worked on the arousal system, the reticular ascending system. It had become clear that people's arousal could definitely be diminished and re-activated again if they were stimulated so that they could function quite normally under the effects of the drug, until they were not stimulated any more. Given this, I wasn't surprised that they were just not very active and that they remained passive. I felt very much better seeing them passive in this way than seeing them the way they were with barbiturates or paraldehyde because I knew that if necessary they could play chess with me just as well and could beat me in chess although they were sitting there apparently completely passive.

I had a lot of personal interaction with patients at the time playing chess and cards and chatting with them. But then a few months after we started the treatment, a friend of mine, a neurologist, and myself, were both looking at some patients and they were walking like typical Parkinson patients and I said 'by the looks of these, it looks like they have Parkinson's'. He said 'it's not possible because there is no way of inducing Parkinsonism'. It couldn't be but there it was. Anyway, we coined the term extrapyramidal symptoms, which hadn't been described before. So we wrote a paper on the extrapyramidal symptoms as side effects and how these effects looked just like Parkinson's – but again not daring to say something that was 'impossible' at that time, when there was no pharmacological way known to produce Parkinsonism in humans.

Were you concerned that when patients began to walk this way that even when the drugs were halted that they would still remain Parkinsonian?

No. Of course we had tried to stop the drug and we found that in a week or so the patient would be alright. We didn't witness them develop tardive dyskinesia; that came very much later. So, we knew it was easily reversible and we also knew it occurred only in 20% or 30% of patients. We wondered how high we could go with our dosage, but then Kinross-Wright in Texas, like a typical American, went up to 2000 mg or about that high.

That early?

Yes. The Europeans made fun of this as being so American, Texan even – you know everything is bigger in Texas. We thought it was fairly high, also, but anyway he went up to over a 1000 mg and I think up to 2000 mg within a year or so.

Deniker came over to Canada then and visited us. We had had two or three cases of jaundice, which they hadn't had with chlorpromazine.

What was Deniker like?

I saw him last about a year ago at the 40th anniversary of chlorpromazine. I went over to Paris and saw him. He had a stroke. He is a fairly typical Frenchman; my wife is a French Canadian and he visited us several times. He was like a Frenchman – they are very sure of themselves; Parisians particularly – they tolerate everyone else, they are very nice to them, they are very polite – he was that type, a real Parisian intellectual. He wondered why we had – and he never had – any jaundice. I remember Hanrahan asking me if we really had to mention that there were three cases of jaundice – it wouldn't be very good in our first publication on the drug. I said 'look, we've got to', but I haven't seen one since then. At that time I think Rhône-Poulenc probably had something or other in the drug that they have eliminated since then. Or what is also possible is that there was a subclinical epidemic of hepatitis which hasn't been there since. In France they didn't have any cases of jaundice.

Nothing happened anywhere that caused people to stop and think perhaps we shouldn't go any further with this drug?

No. Look, you can't imagine. You know we saw the unthinkable – hallucinations and delusions eliminated by a pill! I suppose if people had been told 'well, they'll die two years later' they'd still have said it's worth it. It was so unthinkable and so new and so wonderful. There were all kinds of things happening. Chronic schizophrenics who had been divorced because they had been psychotic for 10 years, now all of a sudden they were symptom free and their husbands or their wives were married again. It was a very strange time.

Anyway, I began to see detail men from the pharmaceutical companies more often and I would tell them 'now we can really do something very dramatically about psychotic symptoms, now its up to you to find something for manic-depressive disease' – because we were always fairly sure this was a physical thing, much surer than we were about schizophrenia. Anyway they came up in 1957 or so with the tricyclics – imipramine.

Strangely, although neuroscientifically we didn't know what was happening with the antipsychotics, when the antidepressants appeared, it didn't take very long to find something out. By 1959 or so the effects of reserpine on neurotransmitters had been noted and hypotheses about antidepressants and neurotransmitters and reuptake and so on were appearing. So we began to have an understanding of how antidepressants worked but it took until about 1965 when Carlsson and Lindquist came up with their Dopamine theory for neuroleptics. So for more than 10 years I was working only with the kind of theory I had that the organism helps itself once it is freed from agitation.

In 1957 there was a meeting of the World Psychiatric Association in Zurich. I remember it. Jung, I think, was still there and one thing I remember was that for several days, until late at night, people, at the congress, would discuss existential psychiatry which only Europeans could understand. I flew back from there with the Chairman of the Department of Psychiatry at Toronto University. He had come from England.

Who was it?

Alwyn Stokes. He asked me, since we were sitting side by side, he said: 'now look, there was so much fuss about existentialism; everybody talked about it until late at night, what is this whole thing'. So I thought, well, here is a captive audience; he wants to hear about it, he is a Professor, he is obviously quite bright so I'll start. Then for about two hours I talked about it – Husserl and Heidegger and so on and so on. He listened carefully and very attentively and at the end he said, 'well the whole thing is really just a symphony of words isn't it?'. So ever since I have given up trying to explain existentialism to anyone outside Europe, although South Americans take well to it. Indians from India take well to it too. I developed a whole theory actually and I gave a few talks on the question of why people who have had an Anglo-Saxon education until the age of 12 or 13, will never be able to understand existentialism unless, like anthropologists, for years they do nothing else but study it and immerse themselves in it. And that is because the English, you know, they had the Magna Carta; they had the celebration of commonsense with Locke and Hume, they had the tremendous scientific breakthrough at the same time as they had Locke and Hume – at the same time, they had Harvey discovering the circulation which must have been like our nuclear developments. Anyway, because of this and because of their moral and political maturity, anyone who had an Anglo-Saxon education would be commonsensable and would view people who would say that suffering is good for something as just ridiculous. My son went to an Irish Anglophone school where we lived until he was about 11 or 12, then he went to a French High School and College then he went to McGill finally and graduated in medicine and I don't think he could understand it.

When I wasn't speaking to this Professor about existentialism on the plane, I read what I had brought with me and that was a paper by Kuhn on Imipramine. He had given a paper there with about 12 or 14 people in the audience. I wasn't there. But I did get (in German), the *Schweizer Medizinische Wochenshrift* (see Select bibliography, Chapter 5), where he had published it, and I read it there. Immediately when I arrived back in Montreal I asked Geigy; I phoned them and said I would like to have some of this imipramine stuff. They said 'what's that?' I said 'well, it's an antidepressant apparently: you have worked on it for years. But people at Geigy in Canada had never heard of it. They were quite embarrassed. But, within a week, I had the stuff and we did the first study of anti-depressants of the tricyclic type in North America, I think — Nathan Kline had already done the first trial of the monoamine oxidase inhibitors.

How did the first trial go?

Fine. There again, they had said about 65–70% would respond. We opted to inject it — it was injectable at the time. We didn't quite know whether that really helped. What we did establish was that if you went over 300 mg it didn't help any more; you just got more side-effects. We also tried the MAOIs and we unfortunately had one fatality, that was with iproniazid. So for a while we laid-off those but kept on with the tricyclics. Because of all that, I was kind of character cast as a psychopharmacologist; we kept on working with the various derivatives of the antidepressants and the antipsychotics — Tom Ban joined me then and we did a lot of this work. But that still didn't really change my philosophy — to me drugs are only adjuncts, very helpful practical adjuncts, but psychiatry is not psychopharmacology. I don't think it ever will be.

Please tell me more.

Well, psychiatry is a medical speciality. Now all medical specialities are there to help sick people to get better. It so happens that in most of the other medical specialties, there is a great deal of scientific background, which is quite solid, evidence based. But I really don't think that internists or surgeons or whatever are great scientists. They use what the scientists produce for them. They have to understand a little, just like somebody who is a pilot of an aeroplane, for instance — he has to know quite a bit about the plane but he doesn't have to know very much about aerody-namics or how to build a plane or how to fix it even, but he has to know how to fly — and flying is quite different. Somebody who is the world's expert in aerodynamics — I wouldn't want to fly with him. Now a psychiatrist ought to be somebody who can use whatever is available to help his patients, but what is most important, as far as I am concerned, is the contact-intensive training that you have to have. You have to have 1000s of hours of contact with patients, regardless of how much molecular biology is behind it when you finally give them a pill. Nor do you have to know too much about the molecular biology of genetics when you have to tell relatives of patients when they come for consultation – but you have to know enough about it to know what to say.

I have often wondered whether it was a good thing that I was instrumental in getting the drugs into psychiatry because now people are increasingly using DSM-IIIR, or things like that, as a laundry list and psychopharmacology as a cook book. I actually know some colleagues to whom I used to send patients but I don't do it any more, because doing the laundry list they are no longer using much of their empathy – they think it is not very scientific. So they aren't as good.

I still think that you have to help as a psychiatrist, not as a neuroscientist. You have to help individual patients and to help individual patients you have to know when to smile and when not to smile, what kind of tone to use and what not to and so on. That comes only after thousands of hours of contact with patients. Now what our residents do is they get, I think, much more than they can digest of neuroscience. They don't have PhDs, which they really would need to understand molecular biology nowadays. I have a hell of a time of just keeping abreast of the headlines, you know, and that's having done it all along. How anyone new coming into it can understand it without being, as I say, a PhD, I don't know. But they are being taught this, hours and hours and hours. There are also still many many hours of psychodynamics and the theories behind that and the supervision of long-term psychotherapy. Now all these many, many hours take away the time for contact with patients.

I never had postgraduate training – it was during the war and there was no way of getting away because they didn't have enough staff to let me go anywhere. But I think I got the best training just by the fact that from 8.30 in the morning, until midnight, I was making my rounds and seeing hundreds of patients for many, many hours every day over many years. So I learned the kind of idiosyncratic, individualized flexibility that you have to get through, I suppose, empathy, and the expertise you get through the experience of being able to relate to individuals rather than to statistical numbers or biological facts.

Now, to me, a psychiatrist ought to be the ideal mixture of a science-minded physician; but still a healer. Let's say a painting has been discovered somewhere in an attic and it's supposed to be a Rembrandt. Somebody says, how would they ever establish it? Eventually it goes to one or two of the experts in the museums. They don't get the answer from books – anyone can get from books what you can learn about the infrared and the X-ray qualities of the paints and so on and so on – but they have seen thousands of paintings and therefore they know whether it is or isn't. That sort of thing just has to come through personal contact and that to me is still the most important thing because the rest you can learn fairly quickly. I can teach somebody basic psychopharmacology in two weeks, if he's really well motivated. And my students, who have never seen a psychiatric patient before, within a week of looking at DSM-IIIR for the first time, they argue with me about diagnoses. So that can be taught very quickly too.

The fine tuning of it takes years and that has been short-changed now because of our progress in the neurosciences. We clinicians have been responsible for all the new treatments from the moral treatments of the 19th century, which was very effective, to psychoanalysis and then the unspecific shock treatments; and then the psychopharmacological treatments, all of this came from the clinicians. Finally, we asked the neuroscientists to help us to find out how they work. They did and eventually after 10 years they came up with some explanations. Now they are going ahead, intoxicated by their own successes but it's research for research-sake, it's not research for psychiatry any more.

I am as excited as everybody else looking at these sexy pictures of the thinking brain – when you think of lifting a finger, this lights up and then that lights up, you know. You can even see what happens in the brains of the obsessive – compulsives when they follow their compulsions or obsessions or whatever; but you don't need to do this because you could see it before in their behaviour. It doesn't tell us any more. Anyway, my fear now is that with that tremendous and really exciting progress, we will get away from the patients and become therefore less competent psychiatrists but great prescribers of MRIs and SPECTs.

Let me take you back, after introducing chlorpromazine, the first series of meetings began and you went to the Val-de-Grâce meeting in Paris. What was that like?

That was two years later, in 1955. I don't recall very much of it except it was a very great celebration. Everybody was very happy. You know what I remember most was flying over from Montreal; Rhône-Poulenc paid for it. In those days, it was before the big jets: you still had real beds. You could really lie down on a bed in a plane. There was a thunderstorm outside and I was lying on the bed and falling asleep and it was just wonderful. I remember a festive atmosphere at the meeting but they weren't going overboard.

I've just come from a luncheon now of previous organizers and past-presidents of the International College and Lewis Judd was saying how well everything was going ahead, and Neurobiology is our basic science now and in another 10 years we'll have done this or that. Well it wasn't that way then. It was very much like having won the lottery, I suppose. I never did, but I think I would be that way if I had suddenly won $500,000 in a lottery. I would be very happy I wouldn't think of the future or anything else. I would just be very happy about it and talk about it a lot. So that's what we did. We didn't think, like we always do now, of the future and what's coming next and what's the cutting edge, or this sort of thing. That frantic kind of thing which I think is counter-productive, we didn't have it then. We were happy and said okay. Now we have much more to work with, let's go on working without making projections of what we should be doing.

Who were the people who stood out for you at that meeting?

Obviously Deniker and Delay because they had called it and they had laid the foundation for our euphoria.

What was Delay like; he has a reputation as a card-playing, novel-writing, flamboyant person.

He was patronizing really. You were happy if you were allowed to talk to him, kind of. Pierre Deniker was much more down to earth although still Parisian. Delay, for instance, became a member of the French Academy and all his students had to heavily contribute to the jewel-encrusted sword that he got. This sort of thing.

Pichot was there as well.

Pichot is very nice. He is also down to earth. You can talk with him and he is concerned with what one has to be concerned with. And he has a good sense of humour, not particularly French. You know I come from Quebec and we aren't very happy about the French; the French let us down in the time of Louis XVI, with their 'who are these people, it's just a lot of desert with snow in it; we won't send any soldiers'. Voltaire even celebrated Wolfe's victory as the beginning of the liberation of all America. So that's how Wolfe and the British could get us and now you know all the troubles we have about autonomy and so on. Politically today it is just all horrible. Anyway we were talking about the French, Pichot is in that respect not very French. The way we look at it in Quebec, Churchill wasn't very English – he was not like an Oxford Englishman. Pichot is not like a Sorbonne Frenchman.

One of the other early figures was Wolfgang de Boor. You called him later to find out why he later lost interest in psychopharmacology – you also reviewed his book on psychopharmacology (de Boor, 1955), which you saw very much as a watershed book?

Yes, the interesting thing about it was that when he wrote that book, we actually already had chlorpromazine but he was not particularly enthusiastic about it. It was a watershed without him knowing it. He kept saying in the book, there isn't really any possibility of having a physical foundation of mental illness. At the same time, he was looking at the physical effects of drugs on dimensions of mental functioning. But he wasn't thinking of actually curing anyone. In the whole book, there isn't anything about curing or even about being significantly therapeutic with any of the drugs. All he proposed we do was to study the phenomenology of the brain being affected by these drugs.

When De Boor vanished, everybody had the impression that there might have been a clash of personalities between himself and Rothlin

He wasn't easy to get on with, Rothlin.

In an article in this book Thirty Years CINP *(see Glossary), Pierre Deniker suggests that at the meeting, when Rothlin was proposed as the first President of CINP, there was silence because he had been hostile to the idea of CINP in the first place and then he emerged as the first president.*

You know in the early days I wasn't there. I wasn't invited and Freyhan and I, we were quite angry because we hadn't been invited although we . . .

Why do you suppose that was?

I don't know. For one thing Ewen Cameron, who was a very important person at the time, Scottish American but teaching at McGill University – he had all kinds of scandalous troubles afterwards with the CIA – well, anyway, he and I we were both in Montreal. He was up the hill in the University Clinic and I was in the mental hospital. He didn't like mental hospitals. And I, since I was five years old, had aspired to become a Professor eventually but there didn't seem to be much chance for it where I was. I had asked him for a job at the Allan Institute where he was but he made some excuse and didn't give me a job. He may have been a little jealous. Chlorpromazine had worked out for me while he was struggling with all kinds of other things. He wasn't much of a scientist. Not a good researcher but very ambitious. I think he was a good clinician. He was a tremendous administrator and at the time one of the world's outstanding psychiatrists. So I think it may have been personal that he didn't want me to get in there. He was one of the movers in the first meeting.

Anything else you can tell me about Cameron – you're probably sick and tired being asked about the man

He was tall – most of his medical staff were too and I am still convinced that one of the reasons he did not accept me at the Allan, when I once asked him for a job there, was that I was not tall enough. I was angry and frustrated then and actually made the tacky 'decision' that when the mountain wouldn't come to Mahomet, Mahomet would have to come to the mountain, meaning that I would have to outprestige the Allan and him, through my work at the little mental hospital on which he looked down so much. That, in 1950, seemed to be as likely as the David and

Goliath story. Of course, I was jealous of Cameron but he became jealous of me a few years later.

As a person, he impressed as being rather cold, aloof, distant, dry and patronising – he called everybody 'Doc' but nobody dared to call him that or by his first name – not much of a sense of humour in short. Rather arrogant. His general rule was never to leave a meeting without having spoken there publicly at least once. I did not like that he thought that accepting the French-Canadian language and culture was unnecessary and expensive. However, he made it a point to devalue politically accepted issues – and that sometimes impressed me favourably. For instance, he publicly ridiculed the concept of 'nice girls' and was scolded in the newspapers for that by the Anglican bishop.

What did you think of his methods of depatterning and psychic driving?

I thought they were original – but ludicrously simplistic. You know in those days, I never thought that what he did was not ethical! I was one of those who thought that Cameron was a very ambitious but incompetent researcher. However, I am still convinced that he was a fair man, of good moral integrity and primarily motivated by clinical concern for his patients – at least consciously. My wife and I never liked him but I would always stand up and defend his integrity. Quite recently, I have heard that he was involved with the CIA. The information is quite credible but I am still convinced of his integrity as a clinician.

There seem to have been problems for the first few years of the CINP – people like Frank Ayd, who had been there at the start, all of a sudden found that they weren't listed as members any more.

Without knowing why! Well, you know it was international and as I told them today at the luncheon, before I came here, I was the oldest past-president there and they asked me to reminisce. I couldn't remember very much of it except that to me it was amusing what went on before I was on the Councils. Who should become president? And in those days, iron curtain and so on, political considerations were very important. The French were too arrogant, the English didn't do this or that, the Americans wanted to do it all, the Germans – oh, for heaven's sake, no, don't let's get them involved, and the Italians were not quite right. So eventually it had to be Canada because, as usual, that's the role we have been playing successfully in the world – being accepted as nice people. And we are more tolerant than everybody else. We don't have any nationalism to speak of because we haven't much in the way to be particularly proud of. That's why I like it very much and I'm afraid of what's going to happen now with Quebec nationalism. But because we didn't have nationalism and heroism, that's why they wanted me in at the time.

After CINP began there seemed to be a point around 1960/62 where it could have fallen apart.

I didn't even realize it at the time, although later I became president. I was kind of drafted into this but I had never been very much interested in politics and I let things pass. It amused me to see this – for me – ridiculous puttering around of who should get what and why and so on. I did realize it wasn't very easy what was going on there. But it could have fallen apart you say?

Yes, it seems around 1960 to 1962, things weren't good. Denber and Rothlin didn't get on.

That was very true. They almost had fist fights. I never was interested enough in the why's and wherefore's. Denber was a little tough and Rothlin was very insensitive. So I think it was almost purely personal in an international thing like that, which was troubling. Later, the issues had to do with the various nationalities but in the early stages it was mostly personal.

You also were involved in the founding of the ACNP.

No. There again they drafted me into it. Several people told me I had to come along and I said I have too much to do, I can't get bothered with another college, another meeting and so on. But they said, well, you know what drafting means: we draft you. So that's how I got into it. But again a lot of it was due to the fact that I was the – what do they call these things the opposite of a catalyst? – something that holds things down, this is what being a Canadian is. Like graphite rods in a nuclear reactor, to slow things down. This was a very hectic thing to start in the States and they wanted a Canadian in to temper it down.

It was quite a powerful group of people; quite a few of them ended up in court on opposite sides of the fence like Saunders and Kline. If ever a group of people looked like it needed a few graphite rods in there . . .

Nathan Kline was one of my best friends. I went to some of the court meetings with Saunders. He was not always easy to get along with – a very determined man. Brill didn't like Nate because he was a bit of a clown but that's why I liked him. But he was very determined and very powerful. He had all kinds of political connections. I had never been interested in and never really been impressed by the political importance of anything. To me only persons matter. But the personal interactions and difficulties were always very interesting and if somebody wanted me to get in to make peace or to keep the passions down – okay, for that reason I would always be available. I certainly never wanted power and I still think it is an ugly or dangerous thing to have power.

Do you recall much of the two day ACNP foundation meeting?

No. Only I still have the photograph of a very long dinner table. No, not of the meeting. The Council meetings I do remember. I don't think anything earthshaking ever happens at meetings. At least that's my perception.

I am thinking more in terms of the people. The two people who seemed to have talked the most at this meeting were Frank Ayd and Bernard Brodie.

Frank Ayd, of course, had a legal training; that's why we wanted him always to be there because that was very important from the beginning. You know he was not very much liked by some of the more orthodox neuroscientists. But on the other hand, and I think this is much more important, we wanted him because he is a pragmatic fellow who is very bright and has legal training. Now Brodie, he was also important then. Incidentally I became president of the American College of Neuropsychopharmacology almost by default.

When was that?

It must have been 1966/67. What happened was that I was president elect. Brodie was the president but he didn't show up in San Juan where the meeting was and nobody knew where he was. He hadn't said he wouldn't come. I think there were rumours that he wasn't well. Something had to be done right away so I had to become president overnight, not being prepared for it and not knowing much about how to run meetings and all this sort of thing. I chaired the meetings with people telling me all the time what to do and that was my presidency. From then on Brodie disappeared altogether.

In 1960, though, he was still very much the commanding figure. Axelrod worked in his lab, Costa worked in his lab.

Carlsson too worked in his lab. But Brodie just disappeared really. We didn't know and as I said he wouldn't let anyone know either that he wouldn't show up. He was very much there and all of a sudden . . .

ACNP began life as a largely clinical grouping. People who were giving these drugs for the first time and wanting to share what they were doing and what was happening and what was the best way to actually look at the new compounds, etc. It's moved a long way from that now almost to the point where clinical people feel excluded and someone like Don Klein has gone and formed an American Society for Clinical Psychopharmacology. How do you read all of that? Is it as you say: the neuroscientists have gone into research for research's sake and they have lost sight of the goal.

I really see them as charging ahead, intoxicated by their own successes and forgetting completely their roots – where they started and why they started. Okay, fine for them but then we must question their role with psychiatry. Today at the luncheon, Lewis Judd was very proud that this was the first time we arranged a CINP meeting 50/50 between basic scientists and clinicians. He said, well, I don't know whether we took risks but then he said there were 2500 people at Eric Kandel's lecture so he said 'okay, we know that neuroscience is the thing everybody wants to go to'. Well, yes, everybody wants to go there but what is it going to do to psychiatry?

I think that everybody would want to go and hear Kandel but not for the neuroscience necessarily but because of who he is and to be able to say they had heard a lecture from someone who is probably going to win a Nobel prize.

That's it. Kandel is an excellent presenter. But you see how you can misunderstand the significance of this 2500. So now Judd thinks that proves it, so now they will have 50/50 and then it will become 70/30 and so on. A year and a half ago, in San Juan, we had a meeting with previous presidents of the ACNP, on just this problem. They said that they would mend their ways and get more clinical but Don Klein who was there wasn't very convinced apparently and soon afterwards he started his own group. But I think even that group, if it is called psychopharmacology, will have to go into molecular science and so on. It means it will go away from psychiatry.

It's not politically correct to even say that today. So I don't know what is going to happen. Recently, I think in the *Lancet*, there was an editorial suggesting that we dissect psychiatry into neuroscience and psychosocial. I don't know where I would go – I'm not neuroscience and I'm not psychosocial. The psychosocial problem is that they don't want any drugs.

Aubrey Lewis, apparently, at the first CINP meeting said that if we had a choice between the new drugs and the social treatments, such as industrial rehabilitation units that have been introduced, we would pick social treatments. And it's interesting that in the UK under Lewis' influence the Maudsley remained very aloof from the new drugs and in the UK psychopharmacology is something that has happened outside Oxford, Cambridge and the Maudsley.

That's not so good either. Somehow we ought to get some sort of an understanding of how to integrate it. You hear people talking about the death of psychiatry and perhaps there will be a death. There will be psychologists and, you know, some clinical psychologists can do psychotherapy as well or better than some psychiatrists. And then, psychopharmacologists and neuroscientists they are not physicians at all. It's very strange almost paradoxical that the more progress we make in psychiatry the more we seem to be heading to our own destruction. I'm quite pessimistic about it. Although I am optimistic about the possibility of helping mentally sick people much more nowadays.

That also came up today at the luncheon. Paul Jannsen asked whether there was anything that we know now better than 10 or 20 years ago. I said, yes, we know we don't have to give such high doses; low doses will do. The discussion then developed around the table and the others said, well, we understand so much more about the brain's pathophysiology and neurophysiology – but that's not psychiatry. The fact that we can explain more is not understanding. The understanding part is the personal part, the interpersonal part, and that isn't even seen.

Can I take you back and explore a further issue. Talking to someone like Frank Ayd, when the new drugs were introduced in the US, at least, people who advocated drug treatment were seen as being in league with Satan – this was the wrong way to treat mental illness. The analysts held the field. I have the impression that the reaction down here was probably a little more vehement than it was up North in Canada.

That's true of everything but actually it's a strange thing. I know more psychiatrists here and I am much more in touch with American psychiatry than I am with Canadian although I was Chairman at McGill in 1970. You see we had three paradigms in the 19th century. In the first phase, psychiatry couldn't develop before Pinel because the philosophy was that the whole cosmos was a clockwork: it was all material and therefore there probably wasn't any soul or psyche or whatever. But even if there is it couldn't possibly be sick, so to speak, of a mental disorder. That was philosophical nonsense – it was not logical. Then Pinel, who at the time of the French Revolution was a courageous young activist and a great philanthropist, he said, 'to hell with all the philosophy, as far as I am concerned I want to get these people out of the dungeons'. That's how it started. Psychiatry was philanthropy not science or philosophy, not even clinical. He wanted to get them out of the dungeons.

Then he and Esquirol wrote the first textbooks on psychiatry and within the 19th century, the three paradigms developed: first the psycho-social with its emphasis on checks and balances of a moral kind. Then Griesinger around 1850 put forward the idea that there are no mental diseases, these are only brain diseases – this was the organic paradigm. And then finally with Kraepelin the, what I call, the agnostic paradigm – 'I don't care whether it's mind or whether it's organic – it's clinical'. And, of course, DSM-IIIR is also agnostic – it's operational and atheoretical, and so on.

Now the psychosocial·bedfellows of Heinroth from the 19th century are the behaviourists, Freud and the anti-psychiatrists – they are all shaped by the psychosocial model. And the Griesinger model was picked up by Meynert, Leonhard and Kleist and so on, and then, of course, also the neurosciences. The agnostic one is DSM III and IV. Then there is what I call the integrative imperative – it's not really a paradigm – Engels' bio-psychosocial model. I don't think anyone can think of all this together, but anyway.

So then, in the 20th century, particularly here in the States between 1930 and 1950, there was an absolute reign of the psychosocial model.

Everything else had disappeared and you just were anachronistic and simplistic and you just didn't know anything if you thought that there might be physical causes or a physical substrate or that anything physical could ever help – I mean that was seen as ridiculous. You just wouldn't do that. It was politically incorrect for anyone who had academic aspirations. I had those but I wasn't very close to academia in those days, so I could carry on my own work.

This was never the case in Europe, in Germany, for instance, they were much more temperate. As you say, though, in England there are almost the two parties still. I hope somehow psychiatry can be saved by having both and saying okay the neurosciences are there to help us to find the tools for diagnosis and the tools for treatment but the treatment itself is not neuroscience.

But in terms of the reaction, though, to the introduction of the drugs during the 1950s and 1960s, it seems clear that even people like Nathan Kline and Roland Kuhn, even as they introduced the drugs, were still thinking very much in analytic terms.

Yes, it was so, but not for very long. I think Kline became much more absolute about drugs doing everything eventually. As I said, I myself thought of the potential self-help powers of the organism and freeing it rather than doing something physically to it. But, yes, in the States, it became hostile almost. That was very understandable because the psychoanalysts had reigned for two decades without anyone even in the shadows threatening them. All of a sudden they were threatened. Their livelihood was threatened. Their academic reputation, their whole ideology, everything. And of course they fought a rearguard action. But they gave up fairly gracefully within three or four years or so. It was interesting to see this rearguard action because they were threatened; they were completely surprised – completely. It took them about a year before they began to believe it and another two or three years before they could accept it.

Which years were these?

Actually, after our paper in 1954. Brill by 1955 had already shown how the rate of the inmates in the mental hospitals went down, how seclusional restraints went down and so on and so on. So by 1957, I think, they began to really become convinced.

It took 20 years after that though for US Psychiatry to change to a more, as you would say, a more agnostic condition.

Yes, that's because for the Americans it was almost a status symbol that you have your analyst and it is still to a certain extent.

Well you can take Prozac now. Take this book by Peter Kramer, Listening to

Prozac (see Glossary). It does mark, at a street level, a change in culture. Whether it is a good change or not is another issue

That's true. But, still, if you go to Hollywood, the well-known writers, they all have to have their own analyst. And in a way this is what Freud really wanted, I think – an educational, guiding kind of technique, not a therapeutic one. So that also influenced people who were not definite psychoanalysts, orthodoxly trained; they still had private practices and then they had to face the fact that private and solo practising would disappear gradually and there would be teams and so on; it was very difficult to take for most psychiatrists because their whole culture had been one of private office practice.

Can I jump and put it to you that before the Second World War, indeed from the turn of the century until 1950, German psychiatry was world psychiatry, but since 1950 German influence has been almost minimal. Why?

I was sitting beside Hanns Hippius at the luncheon today. He said that after the Second World War, there were two stars of psychiatry from the generation born before 1920 and they were de Boor and Matussek – there were two brothers Matussek, one is a psychopharmacologist the other one was the star, he was an analyst. But neither of them became really anything great. De Boor disappeared and Matussek remained as an analyst but didn't get very far, for political reasons probably. So the leading teachers before them had been Kurt Schneider and Kretschmer but apparently that was all the psychiatry there was after them – it only gradually built up around Hippius and so on, later on.

Is there a sense in which the psychotropic drugs have led since the 1950s to an Anglo-American psychiatric culture? Perhaps because these formulations have been drug friendly, they just happened to fit what the drugs can offer.

What also stopped Germany was the complete economic collapse after the War. The universities had to be rebuilt according to American models. No, the Germans accepted drugs. I think German psychiatry has always been more integrated than probably any other psychiatry in the world. They were tolerant to both.

But where Germany clearly led the field before the War, they haven't since.

No they haven't since. Well, now you know there is the American money. You can't produce PET scans without a lot of money and that's what is leading us on now or luring us on. The PET scans and the large trials which are very expensive. The drug companies at first paid for it and then Government grants, NIMH and so on. I think that's where America has stolen the edge.

Did the fact that so many people emigrated from Germany because of the war take the intellectual wind out of German sails?

It took away the intellectual impetus, yes, and the self-assuredness. German medicine was an impressive thing and there is no doubt about it. When we all went away, I don't think that this tradition was transferred to America but it was abolished in Germany.

I just read the biography of Einstein, the latest one that came out, and it is interesting that when he finally came to Princeton, he had got a telegram before he left Germany in 1933 asking him to enter the US very quietly and not give any interviews to anyone. Because the FBI and the CIA didn't like him at all. He was very suspect and the more interviews he gave to journals and newspapers the more suspect he became. So when he finally got into Princeton, it had to be done very discreetly and against the opposition of people like Planck, for instance, in Germany. They stood on their heads to prevent him leaving. I think Planck talked personally to Hitler. But I don't think this brain drain transferred things so much as it did stop an impetus and it also was a blow to their self-assurance.

You wrote a fascinating piece in Thirty Years CINP, *looking back at the Prague meeting about how things have changed. What you say is that we couldn't have foreseen how much would have changed so quickly if PET scans, chronobiology all sorts of things that weren't just there. On the other hand, as you say, when it comes to the actual practice of psychiatry, very little has changed.*

That's what Paul Janssen implied at today's meeting, I think. It's funny, he is not a clinician, but he meant it and it seemed that none of the other clinicians there understood what he meant. Not much has changed in practice. We know how to do it faster and a little better but the modus of doing it really hasn't changed.

Can I ask you about some of the people who have been involved in the past 30 or 40 years, people like Freedman, Klerman, Kline, etc., etc. Who have been the key people do you think that have helped shape the period if one can say that any one has been important enough?

Well, Kline was very important politically. He had a great deal of expertise and instinct and skill and he actually went to the Congress and after he had talked to them, giving a very dramatic and I think very exaggerated view of what was going to happen, Congress gave a lot of money – it was almost forced upon psychopharmacology. Now I was in the study section of the NIMH for 10 years, starting in 1956 or so with the psychopharmacology service centre with Jonathan Cole. He was a very important person. He was very young at the time and I still don't know why they picked him, but he did well in heading the psychopharmacology section. In the early days we had two- or three-day meetings and there weren't enough grant applications. We met three times a year, I think, and at the end of one of these sessions, I think there was about a million dollars left over, which was a lot of money in those days. We didn't know what to do with it. We said what can we do with it, is there anyone who wants seed money? How can we give the money away? This sounds absurd today, bizarre. But eventually I think we had to give half of it back and for half of it we just practically forced it down people's throats. I had never asked for a grant but they phoned me and asked would I please apply for a grant – you will get it but you have to apply. Which again is bizarre as now only 3% of people are getting grants.

So we got a lot of money and we got Congress convinced, almost single handedly by Nate Kline, convinced, that we now could cure mental diseases and really have a handle on it.

Then there was the 'Camelot Times' with Kennedy; Felix was the NIMH Director then and he unfortunately was over-enthusiastic. They created the CMHC, the community mental health centres. They were thinking of prevention and treating the worried well so that they wouldn't get seriously ill. Not thinking at all of where the emphasis now is on the seriously ill and rehabilitation – that's why we have people on the streets, homeless, and so on. Felix, himself, a very enthusiastic fellow, was convinced, not like Aubrey Lewis at all, that it was just a question of time before we could close all mental hospitals – now that we had a handle on it with the drugs and these new community centres. That's it, so forget about it; it's no longer a problem. Well, it was a bit too much and that's why we now have the de-institutionalization problems.

Now Freedman was an editorial restraining influence. He made the Archives *the* journal. Who else? Klerman, we were good friends. He was in charge of, what was it called – ADAMHA or something – anyway, even over-ruling the NIMH – and he felt very strongly, and rightly I would think, that what was necessary here was to establish, if at all possible, the efficacy of psychotherapy. That was a very clever idea but not political, and still isn't political and therefore I don't think he ever got very far. Too bad. He went to Cornell. His wife is the star now, Myrna Weissman. Elkes, has anyone mentioned him to you?

I have a range of views about him, some saying that he was important but important by virtue of his charm and enthusiasm rather than because of anything tangible actually done.

His rhetoric. Yes, he is a very good speaker. That's it. I don't think he influences people because of anything he has written or really done very much, but wherever he goes and talks people are very much taken by him. He has known, particularly in England of course, but globally also most of the pharmacologists and psychopharmacologists. If you can, you should really try to interview him. If you had asked me who to pick I would have picked Joel Elkes.

What about people from Europe, Paul Janssen?

Yes, he is a very bright fellow. He always hits the right note somehow.

He was the first one, of course, who had haloperidol and who got away from the phenothiazines. I asked him several times about this – some sort of instinct – one of his young ladies, technicians, had found something in mice which intrigued him. He got on to it and that's how haloperidol came about and now again they have risperidone. But he has always impressed me as somebody who is really interested in how do the drugs work clinically, which is very nice for somebody who is a pharmacologist and so successful. He has not been lured away. I think he knows a lot about psychopharmacology.

Are you at all concerned about the fact that we don't seem to have any new drugs?

Well, we do have the atypical ones now like clozapine which we had since 1965 but didn't really know we had. I suppose there are a lot on the shelves. My feeling has been, this is again not very politically correct and perhaps not even right, but somehow I feel if we would only stop a while and try to make the best of what we have. We don't even know all the drugs that we have on the shelves. The benzodiazepines were on the shelves for 20 years or so before we discovered their use. We knew clozapine worked and we knew that it didn't cause extrapyramidal symptoms but we didn't know that it was better than the other neuroleptics. We should have done what Kane did eventually to show that it was better than the other antipsychotics. We could have done that in 1970.

What I see in the future of psychiatry are two things, one will be that there will not be any breakthrough with any new drugs but a breakthrough, through the media, in public education – something like the way the media brought about the sexual revolution in the 1960s. So there will be a mental health revolution sometime in the year 2000, or whatever, how to treat and how not to treat children and this sort of thing. And if we could do that, I think we could probably do away with about 25 to 30% of serious mental disorders. If we just knew how to bring up children. But that has to be done in every household not just in an Institute. Genes do a lot but their expression depends greatly on the environment in the developmental stages. Only the media can do that and it might take 50–100 years once it starts.

The other is, because of my age I am particularly interested in successful aging. I have a notion that we can't do anything about neurones that are gone irreversibly but we can probably do a lot more than we are doing now to prevent them from going. Now we have done amazing things in preventive medicine with reducing smoking, exercise, high fibre, low fat diet and vitamins to the point where strokes have gone down and heart disease has gone down – people live much longer. I think we can do the same probably with mental health or with aging if we had a different value system.

Again, that comes back to the media. Our value system now is such that even two and three year olds are learning about money and power.

You have to be successful, you have to be competitive, you have to beat the others and money and power are the manifestations of that success. So when people get to be 65 and they can't get much more money or much more power but they lose some of it, they are completely devastated. What we now need is a new psychotherapy for the generation from 65 to 95. Before this, there weren't any in this group apart from a few who lived to be 80 and so there was no specific psychotherapy for them. The first thing this geropsychotherapy would have to do is to dismantle these life-long primary values of money and power and replace them with autonomy, creativity, knowledge, learning – what have you. All kinds of other real values. That would take two or three years before you could do anything else psychotherapeutically.

But what I immediately would like to see is what we can do about preventing stress. I think there is a lot of what I call latent stress. People are seldom fully aware of being stressed. For instance in the elderly – today when I came up on the street here I met a black fellow, a worker, I don't know what he was but he was wearing work clothes and he smiled at me, greeted me, saying 'Hi young fellow'. Now, ridiculous as it sounds, it gave me a boost. On the other hand to say to yourself, well, I'm over the hill and what can you expect, is a constant latent stress unless you actually can counteract it.

Now we know through the work of McEwen and others, that stress, not only in the elderly, increases corticosteroid hormone output and this produces a cascade of excitatory amino acids. In young people, this can be cut off because there is enough homeostasis but not in the elderly. They don't cut it off and they have shown in rats and in primates as well, that this cascade definitely produces atrophy of the hippocampal cells. That we can't afford. So we have to avoid stress by all means. Elderly people have usually a higher corticosteroid level than younger people. I think it is because they are constantly more stressed and they don't realize it. So we have to discover these latent stresses and then see how to counteract them and in that way prevent the loss of neurones, which can be shown to lead to loss of cognitive function.

We learnt about stress from Selye but what we don't know yet is where stress becomes distress. Stress is not only tolerable but it is necessary to activate us, but distress becomes immediately destructive, particularly if it is chronic, and more so if it is latent because then we don't even know it is there. So we have to do something about chronic stress, finding out what it does if anything, what the latent stresses are and how to counteract them. So I'm looking towards prevention rather than cure. As regards treatment, I think we have probably enough on the shelves to serve us for some time if we learn how to use it.

Select bibliography

De Boor, W. (1958) *Pharmacopsychologie und Psychopathologie*, Springer-Verlag, Berlin.

Lehmann H E, Hanrahan G E (1954). Chlorpromazine, new inhibiting agent for psychomotor excitment and manic states. *Archives of Neurology and Psychiatry*, **71**, 227–37.

Lehmann, H.E., Kahn, C.H. and de Verteuil, R.L. (1958) *Canadian Psychiatric Association Journal*, **3,** 155.

Lehmann, H.E. (1980) Reflections on a career in psychiatry. *The Canadian Psychiatric Association Bulletin*, *12,* **4,** 14–16.

Lehmann, H.E. (1986) The future of psychiatry: Progress – mutation – or self-destruct? *Canadian Journal of Psychiatry*, **31,** 362–67.

Lehmann, H.E. (1993) Before they called it psychopharmacology. *Neuropsychopharmacology*, **8,** 291–303.

8 Hanns Hippius

The founding of the CINP and the discovery of clozapine

There are two people at the moment whom I particularly associate with an interest in the History of Psychopharmacology – Tom Ban and yourself. Why are you interested?

Both of us – Tom Ban in Hungary and me in Germany – joined the field of psychiatry in the 1950s. We joined at a time that has since justly been called the 'psychopharmacological turning point in psychiatric therapeutics'. Therefore, as young psychiatrists, we were involved in the early development of clinical psychopharmacology and took part in the discovery of new therapeutic drugs.

Now – almost 40 years later – it is fascinating for us as participating witnesses of modern psychopharmacology from the beginning to document, to summarize and to analyse this history. Tom is particularly interested in this.

I am also interested in history but the reaction I get from many in the profession is that history is bunk – Henry Ford's view. The field is moving forward, you only need to know what's current. How do you explain this?

I think the position of Henry Ford is not acceptable in our profession. Each psychiatrist has to be interested in history because in our everyday practical work we are occupied with biographies, with the histories of individual human beings.

Besides, for a German psychiatrist, there exists a very serious and special reason to be engaged in the history of our field – the development and situation of psychiatry in my country during the Nazi period. In that time, German psychiatrists were responsible for the most excessive and cruel misuse of psychiatry. How was it possible that German psychiatrists tolerated and some of them even supported actively the killing of almost 100 000 psychiatric patients? This is up to now one of the most important problems for historical research in psychiatry.

Finally, there are some personal roots and reasons for my interest in history. As a boy at school I was for a long time irresolute whether I should study history or medicine. Later, working in clinical psychiatry,

I had the privilege to work in two places with outstanding psychiatric traditions – in Berlin from 1952 to 1970 and in Munich since 1971. For the past 20 years I have worked in the hospital where Emil Kraepelin, Alois Alzheimer and many other excellent psychiatrists were active as both clinicians and scientists. In such an atmosphere under the influence of this 'genius loci' you must be interested in the history of psychiatry. In the library and in the record office of the Munich hospital I discovered a lot of interesting documents. For example, there were the unpublished memoirs of Emil Kraepelin – now edited and published in German and English. I've got exciting letters from Wilhelm Wundt to Kraepelin or a private letter of Sigmund Freud to a patient with the recommendation to continue in treatment in Munich, because treatment in Vienna with Freud himself, with inflation as it was in the early 1920s, would be too expensive. I also found documents on the mental state of King Ludwig II of Bavaria, who died in 1886, together with those relating to the psychiatrist Bernard von Gudden, one of the predecessors of Kraepelin in the Chair of Psychiatry at the University of Munich.

From 1900 to 1950, world psychiatry really was German psychiatry. The leading concepts and the leading people were German. As of 1950, there was this watershed and in a sense no one seemed to replace the generation of Kurt Schneider. That's the way it seems to me; am I wrong?

I am not sure that it is justified to say that psychiatry from 1900 to 1950 was German psychiatry. It was owing to the efforts of French psychiatrists at the end of the 18th century that psychiatry had been established as a clinical discipline within medicine. At the same time, important influences also came from Great Britain in the field of the practical care of psychiatric patients. In Germany psychiatry developed in the first half of the 19th century on two separate fronts. Up to the middle of the century the first professors of psychiatry at the Universities in Germany were more engaged in philosophical aspects of mental illnesses than in the practical care of mental patients. These psychiatrists (*Psychiker*) created the basis for psychopathology and psychology, for anthropolotical aspects of our discipline, and even for psychoanalysis.

More or less independent of these developments in the first half of the 19th century, in all parts of Germany, psychiatric hospitals were established. The medical doctors (*sornaliker*) working in these institutions became the pioneers of the practical care of mental patients. The relations and the exchanges between these two groups of psychiatrists were not very good – sometimes there were even pugnacious arguments.

This unsatisfactory situation changed in the course of the second half of the 19th century by establishing hospitals and chairs for psychiatry in all German universities. A key person for this development was Wilhelm Griesinger. And in connection with this evolution, German psychiatry – or it would be better to say psychiatry in the German-speaking countries

(Switzerland, Austria and Germany) – got an increasing role in psychiatry as science.

But the hegemony, as you put it, did not last up to 1950. I think it was only up to the 1920s or early 1930s. It was finished with the emigration of an enormous number of German-speaking, especially Jewish, psychiatrists, from Germany and later Austria, into other countries. In connection with this pitiable development, the standard of scientific psychiatry inside Germany sank remarkably and international attention on it decreased. The reputation of German psychiatry collapsed entirely in connection with political developments and the misuse of psychiatry during the Nazi time. This is also the reason for the fact that the reception of the scientific achievement of some German psychiatrists who worked and published inside Germany after 1933, for example, Karl Bonhoeffer, Kurt Schneider, Ernst Kretschmer and Karl Leonhard, happened with more or less delay after the war.

The belated recognition of Jaspers' work has another origin. Karl Jaspers only worked in psychiatry for six years, from 1909 to 1915, at the psychiatric hospital of the University of Heidelberg. He left clinical psychiatry very early and had already by the age of 38 been appointed to the position of full professor of philosophy at the University of Heidelberg. Because his wife was Jewish, he was forced in 1937 to leave his outstanding chair of philosophy. After reinstatement in his former position in 1945, he moved in 1948 to a chair of philosophy at the University of Basel. For these reasons, Karl Jaspers was very often classified as a pure philosopher and his fundamental and famous book *Algemeine Psychopathologie* – General Psychopathology – first published in 1912, for a long time did not find an entrance in psychiatry – with some exceptions such as Germany, Austria, Switzerland, of course, but for example Japan too (Jaspers, 1965).

If you talk about a watershed around 1950, I think this year marks a point of time for the start of the reintegration of German into international psychiatry. The situation of scientific psychiatry inside Germany during the first years after the war was a peculiar one. At the University hospitals research was only orientated on the one side on psychopathology and on the other psychoanalysis. The philosophy of Husserl and Heidegger influenced the interpretation of psychopathological phenomena. This was so-called anthropological psychiatry. Immediately after the war almost all prominent psychiatrists were engaged in this while the younger ones were involved in the re-import of psychoanalysis and for them this had priority.

For biological research or even for therapeutic research at all there was little or no interest. This situation changed dramatically in the 1950s with the introduction of the neuroleptics. At this time several young psychiatrists began very soon to investigate the therapeutic effects of the new drugs. Doing this these young psychiatrists became increasingly enthusiastically engaged in this field. But in the early 1950s, the heads of university departments, the full professors of psychiatry in Germany, had decided that therapeutic research could only be a 'side-effect' of basic science in psychiatry. In the German tradition, since the last century through to Karl Jaspers and Kurt Schneider, 'real' science could be psychopathological research only. This situation is, by the way, the background for a pioneering German book on the new therapeutic drugs: the monograph on 'Psychopharmacologie und Psychopathologie' published by Wolfgang de Boor in 1956 (see Select bibliography, Chapter 7). As a pupil of Kurt Schneider, he trained in psychiatry immediately after the war at the psychiatric hospital in Heidelberg. In his book, De Boor reviewed the effects of psychotropic drugs principally from the point of view of experimental psychology; he had much less interest in their role as therapeutic agents.

That tradition in a sense goes right back to Kraepelin who coined the term 'pharmacopsychology'.

Yes, that is right. More than 100 years ago, in 1892, Emil Kraepelin had published his classical monograph 'Uber die Beeinflussung einfacher psychischer Vorgange durch einige Arzneimittel'. Therefore it is justified to call Kraepelin one of the founders of experimental psychopathology.

In a sense, that's the one area of psychopharmacology that, in recent years, we have missed out on − the use of drugs to test cognitive function. Perhaps with the eclipse of LSD this whole area atrophied.

I agree with you but we should distinguish between drug-induced experimental psychology (in the sense of Kraepelin) and drug-induced experimental psychopathology in the sense of Moreau de Tours which had the aim of provoking a 'model psychosis'. This second kind of experimental psychology had in Germany a tradition up to the present time. For example, K. Behringer has investigated the psychotropic effects of mescaline and H. Leuner has written on the basis of his experiments with LSD a monograph 'Die experimentelle Psychose'. Later Leuner tried to transfer his experiences with the application of LSD under experimental conditions into a special kind of psychotherapy − so-called psycholytic therapy. This therapy does not now play a role.

From my point of view, for further scientific progress, we do not need this kind of experimental psychology with hallucinogens and related drugs. Instead of this purely experimental approach we should intensify again the global but more precise psychopathological investigations of therapeutic drugs on the whole − that means including drugs used in internal medicine.

How much do you think the War also influenced things by making the outside world hostile to German ideas? Reading back through some of the archives of the British Journal of Psychiatry *at annual meetings, just after the First World War and after the Second World War, you heard statements being made in public*

meetings, 'well the War has proved we cannot believe anything the Germans say'.
Do you think this kind of reaction delayed the acceptance of the ideas of Jaspers
and Schneider?

Not very markedly. On the contrary – it was an unexpected and surprising
experience for me as a young assistant to be welcomed in a very friendly
way as a participant at international psychiatric congresses in the 1950s –
Paris in 1955, Zurich in 1957 and Rome in 1958. German emigrants
such as Willy Mayer-Gross from the UK, Lothar Kalinowsky and Fritz
Freyhan from the US, Heinz Lehmann from Canada and Hans Hoff from
Vienna who was back in Austria after his emigration time in Iraq.

Mayer-Gross and Kalinowsky later very strongly influenced my development in clinical psychiatry and research during my training in Berlin.
When Mayer-Gross was informed that I had studied chemistry besides
medicine, he stimulated me, with this background of knowledge in biochemical and neurophysiological research, to do investigations on psychotropic drugs. In our correspondence, he had suggested already in the early
1960s that I should investigate serotonin in mental patients. Kalinowsky
invited me to be the co-author with P. Hoch and him in writing the
textbook on *Somatic Treatments in Psychiatry.* I was responsible for all
chapters on drug treatment.

Now to the other part of your question. I cannot explain conclusively
what the reason was for the long delay in the reception of the ideas of
Jaspers and Schneider in the US and the UK. Is it not the general problem
of the increasing influence and expansion of the English language in all
branches of medicine, including psychiatry, with the consequence that
the concepts and ideas of authors that need to be translated into English
have a delayed reception?

Comparing the situation in the USA and the UK relative to the
reception of German contributions to psychiatry in the 20th century,
the UK had a different – if you want, a better – situation. For example,
by the medium of Mayer-Gross and his classical textbook with co-authors
Martin Roth and Eliot Slater, and through the influence of Erwin Stengel,
the contributions of German psychiatry were integrated unconspicuously
in English psychiatry. In contrast to the UK, in the USA for example,
Emil Kraepelin was not .very well known until 1970 and the name of
Alzheimer completely unknown until 10 years ago. Now the situation in
the USA has changed drastically with the result of DSM-III, DSM-IV
and the so-called 'Neo-Kraepelinism' and Alzheimer has advanced to a
term of colloquial language.

I think the reciprocal influences in psychiatry between our two countries in the last four decades were stronger than we will admit. For
example, William Sargent's work on ECT was noted by the book of
Hoch and Kalinowsky. And the Leonhard concept of classification and
the course of the endogenous psychoses – mediated by Frank Fish – was

for some time better known in the UK than in the western part of Germany. Finally, the fruitful and successful development of social psychiatry in Germany after the war was owing to the many stimulations of British psychiatry.

You were at the 1955 Saint Anne meeting, and in Towards CINP *(see Glossary) you mention that it was the first of the large international meetings but also that one of the odd things about it for you it was that it was the first time for you to meet some people from Germany. Is that where you met Wolfgang de Boor?*

You have to take into consideration that I have worked in this time in Berlin which was a very isolated situation. During the first 10 years after the War, travelling and attending scientific congresses – even inside Germany – was almost not possible. In these years German psychiatrists were not allowed to attend international meetings. They were not invited and not accepted as speakers. Therefore in 1950, with the exception of K. Conrad, the professor of psychiatry in the Saar, which at this time was under the French Government, no German psychiatrist was allowed to attend the First World Congress of Psychiatry in Paris. In the following years the situation improved – at first with regard to neurological congresses – for example, the World Congress of Neurology in Lisbon in 1953. But the first important international psychiatric meeting with several German participants was the International Colloquium on Chlorpromazine and Neuroleptic Drugs in Psychiatric Treatment in Paris, in October of 1955.

By chance, I had the opportunity to attend this three-day congress with many possibilities to meet for the first time psychiatric colleagues from Germany such as Wolfgang de Boor from Cologne, H. Kranz from Mainz, Fritz Flugel and Dietmar Bente from Erlangen as well as psychiatrists from many other countries – Delay, Deniker, and Pichot from France, Rumke from The Netherlands, Hoff from Austria, Mayer-Gross from the UK, Delgado from Peru, Overholzer, Denber, and Freyhan from the USA, Lehmann from Canada and Barahona-Fernandes from Portugal.

For me, the very interesting scientific experience of the Paris Meeting was the differences between the conceptions of the few German psychiatrists – De Boor, Kranz and Selback – and the scientific approach of the majority of psychiatrists coming from other countries. For the German psychiatrists, the drug therapy of psychotic diseases was only an instrument for research. The overwhelming majority of psychiatrists from all other countries (including those who came originally from the German psychiatric tradition such as Mayer-Gross, Hoff, Lehmann and Freyhan) saw the enormous importance of chlorpromazine and other neuroleptics in the area of therapeutic efficacy. This experience was decisive for my own orientation to research since 1955 – my efforts I thought should be directed closely to psychiatric therapy.

Why is that?

The influence of philosophy on psychiatry has a long tradition in Germany. I have already referred to the situation of psychiatry in Germany during the romanticism early in the 19th century. And immediately after the Second World War psychiatrists as scientists were again inclined to be engaged more with sophisticated philosophical problems than with such pragmatic and ordinary questions as therapy!

I do not want to be misunderstood: psychiatry as a part of medicine has the function to import philosophical and anthropological ideas to all other disciplines of medicine. Psychiatry is the ideological seismograph of medicine, reflecting many facets of the predominant 'Zeitgeist' – but psychiatry has to fulfil this function without neglecting its original duty: the care and therapy of patients.

I think several psychiatrists as Mayer-Gross – originally Germans but forced by the Nazis to leave Germany – emigrated to countries such as UK with a long tradition of very pragmatic orientated psychiatry. The emigrées became through their fate representatives of a very creative integration of two different psychiatric traditions. In their new homeland, they were proofed against too much philosophical speculations and could not neglect the care and treatment of their patients.

So how did you escape that?

I have studied both medicine and chemistry. After finishing my studies, I first worked in an institute for immunology and biochemistry – then I switched to psychiatry. In my first position, in a department for psychiatry and neurology, I was responsible for the laboratory only, not for patients. But this changed. I got increasingly interested in clinical work. In this field I had the choice between neurology and psychiatry. Initially, I was inclined more to neurology. Finally my ambivalence between neurology and psychiatry was solved by the introduction of the first therapeutic psychotropic drugs in psychiatry. This became decisive for my professional life. I switched definitely to psychiatry with the aim to work also in laboratories (EEG, clinical chemistry). My clinical training was directed from the beginning to therapeutic problems and my interest in research was in the field of biological psychiatry. At this time I read extensively the classical psychiatric literature in German. And of course I studied Jaspers – but I had only very little time to read Heidegger and all the other authors who were obligatory at this time for a young psychiatrist in Germany if he was interested in an academic career

Who introduced chlorpromazine to Germany?

In Germany, chlorpromazine was already introduced in five university hospitals and in several state hospitals by 1953. The background for this early availability of chlorpromazine was the fact that since the end of the

1940s, the first contacts between the French and German pharmaceutical industry (Rhône-Poulenc and Bayer) grew up. Because of this, information on the spectacular therapeutic results in French psychiatric hospitals came to the Bayer Company and then to the directors of the psychiatric hospitals. Surprisingly, the resonance of this information was small. But in five university hospitals – independently from each other – younger assistants were stimulated to investigate chlorpromazine as a therapeutic agent. This was D. Bente in Erlangen, Schmitt in Heidelberg, M.P. Engelmeier in Munster, K. Heinrich in Mainz and J. Hiob and me in Berlin.

In some places the first therapeutic trials with chlorpromazine were carried out without support by the chairmen of the departments – in single hospitals even against the recommendations and orders of the chairman. Only Professor Fritz Flugel, the chairman of department at the University of Erlangen, actively promoted early on his assistants Bente and Itil in their research with chlorpromazine.

In Berlin, J. Hiob was a pioneer with the early clinical investigations of chlorpromazine. He was an experienced clinician already trained in internal medicine. I came from the biochemistry laboratory and was a beginner in psychiatry. We both decided we should start a chlorpromazine trial in a single chronic patient. We had both read the early papers of our French colleagues and were so impressed that we asked the people of the Bayer Company if we could have material for a therapeutic trial. We received the material but the director of our hospital hesitated to allow us go ahead. We regretted this order because we knew that we were one of the first places outside France in a position to investigate chlorpromazine. Because of the hold-up, I began with animal experiments and investigated the influence of chlorpromazine on the EEG of rabbits. Nice results, but not very useful! Hiob on the other hand had no interest in a switch over to animal experiments. He insisted on carrying out therapeutic investigations. Finally our head of department agreed but told us to go ahead, but it would not be successful because all drugs which have been used since the beginning of the century, barbiturates, etc. had not been effective. And in addition 'therapy is not science!'.

In spite of this not very encouraging comment, Hiob proposed to try chlorpromazine with a special patient. It was a female chronic schizophrenic patient with a paranoid – hallucinatory symptomatology. I remember exactly the visit with our Professor two weeks later. He said to us 'please, look, she improves completely independently of therapy! It was very good that I have not encouraged you to treat this patient with chlorpromazine. This is a typical incalculable spontaneous improvement. She has now much less hallucinations than two weeks ago. And I have saved you from a misinterpretation'. Hiob hesitated several seconds and then he stuttered 'Oh yes, oh no, oh yes – but we have treated her for two weeks with chlorpromazine'. That was a peculiar situation. Our

Professor of psychiatry was a little bit angry about all of this. But finally he permitted us to go ahead with further investigations.

After seeing it work, what was the next step?

After our exciting results with chlorpromazine, Hiob and I studied intensely the literature to find comparable drugs. We came across some pharmacological and a few clinical publications on reserpine. This alkaloid drug was already used in internal medicine as an antihypertensive drug. We were able to show that reserpine had in some cases antipsychotic effects comparable to that of chlorpromazine and was in addition even effective in other clinical syndromes (including depressions).

The next step was determined by our interest to discover relations between chemical structure and the clinical profile of antipsychotic drugs. With this aim we investigated tricyclic neuroleptics. Very soon after the investigation of chlorpromazine we had the opportunity to carry out many trials with a lot of different tricyclic drugs, having a chemical structure more or less closely related to chlorpromazine. We found some regular relations between therapeutic effects, side effects and the chemical structure of these tricyclic drugs.

Comparable investigations with drugs chemically related to reserpine were not possible, because the chemical structure of reserpine is so complicated, that the efforts to synthesize related drugs were not successful.

In our investigations with tricyclic drugs we had very early on the opportunity to investigate imipramine. With regards to our results we classified imipramine as a weak neuroleptic. If I am informed correctly, Roland Kuhn in Switzerland, in his first trial, came to the same judgement. But he and his male and female nurses then discovered the unexpected antidepressant effect of imipramine.

I met Kuhn personally at this time. From my point of view the discovery of imipramine as an antidepressant was a special merit of Kuhn. He was trained in traditional Swiss clinical psychiatry and his scientific interest was the 'Daseinsanalyse', the anthropological psychiatry and its points of contacts to existentialism. In spite of a basic orientation in such a non-biological framework, to discover the clinical profile of the first tricyclic antidepressant – that is an achievement.

Of course, he had the support of an excellent nursing staff and the advice of an ingenious industrial product manager from Geigy, Paul Schmidlin – but finally with his personal trials he went beyond the judgement 'equal', 'stronger' or 'weaker' than chlorpromazine. All investigators (me too!) came to the result, that the new Geigy drug was a very weak neuroleptic even in high doses of 1000 mg. Our finding was that in such high doses imipramine resembled chlorpromazine a little bit more than in doses of 100–300 mg. But Kuhn and his staff discovered that imipramine in low doses was an antidepressant.

Besides, the consideration of nurses' observations – as Kuhn has done

– is a reliable indicator for the clinician and it is better to consider them than to neglect reports from nursing staff. I have learnt many important things about drug-therapy, for example on side effects, from the precise observations and descriptions of my nursing staff.

The discovery of imipramine had for me another stimulating effect. With my interest in relations between clinical structure and clinical profile in the beginning I was asking only for quantitative differences between the various chlorpromazine-like drugs – this now extended to questions on qualitative differences with regard to therapeutic and unwanted side-effects between chemically closely related drugs.

Can I move you back to the 1955 meeting? What was the atmosphere at that like? Was it clear to all of you that this was a new era or not?

Oh, I think at least the younger people attending the Paris meeting were convinced – that is, of a new era in psychiatry.

Linford Rees was at that meeting and presented the only randomized controlled trials at the meeting – it does seem to have been a British thing, this idea of let's randomize . . .

If I remember correctly at the Paris meeting in 1955, Linford Rees has presented results of controlled studies with chlorpromazine in anxiety states and these were published in the proceedings of the Paris meeting. Elkes was not personally at the Paris Colloquium. But W. Mayer-Gross, the mentor of Elkes during his time in Great Britain, mentioned the investigations of Elkes in inpatients and outpatients following a scheme for controlled trials which started already in 1954. But I don't know if these studies were published earlier than the studies of Linford Rees.

By all means, I agree with you, the first proper randomized controlled trials have been a British thing. This is but a single example – in fact a great deal of the contributions to methodology in psychopharmacology (including statistical methods of evaluation) came from UK. The development of adequate research methodology is closely connected with the names of British scientists, from H.J. Eysenck and Max Hamilton to Malcolm Lader more recently.

I think for methodology the development in Great Britain was a big influence for the whole world. Another German who was eminent in Britain, at this time, of course was the psychologist Hans Eysenck and he made contact with German academics very early after the War. In this way Great Britain, either through clinicians like Linford Rees, or on the other side Eysenck as a psychologist, methodology came back to Germany.

Let me chase you a bit further and get into Mark Twain country.

I am sure you mean this question in connection with the so-called 'Mark-Twain-Syndrome', which was coined by Tom Ban and me in the little booklet 'Psychopharmacology In Perspective'. Mark Twain pointed out:

'The older I get, the more vivid is my recollection of things that never happened'. If you write something on the history of psychopharmacology on the basis of your memory, you run the risk of being a more or less distinct example of a 'Mark-Twain Syndrome'. This risk is particularly high in the situation of an interview! Nobody is immune against Mark-Twain Syndrome.

But Michael Shepherd was the first to point this out in terms of psychiatry. If you go into the history of psychopharmacology or in other fields you will find that some people remember better and better with increasing age things which have never happened. For instance, I was an editor on the first booklet on the Founding Members of the CINP and I had very critical comments from some people to whom I had to say that we know you were very involved but you were never a founding member.

This seems to have particularly applied to the 1957 meetings. Who was responsible for the 1957 meeting?

I think besides Emilio Trabucchi, head of Department of Pharmacology of the University of Milan, Silvio Garattini played the greatest role for the organization of the Milan meeting in May 1957. At this time Garattini was a young assistant at Trabucchi's Institute. In Italy already in the 1950s the young generation of pharmacologists (for example, Garattini, Paoletti and Costa) were engaged in neuropharmacology and they were interested to have a scientific exchange with clinicians. Being informed that in psychiatry since 1952 pharmacological treatments played an increasing role, Garattini stimulated Professor Trabucchi to arrange an International Symposium on psychotropic drugs. Trabucchi agreed and the idea was realized in Milan (May, 9–11, 1957). And after his role as 'spiritus rector', Silvio Garattini was a very active and successful organizer of the excellent symposium.

The participants were in the first place pharmacologists and other basic scientists from universities and pharmaceutical industry, but clinicians from various countries too. In the course of the Milan Symposium, the pharmacologist Radouco-Thomas and the psychiatrist De Boor came up with the idea of founding a scientific association for neuropsychopharmacology. They were supported by some important people – Trabucchi, Deniker, Denber, but they had some opposition too. And therefore the founding of CINP was delayed till to the World Congress of Psychiatry in Zurich (September, 1–7, 1957).

Why did De Boor get involved in getting the CINP going and then slip out of it so early on?

De Boor had written the monograph 'Pharmacopsychologie und Psycho-phathologie' as a member of staff of the outstanding German psychopath-ologist Kurt Schneider, who was head of Department of Psychiatry at the

University of Heidelberg from 1945 to 1955. With the end of Kurt Schneider's chairmanship, De Boor moved to the University Hospital in Cologne. Under the influence of Kurt Schneider, De Boor worked on psychopathology, the traditional field of German scientific psychiatry and therefore – as I have already said – his interest on psychotropic drugs was narrowed down to their role as tools for research in experimental psychopathology and was not directed to their therapeutic importance.

When De Boor's monograph was published in 1956 he had already moved to Cologne. After changing his place of work, he terminated completely his interest in psychopharmacology and pharmacopsychiatry. The University Hospital in Cologne had been headed since 1950 by W. Scheid. He was likewise a pupil of Kurt Schneider, several years older than De Boor. He had worked as a very successful scientist not only in psychiatry but in neurology too. In Scheid's hospital De Boor was responsible for forensic psychiatry and since that time this branch of psychiatry has been his main field of research. Even after his retirement he remains active in forensic psychiatry. He has enlarged his interest from psychopathological aspects of forensic psychiatry meanwhile to more general historical and political questions as for example, in his book 'Ober den Zeitgeist', in 1993.

What was the chain of events from the Milan meeting to the actual founding of the CINP

The majority of the participants of the Milan Symposium 1957 were pharmacologists and other basic scientists. There was not the clinical orientation that there had been at the Paris Colloquium 1955. If the more clinically orientated Paris Colloquium was the first opportunity for contacts and exchange between clinicians from many countries – the Milan Symposium was the first congress with opportunities for exchange and discussions between clinicians and basic scientists on an international basis.

The participants included such outstanding basic scientists as H. Blaschko, D. Bovet, B. Brodie, A. Carlsson, E. Costa, G. Moruzzi, E. Rothlin and many others. During the meeting, as I mentioned, the idea of founding a scientific body for periodical meetings of basic scientists and clinicians on psychopharmacology arose. But a brake was put on it by E. Rothlin. He was at this time the president of the International Association of Pharmacology and he argued that such an interdisciplinary society should be founded only with consent of the international societies of the mother disciplines. In spite of some contradictions – especially by younger people – Rothlin's advice was accepted.

After that, Rothlin, who was the main pharmacologist of Sandoz in Basel, used the next months to contact M. Bleuler, the professor of psychiatry in Zurich, who was in that time preparing the Second World Congress of Psychiatry for September 1957 in Zurich. The result of these and many other consultations was the foundation of CINP in Zurich in September and Rothlin became the first president.

There were some problems though for a few years – there were clashes of personality almost it seems for the first two or three years with people finding they weren't listed on the membership anymore.

Of course, after foundation of the CINP with 30 people only, there was some trouble. But I think that was overcome very soon, at the latest by the first CINP Congress in Rome in 1958.

Somewhere around this early period, was it because of this discontent, a German society for psychopharmacology began? Why did you begin so early?

You and the Czech's were the first to begin national societies, which in a sense seems odd against the background of a German tradition of not being interested in therapy.

After the Paris Colloquium in 1955, some of the young assistants at five German psychiatric university hospitals, D. Bente in Erlangen, M. P. Engelmeier in Munster, K. Heinrich in Mainz, W Schmitt in Homburg/ Saar and myself in Berlin-West, met periodically for discussions on our investigations and very soon in 1956 to organize joint research. After the Milan meeting in 1957, we met up at annual meetings in Erlangen and Nurnberg. At this time, in Germany, we had the reputation of 'outsiders', because we were occupied 'only' with therapeutic research – and this, over and above, with drugs!

Even our professors remained more or less sceptical on our work. Only Fritz Flugel, professor of psychiatry at the University of Erlangen and boss of D. Bente, encouraged us. Therefore in Erlangen – for example – very early systematical EEG investigations on patients on neuroleptics were carried out by D. Bente and Turan Itil. Itil came from Turkey with a scholarship to Erlangen and became a collaborator of D. Bente. Bente and Itil pioneered the methodological development of Pharmaco-EEG. Itil moved in the 1960s to the USA and made a career there and became very well known. Bente stayed in Erlangen and moved in the 1970s to Berlin, where he died very early at the age of 62 in 1983.

Bente was a little bit of the bavarian baroque type and was, in his time in Erlangen as assistant of Flugel, very productive with a lot of ideas. As early as 1959 he encouraged his professor Flugel to agree with the foundation of a German psychopharmacological association by expanding our Group of Five (the 'Funferclub') to an 'Arbeitsgemeinschaft fur Neuropsychopharmakologie' (AGNP). Flugel supported him. The other five convinced their professors too and in summer 1959 we met together in Cologne. The professor of psychiatry in Cologne, W. Scheid, and the professor of pharmacology in Bonn, R. Domenooz, also became founding members of the AGNP.

The AGNP had the function to prepare on a national basis the German contributions to the international congress of CINP. Therefore we organized the first AGNP meeting near to Erlangen in Nurnberg at the end of April 1960 with 40 participants some months before the second CINP Congress in Basel in July 1960. With consent of the executive committee of CINP, AGNP has since 1959 the function of a 'local advisory committee to CINP'. Because the temporal distance of two months to the international congress was too short, the second meeting of the AGNP took place in September 1961, again in Nurnberg one year before the next CINP meeting. Since that time, the AGNP meetings were organized biannually alternating with the likewise biannual CINP Congress. The Second AGNP meeting 1961 was important for us, because the CINP executive committee, with Paul Hoch as president, accepted our invitation to host the Third CINP Congress in Munich, where the meeting took place in September 1962.

I don't know, if the pharmacological section of the Czech Purkinje-Society was earlier than AGNP in Germany. In any case, we developed very good relations with them and our colleagues from Hungary, Poland and Yugoslavia very quickly. Some of our Czech colleagues (for example O. Vinar, M. Vojtechovsky, Z. Votava and E. Vencovsky) visited us and our meetings regularly and we got permission to cross the Iron Curtain to visit them in their countries. Some years later, Bente organized a Central European Congress for neuropsychopharmacology. The first meeting happened in Karlovy Vary in Czechoslovakia in 1967 and another one in 1971 in Split in Yugoslavia. But the most important event for Central Europe at this time was the CINP Congress in Prague in 1970 under the presidency of Heinz Lehmann.

How has the Germany society gone? Is it still functioning with all these other societies ECNP and CINP? Does it show the tensions between neuroscientists and clinicians that there seem to be in the equivalent American and British societies?

Yes, we have some tensions too – but not so distinctly. We also have in the German-speaking countries a 'Gesellschaft fur Biologische Psychiatrie'. This younger association also arranges biannual meetings so that we have every year either an AGNP or a Biological Psychiatry Meeting. Therefore, there is less competition than in the USA between the two meetings because in the USA both societies have one meeting each year. In Germany the membership is overlapping to a great extent and the themes in the meetings are overlapping likewise. A difference is that the presidency in the AGNP alternates between psychologists, pharmacologists and clinicians, whereas the presidents of the Society of Biological Psychiatry are clinicians. The German Society for Biological Psychiatry has joint meetings with the Societies for Biological Psychiatry of Austria and Switzerland.

Let me ask you about the early days of clozapine. How did it get introduced first?

Thank you, Dr Healy, for this question! Up to now you have asked me only those relating to more superficial historical and organizational points. The question of clozapine is a scientific one and has for me some peculiar facets.

Already by 1953 the extrapyramidal side effects of the first neuroleptics, chlorpromazine and reserpine, had been observed. The majority of clinicians and all pharmacologists were convinced pretty quickly, that there is an absolute connection between extrapyramidal symptoms and clinical effectiveness in psychotic patients. After the introduction of the butyrophenones in 1958 this conception got such a strong support that it developed under the influence of Paul Janssen to a psychopharmacological dogma. The position of Janssen was supported by the prominent German clinician H.J. Haase who confirmed from the clinical point of view 'there is no antipsychotic effect without extrapyramidal side effects'. To demonstrate this Haase introduced the so-called 'hand-writing' test.

If a patient was treated with chlorpromazine, reserpine or one of the other early neuroleptic drugs, they had to write a nursery rhythm such as 'Jack and Jill went up the hill' before treatment and then every day. The idea was to see that under neuroleptic treatment with a defined dose the writing becomes smaller as part of the micrographia that you find in Parkinson's disease. I think the hand-writing test is useful to prevent an overdose with classical neuroleptics. But the investigation with this test does not prove the Janssen − Haase hypothesis of an absolute coherence between therapeutic and extrapyramidal efficacy.

Before the introduction of haloperidol, our group in Berlin had tried to find neuroleptics with weak or no extrapyramidal effects but with equal or greater therapeutic efficacy than chlorpromazine. The starting point for our efforts were speculations on the relation between chemical structure and the profile of effects and side effects of tricyclic psychotropic drugs and the clinical findings − that on the one hand, in single cases, excellent therapeutic effects could be obtained without any extrapyramidal side effects, and on the other hand patients with severe extrapyramidal side effects were often completely therapy-resistant.

In our search for antipsychotics with low or very low extrapyramidal efficacy our first success was in 1957 with the piperacinyl-phenothiazine-derivative perazine. This drug was therapeutically superior and had a lower intensity and frequency of extrapyramidal side effects than chlorpromazine. We published our findings with perazine in 1958, but they had little impact because it was the year of the introduction of haloperidol. Perazine remained a neuroleptic drug used only in Germany, whose use nevertheless spread and continues to spread!

In spite of the overwhelming success of butyrophenones and the prestige of the outstanding pharmacologist Paul Janssen, we searched further for antipsychotics without extrapyramidal effects. To this end our 'Group of five' worked in the early 1960s with the Swiss pharmaceutical company Wander. They had developed the tricyclic antidepressant dibenzepine, which is chemically characterized by a central ring with seven atoms comparable to imipramine. The scientists of the Wander company, especially the ingenious pharmacologist G. Stille, offered us a group of tricyclic drugs with chemical similarity to dibenzepine. We expected antidepressive efficacy but we found an antipsychotic profile. One of these drugs was clozapine.

When did you come across it?

The first publication was in 1966 at a CINP Congress in Washington. This was a very small announcement that we had compared five different although similar structures and looked at which are effective and which have less extrapyramidal effects – we wrote 'less' at this time rather than 'none'.

At first we investigated the five chemically closely related Wander drugs. Then we were informed that Stille had found that one of these drugs had an unusual pharmacological profile. That was clozapine. At the same time some Austrian Investigations had clozapine too and they published an enthusiastic paper on therapeutic results with it. Angst did the first double-blind trial and found comparable results as both our group in open studies and the Austrians had found. From this moment on both the Swiss investigations and our group began to concentrate on clozapine. In all clinical trials we came to the conclusion that it was a drug with a satisfactory antipsychotic profile but without extrapyramidal side effects. So the discovery of the first atypical antipsychotic drug was at the end of the 1960s. Together with Stille, I published a paper in 1971 calling for a revision of the psychopharmacological dogma of antipsychotic efficacy.

But at just this time two events happened which were to delay for 20 years the general acceptance of the possibility of treating with antipsychotics without a risk of extrapyramidal side effects (particularly without the risk of tardive dyskinesis). Wander was bought by Sandoz, lost its independence and became a part of Sandoz. And a short time later information came from Finland about some observations of agranulocytosis in clozapine-treated patients. The conclusion for Sandoz was that clozapine is a dangerous drug.

Sandoz had already reached the decision that this drug they had bought with Wander should be removed from the market and its further development finished. But in Berlin, H. Helmchen and I were convinced that this step would prevent a breakthrough in antipsychotic treatment. I wrote a letter to Sandoz and finally I travelled to Basel and told them 'you must continue'. Their answer was 'but we don't believe it is effective, because Janssen's idea about neuroleptics is correct. We know clozapine has no extrapyramidal side effects and therefore it is only weakly effective and we will withdraw it'. But soon after two Sandoz representatives (H. Berde and H. Buhlmann) were persuaded of our arguments, and clozapine was given a chance to survive!

On the basis of our early investigations with chlorpromazine, perazine and other tricyclic drugs, we were able to prove that clozapine was not unique in introducing agranulocytosis. This happens with all these drugs, with a comparable frequency, and it is not only a danger with clozapine. If agranulocytosis with any of these tricyclic psychotropic drugs is diagnosed early enough a fatal outcome can be prevented. The regular monitoring of blood-picture is the basis for early diagnosis and under these conditions we were allowed in Germany and in few other countries to continue with clozapine for almost 20 years until Herb Meltzer and some other US investigators rediscovered it. Now clozapine is accepted in all countries with all its unique properties. In comparison to classical neuroleptics, it is pharmacologically 'dirty'. It has less effect on D-2 receptors, poses a very low risk of tardive dyskinesia, but it is effective in treatment-resistant schizophrenia, against negative symptomatology and it shows a very high compliance rate compared to classical neuroleptics.

Another way to read the clozapine story, which is something that the industry I guess have been unhappy with, is that they moved on a fairly coherent path from chlorpromazine through to remoxipride getting purer and purer agents and now we get a dirty drug again being better than the pure compounds. Does this say something about the nature of the illness? In a sense, it's a problem for the industry because how do you make the correct dirty drug — it's easier to purify drugs.

On the one hand, from the basic sciences point of view we have made great advances and have been able to produce drugs that are more and more selective. But on the other side the decision about which drugs should go in clinical trials should not only be taken by basic scientists and people in the pharmaceutical industry. I think there must be much more communication between pharmacologists, even the chemists, and clinicians. It should be more like it was in the pioneering days when both worked together more.

You think they worked closer then?

Oh, yes, in the 1950s, I had good, very strong and frequent contact even with the chemists. For instance, in the Ciba-Company in Basel I had close connections at this time with M. Wilhelm, a chemist, who speculated very ingeniously on connections between chemical structure and therapeutic profile of polycyclic psychotropic drugs. His publications reactivated older ideas that I had. Indeed, recently, this approach has a fascinating and promising come-back in the computerized drug design.

Apart from clozapine, nothing has really happened for almost 30 years. We've got some variations on a theme but no new themes.

I don't agree totally. I think in the meantime some new things were discovered. But I agree that in the field of antipsychotics the most important years were between 1952 and the end of the 1960s with the discovery of clozapine. Clozapine is, curiousl,y on the one side a very old drug but on the other side a very new drug. All attempts to imitate or surpass the profile of effects of clozapine, for example, with risperidone, have not so far been successful.

The situations with antidepressants is not much better. But in the last years we have registered a comeback of the monoamine oxidase inhibitors with the reversible selective MAOIs and the SSRIs are a very promising development. One area of real progress has been the development of relapse preventing drug treatment strategies. And there have been the first steps into the field of treatment in addictions and alcoholism, for example, with acamprosate.

On the other side we have to keep in mind that at the end of the 1960s and the beginning of the 1970s in most European countries the pharmaceutical industry was very irritated that the people were being informed in detail only about the dangers of psychotropic drugs and not enough on their advantages and the real progress in treatment of mental disorders. Against this background, the situation with clozapine was not easy for Sandoz. Given what happened in Finland, Sandoz deserve some praise for keeping this drug on the market in spite of all negative press and radio news on clozapine and its risks.

In similar situations we have already lost some useful and promising new drugs, as for example in the case of the antidepressant nomifensine, which was developed in Germany by Hoechst. To this day there is no substitute for nomifensine. Hoechst developed and produced it after hesitating to enter the field of psychotropic drugs. They have developed it through very good chemical, pharmacological and clinical research. They introduced it very carefully. Its presynaptic dopaminergic mechanism of action was unique. It was very well accepted, especially by patients and by general practitioners, to treat outpatients. In a very short time nomifensine became broadly used. But then there were alarming notices in the newspapers about patients who had a thrombocytopenia with it, with a fatal outcome in single cases and almost immediately it was withdrawn from the market.

Too quickly?

From my point of view too quickly. It would have been better to investigate the pathophysiology of this serious side effect with the aim of developing methods for early diagnosis to prevent fatal outcomes. There are now successors to clozapine but with nomifensine there is no successor drug – this line of development was completely stopped.

I think the problem is not that there is a dangerous side effect – we should be prepared to do anything to make the risk from dangerous side effects minimal. The problem with clozapine is not the agranulocytosis, for instance, but death by agranulocytosis. Sandoz does this exactly in the United States – they have the drug monitored in a manner that if it is handled in an appropriate manner, death should be prevented. I see this with other drugs – every year a handful of cases of agranulocytosis but the patients survive and I think that's possible.

You've touched on an issue there which is an issue you've seen develop and it has hit its peak maybe with the question of fluoxetine in the US. With fluoxetine and with diazepam before it, but especially with fluoxetine, the psychotropic drugs have entered a public domain. They've become issues of controversy . . .

In comparison to the US and the UK, I think in Germany the development of fluoxetine has been much slower. Lilly are surprised about this. They had hoped that it will be the same as in the United States.

Why do you think it has been so big there?

In the United States at the time its introduction, they had only few antidepressants and fluoxetine was introduced into an open field. In contrast, in Germany, we have too many antidepressants and therefore the introduction of fluoxetine, even with a very strong advertising activity, didn't have the same impact. In addition, in Germany, we had already the SSRI drug fluvoxamine before fluoxetine came on the market and now there is competition from other SSRIs. For these reasons fluoxetine will never be such a big product as it is in the United States.

Talking about clozapine, nomifensine and fluoxetine and just how these drugs get out into the popular culture, raises the whole question of how the public assess risk and benefit. This must be something that you've had to think about.

I think the fate of nomifensine is an example of how in the public and in the newspapers there can be such a movement against the pharmaceutical industry that the decision to withdraw the drug becomes understandable.

You said that at that time in Germany the pharmaceutical industry was looked on with a certain amount of suspicion: can I pursue that theme? The pharmaceutical industry really began in Germany and Switzerland and it's been possible in those countries for over 100 years to have a respectable career within the industry in a way that in the US and the UK it hasn't been. In the US and UK, if one moved, as a clinician or as a research scientist, over to the industry you were thought as not being a respectable scientist. So it's curious to hear that even in Germany the industry developed problems; what was happening?

I think that there was a general anti-natural sciences movement in Germany. This developed since 1968 and the student revolution, and later on with the ecological movement. For instance, you get reports about the World Congress of Social Psychiatry in many newspapers but about the CINP Congress not a word. In Germany we also have a polarization between social and biological psychiatry and that is not a good development. In the US, the basis for the development of social psychiatry was the introduction of psychotropic drugs.

But in the UK it's almost been the opposite in that the centres of excellence for social psychiatry have always been somewhat anti-drugs. Aubrey Lewis at the first CINP meeting said that if we had to choose between the industrial rehabilitation units we have, and these new drugs, we would choose the industrial rehabilitation units and, in the UK, psychopharmacology has happened outside the main scientific centres

I think in Britain, nevertheless, they were much more pragmatic. For instance, Michael Shepherd took many aggressive positions about various things but in his daily work he was much more pragmatic than comparable people in Germany. I remember his attacks against lithium and its use by psychiatrists – he was almost killing Mogen Schou but on the other hand later on he used it. It was the same with Aubrey Lewis. I think that what happened in the Maudsley at this time influenced Germany. But in Germany, in contrast to this, the polarization is not only in the discussion, but it extends to daily practice too.

In the US, there was polarization to the extent that the analysts would not prescribe drugs. There would be one doctor in the hospital who was termed the druggist, but the therapist wouldn't prescribe. Did polarization go that far in Germany?

Yes, and more. If there was a psychoanalyst as the head of the hospital, then he would not allow any drug therapy to be prescribed. In the US, there was a certain pragmatism so that at least one doctor could prescribe and the first publications about the combination of psychotherapy and drug therapy were published in the United States. In our country it's not possible. The doctors with a biological basis, if they do behavioural therapy, in combination with drug therapy, for instance, they are attacked about this and told that what they do is not real behavioural therapy because they use drugs. I think the polarisation is greater and we take more intolerant positions. We Germans are more abiding by principles than people in other parts of the world. It is a disadvantage.

Let me take you back. Why did you go on to do medicine and why did you choose psychiatry?

I don't come from a medical family. My father was a school teacher in chemistry and physics and his interest was that I should study chemistry. He was a little bit upset when at school my interest was more in biology, history and in all things which could be involved in communication with human subjects. The logical consequence was that I decided firstly to study medicine. But my father was happy when I also studied chemistry later on. After doing medicine I stayed in psychiatry, because I got caught up in the fascinating development of psychopharmacology.

One of the other intriguing things about Europe in particular, which I guess you don't find in the US so much, is that in the different European countries or regions different drugs get prescribed and there are also different nosological entities – such as vegetative dystonia in Germany and Middle Europe. George Beaumont mentioned that some time back, when he was working for Geigy, they were saying that opipramol was marvellous for vegetative dystonia, go and find out what the market would be like in the UK but there was no-one with it in the UK.

There are few issues here – one is 'vegetative dystonie', another is national differences in classification systems and diagnostic procedures and then there are national differences in prescribing psychotropic drugs such as opipramol.

Patients do not change but the diagnostic classification systems have changed tremendously, especially in the United States. At the moment, autonomic symptomatology had been neglected in some countries but in contrast to this in Germany symptoms and complaints on the basis of disturbances in the autonomic nervous system were for a long time overestimated. These differences in diagnostic procedures have led ultimately to different outcomes in treatment. I think these national differences should be subject to real research. I don't know of any results of such investigations in the past. I don't believe there is any research aimed at finding out the diagnostic categories that would be used in countries outside of Germany for patients diagnosed within Germany as having 'vegetative dystonie'. I have to concede that this German diagnostic speciality was used too frequently in my country and its definition was too vague.

The idea of vegetative dystonia came about 50 years ago in connection with intense research on the two branches of the autonomic system – the parasympathetic and sympathetic. The term became a diagnostic fashion related to speculations on the pathophysiological role of autonomic system. The fashion survived a little bit outside of Germany in the concept of 'stress' and stress-related disorders. But we should keep in mind that current speculations on the role of neurotransmitters, receptors and neuro-endocrinological regulations in general pathophysiological conceptions may in due course have the same fate as the exaggerated conception of a 'Vegetative Dystonie'.

At present, we have in the new ICD-10 classification, although not with DSM-IV, within the diagnostic class of 'somatoform disorders' a subclass of 'somatoform disorders with autonomic dysfunction' (F 45.3). Of course, that is not a nosological entity but a syndrome but it is a syndrome with a symptomatology not far removed from that of 'Vegetative Dystonie'. It's possible that we shall have with this new diagnostic term a revival of the 'Vegetative Dystonie'. I am glad about this special diagnostic subclass in the ICD-10 because patients with autonomic dysfunctions are a reality! I think it is a gap in the DSM-IV and, in relation to this, ICD-10 is superior.

Now, finally, some comments on opipramol, which is used frequently in Germany but very rarely – if at all – in other countries. A simple principle of classification of modern psychotherapeutic drugs makes distinctions between antipsychotics (neuroleptics), antidepressants, anxiolytics (tranquillizers) and relapse preventing drugs. This classification of drugs fits very well with a similar simple classification of mental disorders: schizophrenia, affective disorders and neurotic disturbances. The naive but obvious conclusion from these two three-armed classifications was a crude rule for indications of psychopharmacological treatments: one type of drugs are indicated for each class of disorders – the antipsychotics for schizophrenia, antidepressants for depression and tranquillizers for neurotic disorders. This very crude but in practice generally and successfully applied 'psychopharmacological axiom' for differential indications of psychotropic drugs urgently needs modification and differentiation.

There has been an impressive differentiation with regard to diagnostic classification with the new diagnostic systems ICD-10 and DSM-IV but as regards the differentiation of psychopharmacological agents the distinction into three classical groups lasts even now and it is dangerous for a single drug not to fit more or less exactly to one of these 'classical groups' of psychotropic drugs.

Opipramol is such a drug. Other examples are clozapine, buspirone and the benzamide derivative sulpiride. These drugs run the risk of becoming 'outsiders'. Clozapine has overcome this danger and has now a special position as an 'atypical antipsychotic' with unique qualities. Opipramol is until now in the position of an underestimated outsider.

From a chemical point of view, opipramol has characteristics both of tricyclic antidepressants – a central ring with seven atoms like imipramine – and of neuroleptics with a fluphenazine-like side chain. Its clinical profile is between antidepressants and anxiolytics. Because of the requirement to give opipramol a clear-cut position in the system of psychotropic drugs, it was recommended as a tranquillizer – as a drug with an anxiolytic and tranquillizsing profile with advantages in comparison to benzodiazepines – it has no addiction potential or muscle relaxant effect. That is true but does not define the special position of opipramol. Its widespread use in general practice can be explained by its remarkable effectiveness in syndromes which I have mentioned previously – it works in 'somatoform disorders with autonomic dysfunction' and in other kinds of somatoform disorders!

It should not therefore be integrated offhandedly together with the numerous benzodiazepines in the group of 'classical tranquillizers'. Opipramol is an 'atypical' tranquillizer and has an exceptional position – perhaps together with sulpiride. The 'atypical tranquilliser' is an 'autonomic stabilisator' and therefore useful in the treatment of (neurotic!) 'somatoform disorders'.

The rough correlation between the uses of the drugs and clinical states did something did it not to transform US psychiatry and make it Kraepelinian. You could argue that the drugs, which were introduced in two broad groups – the antipsychotics and the antidepressants – seemed to cement the Kraepelinian formulation in place up till now anyway – while the more recent emergence of treatments for OCD and delusional disorder might undo that synthesis.

Your question goes deep into the general problems of psychiatry we have already discussed. I agree with you that the discovery of new psychopharmacological treatment strategies in OCD are another contribution to the necessity to modify the simple three-armed-psychopharmacological conception. Despite being one of the successors of Kraepelin, I have expressed my doubts about the unmodified validity of Kraepelin's conception. OCD and the modern delusional disorders are a comparable problem to that of the somatoform disorders mentioned before. But I think our doubts and reservations about Kraepelin's conception is only justified regarding his early nosological system which was often overinterpreted by his *epigones*.

In the first decade of our century there was a famous scientific controversy in German psychiatry between Kraepelin and A. Hoche. Until this time all Kraepelin's efforts were directed at describing and defining nosological entities comparable to the entities of illnesses in internal medicine. Hoche was opposed to Kraepelin's concepts. He had the opinion that only psychopathological syndromes could be defined exactly. Kraepelin's position prevailed in German psychiatry and has now a worldwide revival especially in the US with the elaboration of DSM-III and DSM-IV. The provocative opposite position of Hoche with his conception that only syndromes were discernible was for a long time almost forgotten. At present Hoche is only remembered because he has published in 1920, together with Binding (a professor of law), a book which was used after 1933 by the Nazis to justify their programme of sterilization by force, and finally the killing of mental patients.

But while DSM-III and IV are interpreted in our time as a revival of Kraepelin in the USA, some elements of Hoche's position are integrated also in the DSM classification systems. Axis-1 of the DSM-IV is a combination of nosological and symptomatical operationalized categories. After the controversies with Hoche, Kraepelin was influenced through Hoche's conception – more than he himself was aware of. In his last years he has recommended as the starting point for a diagnostic process two aspects of the illness: the precise description of symptomatology (ie syndrome) *and* the life-long course of the illness.

My position, after more than 40 years experiences as a clinician is more and more inclining to Hoche's conception – or better expressed – to the conception of Kraepelin after 1910, into which several of the ideas of Hoche were integrated. If I were asked to propose a new principal construction for DSM-V, I would have five new axes:

—Axis-I: (Description of) *psychopathological symptomatology*(syndrome) (an axis 'purified' of nosological terms and speculations)
—Axis-II: (Description of) *course of the illness*
—Axis-III: (Description of) *personality of the patient*
—Axis-IV (Description of) *social surroundings*
—Axis-V: Enumeration of evident (and supposed) *etiological and influencing factors* (from somatic factors to biographical and social determinants registered in Axis-III and IV)

In this figment of my mind, this dream, axes-I – IV are pure descriptive dimensions; only axis-V is an etiological and interpretative dimension. Finally the overview of all five axes is a clinical diagnosis! I have said – this is my dream for the future, but you may register my sympathy for such a conception of multiaxial diagnostic classification as introduced by US psychiatry! The DSMs represent real progress in psychiatry and I regret that the chance of a multiaxial diagnostic classification was missed with the ICD-10.

If axis-I were established as a pure syndromatical axis, then we would also come to a new description of the differential indications of psychotropic drugs to treat patients. The choice and decisions on 'the right drug for the right patient' would be done regarding the symptomatology (axis-I) and the course (axis-II) without neglecting the etiological axis.

Such an unconventional idea would also influence basic research in psychiatry. At present our biochemical, physiological and molecular biological research is directed and orientated on more or less precisely defined nosological entities. This approach presupposes a specific coherence between etiological factors and nosologically defined disorder. Such a concept, for example, in biochemical investigations of schizophrenia, means that the object of research is the dopamine system only or in depression it is the 5–HT or the noradrenaline system only, and in anxiety states, the GABA system only.

I think it is necessary for us to move on from these approaches which presuppose that specific disturbances of only one transmitter system should be the etiology of one disorder. In the new approach, for example, the 5-HT system could be investigated in various disorders such as depressions, OCD, eating disorders, etc.

So, if the major entities break down, what will the rational basis for giving drugs to people be other than giving it to them on an empirical kind of basis and seeing if this drug works for that person?

The revival of the old concept of 'target' symptoms of Freyhan.

Tell me more about Freyhan. A number of people have mentioned him. Why was he important?

Freyhan was a German emigrant in 1939 from Berlin. He has had a comparable kind of development as Heinz Lehmann. They came to the United States and Canada respectively after they had already studied medicine; both were in their middle 20s.

Freyhan worked very early together with Seymour Kety and made investigations on the bloodflow in the brain. Kety was already a distinguished pharmacologist, Freyhan was a clinician responsible in these investigations. The publications together with Kety made him well known. Some years later with the introduction of chlorpromazine in USA, Freyhan was one of the first investigators of these new drugs in the United States, while at the same time Lehmann has introduced chlorpromazine in Canada.

Kalinowsky and Freyhan were good personal friends. Kalinowsky, Freyhan and Lehmann all came back to Europe very early after the war, visited German universities and stimulated younger people to go into psychiatry to do research in this field. From this time on I had very good contact with Freyhan. In contrast to the majority of his American colleagues, he knew all the old German psychiatry literature; he knew Kraepelin and K. Schneider and Jaspers. On the basis of this knowledge of the literature and with his experience in psychiatric research in USA, Freyhan described the concept of 'target symptoms'. He has explained that we need a double accounting system ('doppelte Buchfuhrung') if we treat schizophrenic patients with neuroleptic drugs. In the evolution of Freyhan's publications, in the 1950s the prescription of neuroleptics was orientated on nosological diagnoses only. But then, very early, he said that it should not be on the nosological entity alone, but in combination with the target symptomatology that the decision for the differential use of drugs should be made.

What were the target symptoms for the antidepressants?

Of course in the first place the target symptom of antidepressants is depressive mood.

For the field of depressive disorders P. Kielholz picked up the concept of target symptoms of F. Freyhan. They met at a conference in Montreal (1959) and since that time a personal friendship and close exchange of knowledge and ideas developed. Kielholz suggested that there is not only one target symptom to recognize in the treatment of depressive disorders. He defined a combination of two or more target symptoms which should be the basis for the use of particular antidepressants (depressive mood, reduced or increased motoric activity, disturbances of sleep, somatic complaints, etc.).

Does Donald Klein's concept of anhedonia fit this bill?

Yes, I agree, anhedonia should be recognized as an important target symptom. It is a nosological target symptom. It has a nosological neutral position and therefore it is a typical target symptom, which may be too a very good starting point for the choice of a particular drug in treatment. The accentuation of anhedonia is not the only merit of Donald Klein. His investigations on atypical depression and anxiety states are meanwhile fundamental elements for differential approaches in pharmacological treatment.

In the past, all anxiety states were treated in my country with benzodiazepines. Now we have in drug treatment of anxiety a clear-cut distinction of the choice of the most promising drug if we consider not only the syndrome (anxiety) but the course of the anxiety disorder too. Meanwhile benzodiazepines are used only in therapy of anxiety states with a chronic course (generalized anxiety). in patients with more or less short but time-restricted manifestations of anxiety (panic attacks) the treatment must be carried out with MAO-inhibitors or imipramine. The differential approaches to the treatment of anxiety states is also a good example of the need to consider not only the target symptoms but the course of the illness too.

Do we really have drugs which have an effect on the course of an illness?

Yes, we have but in the classical field of drug treatments in psychiatry we need more therapeutics with an effect on the course of an illness. Lithium, carbamazepine and valproic acid are the first drugs working against periodical manifestations of mental disorders (unipolar depressions, bipolar psychosis, schizoaffective psychosis). this principle has to be expanded. It should be investigated if these already known drugs are effective in periodical manifestations of other syndromes (for example, obsessive syndromes, anxiety syndromes).

Lithium and carbamazepine belong together. Carbamazepine is a fascinating drug. Regarding the chemical constitution, carbamazepine is very similar to all tricyclic psychotropic drugs, but it was developed in epilepsy. Later carbamazepine was found to be useful in trigeminal attacks. And now as a third quality the mood stabilizing effect was discovered. What are the common elements of mood disorders, epilepsy and trigeminal attacks? – it's their course, whether on the one side it is more or less short attacks and on the other side longer waves of mood swing. And therefore I believe that the usefulness of this drug in such different disorders is not an accident. Carbamazepine is a drug which influences the course of an illness with manifestations and intervals.

Another point is that a special therapeutic property of clozapine is its effect against chronification. For the future we need drugs comparable to clozapine active against chronicity and which prevent the progressive course of an illness, especially schizophrenia.

All these ideas are speculations only – but from my point of view speculations are the first step in the direction of discoveries.

Select bibliography
Jaspers, K. (1965) *General Psychopathology* (trans. M. Hamilton and J. Heany), Munich University Press, Munich.

9 Hannah Steinberg

Bridging the gap: psychology, pharmacology and after

By the time of first CINP meeting you had been in psychopharmacology for some time. Can you tell me how you came into it, what you were doing and who you were working with?

My being at the Rome meeting was somewhat to my surprise. I had been in touch with various people who knew of our work, including several Americans, such as Joel Elkes at Johns Hopkins and Jonathan Cole, at the Psychopharmacology Service Centre in Bethesda. I also knew British and European pharmacologists, psychologists and psychiatrists. And so I received an invitation.

Like many people in those days, I came to psychopharmacology in a fairly haphazard way. I had a BA degree in psychology and wanted more science training. I consulted the Professor of Pharmacology at University College London, whom I knew through music, Frank Winton. He was a former Cambridge physiologist and, unusually, an early member of the Institute of Psychoanalysis, and so had an interest in things psychological. He suggested that I should join his department. I said 'oh I don't know anything about drugs', but he laughed and said that I could teach them English in return. I had won a University of London postgraduate studentship in psychology with which I could do a PhD in almost any London Department that would have me. After a lot of heart-searching I did what he suggested.

To begin with it was very lonely because hardly anybody else was working in the field. Frank suggested that I should work on nitrous oxide – laughing gas. So I began by working with humans. In retrospect this seems to have been a brave thing to do. I gave student volunteers and colleagues concentrations of nitrous oxide between 20–40% in oxygen. These doses were relatively small and I tried to establish whether N_2O impaired the performance of cognitive and motor tasks according to their relative complexity – it did (Steinberg, 1954). And also whether N_2O behaved like sleep and could be used to improve memory and to test the interference theory of forgetting – it could (Steinberg and Summerfield, 1957). This is again of scientific interest today because of current research on implicit learning. The memory experiments, done in collaboration with Arthur Summerfield had a high media profile because the *Daily Express* summarized them under the heading 'Alcohol is good for the memory' which went the rounds as far as the *New York Times* and the radio in South Africa and Canada. One of the *London Evening Standard*'s leader journalists reported finding it easier to memorize her shopping list if she had a quick nip after breakfast. I was mortified by the brash publicity, whereas in today's climate it would have been proper to feel gratified. I also collaborated with Roger Russell, Professor of Psychology at University College London, to show that N_2O could reduce experimentally induced 'stress' (by setting subjects a difficult task, an insoluble problem), much like alcohol. Again, stress reduction has become a big topic today.

I had some interesting subjects for my N_2O pilot experiments, for example, the biologist J.B.S. Haldane. He thought that he would fail all the cognitive tests but found the experiments valuable because he compared the effects of N_2O with those of simulated submarine experiments and anoxia in which he had been involved during the war. Nitrous oxide had a vogue during the 1960s and 1970s, when youngsters were supposed to sit around at parties with little canisters strapped to their backs and taking a sniff whenever they thought they needed cheering up. But some experimental subjects did not like the sensations. Have you had it?

No.

It can make one feel rather abnormal, rhythmical and overwhelmingly 'drunk'. I obviously had to try it out myself several times and didn't like it at all. But nitrous oxide is of interest again now because it is in the atmosphere and we seem to have small concentrations in our bodies, and so it might well have slight effects on people's behaviour at times. As well as the drunk feeling it also changed the perception of time.

A scientist whose encouragement meant a good deal to me was J. H., later, Sir John Gaddum who was Professor of Pharmacology at Edinburgh and then Head of the Babraham ARC Research Institute. He asked me to compose a few pages on psychological methods of studying psychoactive drugs for his textbook. I remember once complaining to him that this was such lonely work and that a lot of the time I didn't know what I was doing and he said 'No, no, you must carry on. Finding out about the brain as you are doing is the most important gap left in biology'. Gradually, of course, I was able to work with various interesting collaborators.

By the time I got to the CINP in Rome I was on the staff of the Pharmacology Department at UCL, which for a psychologist was unusual.

You were one of the first academics to be designated a psychopharmacologist. When did they create the post for you?

I was made a reader in psychopharmacology in the University of London in 1962. It was the first university title in psychopharmacology in Western Europe I think and probably the USA too. There were laboratories of psychopharmacology springing up in the States then, but not academic posts as far as I know. We early psychopharmacologists were busily 'networking' and great friends, and I remember trying to explain to my American colleagues what this quaint title of a 'Reader' meant. In 1970 I became the first Professor of Psychopharmacology.

In the 1960s our main research work became known as 'Purple Hearts'. By chance it coincided with a wave of popular interest. I was asked to contribute a chapter to Clarke's *Applied Pharmacology*, and Andrew Wilson, one of the authors, said 'Please do the barbiturates and I wish somebody would find out what these mixtures do'. I said 'what mixtures?', because I really didn't know much about them and he said 'mixtures with amphetamines'. The best known of these was a proprietory preparation called 'Drinamyl'; the tablets were mauve and vaguely heartshaped and scored down the middle.

So my collaborator Ruth Rushton and I gave small doses of barbiturates to hooded rats, who seemed to like them. Their locomotor activity was stimulated by them, which in those days was an unusual finding, since barbiturates, like alcohol, were officially regarded only as CNS depressants. One day we added a small dose of amphetamine to the barbiturate. To our astonishment this produced an enormous potentiation of spontaneous motor activity in the rats. At first we didn't believe it but then we had to because it happened again and again (Rushton and Steinberg, 1963) and other investigations in a variety of experimental contexts found similar potentiating effects. It also worked in man since amphetamine–barbiturate combinations produced a better mood and also slightly better performance of simple tasks than the separate ingredients in students (Steinberg *et al.*, 1988). There was good agreement between dose ratios that worked well in rats and mice and those used in man, especially 1 mg/kg dexamphetamine and 6.5 mg/kg amylobarbitone by weight – which was in fact the Drinamyl ratio which was fairly widely used to help mildly anxious and/or depressed people, especially, it was said, bored housewives. Just about then it was discovered by teenagers to produce 'high moods', especially if mixed with alcohol.

We constructed 'isobol' diagrams (from the Greek *isos*, 'equal' and *bolos*, 'effect') which enabled one to read off equi-active dose combinations, illustrating the agreement between optimum dose ratios in rat, mouse and human. We extended this to other drugs, including benzodiazepines combined with amphetamine, which produced even more pronounced motor activity. Recently we were able to use the Cambridge University computer (all of it for 10 minutes, so that we had to work at midnight) to construct high resolution 3-dimensional isobols in colour.

There were many opportunities to lecture abroad, including at Smith-Kline and French in Philadelphia, where drugs had first been combined to produce Drinamyl. We tried to find out just how they had hit on the particular drugs, doses and dose ratios. Was it just good luck or that there was some special kind of logic. In Philadelphia I met one of the people who had been involved in putting together the two drugs. Apparently what had happened was that the Chairman of the company wanted something relaxing, but not too relaxing, so he put together the smallest marketed tablet of dexamphetamine, which was 5 mg, and the smallest marketed tablet of amylobarbitone, 0.5 grain or 32.5 mg, and that gave this ratio of 1:6.5. So it was really pretty lucky that that turned out to be the best mix. It took us some time to find the best amphetamine chlordiazepoxide combination, and, interestingly, the ingredient dose of dexamphetamine was about the same as with amylobarbitone. It is a pity that amphetamine is no longer much used medically but these combinations remain of scientific and heuristic interest. It seems that combinations of drugs in all kinds of fields, as far apart as cancer and HIV, can achieve better therapeutic effects than single drugs, and this relatively under-investigated phenomenon probably has a big future.

The problem of drug interactions has really pursued me through my career. Our recent work with benzodiazepine/antidepressant combinations and backward walking in mice was again an example of the surprises one can get when one works with mixtures. Elizabeth Sykes, Christine Davis, Claire Stanford and I combined clenbuterol, which is a beta-adrenoceptor agonist and a potential antidepressant, with chlordiazepoxide – in the hope that the combination would lift locomotor activity to some extent, as we had found with amphetamine and chlordiazepoxide. Instead, we got spectactular and prolonged backward walking. The mice walked backwards energetically, for many minutes at a time (Steinberg et al., 1988). This has developed into an effective and simple potential screening test for antidepressants and anxiolytics which we are hoping that an enterprising industry may take up.

Backwards walking mice were reported first in connection with opiates, LSD and mescaline, and some people have suggested that backward walking is really a hallucination of sliding down a hill; if you believe that you are sliding down a hill you would push back with your front paws to stop yourself, and the effect would be to walk backwards. Whether that applies to humans is doubtful, but might be worth investigating.

The only human backward walking we have traced is in connection with Parkinson's disease where it occasionally happens. Apparently patients cannot help walking backwards and when they reach a wall, they press their back into it. The mouse backward walking also happens with combinations of salbutamol and chlordiazepoxide, and it seems possible that some asthmatics who take benzodiazepines get a kick out of their Ventolin inhalers which are very popular. There must however be many people who are co-prescribed antidepressants and benzodiazepines. It might well be worth while studying the combinations deliberately in humans.

Fascinating.

In the 1960s our amphetamine-barbiturate work led to a time of great activity. University College provided accommodation, and together with Professor Arthur Summerfield at Birkbeck College, we got grants from NIMH, which made a huge difference to our progress. Grant seeking is now the order of the day, but then it was still unusual and we felt both pioneering and slightly apologetic that we had more money than other people. But of course nearly all went on salaries. We tended to use simple equipment, such as Y-mazes, hole boards and activity cages, and so our expenditure on equipment was modest. Most of our results were obtained by scoring methods which depended on visual inspection which with experience became very accurate, with high inter-observer reliability but were labour intensive. For example, we developed a simple but accurate method for drug-induced 'ataxia' using measures of footprints. And of course we had no PCs or photocopiers in the 1960s.

Who were the principal people who influenced you at this time?

Well, there was Gaddum and Andrew Wilson who became Professor in Liverpool and who was one of the first clinical pharmacologists in the UK. Roger Russell was here from the USA and we published together. He was a great innovation for this country because he was the first animal psychologist who headed a department. Bill Paton, who became Professor of Pharmacology at Oxford and had discovered hexamethonium with Nora Zaimis, was another. Arthur Summerfield at UCL, who was a very systematic expert at experimental design and statistics, was another. With him I did most of the N_2O memory experiments. He became Professor of Psychology at Birkbeck College.

Then there was Daphné Joyce, also at Birkbeck, who collaborated with us some of the time; her early work on 5-HT has become a classic. Dick Joyce, who was at the London Hospital Medical School, where he did human experiments on, for example, drugs versus dummies; he has been working in Switzerland for years now. Michael Chance was an ethologist at Birmingham who worked with drugs, and Paul Silverman wrote an ethologically orientated book on psychopharmcology, *Animal Behaviour in the Laboratory*, which deserves to be better known.

Channi Kumar from Cambridge and Ian Stolerman from the School of Pharmacy came later as PhD students and worked particularly on drug dependence in rodents, and Roger Porsolt was with Daphné Joyce up the road at Birkbeck and now heads a commercial psychopharmacology laboratory in Paris. David Sanger was a postgraduate student at UCL with us for two years. Michael Besser, a rather grand endocrinologist and now Professor of Medicine at Barts, worked on drug combinations with us, which was particularly helpful because he had access to medical subjects and of course lots of endocrinological know-how. Milos Krsiak, now

Professor of Pharmacology at the Charles University, Prague, spent a year with us and started interesting experiments on how the behaviour of drugged rats could 'rub off' on that of their undrugged partners. There was a great spread of people and skills. I also learnt a lot from many colleagues in the Medical Sciences Faculty at UCL, especially Sir Andrew Huxley, Bob Simmons and Donald Jenkinson, as well as from many pharmacologists, psychologists, psychiatrists and statisticians in and outside the College, and of course Americans, all too numerous to mention, except perhaps for special friends like Murray Jarvik, Gerry Klerman, Conan Kornetsky, Len Cook and Peter Dews.

One of the most important people early on was my collaborator Ruth Rushton who had been a GP but who joined us and was an excellent experimenter. The rat experiments were exacting and minutely timed, and usually three of us would need to get together to do them. We also had a splendid technician called Marian Dorr who married one of my PhD students, David Katz; David was one of the first to show how the social context could affect reactions to morphine. Philip Harrison-Read now a successful psychiatrist with a special research interest in lithium was also of that generation.

Much later I collaborated with Elizabeth Sykes who had done classical work with John Smythies in Edinburgh on structure – activity relationships of mescaline in rats in the hope of locating the hallucinagenic fraction of the molecule. She and I had many discussions during the period when people were trying to make experimental sense of the hallucinogens. Nora Zaimis, by then Professor of Pharmacology at the Royal Free, gave LSD and mescaline to day—old chicks and demonstrated that they almost immediately behaved oddly.

Philip Bradley, who was Professor of Pharmacology at Birmingham, was influential, as was Michael Shepherd, a Professor of Psychiatry at the Maudsley. They and I did not actually collaborate, but we discussed many topics and problems over the years and contributed to symposia and other meetings.

What was the feeling about what all this work might actually reveal? Did you have a feeling that this was a new frontier? Merton Sandler for instance talks about having been in the area for years without having realized that it was a new area but you seem more clearly to have been aware that it was a new area right from the start?

Yes and no. It was certainly new to me. But I did know what German scientists like Kraepelin had done, and I did know that there had been Grace Eggleton at UCL, a physiologist, who had shown before the war in a rudimentary but correct way, that the same blood concentration of alcohol was more potent if the concentration was increasing than decreasing, and if it was increasing quickly rather than slowly, which are useful principles to bear in mind. So I knew that there had been isolated antecedents but I also believed that what my collaborators and I were discovering was new, and I found drugs and their power and of course the discovery of new ones intensely interesting.

Between 1962 and 1974 when the BAP began what were the main forums for you to talk about your work?

We gave papers or took part in symposia on aspects of our work at many different societies. For example, there was the Association for the Study of Animal Behaviour for whom some of the rat exploratory behaviour work was relevant. The British Pharmacological Society was very welcoming throughout. Two symposia under the auspices of the Biological Council and the British Pharmacological Society had me as secretary, and I edited the proceedings, jointly with the Ciba Foundation in one case. Both these books, *Animal Behaviour and Drug Action* in 1964 and *The Scientific Basis of Drug Dependence* in 1969 became well known. I saw copies of them on students' desks in the States which was a surprise since I had no idea how far anybody in the USA read what we wrote in the UK. The British Psychological Society and the RSM also invited us to take part in Symposia, as did the Biochemical Society, International Congresses of Psychology and the CINP. I even gave a paper to a special meeting of the British Adlerian Society and at various other somewhat unexpected bodies, as well as talks at many pharmaceutical companies, research institutes and universities and colleges in the UK, the USA and Europe. Though hard work, this kept one's mind elastic and one exchanged ideas with a great variety of students and experts. Once you have got your own specialist society, this can confine you a bit and you need to make greater efforts to keep outside contacts.

A point you made earlier is that you think that in the early years because you all knew each other, and got on well, it was possible to get things done. What impact do you think the sheer scale of things now has on development?

It seems to me that sometimes quality has not been as good and findings have not been as novel. It is much easier to produce novelty when there is not yet a huge corpus of findings, as there is now. Sometimes now, when I listen to communications I find myself thinking, well it is good for you people to have done this work, but if you had made a few searches and read a few papers you would have found that this particular point has been discovered before. On the other hand, young scientists profit from repeating and checking their elders' work, and this is one of the best ways of learning.

Also nowadays, with such a large psychopharmacology population it is almost inevitable that there are people who are 'in' and other people who are 'out', and those who are in speak in symposia and get kudos and the rest feel excluded. And so you sometimes hear the same people going over more or less similar ground. Many things do of course need to be said more than once, but I also think that people have become less willing to talk informally about current work and ideas because of our intensely competitive climate. Priority seems to be vital these days. Everybody struggles to fulfil targets and justify themselves. These problems can also arise with industrial collaboration. But there are examples where open exchange of views and information have worked to everyone's advantage.

When the BAP was born you were one of the most prominent non-clinical people, the only non-clinical person on Council?

Yes. That was also a bit of an accident. I saw the foundation announcement in the BMJ and went along, and someone from the floor (I think it was Paul Silverman) proposed my name, and there was a ballot and I got elected. Then I realized that other people felt that it should all have been organised differently. I was surprised at the strength of feeling, but strange things can happen when new societies are formed in a new area; many people want to be involved. In the end it was all sorted out. In a sense I suppose that most societies start with a group of friends.

You mentioned secrecy. What role do you think industry has had on the development of psychopharmacology?

Mixed. The unique advantage of industry is of course that scientists get exciting new drugs to work with, backed by big resources if success is in the offing. Sometimes you can find someone in industry, as we have done more than once, who is interested and the time is right for them – you can do very well then. They support you financially and give you your head. Maybe you won't get very much feedback from them but it does not matter because you can do the work and publish it and they can use what they want of it and they do. For example, we had excellent collaboration over a number of years with the late Maurice Shapiro who was research director at Ward Blenkinsop later taken over by a big German company. A drug, a benzodioxane, which was being tested as a centrally acting muscle relaxant, had been found by accident to increase mounting behaviour in male rats and we were asked to investigate. We were able to confirm this increase in mounting in otherwise sexually fairly inactive male rats and Professor Ian Russell at the MRC Unit at UCL found that the drug produced erections for several hours in singly housed male monkeys.

It was decided that I should test the drug more extensively in monkeys. I managed to arrange facilities in the primate station of a high prestige American university. So, armed with my white powder and a carefully-phrased technical memorandum, I set off to test pairs of 'pigtails' (*M. nemestrina*) for sexual activity, precisely defined. Despite the fact that only highly potent male monkeys were available, who presumably exhibited a ceiling effect, there was no doubt that it was an interesting and powerful drug. Immediately after being given the drug the male monkeys showed marked muscle relaxation. This wore off after a few minutes and they became active, cooperative and helpful, even allowing the females to help themselves to raisins before they did – which was unheard of in undrugged males.

This lack of aggression seemed to us even more interesting than the subsequent sexual stimulation, but the German company felt that a sexual stimulant with potential use in man was too risky and the project came to an end. For years afterwards we received enquiries from interested scientists and practitioners about the drug, and I suspect that if work on it were resumed now, it might be a great success. Drugs that reduce aggression are of at least as much interest as drugs that stimulate male sexual behaviour, and this drug apparently does both!

Apart from a few people in the early days psychologists have been .very reluctant to go anywhere near drugs at all – as though that would compromise them.

I'm not sure that I entirely agree that psychologists have been reluctant. I seem to remember that in the early days almost anybody who was interested came to meetings and collaborated in research and there were a number of psychologists in this country who worked with drugs. Nowadays there are, quite rightly, ethical guidelines for giving drugs to human volunteers or to animals, including rodents, but this has also increased expense and hassle and deterred some institutions and individuals, as of course has the occasional bad press and drug misuse.

In terms of the first CINP meeting or two, what were the issues that come back to you as being important?

One of the main administrative issues I suppose was who was going to be on the committee and run the show and how different nationalities and disciplines could be fairly represented. The main scientific issues centred around drugs and schizophrenia, in the broadest possible sense: neuroleptics, comparisons with other methods of treatment, psychotomimetics and their role as tools for research, different methodologies and approaches. In the index of the first CINP Proceedings book, the largest number of entries was under 'chlorpromazine' with reserpine, LSD and serotonin not far behind. There was also growing interest in instituting research collaboration between different countries and disciplines. There were quite considerable communication difficulties, partly language and partly ethos. For example I was by then working with both animals and humans and that was considered by some colleagues very unusual and undoable. And when they had a discussion panel, on the whole people gave mini-papers rather than discussed. I was sitting on the platform waiting to say my piece when I had a note from Joel Elkes, the chairman, saying something like 'do please discuss and do not give a paper, we'd be very grateful'. So I discussed and was praised by Aubrey Lewis. Aubrey Lewis was another influence. He was rather terrifying.

Why?

He was Mr British Psychiatry and had a formidable reputation. I knew him semi-socially through work and he was always very interesting to talk to. But I gather that, for example, there was a famous Saturday morning journal club at the Maudsley which he ran and which made everybody who had to give a talk very nervous.

You mentioned Joel Elkes. People seem to be split on whether he was important or not. Some say that he was because of the enthusiasm and ideas he brought to things, what's your impression?

He certainly was very skilled and helpful at meetings. I am still in touch with him now. His work with Philip Bradley on LSD quickly became well known. I think he was actually a nice sort of outgoing person who had many ideas and at the CINP meetings we had in Washington and elsewhere, he was very much a presence.

What did you make of Max Hamilton? He seems to have influenced the field at two or three distinct points. He came in with the rating scale in the 1960s and came back as the BAP President.

I don't quite know why he was president of so many organizations because basically he was not an institutional type at all. But he was willing to give quite firm opinions on subjects such as how constitutions should be worded or how high subscriptions should be. Of course the Hamilton Depression Scale became very well known. Maybe people were grateful to have someone definite even if they disagreed with him. When organizations are being set up it needs someone who says loudly and clearly how things ought to be. Max was also involved in the foundation of the European College of Psychopharmacology.

Looking back at some of your early work on nitrous oxide, one of the striking things for me about this is that you were aware of Kraepelin's earlier psychopharmacology work. It shows an interest in history that is unusual.

Well, we had to find decent references for our own work and he was one of the first psychopharmacologists. I went to the Wellcome Library and looked out what I could of the early work. I remember that he described a test of manual dexterity which involved threading needles under the influence of caffeine. The interest in history was partly due to the training of Sir Cyril Burt. We realized that Germany was a strong source in the early beginnings because Burt was very scholarly. That's really how I came across Kraepelin; I don't know why so few people know about him. Then there were hallucinogens.

As in mescaline?

Yes, there's a long history of mescaline that goes back to about the 17th or the 18th century. I had a big bibliography on this. That was probably one of the earliest psychoactive drugs apart from alcohol and opiates. Opiates are particularly interesting at the moment because of the link with endorphins. To begin with I kept well away from the huge, complex and largely biochemical literature on endorphins but they have turned out tremendously appealing. Some people think it rather miraculous that we should make our own opiates but to me it seems quite natural. After all, we make our own adrenaline and 5-HT, and so why was it such a sensation?

Any thoughts?

I don't know. At the time, 1975, we went off and bought *Nature* and there was the first article. When I looked at it later in the College library most of the page had been worn away by numerous thumbs. To us it was particularly interesting because we knew Kosterlitz and Hughes, although not well. Kosterlitz had been host at a symposium on opiates in which I took part a few years before. It's not so amazing, though, that painkillers should be made in the brain. Would you be surprised if LSD were found in the brain?

After the discovery of endogenous opiates, no, but that was really the watershed and the question is why did it cause such surprise? It made sense of pharmacology in a way that a compound like LSD – a fairly exotic compound, alien to the brain – didn't.

Well, is it?

Perhaps not, but until opiates were actually found in the brain you had people like Jaspers and so on talking about drugs like mescaline in terms of them being poisons. After the discovery of the endorphins, drugs were not quite the same poisons – they are actually there in us to begin with so you're not actually corrupting some spiritually pure thing. You are altering the balance.

Altering the balance. I think that's actually the most useful way to look at it – to say that one is altering the balance or improving or restoring the balance. It is a better approach than expecting a particular drug to do one particular thing exclusively.

Now that one knows more about the brain, it makes more sense to look at it as a highly complex and constantly shifting network. It may be unrealistic to expect one single drug, unless, it is a multi—faceted drug, to 'cure' something. Whatever you administer you may disturb something else as well. The drug companies on the whole don't like that concept.

But, for example, if there had been more discussion about what used to be called 'autopharmacology', something like the endorphins would not have been such a sensation – when you think about it, it becomes fairly obvious that all sorts of substances we call 'drugs'' are actually variants of naturally occurring endogenous substances.

Autopharmacology is not a term you find around much really.

It is not in every textbook but it was in some (Greek *autos* = 'self'). Often it is words that determine what happens. I can give you an example from our own work. We published a paper on drug dependence in rats who were used to drinking solutions from a bottle. The paper was called 'Development of morphine dependence in rats: lack of effect of previous ingestion of other drugs' (Stolerman, *et al.*, 1971). We asked whether rats, given the opportunity to drink amphetamine or benzodiazepine solutions would become dependent on these drugs and would then more easily become morphine addicts. And the answer was no. There was no connection at all. Now, in the USA, there was something called 'the stepping stone theory' which says just that. You graduate from cannabis to heroin. If we had called this paper 'The Stepping Stone Theory Rejected' instead of the boring title we gave it.

You'd have had much more citations . . .

. . .

and more impact.

I'm sure you're right. Some people coin the right phrase. People like Tim Crow with Type One and Type Two Schizophrenia, which is all wrong, but the marketing principle works. Merton Sandler had the same point that he and Michael Pare in effect produced the amine theories of depression seven years before Schildkraut but they didn't quite call it something catchy like the catecholamine theory of depression. Now you began working on humans with compounds such as nitrous oxide but later moved onto animal work. Why the change from human to animal?

I think in those days animal work, especially rodent work, was regarded as much more basic than work with humans. It was 'real' science. One felt it was more controllable than experiments with human subjects, and of course much of experimental psychology was based on rodent behaviour and so there was good background information, and one could test many more mice and rats than humans in the same time and devise ingenious animal models. To begin with our animal work was very restricted because we had little equipment and used semi–naturalistic methods of testing, which was actually good. They were very gentle and meaningful situations for the animals.

Could you argue that to some extent that the animal work today is less sensitive because we have these high powered animal houses and people have lost a feel for animal ethology?

I would agree with that. Some current work seems to me too mechanical and routine and probably doesn't tell us much about animals or about drug effects. It may tell us something about underlying processes but even then I'm not sure about that. But there was a lot of pigeon pecking and rat bar-pressing at that earlier time that was in many respects not much more sensitive.

You mentioned Roger Russell as one of the people who helped to develop animal work.

He not only developed animal work; he set up the laboratory and enabled the rest of us to have this facility. Until one actually works there one does not realize how much work it is to get an animal lab going. The work I did with Roger was actually human work. But he had set up a small animal lab at UCL with Ralph Watson as a permanent member of staff and he and I were able to show that male rats stopped growing if you changed their habitat, for example, their home cage, but if one restored the normal environment they started to grow again. This paper was listed by the Royal Society in its recommendations for implementing in the Home Office Act in 1986 (Steinberg and Sykes, 1985).

So, you're saying that before, possibly, the middle 1950s it would have been quite rare for any pharmacology department to have much in the line of an animal house for . . .

For behaviour work. There were many animal houses for medical sciences but not for behaviour studies. Roger Russell set up behaviour laboratories, first at the Maudsley and then at University College where it started with just two small rooms in a basement. It was said that the space had been condemned as a book bindery but it was all right for psychologists and rats.

What kind of things did you hope to tease out with the animal work?

We devised 'animal models' which mimicked in some simple way what happens to human subjects. For example, we subjected rats to mild and simple forms of 'stress', such as changing their environment or diet and gave drugs to see whether they would reduce the effects of stress, measured mostly by loss of body weight. Both chlorpromazine and alcohol reduced the weight loss effect. This was a simple and useful measure. We also measured blood sugar and again the drugs reduced blood sugar rises in response to stress.

In the late 1950s there would have been people who were using animals to test what the drugs did in the brain and you also had people working with animals and their behaviour per se, but was there anyone before you interested in the actual impact of drugs on animal behaviour? I can't imagine there were terribly many.

No, there weren't many. I suppose Roger Russell, although drugs were not his main theme. There was Malouka Khairy – she was Egyptian. She worked in the UCL animal lab and did work with dieldrin and showed it did impair muscular performance. Ralph Watson who was in charge of the laboratory often collaborated with me at the time. Gradually most of the major psychology departments in this country established animal laboratories and many of them worked with drugs.

If one tries to get a picture of how over the years psychopharmacology has developed, it probably is still as it was at the start, with scientists and practitioners trying mutually to reinforce each others' skills. It is one of the strengths of the BAP that it continues to bring them together. When I started out I had many contacts with psychoanalysts and psychotherapists and used to listen to their papers and try to work out how one could transform their statements into experiments. It was not always easy.

In the early days, looking at the question of drugs and how they may be used to actually investigate behaviour, Eysenck was a big name . . .

Yes. He wrote a book called *Experiments with Drugs* in 1963. It was very much linked with his theories of personality – stimulant and depressant drugs causing opposite effects – later expanded to include parallels between the effects of different drugs and personality type, some of which have stood the test of time.

Was this work eclipsed because of the cloud over LSD made it seem like a bad idea to give drugs to healthy volunteers? People like Gordon Claridge, for instance, pursued Eysenck's work through the early 1970s and then it stopped. But you don't really hear of Eysenck's theories being conclusively disproved?

I do not think that Eysenck's ideas were dependent on LSD. Since that time we have had to come to terms with the fact that drugs which act on the CNS mostly have highly complex actions. It has also progressively become more difficult to do experiments with human volunteers for justified ethical and practical reasons. LSD did have an impact partly because its effects could be spectactular and because people used it illegally. It slowly became realized that it was not a safe drug to play around with, and Sandoz stopped making it.

One did hear awful anecdotes such as people throwing themselves out of windows under the impression that they could fly. It works in very small ·amounts, thousands of a milligram, which is pharmacologically interesting because it suggests a naturally occurring substance, but this makes it extremely poweful and far too risky to use. In addition to the general ethical tightening up on human experiments more and more substances are now available, and experimenters cannot really try them out on themselves as they used to.

Are you saying that during the late 1950s and 1960s you or anyone else working in the field would try out most of the things themselves?

Yes, if one worked with volunteers such as medical students, or at least be willing to. And that is partly why I never worked with LSD because I would not take it. At one time as you know it was thought that it might give special insights into psychotic behaviour.

So what happened to Eysenck's approach. He was an invited speaker at one or two of the early CINP meetings.

He was certainly at a symposium in Bonn where he and I spoke and even argued on the same platform, but I think this was an International Congress of Psychology. How far his way of looking at drugs in terms of a theory of stimulation and depression and personality types, and what this meant personality and brain-wise ever fitted into the mainstream of thinking, is hard to say, though this does not mean that he was wrong. On the whole, receptor and neurotransmitter ways of thinking are very remote from human behaviour ways of thinking. Silvio Garattini mentioned recently that in his opinion there was still a big gap between what drugs did clinically and what they ought to do according to their biochemistry, and that it was still possible to talk about these two aspects quite separately. People sometimes drag in receptors because they feel that it is expected of them and it makes their work respectable, but I don't think that there is necessarily a close connection.

If you think of Eysenck you think of learning theory. One of the interesting things about the early days with neuroleptics were that people were looking at the effects of chlorpromazine on conditioned reflexes and on the rope test. What was the rope test?

It was a conditioning test where a rodent could learn to avoid a shock by climbing up a rope that hung down in the middle of the cage. There were actually two strands of research. There were the psychologists who were using mostly established tests like Skinnerian type responses to map what drugs did for responses to different schedules of signals, and then there were the other kinds of test which were mainly devised or dusted down by pharmacologists who wanted quick returns, a simple method which gave big effects. And there they devised a host of tests from antagonizing body temperature falls to rather more behavioural tests, such as food intake, mouse 'waxy flexibility' or ataxia, sleep measures, etc. but usually fairly gross behaviours. They hoped that these could distinguish between several related but not too similar substances by this means, largely on an empirical basis.

When we did the backward walking experiments, we moved from an interesting interaction between drugs which had not been expected and which could be obtained very reliably to a potential method of screening. This is much more the sort of pharmacological type of behaviour, that is, an empirical test which happens to discriminate, for whatever reasons, between clinically different drugs. We have discussed it with many scientists including ethologists, and I suppose you could say that walking backwards might be a fear response but there isn't much evidence of that, from careful observations of the behaviour, as in the films we have made.

There are problems with animal work these days. The whole question of the animal liberation movement and all that has come to the fore in the last 10 years. Do you want to comment on why these things have happened?

Some of it is justified. I have myself seen, not in this country, unnecessarily strident animal experiments. But it would be a great loss to medicine and to science if all animal work were stopped. At the same time it is right that work should only be carried out on important medical and scientific problems and should be subject to regulation. It should be done with the minimum number of animals, and should be competently done. And scientists and physicians should realize that you can extrapolate from animals to man. If you could not it would be fairly unjustifiable to do these experiments at all. In the past I have often found a good deal of resistance to the idea of extrapolation. People may feel that man is so much more complex, special and interesting than animals. I don't think so. If you do ethological work as I have been involved in you realize that animals actually have an enormous behaviour repertoire. They can be very pleased and stimulated to explore the environment or scared and disappointed. To deny this seems to me unrealistic.

You became very interested in the whole area of substance abuse and the big thing for me reading through your articles is the emphasis that you had on the interaction between the drug and learning or the drug, learning and the environment. Do you want to tell me why you got into that and what do you think the outcomes have been.

This came from work with Ruth Rushton on drug combinations where we found differences between habituated and naive rats. Naive rodents showed the highly stimulant effect of drug combinations but rodents habituated to the test environment didn't. It seems pretty obvious that there must be interactions. But some people, particularly pharmacologists, wanted to look at the 'pure' drug effect irrespective of any other factors such as the internal and external milieu, and basically I do not think that you can do that.

Would you go so far as to say that there's no such thing as a pure drug, or if there is it's an artefact almost?

Almost. Certainly with psychoactive drugs I would have thought so. Because you can only test a drug on manifestations of overt behaviour. The manifest effect is a compound of drug plus personality plus environment plus suggestion and so on. Therefore, I think for example that double-blind clinical trials may often be misleading because there again there is a search for a 'pure drug' effect compared with a placebo but in real life drugs aren't given without any suggestions. In real life you say to the patient 'this is going to help you' and that is a reinforcement which may work very well with some drugs, for example, those that *inter alia* increase suggestibilty or which are prescribed by a confident doctor but not so well with others. Therefore it is quite important to vary not just the drug dose but also to vary the environment and vary the personality as far as you can.

Vary the personality?

By that I mean one should test drugs on different kinds of personality to discover which drug suits which kind of individual. To get the optimum drug effect in a patient you ought to look at their personalities and the environment quite specifically. But why is there such keenness to find this pure drug effect?

I guess that's the way science goes forward, you try and get it as close to a pure effect as you can and in so doing you find out the other influences on what you're looking at . . .

But is this really helpful if you're trying to develop drugs for practical use because you're actually taking away the practical use. Now it may be that that this teaches you something else which you can only learn that way.

In the field of dependence on drugs I guess the interactions between the environment and drug are more obvious than in any other area of psychopharmacology. There are people like Jane Stewart working in this area now.

Yes, and others who moved this forward also. There was a USA scientist called Ross I think, who gave drugs such as amphetamines and barbiturates with opposite instructions, for example, that amphetamine would make subjects sleep but that sort of research isn't very strong at the moment is it? Maybe I am wrong.

The curious thing about it is that there's been so much good animal work done in the whole area of interaction between drugs and learning that hasn't translated it seems into the clinical situation. Have you any ideas why that's the case?

Maybe psychiatrists deep down still don't think that animal work is relevant to man. And I suppose another reason could be that it's easier to ignore animal experiments if you are working as a practitioner. It's easier to say 'oh drug X does so and so' and not to get too involved in the often equivocal evidence on drug – environment interactions.

I guess politically it's always easier to just give a drug than to try to change the environment?

Absolutely. On the other hand did you see a recent newspaper report that people in hospital got better more quickly if they had a view of trees than if they had nothing much to look at. This really seems to be pathetically obvious but even so it has to be demonstrated.

Malcolm Lader worked with you.

Yes, he did, on amphetamine-barbiturate combinations in medical students. He has been very consistent in evaluating different drugs and experimental and clinical situations. I am not sure how far the dependence problems with benzodiazepines are as fierce as the media maintain. I suspect it's like so many drugs. It becomes known that there is interest in a particular somewhat dramatic effect and then it becomes a self-fulfilling prophesy. It's rather like amphetamine becoming completely proscribed and naughty in the 1960s when for many years it had been helpful with not much trouble for middle-aged housewives or whatever. On the other hand, the longer a drug is successfully in use, the more over-prescribing is liable to occur.

It's awfully curious isn't it that people can go along quite happily for 20 years with no problems really and then all of a sudden things change and it seems like the end of the world if you have these terribly nasty drugs.

I wonder why? Maybe somebody publishes something which gets taken up or somebody is on an influential committee. I'm not sure that it's always justified. On the whole I feel that drug addiction has been made too prominent in the media and for some reason which I do not fully understand they have made it seem extremely interesting. If you are at a party and say you work on drug addiction you are immediately an object of curiosity.

Addiction of course has repercussions way beyond drugs, in the sense that there are all sorts of dependencies which seem to be quite as strong as drug ones but somewhat different because they don't involve ingesting anything. In our present society there seems to be a high place for activities which become compulsive and very central to people – gambling, collecting, shopping, eating, computer games, physical exercise and whatever.

In the middle 1980s, you became very interested in the whole idea of people becoming addicted to exercise. Can you tell me why you got into this area? You must have been one of the earliest people to start talking about exercise addiction in this country.

Yes, I suppose so in this country; David Veale was another. Elizabeth Sykes and I wrote a review article which was pretty early in the field (Steinberg and Sykes, 1985). Exercise is relevant in psychopharmacology because it seems to release endorphins into the bloodstream and endorphins are very interesting substances. We had a postgraduate student who wanted to do a PhD on exercise and depression and she was an aerobics fan. Then came an invitation to chair a symposium on psychological aspects of endorphins. In order to do this I thought I'd better bone up on endorphins. Exercise was discussed and the favourable mood effects of exercise were stressed, and so I built my introduction to the symposium around exercise. The meeting was held early in the morning, about 8.30, just after summer time had started, so it was really 7.30, and we thought nobody would turn up but in fact it was very well attended. Eventually it led to publication of the review article in an American journal on the possible role of endorphins in the mood effect following exercise – at its extreme the controversial but well known 'runners high'. We found some literature on this, mostly American. The review we published was apparently very successful – people wrote from all over the world for copies, including The Japanese Horse Society. We were pleased since it had been a terribly hard job to get it written because it compressed large quantities of scattered work into a small space, and we had as yet no PC.

Because endorphins are interesting in the same way as drugs are interesting, one went on to do more work on exercise and its psychological benefits. Although there is plenty of evidence, it is still not widely known that physical exercise has favourable psychological effects on mood and self worth. I think that for anyone interested in well being it is a very interesting topic. People have also done animal work since you can get animals to exercise spontaneously, for example, by giving rodents activity wheels. Rats will cover several kilometres a night if given the chance. And because the public interest in physical exercise is quite great it does bring with it media attention, which these days is probably very valuable. We were fortunate to get a grant from the Wolfson Foundation for this sort of work and a research assistant. Elizabeth and I were keen to determine how long the mood benefits last and whether benefits differ for different kinds of people and circumstances (Morris et al., 1990).

Can you give me some outline of what kind of findings seem to be coming out?

Habitual human runners will become anxious, depressed and generally unwell if deprived of their habitual running for even a fortnight. Experienced exercisers have a different mood response before their weekly exercise session, as compared with beginners, the advanced class feel much less well and happy than the beginners. On a scale from positive to negative feelings the advanced ones do rather badly pre-exercise but do pretty well post-exercise. The beginners are much better pre-exercise and about the same as the advanced post-exercise. So the end point is the same but the beginning is different. It does seem to us that the advanced class is much more dependent on exercise and miss it much more.

What about the impact of exercise on mental state; quite apart from it making you feel good, do you think it has any further effects? If you go back 100 years or so, before we had drug treatments or psychotherapy, people like Pierre Janet talked in terms of lengthy hikes in the mountains being therapeutic for people who've got mental problems.

There is a good deal of work, some of it carefully controlled, which shows that physical exercise relieves anxiety and depression provided that they are not too severe. If depression is really severe, one probably cannot get people to exercise. But there is now growing a consensus of evidence for mood improvement in patients. And deliberate exercise prescription by GPs is beginning, but it's not happening yet, I think, in psychiatric hospitals.

No, it's a thing that I actually feel quite strongly about. We take people in and we immobilize them which cannot be good. Is there anything that could be done?

It has been said that hospitals are not places for sick people. You could build exercise into a structured programme so that patients have the exercise to look forward to. Also I think that you want to be very supportive very early on, so that they get praise and feedback for doing it – to get them off to a good start. And then with luck exercise will acquire a reward value of its own. To begin with one probably has to make it a group activity and take them out, which in psychiatry may be difficult.

I don't think so really. What kind of exercise programme would you do?

It would depend on what people like. Some like aerobics and some like aerobic dance, which are energetic activities. Some like swimming but that's not very social. And running is not very social either. Brisk walking can produce good results. Anything that people like, probably.

Actually, the evidence for patients is somewhat better than for normals. The reason I think is that it's easier to test patients and therefore more controlled work can be done. One problem with all this exercise work is control groups and the comparability of exercise regimes. You will find that often not enough detail is given in publications. When trying to draw conclusions, it would be useful to be told what the exercise was like and the structure of the session but mostly papers just say 'subjects did aerobics for an hour'.

You also need a very good teacher. We have one at Middlesex University who is very enthusiastic and dedicated and so she can adapt herself to our experimental needs. But there have hardly been any trials in which, for example, antidepressant drugs and exercise, or drugs combined with exercise were compared.

As I said, it seems crazy we just sort of immobilize people. They are left to wander up and down this ward and perhaps go along to the day hospital and make some baskets. I'm sure they need something more active.

Quite so. People think when they send somebody to a mental hospital that they will be fixed up but often the treatment seems to be rather haphazard. I also think that exercise might be an effective, cheap and relatively pleasant treatment for drug addicts, since endorphins might substitute for methadone.

For the last 30 or 40 odd years, for the first time in human history, we've been able to tease apart elements of human behaviour by using drugs; what in your view has the whole effect of psychopharmacology been on culture – on what we understand of ourselves?

Drugs have become part of society. But even the word drug itself has changed its meaning from meaning medicines, which make you better, to psychoactive compounds, which are used 'socially' and this is not so good. As for what psychopharmacology as a whole has found out, as I have said, probably most psychoactive drugs will turn out to be available in the brain naturally and to that extent I think psychopharmacology has been hugely influential because it has suggested new ways into the brain which nowadays with modern scanners can actually be checked and taken further. As a subject, psychopharmacology is rather more socially useful than many others. It is more interesting and challenging but it's also more rewarding because you do have the possibility of dramatic effects which you don't have in many subjects. With, for example, psychotherapy, people sometimes have to struggle hard to get an effect, but with drugs it is intrinsically easier.

Yes, huge effects which are too big to control.

But that is one of its attractions and I think drug companies could do much more than they do. To give more emphasis to new methods and new drugs and to encourage innovation.

You've commented on a great number of women who have worked in the field – why have they been hidden from view so much?

Certainly, I always understood that I would go to University and that I suppose was even in those days fairly unusual for a woman. At the time, when I started in psychopharmacology, I was probably the only woman who had any sort of established university position, then Daphné Joyce went to Birkbeck. And later Elizabeth Sykes worked in Edinburgh and Bangor. More recently of course there have been several prominent women in this country, Sandra File, Sheila Handley and Susan Iversen.

Nonetheless, women are still expected to be assistants and agony aunts rather than independent scientists, let alone heads of departments. I also think that some male research students may find it harder to be supervised by a woman, which is understandable, if not desirable.

Why?

Because women for a long time have not been taken very seriously. So, while I didn't think it was odd for me to do science, other people must have been very aware that here there was a female. Somebody once said to me that women can do quite well in new and unusual subjects and that again I hadn't thought of.

Once it becomes mainstream the men tend to move in and take positions . . . It's always been a puzzle to me since women are obviously much more intelligent than men.

Are they?

I hate to admit it but exam results show it clearly.

Perhaps women are more adaptable and innovative because they have to be, and there is evidence that they are more verbal. I know that I felt that I must work harder than men to justify myself. To begin with I did everything myself which teaches one a lot, but is very hard work. Maybe men are actually better at getting other people to do things for them. If women are more intelligent than men, then why are men so dominant?

Well, women, as you say, have been tied to the house. They haven't had the opportunities, but give them a level playing field and they'll win any day of the week.

In some ways I think yes. I have been involved with academic women's affairs for some years. The number of women professors has recently gone up at UCL – to something like 20, from 4, 13 years ago – this is about 3 times the national average but still only 9% of the total professoriate at the college. In clinical subjects according to a recent report there seem to be hardly any women professors and things are unlikely to improve overnight. There is still a feeling that women's work is not taken seriously and as a result they don't have the confidence to put forward new ideas, no matter how potentially fruitful, and the current hyper-competitive climate makes it harder for them. So, women on the whole do less well in contributing to a subject. This is a pity and a loss to science, and something that I should very much like to see improved.

People said that my own work was 'pioneering', and it is certainly encouraging to know, for example, that some of one's findings and methods were of interest at the time and are, in some form or another, still so now. But if what I experienced is typical of 'pioneering', it was above all extremely concentrated and demanding work, with luck and success outweighing disappointments. And this is how my scientific life seems to be continuing today, and I would not have it otherwise.

Select bibliography
Morris, M., Steinberg, H., Sykes, E.A. and Salmon, P. (1990) Effects of temporary withdrawal from regular running. *J. Psychsomatic. Res.*, **24 34,** No.5, 493–500.
Rushton, R. and Steinberg, H. (1963) Mutual potentiation of amphetamine and amylobarbitone measured by activity in rats. *Br. J. Pharmac.*, **24 21,** 295–305.

Steinberg, H. (1954) Selective effects of an anaesthetic drug on cognitive behaviour. *Quart. J. Exp. Psychol.*, **24 6,** 170–80.

Steinberg, H. and Summerfield, A. (1957) Reducing interference in forgetting. *Quart. J. Exp. Psychol.*, **24 9,** 146–54.

Steinberg, H. and Watson, R.H.J. (1960) Failure of growth in disturbed laboratory rats. *Nature*, **24 185,** 615–16.

Steinberg, H. and Sykes, E.A. (1985) Introduction to Symposium on Endorphins and Behavioural Processes: review of literature on endorphins and exercise. *Pharmacol. Biochem. Behav.*, **24 23,** 857–62.

Steinberg, H., Davies, C., Stanford, C., *et al.* (1988) Immobility and backward walking induced by co-administration of clenbuterol, amitriptyline or imipramine with chlordiazepoxide in mice. *Pharmacopsychoecologia*, **24 1,** 15–22.

Stolerman, I.P., Kumar, R. and Steinberg, H. (1971) Development of morphine dependence in rats: lack of effect of previous ingestion of other drugs. *Psychopharmacologia*, **24 20,** 321–36.

10 Jonathan Cole

The evaluation of psychotropic drugs

You became involved somewhere around 1955/56, on the back of all the funding that came from Congress, which was put into the psychopharmacology service centre.

Back up a bit. I got into psychiatry because my mother had a manic-depressive illness and maybe into research because I read *Arrowsmith* by Sinclair Lewis at an impressionable age, but anyway I went to a medical school where one of the clinical pharmacologists was doing double-blind studies with placebo fairly prominently.

Now that was early. Who was doing double-blind studies at that point?

Yes, 1945–47. Harry Gold was his name. It was Cornell University Medical College. But this wasn't in a psychiatric disorder. He was doing double-blind studies showing that placebo was relatively effective in pain – in angina. Actually I think a psychologist, called Hollingsworth, who did a double-blind study of caffeine for the Coca Cola company back in 1920 or something like that, was the first. I have never actually seen the reference but I believe this to be true.

Anyway, I got drafted into the Army with the doctors' draft, after doing a residency in psychiatry at Payne-Whitney, part of New York Hospital. When I came out of the Army, the National Academy of Sciences needed a doctor to be executive secretary of five committees that they had. They sent a notice to all the doctors getting out of the military that summer. I responded to it and got hired.

What was the National Academy of Sciences

It was created, I think, in the time of Lincoln, to advise the Federal Government but not be part of it. It's the National Academy of Sciences – National Research Council and it's at 2101 Constitutional Avenue Washington, in a beautiful marble building. It's a sort of a quasi-federal agency and it prides itself in not doing any one activity for a prolonged period. They were doing all the reviewing of grants for the American Cancer Assocation, when I was there, but stopped that after a few years, and they used to run the Committee on Problems of Drug Dependance for several years. They had a small pot of money from the Rockefeller Foundation to distribute for sex research. Kinsey had originally got this money from this Committee and then the Rockefeller Foundation gave it directly to Kinsey.

While I was there Congress got upset at Kinsey for his study on the sexual behaviour of the human female or something or other and decided that the Rockefeller Foundation might lose its tax free status over the sale of the book and their relation with Kinsey. The Foundation ordered the Committee, that I was executive secretary of, not to give grants to Kinsey. Kinsey put in for a grant anyway and the Committee looked at it and said 'oh Shit'. He'd asked for money to import erotic Peruvian pottery! He may have done it to keep the Committee either amused or out of trouble. If he'd put in for a grant on abortion or homosexuality, I think we would awarded him the money and who knows what would have happened after that.

There was a small amount of money from the Licenced Beverage Industry to support alcohol research. I had the fantasy that this money was given mainly so all of the companies that made a lot of whiskey and the like could say 'go see them – don't ask us – ask the National Academy of Sciences'. The Academy's total amount was like £350,000 a year, so we would say we've spent all our money. I think it was something of a run around. Some people got some money.

Then there were two Committees – one on sex and one on psychiatry – who were supposed to advise the Army. When the new drugs came out, the Psychiatry Committee was having real trouble finding a focus. The reason I got hired was that I'd interned at the Brigham, where the head of medicine was a guy named George Thorn, who was an expert on stress and the adrenal gland. He was Chairman of the Committee on Stress and I think I got hired because I was an old intern of his and I knew something about psychiatry.

Anyway, reserpine and chlorpromazine began to be mentioned. There had been a few meetings and I went to a couple of them. The Committee was having trouble advising the Army because the Army wouldn't tell them what they wanted to be advised on – in fact, I inferred that they didn't·want to be advised on anything. And so the Committee really didn't have a role. But I went out to NIMH to find out what they were doing and found that they were about to give a grant to an eminent psychopharmacologist named Ralph Gerard on how to evaluate drug treatments in psychiatry. I turned up just in time because they gave the grant to the National Academy of Sciences and I was the staff member employed on the grant to do all the leg work.

At that stage had anyone any idea how to evaluate the drugs?

Well, I think it was pretty clear that you ought to do double-blind placebo-controlled trials and in fact the Veterans' Administration was getting organized to do such a study and they did one comparing reserpine, chlorpromazine and placebo. At this time, the VA had already done some multi-hospital studies – whether you'd call them trials or not. They had done some work on lobotomy across a number of facilities and they had done multi-hospital trials in tuberculosis. So they had the model already working well before that.

That's interesting because if you look at the UK for instance psychopharmacology didn't begin in the main classical centres – Oxford, Cambridge or the Maudsley . . .

Exactly the same here. The people involved – Heinz Lehmann – at what is now the Verdun, it's the Protestant State Hospital in Quebec. Henry Brill, who was coordinating things for a number of researchers in different New York State Hospitals. Nate Kline, as a crusader in his own right, I think funded by Mary Lasker, with the help of a reporter named Mike Gorman, who was completely funded by Mary Lasker were going around making noises about how everybody must do such and such. At that point Frank Ayd was a private practitioner with what could be called a dubious reputation in the Baltimore. He was viewed by people at Johns Hopkins as possibly unethical. Whenever a new drug came out he would have treated 120 patients with it and come out with a paper within a month after the drug came out. To his credit, his observations were usually quite correct. The bottom lines were all fine. And he provided free treatment to every religious grouping of any spectrum you want, in Baltimore. I just never quite understood how he could see so many patients without much of a hospital base. There was a guy named Bill Winkleman who ran an outpatient clinic for some Unions in Philadelphia and he was the first person to try Thorazine in outpatient anxiety.

They were mainly State Hospital types. Al Kurland, who was probably the eighth person in the United States to try chlorpromazine, was research director at Springfield State Hospital in Maryland and he tried it on six or eight patients and said 'gee, this stuff does something I've never seen done before'. He put a second mortgage on his house and bought stock in SmithKline and French and made a fair amount of money out of it, as a matter of fact. In these days, when you get patients who have been admitted for the 17th time and are still failing on the drugs that we've got you can begin to think the drugs don't work but I think the Kurland story gives you a better idea of the impact of the drugs on a naive patient population.

How much influence did the clinical trials that were happening in the UK have, because there is a little bit of controversy . . .

My vague memory is that Charmian and Joel Elkes had done a small double-blind trial on thorazine and that came out positive. Other than there were the Delay and Deniker papers from St Anne's in Paris and

and there was somebody in Lyon who had done an earlier study of chlorpromazine.

There was also a trial done by Linford Rees in people who are anxious and . . .

Yes, I think I read about that at the time. The principle was clear from tuberculosis and other things and I had, at least, had experience with Harry Gold. We had actually done a study of one of the early anti-hypertensive drugs in anxiety, a double-blind trial, while I was doing my psychiatric residency. That was probably around 1950/51. So that wasn't unheard of, when we got around to organizing the conference with taskforce committees on how to study drugs in animals, etc. and what about their effects on psychological functioning and how do you do clinical trials. The meeting was held in September of 1956 and by that time Congress had already appropriated $2 million for psychopharmacology.

Why did they come up with such a huge amount of money?

Well, Nate Kline and Mike Gorman testified to Congress. Nate actually proposed a $2 million study – his idea was that there would be 10/12 State Hospitals, each of which would have a research team derived from some not too far away medical school and the whole thing would cost $2 million. He had the whole design printed in the Congresional Register. Bob Felix, who was Head of the National Institute of Mental Health, and was recently recovering from psychoanalysis, was opposed to ear-marked funds and felt the funds weren't needed because NIMH was doing some things anyway. But they got the money shoved down their throats whether they wanted it or not. I think they offered the job to Joel Elkes, who came over to run a branch of the NIMH, at St Elizabeth's Hospital – the other side of Washington from Bethesda, and probably they offered it to other people, I don't know. I was the only live body, aged 31, who knew something about research, something about running committees and grant review – and the money was to be used for grants.

Part of my job in the first year was to defend the NIMH portfolio in grants in psychopharmacology, which was pretty lousy. I was doing things like claiming money given to somebody who was studying carbon dioxide effects on cells and vessels and what not – you could argue that in humans carbon dioxide was a form of biological treatment in psychiatry, so that got called a psychopharmacology study. The person doing it had absolutely no interest in psychiatry that I know of. There was a grant to a guy named Carl Pfeiffer, which included one paragraph in which he said he might give some drugs to some schizophrenics to see if they made them worse and thereby learn something about the disease. There was a study of aftercare in schizophrenia that happened to mention that some of them might be on thorazine – there were essentially very few studies that would come close to what one might think a clinical psychopharmacology progamme should be supporting.

There was a feeling from the literature, that I've read, that it wasn't possible to evaluate the drugs in the sense that these new-fangled scales couldn't capture the complexity and richness of clinical reality and to pretend that they could might be a serious mistake.

I didn't have that feeling and nobody was telling me that you couldn't do it. But yes, there is a constant flow of review articles, written by psychologists, saying, that with the antidepressant drugs in particular, but it will apply to any of them, that you can break the double-blind by the side effects and therefore the study is invalid and therefore you cannot prove that the drug is better than placebo. I don't know what you'd do with that one because by the time you have a placebo that has the same side effects as the drugs, you may have a drug that may very well work in the illness. I think this is one of the limitations of the world. I'm prepared to say that if there are nice sizable differences between drug and placebo and people are getting better: the fact that you are likely to guess a drug that made people better well that's one of the things that you are tending to have happen. This isn't a reason for breaking the double blind.

No, I think the real problems to be sorted out were that I don't think any of us thought that Nate Kline's plan was workable in any sense. Relations between State Hospitals and University Medical Centres were on the order of non-existent and most of the University psychiatric facilities had psychoanalysts as Chairmen and no experience in doing new drug evaluation. There really wasn't a cadre there – there wasn't really anything other than the VA that was set up that could do double blind studies at all easily. I had the good luck to pick up at a meeting a consultant named Sherman Ross, who was a Professor of Psychology from Maryland, who was on sabbatical at the time. He worked with me for the first year and taught me a lot about research and psychology and recruited for me two or three psychologists, including one guy who was very good at computers, and so by the second year, we were beginning to get into shape to actually think about the logistics of how we would do the study. Gerry Klerman had come on board for two years to do his doctors' draft requirement.

How did he come on board?

There was something called the Berry Plan. It was required for a number of years that if you had gone to medical school and weren't physically unfit in some sense or the other, you had to do two years in some branch of the Armed services. A number of people had figured out that the public health service was a branch of the armed services and that, if you were a bright young resident from a good programme, that could get the National Institute of Health to pick you up and you could do your two years of required military service doing research in Washington, which struck some people as good for their careers. There was some risk that you might end up on an Indian reservation or at a prison but most of them ended up in Washington.

Gerry Klerman had trained in Massachusetts at the Mass Mental Health Center and came and worked with me. I had hired a social psychologist named Sol Goldberg by that time and he and Gerry combined to go out to get the study on chlorpromazine up and started. This reported in 1964. It was a nine-hospitals study of three antipsychotic drugs and placebo. We just went to an APA meeting and figured out places we thought we knew somebody who we thought could do the study. We didn't put it out on competitive bid the way you'd have to these days and we didn't get approval from anybody. We just asked 10 places to put in grants, with a common protocol and a couple of paragraphs describing what their patient flow was like. One of the 10 places got disapproved because we didn't think they could get enough patients to meet the study needs in the time required.

So we ended up with nine hospitals, mainly public. The Institute of Living at Hartford and the Payne-Whitney Clinic at New York Hospital were I think the two private hospitals in the group – a couple of city hospitals in DC and St Louis, and State Hospitals in places as diverse as Danville, Kentucky and Sykesville, Maryland and Rochester, New York, and Manhattan. Anyway we got up and running reasonably well and, in fact, we came out with the kind of results you would want – anything that could come out significant did. It was clear the drugs worked – even with the dropouts you could discriminate placebo from the active drug. There were no significant differences between any of the drugs, Thorazine, Mellaril and fluphenazine, on any of the outcome measures. There were clearly differences on side effects – we had recorded them but we didn't know how the hell to score them. We could describe percentages but we didn't have, and nobody still has, a really good apples and oranges comparison system for describing whether the side effects of drug A are worse than the side effects of drug B when they have different side effects. But other than the side effect area, the drugs seem to be really remarkably similar.

Did this come as a surprise that the three drugs were so similar?

It didn't seem to be at the time. The people, who had studied the drugs in open clinical trials, didn't have any strong views. Doug Goldman, in Cincinatti, felt that perphenazine was, in fact, the best of the available antipsychotic drugs in terms of the balance of side effects and clinical effects. We hadn't included it so we couldn't prove that. I still think it's a good drug. He may well have been right, but I don't think it's a big enough difference to pick up without a very large study.

Because the French have always had this idea that this group of drugs aren't all just one group of drugs: there are activating neuroleptics, sedating neuroleptics . . .

We were either blessedly or ignorantly free of that preconception, other than sort of thinking 'gee we ought to study several drugs because they might be different'. We studied three drugs mainly because we wanted to generalize and we were looking to see if there were differences but nobody had any clear hypotheses that there would be. We did work out some predictors of which kind of patients did well on which drug. We tried to replicate some of the differences in a second study without placebo and they didn't replicate, so we gave that one up as a bad job. And, in fact, until clozapine came along, I don't think anybody had found a reliable, in the sense of repeatable, significant difference between drugs, other than on side effects. The French may well be right but I don't think they can prove it.

We couldn't even find a difference between depot and oral fluphenazine. We ran a study of that and failed to find a difference, I think because we had such good research nurses, making sure everyone took their pills. Everybody got placebo shots and active pills or vice versa and there were nurses dropping by once a week and calling up once a week saying 'are you taking your pills?' Under that system everybody took their pills and the relapse rate was identical between the injections and the pills. You wouldn't have expected it to be if we had done it under battlefield conditions in outpatient clinics, with nobody bothering whether people took their pills.

The other big thing that came of the 1964 trial was the idea that the drugs weren't just tranquillizers, they seemed to be actually therapeutic for some aspects of the illnesses . . .

Well, they certainly worked on almost anything that was wrong with schizophrenics. In fact, if my memory serves right, among other things if you looked at symptoms, that weren't present at hospitalization and turned up afterwards, the drugs were better than placebo on that. The placebo patients developed more new symptoms, after admission to the hospital, than the people on drugs. And it didn't look like they only worked on patients with hallucinations and excitement. They worked fairly broadly across the field.

We weren't studying a population of back ward hebephrenics – we did do that a year or two later. Eventually, we did a high dose/low dose placebo study in chronic schizophrenia, plus a doctors' choice group, and you could interpret the results any way that you like. At the time, we said that in the less elderly, chronic schizophrenics, the high dose did a bit better than the standard dose. Viewed another way you could say that the high dose caused a lot more side effects and hardly anybody got discharged and it wasn't all worth all the trouble, which I think is probably the correct inference.

The only other interesting thing to come out of it was that whatever class of drug activating versus sedative, that the patient had been on at the

State Hospital, before they even started the study, there was a bigger difference between high and low dose in those patients on that class of drugs than there was in patients who had been on the other class. So whatever the State Hospital doctors were doing they were guessing right or something or other. People who had been on stelazine before were more likely to do better on high dose stelazine and people who had been Thorazine or Mellaril before were likely to do better on high dose Thorazine. But there may be other explanations for that.

Did Nate Kline and Mike Gorman get in beneath the analytic radar as it were?

Oh yes, they got directly under it. I don't think the analysts were capable of organizing to prevent anything happening even if they had so wanted to, which I'm not sure they did. I think their position was more of armchair doubt or disbelief or something or other. Within two or three years, I had a very small private practice, I was getting calls from analysts saying 'can you please prescribe drugs for Mrs Jones'.

Why wouldn't they actually prescribe them themselves?

Well, there was a period of time and a group of analysts who felt it was unclean. There were also odd beliefs that you shouldn't mix administration with therapy in some form or other and a number of hospitals were run on a therapy/adminstrator split with one doctor being in charge of ground privileges and so on and somebody else purely talking to the patient and examining their psyche. But really it wasn't like a political contest. The analysts tended to be aloof, and not awfully talkative, and they certainly didn't picket Congress saying 'don't give money for these drugs'. I don't think most of them cared much what happened at the State Hospitals.

Was that, do you think, because they didn't see the ultimate threat to their livelihood as it were?

No, I don't think they did. About three years after that, let's say 1960, I went to a meeting of the Association for Research in Nervous and Mental Disease on psychopharmacology, and I sat next to a very talkative biological psychiatrist named Ted Robie. He was not a research figure but he knew all the analysts in New York and he would keep leaning over to me and say 'there's another one – they're running scared, they're running scared'. I think that's more of the flavour of the thing. They were quietly going to meetings about psychopharmacology to find out what was going on and wondering a little bit about whether the drugs were okay. I think it gradually became clearer to almost everybody, after the VA study first and our study second, that Delay and Deniker were actually correct and that the double-blind trials are the only useful way of proving it – even though one could argue that very little new has been found since Delay and Deniker reported and what they observed in an open study turned out to be pretty much correct.

What role did John Overall and Leo Hollister play in all this – they ran the VA study and helped to actually devise the rating instruments and all.

There were really two or three people doing rating instruments at that point. John Overall developed the Brief Psychiatric Rating Scale, which proved to be the handiest and the longest lived of the rating instruments for schizophrenia and it was widely used in the VA. Jim Klett was the psychologist statistician in the VA who actually analysed the data from the collaborative studies – he was a friend of Overall, but Overall was in Texas and Klett was at Perry Point, Maryland, North of Baltimore.

Leo had his own research operation in Palo Alto and he used Overall as a consultant. Leo was an internist not a psychiatrist, so he may have had less impact than he would have had as a psychiatrist. These things tended to be run out of a central office with advice from other people rather than run from individual hospital stations, as they were called. Leo with John Overall certainly did a lot of interesting studies on a variety of drugs in that period of time. The first evidence that Librium and Valium caused physical dependance came from Hollister, in fact.

This was extremely early wasn't it? He picked it up about 1961/62.

Yes well he gave a lot of it to chronic schizophrenics and stopped abruptly and by God some of them had seizures. I've never talked to him about what he thought would happen, when he did it – these were the days before you had to get informed consent, which probably made life a good deal easier.

Viewed another way our study and probably the VA study, probably included an unknown proportion of people who would now be considered to be bipolar disorder or amphetamine psychosis or something or other. All of these conditions responded to anti-psychotic drugs, which makes the study less precisely relevant to schizophrenia. John Kane said recently that our improvement rates for schizophrenia have been dropping over time. We got better improvement rates back then than they are getting now. Part of it may just be that if you've got a chronic schizophrenic and he stops talking his pills and he ends up back in hospital, and therefore eligible for study no. 17 in 1993, it's a lot harder to get the worms back in the can. Somebody, who was doing fine on 200 mg of Thorazine before he stopped taking his pills and then relapsed, may require 1200 mg and 8 weeks before things begin to finally settle down. One of the problems with managed care is that they expect psychotics to get better in three days and you barely have time to establish a relationship and set up some kind of an aftercare programme in that period, you don't really get them better – you may get them sleeping better at night but you aren't going to really knock much of the psychosis down.

Phillip May also came out with a trial around 1964 which is, who was one of the first to report using chlorpromazine without any therapy input.

I think probably in most of the studies with chlorpromazine nobody would consider using therapy input because the State Hospitals didn't much have staff to do that anyway. But Phil May is an interesting story. He got support originally from NIMH to compare psychotherapy, supervised by trained analysts, with drug therapy versus psychoanalysts alone or drug alone, ECT alone or milieu therapy – meaning none of the above. He got the study done but he got turned down for more money for the analysis. The State of California's Research Department wouldn't give him money because they believed that he was biased in favour of psychoanalysis because his wife was an analyst. I managed to figure a way of getting him a contract out of NIMH, without going through the grant procedure, to give him enough money to finish the damn thing and write the book.

It turned out psychoanalysis was really quite ineffective in this study. So much for the biases he may or may not have had because of his wife; I think he was interested in finding out the truth. His was the first study to tackle the psychotherapy question relatively head on. Various people complained, probably correctly, that the therapy was done mainly by advanced residents and junior staff and that they weren't really psychoanalysts – that was because there wasn't enough money in the world to hire enough analysts to get out in the State Hospitals to do the therapy.

Jack Ewalt had the same idea. What he did was, he took a bunch of chronic schizophrenics in Boston State Hospital and transferred them to Mass Mental Health Centre, which was then called the Boston Psychopathic Hospital, and he gave them an intensive treatment with daily psychotherapy and rehabilitation and group therapy – you name it. His idea was you can give them a lot of everything and then when you've proved that that's good, you dissect it out and try to get at which part is more essential than which other. In fact, what he provided was a toxic dose of interpersonal contact. Patients off drugs got a lot worse at the Mass Mental Health Centre; they blew apart at the seams under all this. John Wing, at your end of the world, had a theory which I think is quite correct, that if you overstimulate schizophrenics they go actively mad, and if you lock them up in an attic they go catatonic. The ones at Mass Mental got overstimulated and got substantially worse if they weren't on anything. You wouldn't do the study quite that way these days but it fairly clearly showed that you didn't get people a lot better by giving them a lot of psychosocial therapies all at once.

Let's hop back a bit. Because gearing up to the NIMH study, you'd begun to run the early clinical drug evaluation, the ECDEU programme.

That was sort of a parallel event. It seemed to me as I wandered round talking to people that drug companies were perfectly good at giving money but they didn't give it in a consistent fashion. The people who were doing what I saw was a good job of evaluating new drugs for the drug companies, could certainly use some kind of continuing sort of baseline support. You know, a secretary, a nurse and a half-time doctor and it would be good to have a programme, whereby the better people doing this kind of stuff, got five-year grants to do studies, and would meet together and tell the psychopharmacology programme, namely me, and each other what they found out. I managed to sell that to the National Institute of Health because we had enough money going around and, I think at one point, we had 15, 16 or 17 program grants of this sort going. The grants gradually died, mainly because review committees don't like that kind of support. They like hypothesis-orientated research and most of the people weren't doing that. Maybe they didn't deserve it any way, I can't judge.

However, the early clinical drug evaluation programme had then developed a life of its own and now meets yearly as the New Clinical Drug Evaluation Programme. It's sort of parallel with ACNP, only you don't have to meet criteria to be a member. It meets in Florida in early June. It was under 20 investigators when it started. The meeting is attended by over 300 people now. There was an argument about whether drug company representatives should sit in or not and after a while we let them sit in and its now evolved into something rather parallel to the Committee on Problems of Drug Dependence which I had already been exposed to. I had gotten the model from them. There really is a value in having a meeting where clinical investigators and basic scientists present research and the company representatives come and find out what's going on and do a certain amount of bartering over who's going to do studies and the Federal Bureaucrats with an interest in the area also are present. If everybody is at the same meeting, they can hash out things that they might not do otherwise.

In the Committee on Problems of Drug Dependance, they used to and I think still do, pass the hat to the drug companies and get some unrestricted funds out of the companies. They supported a programme where a guy named Nathan Eddy would review new chemicals that might be used for analgesia and do simple stuff in mice and then he'd send them on to Michigan to be tried out in monkeys, dependent on morphine, to see if the new drugs would substitute. And then they would go the Addiction Research Centre of the NIMH to be tried out in man and other people would see if they were effective analgesics. Anyway, this programme is a little bit like that. It's a nice four days in the sun in Florida. We have training sessions on how to use some new instruments and a general review for people from outlying places, who don't get to get to that kind of meeting very often.

It seems to me that you have been a person who has tried to bring people together. Now not everyone else in the field at the time would have been in the business of doing that. Yale or Harvard wouldn't have been in the business of bringing people from the public hospitals in. The NIMH as such, if left to Bob Felix, wouldn't have been particularly in the business of . . .

Probably not. He had a special programmes branch. The NIMH idea was one study of industrial mental health and one study of child development and another study on adoption and one for each thing some staff member had a special interest in – it risked being a bypass route for flaky projects – that may be a little harsh.

I wasn't conscious of it at the time, it just seemed to happen but I turned out to get along well with people. My other role was to hire people to do the research and the analysis, while I answered all the nasty letters from Congress and wrote all the annual reports. I happen to write easily. So I did a lot of the basic crap you have to do to keep a programme alive – defend it and go to meetings and write documents. I actively enjoyed the review committee process and had a good enough relationship with the review committee members that I could speak up and say if I felt they were going off the deep end on something or other. I could occasionally change the course of the grant's review by saying something.

It all seemed to work out very well and I enjoyed going to State Hospitals. In fact, I enjoyed it so much that when I got frustrated with some things happening in the NIMH, and I got offered the job of superintendant at the State Hospital in Boston l took it because I thought it might be fun. It was fun for about five years until I began to feel I was burning out and thought I better go and do something else.

Who did you see as being the key people in the field, between 1955 and 1965?

Oh goodness, I guess at the advisory level people like Danny Friedman, who actually didn't do any of this research but was really excellent person to have on a committee and to talk to about both political and other problems. He was probably the person I felt closest to as a general person to rap with in the late hours of the evening as to how things were going. Louis Lasagna was another. He wasn't a psychiatrist but he knew a lot about the FDA and about clinical pharmacology and he was a very useful review committee member. Heinz Lehmann I used a fair amount and Henry Brill and Phil May and Gerry Klerman.

Seymour Kety?

Yeh, he was sort of so senior that I wasn't quite sure how to use him. But again he wasn't a psychiatrist. He and I were both at McLean for 10 years and I think I saw him about 4 times. He had a big centre grant in schizophrenia and they never included me in it. I don't know whether I'd have contributed anything. I never could tell whether they were paranoid or whether they just didn't think about it.

There was a guy named Neil Waldrup who was over at St Elizabeth's who I knew fairly well – actually the reason I left NIMH, at least on paper, was the people at St Elizabeth's wanted me to take over a research ward over there and it seemed like a great idea to have a pilot plant. The money was probably going to dry up anyway, so maybe it was just as well the move didn't happen. But having a ward where my staff could try out instruments and we could do some pilot testing of study designs seemed like a great idea and I said fine. Two years later, it became clear that they hadn't cleared it with anybody higher up in the hierarchy and when it got up to the then Stan Yolles level, the Director of NIMH, he said 'no, he's over-committed already'. I was moderately pissed at that.

About the same time, drug abuse was beginning to get hot and a guy named Roger Meyer, who had come down on this two-year plan to work with me and handle the drug abuse end of it, got split off from me and ended up in what eventually became the National Institute of Drug Abuse, which was run outside of the psychopharmacology programme. It probably made sense but if it had been inside my programme, I probably would have been too busy to think about going anywhere else. With those two things having been not given or taken away, I got offered this job in Boston. My parents lived in Boston and I was raised there and it seemed like a good time to go try being superintendant at the State Hospital.

With the ECDEU unit actually running by 1960, why was there a need for ACNP?

Well the ECDEU was really a pretty restricted format; it wouldn't have included people like Julius Axelrod, wouldn't have included Phil May, wouldn't have included Danny Friedman and a variety of people, because it was really designed only for studying investigational drugs and the people who do that tend not to be the leaders of science. A few people were exceptions, like Leo Hollister. But I think people, also, thought that we needed a broader organization and model. I think the CINP came first and I think we were sort of modelling it after the CINP. There was a meeting at the Barbizon Plaza. Nate Kline and I and Paul Hoch took the leadership in this – Paul Hoch died two or three years later. He was sort of the autocratic Prussian type and tended to run things.

Ted Rothman was very heavily involved wasn't he?

Yes, he ended up being the guy who did a lot of the work. Ted offered himself. I think he was a private practitioner in LA and he had the time and the interest and was getting older. Anyway, he took over and did a lot of the organizing and was a good example of a practising clinician who decided this was a good way to spend his time, which I didn't have and Paul Hoch didn't have. He ended up carrying the organization on his shoulders for the first three or four years. His main area of research had been giving intravenous speed to people to help them talk in psycho-therapy.

Quite a few of the people in the group were interested in giving drugs to people to abreact them.

Yes, there was a wave of LSD interest going on and we supported some research in that. There were some Josiah Masey conferences, for instance, on LSD that were really pretty wild that I went to. It was certainly an interesting area. I suspect it works in some people, some of the time, but it's damm hard to prove. Drugs that do fabulously in 15% of some unknown number of people pose a terrible problem. I think everybody knows patients who do remarkably well on something or other. You hate to take them off of it but it's hard to convince a drug company to keep something on the market on the basis of it. Short of taking people who you already know are responders on and off a drug, it's hard to think of a design that will pick them up.

ACNP has been run by your secretaries. Oakley Ray has been there for a lifetime really and he almost is ACNP . . .

Dick Wittenborn was there for six years before that and Ted Rothman before him. I think we figured that having an enduring secretary makes a lot of sense so I think we set it up with three-year terms and tended to re-elect people if they wanted to be re-elected and things were going along all right. We've had a backup in case somebody dropped dead or broke a leg or something. But it's worked reasonably well as an administra-tive device. Presidents come and go each year and one year spans a time when, unless you did something remarkably notable like make the organization go broke or pass a law, or get the Nobel prize or something or other, it tends not to be remembered.

How much of an impact did the antidepressants have on the Psychopharmacology Service Centre? You were geared up to look at chlorpromazine, then the anti-depressants began to . . .

Yes, and we did some studies of Librium and Valium without anybody telling us to and when the antidepressants came along we set up a multi-hospital study of antidepressants which got published. It turned out to be very hard to prove that imipramine did anything. We did imipramine, placebo and chlorpromazine and then we did phenelzine, diazepam and placebo − in hospitalized depressions, mainly but not exclusively private hospitals. A guy named Al Raskin, who was a psychologist, did most of the work. We ended up having too many instruments and we ended up factor-analysing factors and we either died of data poisoning or by that time the patients you got in inpatient wards were a mix of people with bad personality disorders or people who had failed on the drugs on the outside. Our dosing scheme was, I think, irrational in retrospect. We ran up to a peak dose on the third and fourth week and then started coming down again and we probably should have run for 12 weeks and kept everybody at the top dose.

So we were able to show that imipramine was better than placebo and that non-retarded depressions did better on chlorpromazine than retarded depression and that was nice. But it was less clearly positive compared with the antipsychotic study.

What about phenelzine, diazepam and placebo?

That didn't show much of anything either but we didn't keep them on a high enough dose and we didn't keep them on it for long enough. Some time thereafter, we supported Don Robinson, who showed that you've got to give at least a mg per kg and probably keep it up for 6–8 weeks or something like that to get a decent response out of phenelzine. But we didn't know that much at the time. We knew about the cheese reaction, because I remember a patient overdosed on cheese and related edibles and in fact got a hypertensive crisis because she turned out to be on phenelzine. Anyway, it was not a great success and we didn't try again after that. About that time money was beginning to get tighter and I think I left while the study was still ongoing or about to be published.

Jerry Levine who had been my deputy took over and he was interested in the NCDEU business and went through a phase of inviting data from a variety of investigators who weren't necessarily funded by us. Jerry got interested in using the dataset and he actually was responsible for setting up the blips system. Jerry was much more organized than I was.

When did the need for operational criteria begin to become apparent?

We felt it from the beginning but we didn't really do a lot of work on it. Criteria like a score of 18 on the Hamilton scale were fairly easy to come by. I guess it was Bob Spitzer, 20 years ago now, who began to really get into diagnostic interviewing. In fact, the Present State Exam I think was in advance of anything sensible over here. There was the Diagnostic Interview Schedule, which turned out to be rather inadequate instrument, at least when administered by ordinary people, without any clinical training. But that was the first standardized interview that I can remember and then Bob Spitzer and various other people in Columbia went on to develop better instruments.

I guess these probably grew not so much out of my programme as out of the US/UK diagnostic study, which was run, in the US, out of Columbia. Spitzer was involved to some extent. That showed that us crazy Americans were over-diagnosing schizophrenia to a large extent. Up to that point, we were allowing for clinical judgement and the training of the people doing ratings and hoping for the best. Certainly, when we were doing anxiety studies, which is another area – the whole idea of panic disorder grew out of Don Klein's work and I think he was actually grant-supported by us.

He and Max Finx at Hillside had done this wild study, which was a wonderful commentary on the analytic view of the world. Hillside was primarily an analytic hospital and Max Finx and Don Klein were doing all the shock treatment. When the drugs came along, the head of the hospital said 'well if somebody isn't better after a month of analytic therapy, they can get sent to Fink and Klein and they can put them on drugs'. They were the only people allowed to do drug therapy in the hospital, so they randomized almost everybody to Tofranil, Thorazine and placebo independant of what symptoms they presented with.

Yes, and actually got some interesting results . . .

I don't think they reported it but the nicest study was that Don had made research diagnoses on a large number of patients at Hillside. They weren't doing formal diagnoses quite the way they are done now, but they had criteria and they were making criteria-based diagnosis. So they had a group of patients that his staff thought were not schizophrenic and the Hillside regular staff thought were schizophrenic, and another group where they both agreed they were schizophrenic, and he made the prediction, that if a patient ran out of money and was transferred to Creedmore State Hospital, which was not uncommon, that the real schizophrenics would stay at Creedmore for a long time and the non-schizophrenics would get discharged rather rapidly. He checked it out and the results were significant at the 0.001 level. The people his research staff did not think were schizophrenic, I think had a mean stay of like three weeks and the real schizophrenics had a mean stay of nine months. There was a whopping difference and that was the first story I remember of the power of diagnosis in actually demonstrating something tangible. That and the prediction about drug response.

We deserve a little credit for introducing lithium to this country because we gave a big grant to Ralph Gerard to run a study of chronically hospitalized patients in the Ypsilanti State Hospital, near the University of Michigan, Ann Arbor. They had research wards there and used every test known to man. One of the people on the grant was Sam Gershon, who had come over from Australia for a couple of years, and brought lithium with him and the first papers on the use of lithium in American patients was done by Sam at Ypsilanti under that grant.

And it worked?

Oh yes. At the time, you'd go buy the pure chemicals, lithium carbonate, by the kilo from a chemical supply store and then you'd get a drug store pharmacist to put it into capsules for you. And then Rowell Labs, a company in Minnesota, got interested in it and began making it for some investigators and then, eventually, SmithKline and French and Pfizer got interested. The FDA was giving out INDs to all kinds of people who wanted to use lithium. Almost anybody who said they wanted to treat patients with lithium, they'd get an IND number. When I was superintendant at Boston State it wasn't on the market and yet I had about 15 patients on it.

What was Boston State Hospital like when you went there? The drugs had been out over 10 years . . .

Milt Greenblatt had been running it for 5 years before and Walter Barton was the notable superintendant for 10 years before that, so the population had dropped from a maximum of 3000 down to about 1600 by the time I had got there. The nursing supervisors were throwing beds out of windows to dramatize the fact that the patients will never come back. The catchment area idea of breaking the city down into geographic areas, each of which would be responsible for its own patients, had started, and they were beginning to work out how to divide the hospital up into defined catchment areas to meet the needs of the new plan.

Where the catchment area idea come from?

Jack Ewalt. There was a commission on mental health and illness that was funded by Congress and Ewalt was chairman of it and it came out with a report strongly recommending community mental health centres. There was some underlying idea that even elevator operators can give therapy and you don't need high priced professionals all the time and you've got to treat everybody and there should be federal grants to support staff and improve liaison between the state hospitals and the community. And it sort of worked – you can argue it both ways. Boston State Hospital went out of existence about four years after I left. We peeled off into mental health centres. The state built buildings for some of the mental health centres and we moved patients to pre-existing buildings in their catchment areas for others.

   Whether it was a good idea in the long run, I tend to think not in retrospect. I think the State hospital had a place and now a major problem in Massachusetts from my viewpoint is that we've got very few places where we can serve the kind of patient who takes a long time to get better and where real rehabilitation is done. We tend to have more people who are home and crazy than we should have and nobody's going to pay for their treatment. We've closed most of the State Hospitals although not all of them. But the procedure to break up into community mental health centres had already started and when I took over as superintendant we continued along that. We had a grant to improve community services for the catchment areas that the hospital was supposed to be getting and we did a number of things but most of the innovative things we did were done before we broke up into catchment areas rather than afterwards.

   For instance, we worked a deal with the Department of Welfare whereby we could put five chronic patients in one apartment, in a three-decker. Boston is littered with buildings with three apartments, one above another, and the landlord would usually live in one of the apartments and he got paid a little extra to keep an eye on the patients. The Welfare Department provided the funds to pay the rent, so we didn't have to deal with it. The landlord showed the patients where to buy groceries and our staff went out to fill up the chinks and provide some education. We had a home treatment service, which was sort of crisis call-out in the home. The psychiatric resident and the nurse would go out to the house, if they heard there was somebody crazy out there. They would drive out to the house, park the car in front of the driveway so the patient couldn't escape on wheels, go in, often backed up by the police, and offer to give the guy a shot of depot prolixin, if he didn't want to go to the hospital with that nice man in blue standing right behind.

We started day hospitals and we did cognitive training of pre-school black kids who lived in the surrounding area. I even did a study of dexedrine in over-active kids in the schools adjacent to the hospital. I published it in *Psychopharmacology*. I knew it would work fine. I needed some money for helping fill out the cracks in the grant for the Outreach Programme and I got $10,000 from SmithKline French for doing that study and used that to help pay travel and buy stuff for community centres we were trying to set up for the community.

Where did you do your clinical training?

I was trained by Oscar Diethelm, who was interested in psychiatric history. He was Adolph Meyer trained, so he believed in distributive analysis which was talking about your mother today and arriving at some kind of conclusion as to how that influenced your life and you talk about daddy the next day and your brother and sister the third day. Distributive analysis was a somewhat more superficial therapy, with life charts – Meyer was interested to relate somatic and social and intrapsychic things and trying to see how things interacted with each other during parts of the life span of a patient.

How strong was the Meyerian strand in US psychiatry?

I wasn't conscious of it as a strand. The place was eclectic. You'd got patients whose average length of stay was three months and you saw them three times a week and tried to do what you could with them. We did shock treatment and insulin sub-coma. If you asked me, was I Meyerian? I would have said no. But it struck me as sensible. You met with Diethelm once a week to go over all your patients. He would come round and visit each of your patients with you, once a week, and Tom Rennie, who was the other guru on the staff, did the same thing. We had two supervisors for each patient, which is a little odd in present day psychiatry but it certainly felt like your patient was being attended to. Diethelm would take notes on those little 3 × 5 cards and I'd get a few patients who had been in the clinic before and he would pull a little 3 × 5 card and tell you all kinds of things about these patients.

So it was a nice comfortable place. All the patients were locked up so they couldn't fail to come back for their interviews. There was almost no outpatient experience. It was probably good training for my future because you had to write a five-page single spaced case summary, which you'd get typed, on each patient. If it was too long or too short you'd get yelled at and then you had to present it or if you weren't presenting you had to comment on the patient and he would start with the most junior resident and work his way around the room and everybody had to say something about the patient. So you got used to talking in public. You probably got more experience in writing under pressure than people do in this day and age, where they tend to write illegible $1\frac{1}{2}$ page admission notes and the occasional progress note but nothing else.

On the history issue, in Josephine Swazey's 1974 book on chlorpromazine, she cites you a lot, do you think she had the picture right?

Yes, she talked to me at some length. As I remember the book, I thought she had it right. There's also a book on the history of psychopharmacology by Anne Caldwell, who was in the National Library of Medicine, which was too full of Laborit worship. I think Laborit had a real role but she thought he walked on water. My comment after was the reason nobody ever got a Nobel prize for this was that one it was a company drug, and who the hell did you give a prize to, and second that the principal person in getting the drug into man was the equivalent of a Head of Anaesthesia at the Naval Hospital in Virginia. He was not a prime mover in French academic medicine and he had an oddball theory of stress which may, in fact, be right but I'm in no position to judge one way or the other.

After Boston State Hospital, you did what?

I got offered a Chairmanship of Psychiatry at Temple University in Philadelphia and my then wife, who has since died, said to try it for a year and if you like it we'll move. At the end of a year, we were losing beds and psychiatry had been kicked out of the planned new teaching building. I figured the medical school was going broke and I didn't like Philadelphia much anyway, so I went back to Boston. I ended up at McLean because they seemed glad to have me and I ended up running a psychopharmacology consultation service. I've been doing that more or less ever since.

We set up an affective disorders clinic with Alan Schatzberg, who's now Chairman at Stanford. The hospital is now quietly going down the tube. We've managed to lose money, even when all beds are filled, and we've got things all re-organized, practically like the way I had in Boston State, with triage, etc. – keep them out of hospital at all costs, provide some place to sleep for the night if they really need it, a day programme, give some of them a therapist and a case manager. Trouble is nobody wants to pay for that in this country. There's no way of funding it, whereas at Boston State I had 1800 employees and if I freed up some employees by closing or emptying a chronic ward, I could then use some of them to be case managers in the community so it worked. It was a lot easier to do then than now. So I'm not sure it's going to survive.

I know you worked with Joe Schildkraut. How much of an impact do you think his amine hypothesis had? It seems to me that things like that helped to bring psychopharmacology into the public domain. People could understand the idea of low chemicals and that treatment was aimed to restore that . . .

'I have a chemical abnormality'. Yes. I think some of it's pseudo science and some of it's real. For 15 years or so, Schatzberg and I got most of the patients that Schildkraut studied. We could get drug-free patients from McLean, collect urines and do ratings and send the stuff to Joe to run all the chemical analyses and so forth. Most of his work for the last 15 years has been based on McLean patients. It was a generally interesting collaboration and there clearly is something about MHPG – people with high MHPG are different from those with low MHPG. I'm not sure whether we're measuring the right thing of course. If you compare Prozac and Tofranil, you get pretty much the same predictors of improvement. Low MHPG people do better on Prozac, they also do better on Tofranil. You'd think there would be something different about them, given the different mechanisms of action. I don't quite know what to make of it.

Talking about fluoxetine and its impact in the US – how do you account for that?

One pill a day for ever. It's very easy for internists. I think primary care docs really never learned how to manipulate tricyclics well – the side effects, waiting, etc. Fluoxetine at one pill a day for ever is the ideal primary care physician's drug. I think part of it was that there is something like 5–10% of patients on fluoxetine, who get remarkably better. Like the 'Listening to Prozac man', at McLean I treated 100 or so patients before it came on the market and a handful of them really were astoundingly better. They had been sick for 10/15 years and were clearly better than they had ever been before in their lives and there were just enough of them to make a difference. You certainly got a small handful of people who said 'wow am I better'! and went on television and said they were better. At the other end, you see people who have been on Prozac for two years and are still waiting for it to work. So it doesn't do that to everybody but it does it to just enough to hit the talk shows and get a lot of sales going.

What about a group of patients who may get worse on it?

Yes. I'm one of the authors of the suicide paper . . . I didn't realize it would be quite that famous. I don't know whether Teicher or I would have published it, if we'd known, although I guess we would have done. Yes, I have seen people, at least a handful, that clearly got more agitated and got weird thoughts and suicidal drive. Tony Rothschild, who has taken over my depression programme in McLean, found three people who had jumped off something while on fluoxetine, who didn't kill themselves, and agreed to take it again. He re-created the same desperate driven quality with fluoxetine.

Is it a form of akathisia?

I think it probably is but whether you get the neuromuscular form or whether it's purely psychic I don't know. One patient I followed through it was so distressed by thoughts telling her to kill herself over and over again, that I never got around to asking her whether her muscles felt funny. The psychic end is so predominant that you forget to ask about the muscle end. I told her to take some Ativan and go to sleep and she did and within 36 hours it had passed. At the end of it she said 'gee, I've been depressed for 21 years, and suicidal a lot but that was ridiculous'. She thought it was clearly different than anything she had ever experienced before which is why I put her case and my name on the paper. Lilly doesn't believe it.

Sy Fisher, who is now at the University of Texas in Galveston, does prescription surveys and he did a study in which a big chain of drug stores in the South and South West participated, where if you filled a fluoxetine prescription you got a thing saying that 'if anything unusual good or bad happens to you on this drug, please call this 800 number'. They did the same thing for everybody who filled out trazodone prescriptions. I would have preferred another drug because who knows how many people get trazodone for insomnia. What they got were all the usual side effects of both drugs, in about the expected proportions. Plus about 1–2% of the people on fluoxetine, and none of the people on trazodone, called up and said I've got suicidal ideas that I haven't had before and another 1–2% phoned up and said I've got crazy ideas that I hadn't had before.

So I think it does happen but I think it's rare. I think now most people have heard about it. Propranolol reverses it quite nicely. Two of three patients that Rothschild re-created it in, he added propranolol and they left the hospital still on fluoxetine, happy as clams. I think it is now known enough that the FDA didn't need to put a warning on it. So I think it's rare and the drug has certainly prevented more suicides than it's caused. I don't think it's a bad drug, I just think it does funny things every once in a while.

We've got much fewer drugs going through now because they say the costs are so big and the industry stands to lose so much if the drug goes wrong. How much has the climate changed in which drugs are brought out?

Yes the risk:benefit ratio for the drug company has changed. I haven't heard of a new antidepressant in the last nine months and I don't know whether it's because there are so many antidepressants out there now that how can you hope to gain any decent proportion of market share no matter how good your drug was or whether it's because the cost is so much. When I've been asked, I've told people I wouldn't mess with an antidepressant unless it was clearly faster acting than existing drugs. If you've got a three-day response, at least half the time, and the side effects are no worse, I'd try it, but I'd throw it out if it took an average of three weeks to handle depression. I think you need some kind of compelling and striking difference. I think you need something more than 'gee, this works through receptor no. 17'.

That's neither here nor there.

Yeh, it's interesting, it may even be relevant but it certainly doesn't make or break a drug. I wouldn't go to market just because it worked on one receptor and not on another. I would love somebody to get one of the rapid reversal MAO inhibitors on the market but I gather they're all being killed by the companies. They may be right. Doctors are peculiar beings. You say the word MAO inhibitor and they think hypertensive crisis and don't prescribe the drug, I think.

That had a huge impact didn't it? Mythologies develop, don't they?

I got so pissed about Lilly saying 'don't you agree that all the doctors know that fluoxetine doesn't cause suicide' that I did a survey of everybody in the Mass Psychiatric Society, who'd answer the telephone about whether they had ever had or thought they'd had a patient who had been made suicidal by fluoxetine, or whether they had heard of anybody, and if they had, did they think they were prescribing less now than they were before. You could make a case that if they had some personal experience with fluoxetine in a patient who they thought got suicidal, they were more likely to warn patients and be a little more gun shy. Not a lot but a little bit.

But I threw in priaprism and Trazodone and seizures and buproprion, at the same time. Now, particularly with buproprion, they might never have heard of anybody ever having a seizure on buproprion, except for the package insert, but they wouldn't touch it with a 10-foot pole. It was really the kiss of death for buproprion. I don't know whether I think seizures are all that bad. I'm not in favour of them but compared to whatever else! It's like the MAO issue, which is the only reason I am raising it. I think that buproprion is a good deal better drug than its use suggests − I've been paid as a consultant by the company so obviously I should state that somewhere. But the idea that it might cause seizures, has caused doctors to avoid it like the plague. It's the same with the MAOIs.

I think we should call this perversity of prescribers the Cole Effect. It's curious how these things happen. Sometimes, ideas just get into popular consciousness and other times they don't. You would have thought that suicidal ideation would have killed off fluoxetine but it hasn't.

But the company probably did exactly the right thing which was to stone wall and the FDA didn't do anything. The company was publishing meta-analyses of everything in the world – 8000 patients in 6-week trials with no increase in suicidal ideation . . .

But you could argue that Upjohn did the same with Halcion but it hasn't been as successful. It's . . .

One of the things is that diazepam and then alprazolam were the bad drugs in this country. I gather lorazepam is the bad drug in England and Serax is the bad drug in Australia. Whichever benzodiazepine is the most widely used is the one that causes the problems – probably because whatever is used most widely stands the largest chance of being taken by murderers, rapists or whatever. I don't know whether that's a reason or not but I don't think the drugs are significantly different from each other.

We haven't really got a handle on all this on just why these things play the way they do in public. Talking of which, Listening to Prozac *seems to me to mark a point where American psychiatry went biological at street level, would you agree?*

I guess that's probably true. Peter Kramer can be somewhat foggy but he makes valid points and he certainly popularized the whole idea. He did an editorial for a throwaway newspaper called *Throw Psychotherapy from the Train.* He said that the rates that were being paid to do psychotherapy by third party payers were just ridiculous and we've got to refuse to accept them. Let's just do psychotherapy like they did in the old days, namely if people can pay for it fine, and if they can't, fine. We won't take $27 per hour for doing something which we think is worth more than that and if people go without, it's just too bad.

The other wave I detect is that cognitive – behaviour therapy is rising in competition to drugs with somewhat more force. There's now been the three hospitals' trial comparing cognitive therapy, interpersonal therapy, tofranil and placebo. Tofranil is better but I keep wondering whether they didn't do something wrong, somewhere. They tried to train social workers to do these therapies and I think there is a problem in skills transfers and because of this I think the non-drug therapies didn't do as well as they might have if they had been done by people who had been trained to do them, who thought it was their favourite therapy. Imipramine worked a little less well than I would have thought and there was a funny business about the psychotherapies doing no better than placebo and then in the last two weeks everybody got better – like they had to please their therapists. I don't know quite what to make out of that one. There have been enough other studies of cognitive therapies that I'm prepared to believe it works, whatever the NIMH study shows. I think, having watched patients, it doesn't work in the very agitated depression, the kind you are seriously thinking about ECT with. You've got to be able to understand what you're there for and do homework to be able to do these therapies and the kind of hand wringing, oh-my-god-doctor-help-me-I'm-dying type of patients, simply can't do the work necessary.

The other thing that I heard from the analysis of the results, which seems to me to be both unfortunate but probably correct, is that with interpersonal therapy, the better your interpersonal relations were at entry to the study, the better you did on interpersonal therapy and with cognitive therapy, the less bad your cognitions were at the beginning of the study, the better you did on cognitive therapy. So each treatment worked better in a way like the Meninger psychotherapy study, which, as Don Klein said, the only finding was that the less sick you were to start with, the better you were at the end. It probably is true that you could learn how to improve your interpersonal skills if you're fairly good at it to begin with and it's easier to correct your cognitions if they're not so screwed up that you can hardly hear the therapist to know what they are talking about.

Are the drug therapies in a permanent advantage vis à vis psychotherapy because they've got a company behind them to market them?

Probably yes. The real question which is not well answered is whether the psychotherapies, which are supposed to teach you something, are any better at preventing you from getting sick again. We are trying to keep people on antidepressants for rather long periods of time and the relapse rate goes up if you stop too soon so you wonder whether . . . There's an old article on imipramine in the *Canadian Journal of Psychiatry,* around the time of the first conference with imipramine in Montreal, saying imipramine is an addictive drug because if you stop it you get depressed again, therefore you are addicted to it. The same model would say that diabetics are addicted to insulin. But there is some truth to it and the question is even more acute with Xanac and panic disorder so I don't know how it's going to work out in the long run.

If the behavioural therapies were able to be shown to give people increased, inner strength to deal with life in the future, I would be impressed and be inclined to refer patients more often than I am now. On the other hand, behaviour therapies are not cheap and not always readily accessible. They end up being more expensive than pills. Pills are not cheap but they tend more often to be paid for by insurances.

Select bibliography

Cole, J.O. and Gerard, R.W. (1959) Psychopharmacology: Problems in Evaluation. National Academy of Sciences/National Research Council, Washington DC, Publication 583.

Cole, J.O., Goldberg, S.C. and Klerman, G.L. (1964) Phenothiazine treatment in acute schizophrenia. *Archives of General Psychiatry*, **24 10,** 246–61.

11 Alec Coppen

Biological psychiatry in Britain

Let's begin with how you came into the area.

I came out of the army in 1946 with no particular idea about what to do with my life and then after I read a book on abnormal psychology (*Outline of Abnormal Psychology*) by William MacDougal, I thought this area would be very interesting. So I thought well this is what I'm going to do, knowing absolutely nothing about the area, and then I found out that if I was going to do psychiatry I'd have to do medicine.

So, I looked around the medical schools and of course in 1946, everyone was trying to get into University – if you'd been in the forces you could get in if you passed the matriculation and then they would select again after the first year's results. I couldn't get into London because that meant waiting an extra year, so I decided to go to Bristol which seemed to be quite an agreeable place.

The first year was probably the most difficult academic year of my life really because you had to take your first MB and they had to weed out up to 60% of our year. But it was a very interesting year because you know everyone had been in the services so you had quite a lot of interesting people there. After that it was a straightforward medical degree – again a very mature year and an interesting time. I think at that time everyone who had been in the army got free tuition and I think something like £350 a year to live on. Then we did a house job but only had a very meagre salary.

After that there was only one place to go and that was to the Maudsley. As I was going on holiday I decided to ask the Dean if they would interview me early, which I suppose was a bit of a cheek. Anyway they interviewed me and I obtained a job at the Maudsley. After my general psychiatric training there, I went to the metabolic ward, which was ward 7, which I think is still probably there.

Who was there at that time?

Well, there was James Gibbons, Gerald Russell, John Hinton and others. My particular interest then was in the blood – brain barrier. I was using sodium[24] as an index of transport and I found an impairment of transport but it subsequently became difficult to do these sort of experiments.

This was on people who were depressed . . .

People who were depressed and after recovery. We found a decrease in sodium[24] entering into the cerebrospinal fluid from the blood. Using blood – plasma sodium ratios, I worked out some sort of transport parameters. It was difficult to do but it fitted my ideal experiment, where you examine a group of normals and then a group of depressives when they are depressed and depressives after they recover. I might say that right from the beginning I was interested in mood.

Why?

Well, clinical research is a matter of practicalities. I thought neurosis was too difficult, too ill—defined. I thought schizophrenia was probably the same but depression and what we now call bipolar illness was interesting because people got ill and then they got well, so I didn't think there was any tremendous irreversible brain damage. I think it was a good choice actually.

Who else was working in this area?

There was James Gibbons, looking at body electrolytes. When I joined the MRC unit we continued using exchangeable sodium but then we could also measure total body sodium and potassium. We got measures of intracellular and extracellular sodium and the results were amazing. To summarize it, David Shaw and I found that, during a period of illness, residual sodium which is exchangeable bone sodium plus intracellular sodium actually increased and when they got better it decreased. In mania we found the same thing but to an even greater extent. We also had measures of total body water using tritiated water, radioactive bromine to measure extracellular water and body potassium using the body counter at the Royal Marsden in Surrey (Coppen and Shaw, 1963).

At the same time in the 1950s, I was also working on stress. In those days I think stress was just going out of fashion. You know these things are cyclical and stress is back now. But certainly in my time at the Maudsley, people were getting a bit fed up with the concept of stress. It could either mean the disturbances you feel or being exposed to disturbances in the environment. Obviously, therefore, there are two quite different things. I did my share in that area, looking at environmental influences on pre-eclamptic toxaemia. I did a study in Croydon at Mayday Hospital and we showed that primiparae with a lot of environmental distress like being chucked out of their lodgings because they got pregnant, were more likely to get pre-eclamptic toxaemia. My conclusion was that environmental factors played a small part in the picture but there were also constitutional factors. They were more neurotic, had more sexual difficulties and a variation in body build.

That was work Linford Rees had begun.

That's right, I've been a great friend of Linford Rees since 1954. Another person I met then was Valerie Cowie, who has made great contributions to genetics. She became a long-term friend of mine. She's a brilliant lady. Then there was Elliott Slater who I think was one of the great people of British Psychiatry – the number one for my money. I've worked with him and I found him very stimulating. One of the best minds I've ever met.

So I was interested in body build and the androgeny index. Androgeny was based on the non-genital differences between men and women. The most common index used was the shoulder to hip measurement. Before puperty you cannot differentiate between girls and boys on this but during puberty under the influence of the sex hormones this changes, so it is obviously a sort of record of the endocrine development during puberty. What I found was that certain schizophrenics have an abnormal androgeny score. They approximated to a rather neutral build; depressives showed that a little bit but not as much. Homosexual men were perfectly normal. But the schizophrenics certainly had an abnormal body build. We took that as far as we could and looked at other factors like calf X-rays. I don't know if you know but you can sex someone's calf X-ray with 70% accuracy. So we looked at that. The idea was to get some idea of someone's endocrine development during puperty.

Did this fit in much with Eysenck's models of temperament and personality?

Yes, it did but a better dimensional model of personality I think is that of Sjöbring, the Swedish psychiatrist in the 1930s and 1940s and his successor Essen-Möller. Sjöbring had three dimensions of personality and in fact my wife and I translated his personality questionnaire into English – I had a Swedish wife and therefore I used to go to Sweden regularly. One of Sjöbring's dimensions is validity, which translates as energy. Another is stability, which has to do with introversion – extraversion and the third is solidity, which is psychic organization. He called them by these funny names because he didn't want them to have any values attached to them. But the result that came out of our studies is that the unipolar depressives have low validity even when they have recovered – they don't change on recovery.

Validity, the energy dimension, I think is very important. I think it's a vital thing in personality and high validity is very useful. I think I've got high validity. My solidity in organizing things is average and my stability, extroversion – introversion, is average also. I could tell you the profiles of very distinguised people but that's obviously confidential. But the characteristic that everyone has who's achieved anything is energy. If you haven't got energy, however much intelligence you've got, it doesn't do you any good. This is why some people don't make a very positive contribution – because they are so critical they are paralysed. You know you've got to be naive to do research.

You think so?

Oh, yes. You've got to be critically naive. You've got to put your hypotheses forward and see what happens. I think what I can do is I can ask questions that are answerable. They've got to be interesting questions of course and they've got to fit in with the fashion. As I said stress went out and stress came back.

Stress has only come back in the last five years.

There are a lot of unsubstantiated statements made about stress and illness even from the WHO. For example, look at hypertension in people with severe depression. There's no one who's more disturbed emotionally than someone who has a severe depression but there is no evidence that these patients have hypertension and no evidence that stress reduction would have any impact on the morbidity of hypertension. But these things come back insidiously. Psychotherapy is another example of changing fashion. When I went to the Maudsley, there was always some American coming along to talk about the definitive research as to whether psychotherapy is effective or not and we used to troop along to listen. Robert Cawley was going to do a study of the effectiveness of psychotherapy but at the end of the day I think he felt it couldn't be done. In the end, I don't think anyone has defined the issues in terms of things you can measure. Psychotherapy went out of fashion and then counselling came in – marriage guidance and things like that.

Your early work culminated in the 1967 article which had an immense impact. What kind of feedback did you get for the 1967 article – it was very much the British equivalent of Joe Schildkraut's article.

I got a very good feedback (Coppen, 1967). It became one of the first citations classics in the area of biological psychiatry. You still see it cited by people who want to show a historical perspective. Some people find it very hard to think anything of importance might have happened more than 20 years ago.

One of the differences between here and the US, when Joe Schildkraut was doing his bit, was that they didn't have the tradition of biological work in small little places that there was here. They didn't have the Archie Todrick's working up in places like Dumfries.

I think small groups actually are quite a good thing. The old MRC tradition was that once you were accepted, you were more or less in a tenured position. Once they picked you, they backed you. I think it must be awful working for five-year grants and so on. I used to put in grant applications for what I had already done and I found that was a quite good idea.

It depends on who you have with you. The people who worked with me in Epsom included Art Prange and Peter Whybrow, who were both interested in thyroid activity. The thing I've learnt from a lot of this is that to have a good response to antidepressant drugs, first of all you've got to have a normally working thyroid and you've got to be well nourished, you've got to have enough folic acid. Ted Reynolds opened my eyes to folic acid. I've done a lot of experiments on it since then. Brookesbanks was our steroid investigator. He was very good. But really we were always a small group, never very big.

Now, in contrast, I think what we lack and what they've got in the States are opportunities. If you have problems in the States you can go off and start again in another State. But what can you do in this country. Everything is done by small groups of people. The MRC is a small group of people with a basic representation from psychiatry and most of those were social psychiatrists so they were very, very conservative. People who did come from biological psychiatry didn't have much influence.

What about endocrine work. In the mid-1950s there were people like Hemphill and Reiss and Harris at the Maudsley.

Yes, Harris was very distinguished and he did a lot of work on the portal circulation of the pituitary but he wasn't a clinical researcher. It's always been hard to be a clinical researcher. People escape to animals or to administration. A lot of people who did the initial work stopped doing any more, you know, once they became editors or heads of department and so on. If you do ten years in clinical research, that's a pretty good average. I've kept doing it till today but that's unusual; most people give it up much sooner. Also, I think, a lot of people have a limited amount of research in them. You do it when you're a young person and that's it.

In a sense the unit with Derek Richter and yourself was one of the few places were the marriage of neurochemistry and clinical research actually happened. Can you tell me about your move to West Park?

Well, we moved first to a hospital around here called St Ebba's but they decided to change it into a hospital for mental subnormality. Then Derek Richter and I went to West Park to see Theo Schlitt, who was the medical superintendent, and said what we wanted to do and that was it. We got an architect from Brighton, who constructed a laboratory adjacent to one of the wards which became our clinical investigation ward. John Bailey was working with me at that time. He was a very important person in the unit actually because he was the chap who could arrange the practicalities of a study. You've got to have a person who can make up for your lack of organizational capacity. John Bailey was that for me. We sat down and drew up plans for the architect and the whole Unit was up and going in six months.

I always say that the first thing you must do when you start research is to have an idea and be doing it. Everything else is rubbish. If you spend all your life waiting for the right grant you'll do nothing. The only thing you and I haven't got much of is time. So even in St Ebbas' where basically the only thing we had was a corridor, we were doing whole body measurements with a bedrest I pinched from my wife and a radio-active counter – that was 1961 and 1962. It's important to get things working. It doesn't matter about the environment. It doesn't matter if you've got a secretary or not or a nice desk.

My idea in West Park was, as Claude Bernard said, to bring the bedside to the laboratory. We had the laboratories tacked onto the ward. We designed a ward that would hold men and women. I think 16 was the maximum but we very rarely ran it full. My principle was that you should give a very good clinical service to the patient. They shouldn't suffer because they've been investigated and from the beginning that was our philosophy really. So we followed up our patients which led us into lithium. We felt it was good that we should continue to see the patient but we also learnt that seeing patients long term is very educational. Very few academic people do that actually.

You produced some very interesting electrolyte results that have never been refuted in any way and arguably the mode of action of lithium could be seen to fit in to that, why did that kind of idea all of a sudden go dead. Why did it not . . .

Well, lithium and electrolytes didn't fit together very well to be quite honest. Lithium had few effects on electrolytes that we could detect in our whole body measurements. The effects of lithium on 5-HT were much more marked. We found that it normalised 5-HT transport in depression. Work on lithium also led us to the 5-HT hypothesis.

How did that come about?

That came out of one of the crucial experiments of 20th century psycho-pharmacology! (Coppen, Shaw and Farrell, 1963). You have to remember how incredibly little knowledge we had in 1960. One idea was that amines were important and most people, particularly the Americans, had put their money on noradrenaline. We thought it was worth looking at other compounds and I was impressed by a paper that was published by Kety and associates, who gave monoamine oxidase inhibitors plus trypto-phan to schizophrenics. It didn't do anything for schizophrenia but they thought the patients felt better on it and were less depressed. It was a very good example of the importance of careful reporting of clinical responses.

I said well, okay, 5-HT may be important in depression. So what we did was we got a selection of people with severe depression and put all of them on a monoamine oxidase inhibitor and to one lot we added a placebo-tryptophan and to the other we added the active form. This was done on a random basis and the trial was double—blind. The difference in response was dramatic. If you look at the data, it wasn't a small difference, there was a big difference between the two groups. These results have been replicated several times. This combination of an MAOI and tryptophan was really the first 5-HT treatment. I claim that it was the first observation that suggested that 5-HT was important in depression – an idea that is now the centre of a multi-billion pound drug market. For many years, people said yah-boo sucks – there's nothing in this and, as I said, fashions are everything in medicine and 5-HT was not in fashion.

When we tried to get people from pharmaceutical companies interested, they didn't want to know. In fact, in the 1970s, Eli Lilly had a conference, about a drug they had called fluoxetine which they didn't know what to do with. So they had a conference at their base in Surrey and they asked me to make a contribution. Of course I was enthusiastic about 5HT and the possibilities in mood disorders. I always remember the Vice President of Research saying 'I thank Dr Coppen for his contribution but I can tell you we won't be developing fluoxetine as an antidepressant'.

Really?

Yes. That was a bit like a person saying 'people are fed up with these boys from Liverpool, they'll never go anywhere . . .'. In fact they must have made billions of dollars out of it now.

So, at this time we had three horses. We had the amine horse, the electrolyte horse and we had the endocrine horse. My hypothesis was that maybe one of those things upsets the balance. There could be too much cortisol, which might affect the distribution of electrolytes and 5-HT. This interesting research on electrolytes we couldn't take any further because my philosophy has been if you find an abnormality try and manipulate it and see what happens to the patient . . .

But there was no easy way to manipulate electrolytes.

No there wasn't. We tried diuretics and steroids but that didn't do it. So we left this area because we couldn't really take it any further and as I said lithium didn't seem to be working through anything to do with electrolytes.

Where did your interest in lithium come from?

Well, the world of biological psychiatrists was very small in the 1960s. Everyone knew everyone. You're asking me about people in this country, you can easily ask me about people in the world. I've known Mogen Schou since about 1959 I think. I knew about his work and that's why we got onto lithium because I thought ho, ho, here's an electrolyte – so we looked at this but on the whole it was fairly disappointing.

What was your view on the controversy that blew up between Mogen Schou and Michael Shepherd?

Well, Michael Shepherd himself never took part in any of the debates about it. I remember, at great cost, I got a very nice meeting together at the Royal College and we booked Michael Shepherd to debate with Schou but he never came along. This was about 1967. He would never talk to Schou about it. You know, Schou's first experiment was the mirror image approach looking at patients before and after lithium and, of course, you can criticize that because it implies something about the natural course of the illness that you couldn't properly define. Then he did a random discontinuation study, which was pretty convincing but you could say that the relapses were lithium withdrawal, which it may be with bipolars. Anyway we were meeting in the 1960s in a group called the Denghausen group.

Yes, tell me about that.

That was very interesting. It was promoted by Nate Kline who was a great entrepreneur, a very flamboyant character and he collected people who he thought were good and interesting. He got some good people along there from Europe. We had Arvid Carlsson, Linford Rees, Merton Sandler and Julian Mendlewicz and we had various Americans, who were all people of great standing. The idea was to have a meeting without the impediments of having to read papers. The idea was just to have a meeting of people who could discuss various subjects in depth. We would sit down in the sunshine on some Caribbean island – the only visual aid was the blackboard, which would usually get blown over by the offshore winds – and have three days of discussion. They were very, very good.

Schou was a member of that group. We all used to discuss the various problems he was having with his data and I thought at this stage, it must have been 1967, that we would have to do a prospective study. Our 1971 study, which I think was one of our best studies, was a result of that. In those days, you met in a pub and hammered out a protocol. So we got I think Michael Shepherd and Edward Hare, who was a great sceptic about any treatment, and Ronnie Maggs, who was a most charming man, and Bruce Burns from Belmont and Ramon Noguera (Coppen *et al.*, 1971).

It was a very interesting design – the idea was that we keep a group of patients on lithium or placebo lithium for two years. The psychiatrist looking after them, who was blind to their lithium status, could give them any other treatment they needed. What I wanted to do was to mimic the everyday clinical situation. The results that came out were absolutely staggering. We found that the morbidity in patients on lithum in terms of rated illness was very much lower and the amount of other medication needed was very much decreased. I always remember Ted Hare coming along with his colleague Ramon Gardner and he said that this can't be right. He and Gardner went through the results but they couldn't find any fault with them.

We looked at unipolar as well as bipolar and we found a very good result in both. I didn't like that but it showed a number of things. One was that the outcome of treating depressive illness is very bad when you follow people up but that you could change that completely by proper long-term treatment. After that we decided to set up a lithium clinic because this was obviously a service we should offer our patients. Recently, I have followed up these patients, some of whom have been on lithium for twenty years and using the outcome measure of death by suicide, I found that the outcome of long—term treatment with lithium and other drugs is staggeringly good. Instead of having a suicide rate of seven per thousand, which is the norm, we had a suicide rate of less that one per thousand.

People have said that this is just our selection of patients and so on. In fact it's not. We had the same sort of patients as everyone else. The only thing I would say is that we didn't have much co-morbidity with alcoholism because we had an alcoholic unit and alcoholics tended to go there. So we had fewer than most psychiatrists coping with bipolar depression but then we had more patients referred by people, who would say 'oh, you must be interested in Mrs Bloggs, she's terribly interesting' – but which was code for . . .

We haven't been able to treat her . . .

That's right. Anybody who has a research unit is familiar with that. So they were severe cases. There was very little dropout in the first year, partly, I think, because we had this instant feedback of the lithium level which is very good and makes for good compliance. And we have always given it once a day at night. There's no justification whatsoever in giving lithium more than once a day. And, secondly, after our 1983 paper on dosage, we concluded that 0.6 mmol/litre was the optimum dosage – that the higher levels, in fact, were not so good as 0.6 (Coppen *et al.*, 1983). Our hypothesis for that was that the higher levels were cutting into the thyroid and you need a good thyroid activity for the best clinical response. So we actually shifted everyone in the lithium clinic to low doses in 1983. In fact, we have shown in our series that the morbidity actually decreased in subsequent years after we switched them all to low dosage.

So I think lithium is a very good, safe treatment. We now have 16 years of outcome data and our death rates by suicide per thousand patients is less than one. There's a study from Gothenberg due out this summer with rates of 1.5. This was not done in a lithium clinic but there was regularly monitored lithium compliance data. I would say if you don't have monitored lithium levels you don't know what you are talking about. There is also Muller-Oerlinghausen's four-nation study. In contrast, one of the most important recent studies on suicide is the 1988 one from the

Maudsley and I worked out their suicide rate per thousand patients at about six. The WHO trial from Heinz Lehmann worked out at about eight per thousand and Keith Hawton and his colleagues in Oxford last year showed that the suicide rate of patients discharged from a psychiatric hospital in Oxford was something like ten per thousand patient years. Horrendous. People are obviously not getting continuation therapy, not getting treatment which has been well established for twenty years. Our data showed an 80% reduction in suicide rate compared with these figures which is fantastic.

I think suicide is a good proxy measure of morbidity. Most people don't have morbidity data but they have the suicide data. I think this is one of the big findings in medicine actually but in spite of this most psychiatrists don't treat depressions very well, they don't give continuation therapy. My big concern at the moment is trying to get people to take some notice of this. The Department of Health in their recent White Paper want to reduce suicide rates but they don't give any idea of how it can be done. And despite the fact that we have now an established method for doing this – which is treating depression, which is responsible for 70% of suicides in the general population – some members of the psychiatric profession are saying these targets cannot be met. They can. Treating depression properly means treating the episodes and giving continuation therapy.

Why do you think people haven't taken as much notice of this data as they should? If this were tumours, there would be a big fuss – it would be a media issue. Why is it you think?

I don't know. I think the *Zeitgeist* is a bit against this. Psychiatric illnesses are seen as a sort of social illness, or depression and suicide are anyway – a social illness that should be treated by social methods. I think this is out-of-date science dating back to the 1950s or earlier but it persists in psychiatry. A lot of people who are in psychiatry are not really interested in the medical model. They went into psychiatry to get away from it. That's one reason. Another is that lithium is very cheap. There is not much money there commercially. But I think the next big issue is going to be the question of long-term treatment of a depressive illness. I think what will happen, and it has already begun to happen in the United States, is that patients are going to start suing doctors who haven't informed them of the course of the illness. There is a general agreement about the course of the illness now – it's pretty bad – so everyone should be told about it.

In the States, long-term treatment is getting a lot of publicity – much more than in this country but in the recent advice to general practitioners from the Royal Colleges, there was very little about long-term treatment, although it did emphasize the importance of continuation therapy. Now I am happy with any sort of long-term treatment as long as it's been shown to work. If you think cognitive therapy is useful okay you should offer them cognitive therapy. But not to offer patients long-term treatment I think is very bad medicine. But this view is not fashionable. I'm a very unfashionable person in British psychiatry at the moment.

You feel that.

Oh, yes. I think things are probably changing. I think the Maudsley under Aubrey Lewis was essentially socially minded and it stayed that way under Dennis Hill even though he started in biological psychiatry. I think biological psychiatry hasn't been popular in this country, even though the big revolution in the management of schizophrenia is tied to psychopharmacology. I can remember just before the chlorpromazine revolution, if you went into a schizophrenic ward, you really were going into quite a terrible place. It was really quite sad really. People have got no idea about that now. Psychiatrists seem to feel that they are going to dirty their hands somehow, if they do follow-up clinics. They get nurses to do it or someone else to do it. But a change will come. It will come from patient groups as well as professionally.

Let me move over to 5-HT, which has become a big issue since the 1967 article.

That stemmed from the 1963 experiments I have already mentioned. Having established the clinical evidence, we decided first to look at tryptophan levels in plasma because that's something you could get at. So we developed a method for looking at free and total tryptophan levels – which is quite difficult really because it changes very rapidly and you have to standardize the time of day and all sorts of things are very important. Anyway, we came up with some findings, which are still a bit controversial, that there was a deficiency of free tryptophan in plasma. This fitted in very well with the 5-HT hypothesis. We then got on to the platelet which is a very nice accessible organelle. The other thing we looked at in the early 1960s when people did cerebrospinal fluid studies, was CSF concentrations and we found a low concentration of 5-HIAA, the 5-HT metabolite, in depressed patients. That was about 1963.

Who else was working in this area?

George Ashcroft was and the other was Herman van Praag. We were the first actually to show an effect on mood. Then there was the probenecid story, which gave us the idea about the rate of synthesis of 5-HT. Herman van Praag was very active in that. He was subject to a lot of abuse in Holland because of it. You know, left-wing politics in those days meant you were antiscience as well. I remember we had a meeting there and the demonstrators were all letting off smoke bombs and things outside which was quite interesting. Nice young men actually. There were these banners up and I asked one of the demonstrators to translate it for me because I didn't speak Dutch. He was very nice and pleasant although he'd just been threatening to kill Herman van Praag but it was just a sort of phase.

That was when?

It was in the 1960s I suppose. Poor Herman had a bad time. We get these various clusters between left–wing politics and green issues. When we were measuring body potassium, every so often the radioactive count would go up because the big powers were letting off bombs. We could pick up Russian and American bombs this way. The thing about radioactivity is that it's very easy to measure, whereas with lots of other pollution you can't. You don't know what pollutants there are in the atmosphere because there's no way of measuring them.

Who else was with you in the Unit?

Well, Eccleston was, he was a good chap. Karabi Ghose, who was a very bright person, who was interested in the alpha receptors. We've never been a very large unit at any time. Art Prange had gone by then I think. Peter Whybrow had gone to a very distinguished career in the US. Stuart Montgomery came to us then and Maryse Metcalfe was our psychologist.

We've always had more ideas than we had people really. But I think you can do multiple investigations at the same time. It's just boring doing one thing. If you're doing clinical research the limitation is the number of suitable patients. Everyone who does clinical research comes across this problem. My idea has always been do as much as one can. I think if any unit produced more than 15 suitable depressives a year they are cooking their books somehow. It can't be done.

Platelet 5-HT uptake had a funny career; it got overtaken by radio-labelled imipramine binding which has been fools' gold as it were.

That's right. We never went into that area ourselves but I knew Sol Langer and he did a very important study and then there were some contradictory reports and since then the controversy has raged on a bit, hasn't it. What would you say the state of play is now?

People would say that there are too many methodological problems with it.

What·you find in science is that in the end you never convince anyone. You just get a silence – which means that people have decided to drop the issue. No one stands up and says I was wrong and this was a stupid thing to have done. They just don't carry on with it.

You think it would have been useful if one or two people stood up and said that they were wrong.

Yes. In a way I did that. Although I didn't say it in so many words. Again, digressing to plasma level and clinical response and the therapeutic window and all that. Some Danes said if you get the plasma concentration of nortriptyline right there will be 100% response. So we had a look at amitriptyline and our initial study which was published in 1972 was confirmatory. We thought oh boy, psychopharmacology is going to be dead simple now. Just give enough to get the right concentration and that's it.

Stuart Montgomery came in on this didn't he? Tell me about how he came to you.

I think he'd been with Linford Rees. He hadn't been in psychopharmacology very long at this stage. He had quite a varied career – he was a poet and a few other things. He was a very interesting chap, very enthusiastic and immediately took to psychopharmacology. This was at the time of the therapeutic window. And we did a study which actually didn't confirm our original findings and then I said well let's set up a WHO study which I think in a way was one of the decisive factors. We showed there was almost no correlation when we had large groups. We published that in the *Lancet* (Coppen *et al.*, 1978).

But, of course, you have the therapeutic window chaps still going on saying that there is a therapeutic window but in fact mainstream interest died a death. So we had one very positive finding which we never explained – there was no collusion; the ratings were independent and the plasma levels we got from Guy's. We just put the two together and we found this fantastic correlation. So you do get correlations purely by chance.

Let me take up your third horse, the endocrine one. Tell me where that came from.

Yes, well, that was terribly in the air in the 1950s and 1960s. Besser at Barts was the first chap to do the dexamethasone suppression test, the DST. But because he used large doses of dexamethasone every patient with depression was suppressed. You had to find the optimum dose and then . . . And then of course there was Barney Carrol.

Now what happened there? One of the ways to read all this is that really an awful lot was happening here in the UK from the 1950s onwards but all of a sudden the US flare for propaganda commandeered the field.

If I may go back to 5-HT. 5-HT never really became respectable until the Americans accepted it more or less in the middle 1970s. Then it seemed as though the 5-HT hypothesis had been invented in America, although they had for years fought with us about it. Joe Schildkraut was one of the great protagonists. I used to be on committees with him. So we knew each other's arguments backwards. But if it hasn't been invented in the States, it doesn't count.

So Barney Carroll invented the Dex Test.

He's a great enthusiast and basically we were all agreed that it was a quite a sensitive way of detecting a depressive illness. Now at this stage it was getting such a big thing so I said we'll have to go into this but we must do other groups. So we tested normals, and schizophrenics, and dementias and neurotics too and the thing that came out was that its sensitive to depression but it was not specific.

You ended up heading up the WHO study on this — how did that come about?

Well, I was invited to join the World Health Mental Illness Centre in the 1960s and I found it very interesting. I used to go to Geneva and meet people in the same field. I always felt we ought to have a practical scheme that we were working on because as I said earlier you must be doing something, not talking about what you would do if you had enough money. The only thing no one has got is time. Having come out of the army and going into medicine I always felt that I hadn't had enough time anyway.

Anyway, it struck me that to test the DST in depression was an investigation the WHO could do. So we constructed a protocol. The cortisol was measured in Epsom and all the different centres had to do was to follow the protocol and send us the blood. It was a very standardized trial. With these international studies, if you do a collaborative study, it's a serious business. Because if one centre does it badly what do you say, you have to include it. There was one centre, if you read the article, which gave us problems. However, the other results were conclusive and I think it really killed the Dex test (Coppen *et al.*, 1987).

I think that's one of our major contributions to that area. When I say killed it, we killed it as a naive diagnostic test — you see it was sensitive but not specific. People are still using it but the truth is that it's no good hanging on to dead ideas once they're dead. I think it had a good run for its money. There used to be psychopharmacology labs who were offering it as a service and charging so many dollars for a Dex test and so on.

Coming back to your idea that these things go round full circle, and the idea that you mentioned which was that cortisol might have an effect on tryptophan and thereby on 5-HT, this was around in the 1960s but I've recently heard it put forward as though it's just being proposed for the first time. Gerald Curzon is another name to mention in this connection I suppose.

Oh, yes. Gerald Curzon did a lot of first-rate animal work on tryptophan and on the interactions between cortisol and tryptophan. It makes a lovely story doesn't it. You get emotionally disturbed by the environment; this causes a burst of cortisol and this interferes with amine synthesis and it goes round in a vicious circle. There may be something in it.

But people now aren't aware that it's been around before.

Well, I think basically we are still living on the intellectual capital of the 1950s .

Do you want to expand on that?

Well how were psychotropic drugs discovered. We all know they were discovered by accident. People doing funny things because they had a bright idea and they tried it. Now I think I was probably one of the last to do that with tryptophan and monoamine oxidase inhibitors. The way to discover things is actually to try things out. This is what we did in the 1950s and 1960s but of course we can't do that now because we're so heavily regulated. You can't have these ideas and it's notable, isn't it, there haven't been many new ideas in psychopharmacology in the last decade.

What about the origins of the BAP?

This really came about because a few of us thought it would be a good idea and we wrote a letter to the *Lancet* in 1974.

The first thing I knew was from old Max Hamilton because I knew him and I knew David Wheatley – he was a general practitioner. I suppose what it all revealed was the sort of problems between specialist pharmacologists and people in clinical situations like David Wheatley.

Yes there was this big row; how do you read it?

Well, I never really knew. I know that people like Malcolm Lader, Philip Bradley – they were professional pharmacologists and somehow it seemed to them it was the clinical people who were trying to take it over. I don't think that was ever anyone's intention. As far as I know, they just wanted to simply get it going as a multidisciplinary forum. That was certainly my idea – a CINP-like group really. And as you know there was a fuss about it because we didn't put the letter in *Nature* and we did put it in the *Lancet* and obviously clinical people are more likely to read the *Lancet*. All that sort of thing but I think there was just a bit of paranoia. But Max really helped to diffuse a lot on that famous Saturday morning meeting at the RSM.

Tell me about that.

Oh, it went on for a long time. Max was a very good Chair because he had a lot to do with trade unions and he knew how you should put motions and amend motions and that sort of thing, which by the time anyone figured it out, it had taken the steam out of the situation. I remember Philip Bradley was very against it but I think he and others were pretty reassured at the end of it and in a way because of the suggestions that they had made we became a very democratic society. No one was allowed to be in Council for very very long. So, it was a very transitory Council. You go on, you do your bit and you're kicked off. I think it's one of the most successful organizations I've been associated with. I think the problem is going to be getting the balance right because I don't know how you see clinical research in this country but I feel that the interest is declining among psychiatrists.

By clinical research do you mean clinical trial work?

Not only clinical trials but clinical pharmacology and basic biochemical pathology in patients; I think that's the most important thing. I think as I say the use of drugs is very important. People like to smear drug trials but in fact good drug trials, good evaluation of therapy, is extremely important. I've been really impressed by the ISIS trials in cardiology. They're wonderful, aren't they. Could one do that sort of thing?

We need it but these haven't been industry run and I think there's a failure to appreciate that we need trials other than the ones that are being done by the industry. The MRC at one point during the 1960s did that kind of thing.

The MRC trial was actually a very bad trial. I was in St Ebbas' and I always remember seeing these yellowing piles of forms going round. I suspect the most junior psychiatrist in most places was told to do it. It wasn't carefully done. I think there should be properly established ways of doing these. But it's not being done in this country. I think in the United States they are more aware of this need.

Yes, but even there someone like NIMH should be taking on this but they are not.

Well, the NIMH has its advantages and disadvantages. It's a very bureaucratic place. A place I have great respect for is the Cochrane Centre at Oxford. Everyone should be looking at their outcomes. It's not difficult to do now, with the NHS central registry, all computerized now. You should be looking to see what's happened to your patients say in 10 years time. In mood disorder trials, you've got the acute trials which are not difficult to do but there are also the continuation trials, which some drug companies are doing now but there are also the long-term trials. The most urgent thing to investigate is the proper long-term treatment of depression and no—one is doing that at the moment. Drug companies I think find that maybe the dangers of doing it are too great – some awful thing might come out and they think well why should they risk their short-term profits.

I think the SSRIs could be the good long-term antidepressants. David Kupfer's trial was interesting. It cost a lot of money to do but at least one has some idea of the three-year outcome. The short-term six-week trial, of course, is still necessary but it's the long-term trials which are now important. The results of six-week trials are more or less the same for most drugs but in continuation trials, there's this enormous difference and I would think that a five-year study would be even more clearcut.

One of the curious things about the BAP has been that it was an organization of small groups. It hasn't been dominated by the Maudsley. Somehow the Maudsley didn't really contribute to British psychopharmacology.

A lot of the questions I've been interested in the Maudsley hasn't contributed to. Malcolm Lader has contributed a good deal to the anxiety area but on a lot of the big questions I think the Maudsley hasn't been there, although they have contributed to genetics.

Why did they miss out on a revolution?

They went very heavily into social psychiatry and actually what has social psychiatry shown that reduces morbidity and mortality? What social psychiatry has done is that it's shown that you if send schizophrenics home to a place where people are unkind, they don't like it very much. I don't know how important social events are in depressive illness. Maybe for the initial episode. I did a study with Gene Paykel, which I never published, on life events in patients on long-term lithium. The bottom line was that even big life events don't cause a relapse in a patient on long-term lithium.

You've risen to the top of the CINP as well. Do you want to chart your career through that?

Well, I've been on the CINP for a good many years. Early on the most dramatic thing I remember was that we were going to have meeting in Prague but when the Russian tanks came in, we had to decide whether we should carry on having the meeting there or not. At that stage it wasn't possible to change the venue so we would have had to just cancel it altogether. Our Czechoslovakian colleagues begged us to go and we went actually and I've asked them since then whether we did the right thing and they all said yes. We weren't going there to prop up any regime. We were there as scientists meeting other scientists. It was a very sad place too. But I think we did the right thing.

I was on the Scientific Programme Committee of the CINP initially and then I was asked to become President-elect. It must have been 1986. I enjoyed it actually because I never canvassed for the job or even thought about it actually; they just asked me to − the nominating committee − and I said yes and I found it a very interesting job to have.

Why?

Well, I was interested to get the best people in the world together and where else to do that but at the CINP, which is a world meeting. Secondly, I had the opportunity of taking CINP to Kyoto − I felt, as a world organization, it was an omission that we hadn't been to Japan. So I put all my weight behind it and it was a very good meeting. It was well attended considering it was so far away for a lot of people and also we had a lot of Japanese contacts. It's very important to realize that America and Europe are only part of a world science club.

I started two new initiatives in the CINP when I was President. One was to start a programme of postgraduate teaching in developing countries. This we did in conjunction with WHO. I asked Brian Leonard to be the Chairman of the Education Committee and he has organized a fantastic programme in Africa, the Middle East, Indonesia and Korea for example.

My second initiative was the President's workshop. The idea was to discuss a subject in depth for two and half days with a number of fairly brief papers and lots of discussion. The CIBA Foundation meetings were our model. As it was my workshop, the first one was on 5-HT. The discussion was recorded and a very good volume was sent to all our members. Merton Sandler was very helpful in the organization and publication of this meeting. I am glad to say that both these initiatives have been built into the cycle of CINP programmes. Since the CINP has become so busy, I felt it was necessary to have an office with an Administrator and Gill Houston has filled this post with distinction. I think the CINP has now become more useful and stimulating.

Can I just ask you about that. A point that can be made is that in a sense psychopharmacology has been a means of spreading US/UK cultural imperialism where psychiatry is concerned. Because of English becoming the language of psychopharmacology all the major journals in this part of the world have had to adopt it so that whereas before the War German psychiatry had been dominant; now it has become an Anglo-American thing.

I think a lot of it was the European actually. I always thought the 5-HT theory of depression developed around the North Sea in a way. George Ashcroft up North, us, even though we're not quite on the North Sea but we're not far away, and Herman van Praag. People say this sort of thing but I don't think it's true. The French publish in English now because they realize this is necessary in order to be read. The British scientific paper has become the normal way to report science.

Yes, but you could argue that the creation of things like DSM-IIIR, etc. have formed a mould in which all of the other cultures have fitted. Japan in particular. You've got these pharmaceutical companies over there now having to make drugs for indications that culturally aren't theirs.

But the Japanese say they are. I mean I agree the Americans are trying to push their DSM-IV but I prefer the ICD-10. Its a bit annoying but I've been surprised how well these things do fit into other cultures. Not relying on our own judgement but that of other people. You know we all say the orientals are very calm and so on but you know they suffer from psychiatric illnesses similar to ours. I've been out in the Middle East, talking to Royal Princesses, and their problems are very much like the ladies of West Ewell actually. Exactly the same – unsatisfactory spouses, boredom, etc. I think it's universal. But, one of the things you have got to realize about oriental peoples is that they have a different metabolism so their dosages may need to be quite different to ours. We had a bit of a problem about a 1 mg dose of dexamethasone in the Japanese, when using the Dex test, and I think they've probably reduced it to half a mg. Their dosage of antidepressants is also less. Another thing is that other cultures may not have our high intake of food and so on. For example, to get a proper response to antidepressants, you've got to have a normal folate and this isn't so in some countries. So I don't think it really is scientific imperialism. I just think that it's evolving. But I think the Europeans and the Americans got there first on this one.

Talking about psychiatric nosology − you've left your mark there in the form of the premenstrual syndrome.

Yes, Neil Kessel and myself looked at this (Coppen and Kessel, 1963). We certainly didn't invent it but we put it on the map. We carried out the work in the early 1960s, which was before the pill, which has made all this kind of work unrepeatable since. Or sample was a group of 500 women randomly selected from their general practitioner and we sent a questionnaire to them. We tried not to suggest that there was a pre-menstrual syndrome but we asked about pain, irritability, depression and other symptoms and whether they occurred before, during or after.

What came out very clearly was that pain occurred during and depression and irritability and all the rest of the symptoms occurred before. It was associated with neuroticism. There was no difference between North and South of England or between country and town. Parity made a difference to menstrual pain but it didn't make any difference to the pre-menstrual syndrome. I can tell you that in those days people didn't talk about menstrual periods. Women could never discuss with men whether they had a menstrual period or not because they found it terribly embarrassing. Your generation probably can do that but I can assure you it wasn't the thing then. Anyway when the results came out there was a lot of interest in them. The *Sunday Times* did a big spread about them but at the last moment the medical editor rang up and said 'Well, the editor doesn't feel the public is quite ready for this'. But at least it got around. It got on the news and I think onto radio as well. The reaction was actually that I had a lot of letters from women saying well thank God someone's described it, because it was common even though it was not recognized at all.

There had been Franks in the 1930s and some work by Katerina Dalton, Raymond Greene and Linford Rees. Katerina Dalton's studies were fascinating. She used to go to boarding schools where they recorded the menstrual periods and girls did less well in the exams during the pre-menstrual time. But ours was first epidemiological study. We found that 10% of women complained of severe pre-menstrual syndrome. But it could never be repeated because people went on the pill and you can no longer get the natural history. Then we looked at the premenstrual syndrome in psychiatric patients. There wasn't very much difference actually – they were like other people. Then we got to nuns, who presumably didn't have much to do with men and they were much the same as anyone else. I also helped to organize a study in Spain. At that time, in Spain, upper class girls were very virginal and they were also the same as in Britain. So we weren't bringing any menstrual imperialism into Spain.

You said that the field has been very small in this country – if I was to ask you who influenced you, would it be more useful to ask a question on a world scale?

Well, let's see. I think of Mogen Schou, Herman van Praag, Biff Bunney, Fred Goodwin, Ed Sachar, who's dead now – a very good friend of mine, I think his death was a great loss. Who else. Well I suppose people like Joe Schildkraut – we were old sparring partners – and a man I have great respect and liking for is Arvid Carlsson.

I don't think we've been inferior to any group actually. We had this habit of doing several things at the same time, which always used to irritate some people, but I never felt over–stretched. I think our 5-HT things were a success. I think our long-term treatment studies were a success. We certainly drew attention to the pre-menstrual syndrome or whatever they call it these days. I think we contributed quite a bit to psychopharmacology as regards plasma levels and therapeutic response and the development of new drugs. I think we were the first to demonstrate that mianserin had some antidepressant effects.

I think the Maudsley has really been a bit a disappointment in the last 20 to 30 years, especially in the field I've been working in which is the biochemistry and the management of mood disorders. It raises the question of which is the best way of conducting research. I think there's a lot to be said for the old MRC idea of selecting a Director and backing him for a good period of time. I think, though, that our small Unit which never consisted of more than a few people at any given time bears quite reasonable comparison with any other unit. I think the thing that is most important, the only things that are important, really, are ideas and the ability to promote those ideas and to put them to practical use in research terms.

Picking the right people also helps.

Picking the right people, and that's a matter of luck really. You know you get awful people, you get good people and some people are shy and don't show themselves. I must say that most of the people with whom I worked were very good and we had a lot of fun. The best days have been when one's just sort of sitting down talking with a bit of scrap paper in front of you putting forward ideas and so on. I think it must be very difficult to work up long term programme ideas because you stumble on all the really new and really good ideas as you go along.

In a sense psychopharmacology really doesn't lend itself to long-term programmes – new drugs are turning up new phenomena and you've got to change to accommodate the phenomena rather than . . .

Yes, you've got to change your ideas in view of what is happening. I gave a talk in France at the Pasteur Institute some time ago and I said that since we can no longer try new things so easily, we need to keep an eye on the side effects of drugs in other areas. They say the best way of finding new oil reserves is to sink oil wells – I mean geology studies are one thing but the main thing is to be sinking lots of wells and see what comes out. But we can't do that so easily anymore.

Ole Rafaelsen used to say that all movements are over in 30 years whether it is Elizabethan or Jacobean drama or painting. The whole thing happens in the first and second wave who have the exciting ideas. After that something dies and something else has to take its place. I think maybe with research projects if you get a very large organization you get into the problem of self-promoting bureaucracies and so on which maybe doesn't produce very much work.

It would be nice really for something really new to turn up but in the interim we must stop research being very conventional. I think I was very fortunate in being in the work at this time. All my colleagues who went into the research side say it would be so awful to try and do that again, given the present circumstances. People today, though, don't realize what a tremendous impact the antidepressants, neuroleptics and lithium have had on the terrible morbidity of mood disorders and schizophrenia, however imperfectly these drugs have been applied by clinicians. When I go to West Park now I find about 400 patients suffering from dementia. What a contrast to 40 years ago when there were 2000 very disturbed young and middle-aged patients, many of whom are now leading ordinary and rewarding lives thanks to these advances.

Select bibliography

Coppen, A. and Shaw, D. (1963) Mineral metabolism in melancholia. *British Medical Journal*, **24 ii,** 1439–444.

Coppen, A. and Kessel, N. (1963) Menstruation and personality. *British Journal of Psychiatry*, **24 109,** 711–21.

Coppen, A., Shaw, D. and Farrell, J.P. (1963) The potentiation of the antidepressive effects of a monoamine—oxidase inhibitor by tryptophan. *Lancet*, **24 ii,** 61–64.

Coppen, A. (1967) The biochemistry of affective disorders. *British Journal of Psychiatry*, **24 113,** 1237–264.

Coppen, A., Noguera, R. Bailey. J, *et al.* (1971) Prophylactic lithium in affective disorders. Controlled trial. *Lancet*, **24 ii,** 275–79.

Coppen, A., Ghose, K., Montgomery, S., *et al.* (1978) Amitriptyline plasma concentration and clinical effect. A World Health Organisation Collaborative Study. *Lancet*, **24 i,** 63–66.

Coppen, A., Abou-Saleh, M.T., Millin, P, et al. (1983) Decreasing lithium dosage reduces morbidity and side effects during prophylaxis. *Journal of Affective Disorders*, **24 5,** 353–62.

Coppen, A., Metcalfe, M., *et al.*(1987) The dexamethasone suppression test in depression: A World Health Organisation Collaborative Study. *British Journal of Psychiatry*, **24 150,** 459–62.

12 Jules Angst

The myths of psychopharmacology

You began training in Zurich when Jung was still there.

Yes, C.J. Jung was in Zurich. He lived with his wife in Küsnacht at the lake of Zurich. He had a wonderful villa, which I believe was built with the money of his wife, who came from a wealthy Schaffhausen family. Jung's father was a clergyman in Basel. His academic career took him to a Chair in Psychology at the Zurich Institute of Technology, but he started out at the hospital where I am, at the Burghölzli in Zurich, where he became, under Eugen Bleuler, PrivatDozent, which corresponds to Reader in Psychiatry. I knew him personally of course.

What was he like?

Well, he was very much as his biographers describe him, a big bear. A very tall, strong man, always surrounded by a multitude of women. There were very few men around him – one was C-A. Meier, who was one of his most important students. He was admired by everyone and I too admired him for his encyclopedic knowledge. He had such a brilliant, wide scope of interests covering all aspects of culture, the history of religions and anthropology and this attracted many sophisticated experts from all over the world, experts in Egyptology, Taoism, Zen Buddhism, mysticism and cabbala. I attended his lectures and was also a discussant at them; he was always very brilliant, able to relate esoteric concepts to his theory of archetypes.

I was a student of Jungian psychology over many years. Originally I had started by studying Freudian psychology when I was in the gymnasium at age 15 or 16 but then I went on with Jung and with Adler and others. The Jungian school was quite strong at that time in Zurich. In the second year of my medical studies I began attending presentations on psychotherapy by psychotherapists: Boss, Banziger, Bjerre, Brun and Herbert and Kurt Binswanger. Then I underwent a Jungian analysis and attended lectures in the Jungian Institute, which had been founded by then. Interestingly enough, Jung did not sympathize at all with the Jungian Institute. He did not attend either its foundation or its opening. He was very suspicious of a school being made out of what he did. I find that rather a healthy reaction, because the more scholastic a movement becomes, the more rigid and less productive it gets. I think that may have been his concern, too. Later, of course, he was not at all hostile to the movement. Anyway that was how I came to study psychology.

Later, I was a guest member of the Psychological Club for many years. The Psychological Club was an interesting idea. Jung founded it because he wanted to organize social events for patients together with their analysts. Papers were presented in the Club by good people from all over the world and these talks were attended by both patients and therapists. There was also another group, the SGPP, the Swiss Association for Practical Psychology, of which Jung became President. The SGPP membership consisted of psychologists and psychiatrists. Jung's aim was to provide a special forum to bring the two groups together – this goes back to the old development of psychoanalysis by Freud. The SGPP was in existence until 1994. Jung was its first President, Meier the second and I was the third. I was also a founding member of the Jungian Analytical Society.

Originally, then, I was a Jungian analyst to a certain extent; later I was also trained in existentialism and psychoanalysis by Medard Boss and Gustav Bally, in supervision groups mainly. With time, I have become increasingly eclectic and when I became Professor of Psychiatry at the University of Zurich, I didn't stick any more to schools. But I continued to give psychotherapy until very recently. I have never given it up completely.

How did Jung react to the introduction of the first psychotropic drugs?

That I don't know. I was a young hospital assistant at the time and I remember that Jung invited the young hospital psychiatrists to his home, in order to discuss psychotherapy and schizophrenia. He still maintained his original hypothesis that schizophrenia was an inner intoxication – an idea which was not in itself absurd. Nowadays it might be expressed as a disturbance of dimethyl-tryptamine (DMT) metabolism, which was also one of my hypotheses for a while. Although he thought that schizophrenia had some organic background, he was convinced patients could be treated by psychotherapy; whereas my experience with the psychotherapy of schizophrenia had convinced me that it was not very efficacious and had led me to abandon it. Indeed that was my main reason for giving up being an analyst in the hospital. The psychotherapy of schizophrenia was carried out under Professor Gaetano Benedetti in Zurich, and I was one of Benedetti's students at the time. Follow-up studies of the results were published by Christian Müller and showed no difference in course and outcome between patients given psychotherapy and the non-treated sample described by Bleuler in his monograph on the course of schizophrenia. So I think Jung was wrong in his psychotherapeutic optimism. He expected too much originally, as many other analysts did, I think.

But I never heard him comment on drug treatment. Jung attended the

1957 World Congress of Psychiatry in Zurich at which he gave a presentation on schizophrenia; this dealt with its causation by strong affects inducing an endotoxin and resulting in psychosis and he also spoke on the psychotherapy of schizophrenia. At this Congress he was also Honorary President of a Symposium entitled 'Chemical Concepts of Psychosis'. I helped edit the four volumes of the Congress report, which was an enormous job and took me about a year.

What was the mood of that conference? Because that was the time . . .

I did not attend the conference itself because I was in the Army. Nathan S. Kline from the United States helped organize a big symposium on psychotropic drugs, the first of its kind to my knowledge to be held at a general psychiatric Congress. The report was later published by Rinkel and Denber (1958). Nathan Kline became a very close friend and told me something about that conference. I can only speak about the attitude of Manfred Bleuler, my teacher, because he organized the congress. He accepted the offer to host the meeting, but his main concern was how to sponsor it. Of course Nathan Kline was an expert in fund raising and had no difficulty financing this symposium.

But drug treatment won through and of course became very important. Bleuler, himself, had played an active role in the field of psychopharmacology from the very beginning. The Burghölzli Hospital was the first to test reserpine in 1953. So by the 1957 Congress we already had four years of intensive research behind us in the field; but we didn't do primary research on chlorpromazine. That, as you know, was carried out in France by Hamon and colleagues and by Delay and Deniker in 1952.

There were quite a few people from Switzerland who were involved in the early days – Kielholz, Staehelin, Poldinger. Was that because the companies who introduced the compounds were largely Swiss?

Yes, in Basel there were John Staehelin, Paul Kielholz and Felix Labhardt, who was one of the first investigators on chlorpromazine in Switzerland. In Zurich, there were Bleuler and Mielke. Mielke, who is probably less well known, conducted the first very large studies on reserpine in schizophrenia. All the trials at that time were open but were as conclusive as double-blind studies, as history has subsequently shown. The development of reserpine, and later of tetrabenazine, a derivative of reserpine, was quite interesting. At that time, the idea was that these drugs worked by inducing a kind of a curative sleep. So patients on reserpine were kept in large 15 to 20 bed dormitories, where earlier the insulin shock treatment had been carried out. The curtains were drawn to encourage sleep. This strategy of keeping patients rested in bed was in contrast to later ideas. We now know we shouldn't keep patients in bed because of the danger of thrombosis. We lost quite a few patients by this treatment at the beginning. We also had sleep therapy with high doses of barbiturates, sometimes together with scopolamine, which was very dangerous, especially in females. I saw patients who had died in the night from an embolic disorder.

That original strategy was later reversed to one which aimed merely to repress the psychotic symptomatology and to activate patients as much as possible, giving them all sorts of occupational or work therapy. The earlier strategy probably arose from the way in which chlorpromazine was discovered. Chlorpromazine was detected in anaesthesia where it was used as part of a cocktail, originally in the sedative treatment of manic patients in France by Hamon even before Deniker and Delay. The underlying concept was that of inducing a kind of hibernation sleep, which is healthy. Now this was obviously a myth, which hasn't been confirmed by subsequent developments.

Were you able to get to any of the early CINP meetings with your Army duty?

I was not at the first meeting. The first one I attended was in Basel in 1960. I became interested in the CINP because Werner Stoll, an associate professor of psychiatry in our hospital, was the son of A. Stoll, a great collector of paintings, who as the Director at Sandoz was involved in the development of LSD. Together with Rothlin, also from Sandoz, he had founded the CINP in 1957. So drug companies played a major role in the CINP's foundation. I was invited by Stoll to present on imipramine at the CINP in Birmingham in 1964. In 1974 I became a member of the CINP executive committee and was the secretary under Pierre Deniker and Leo Hollister. For a while I was very active in testing drugs but then delegated the task to one of my co-workers, Brigitte Woggon. Lately I have become more active again in the field.

I remember one CINP meeting, in Munich in 1962, at which Mogen Schou stood up in a discussion dominated by talk of neuroleptics and antidepressant drugs and spoke about the prophylactic properties of lithium and was greeted with loud laughter. People simply didn't believe that lithium was active. Schou stressed the efficacy of lithium very early on, on the basis of his own experience, but his view was not accepted. There was also no support for the development of lithium because it was not produced by a drug company at the time. In the early days there were no tablets available on the market. When we prescribed lithium it was as a natural product in powder form, which had to be made up by the pharmacy. It was of no financial interest to the drug companies, because it couldn't be patented. Mogen Schou was in an uncomfortable position and showed considerable courage. Lithium is very interesting. You may have heard of the Denghausen group.

I have, yes.

The sculptor Denghausen, whose wife suffered from a bipolar or schizo-bipolar disorder, sponsored many meetings in the Caribbean. The first was in Haiti in 1966 and was organised by Nathan Kline. That was where Mogen Schou and I met. He hadn't yet published his paper with Baastrup on lithium. I had been invited by Nathan Kline because of my mono-graph on uni- and bipolar disorder and my studies on the course of affective disorder, using multiple regression analysis. When Mogen Schou presented on lithium, I offered to do the statistical analysis of his data, which were purely descriptive. He had an impressive number of single cases, before and after lithium treatment, but no statistics. So we did intra-individual statistical analyses, which became a point of controversy, because when Blackwell and Shepherd in 1968 tried using the 'mirror method' they didn't obtain the same results on the spontaneous course of depression as I had.

I'm a strong believer in intra-individual comparisons in disorders, such as schizophrenia, which are known to have a poor prognosis. If you had a drug like lithium that would change the course of the disorder dramati-cally, you wouldn't need many statistics. Intra-individual statistics would be sufficient without any control groups, as in carcinomas with a pure outcome.

So Mogen Schou, Paul Grof, Baastrup and I published these papers together, analysing the data we had collected in Denmark, Czechoslovakia, Germany, Canada and Switzerland. It was a wonderful collaboration. We published three papers on our results in the *British Journal of Psychiatry* and received the Anna Monika award for our work, as it was considered to be good evidence for the efficacy of lithium. But the point I want to make is that we didn't operate with control groups. All these major drug developments in psychiatry came about without controlled trials by using accurate observation, by open trials with good observers and by intra-individual comparisons. There is a comprehensive historical review of the development of lithium written by Gattozzi for NIMH which includes early interviews with several investigators in the field.

You've also been involved with the development of clozapine?

Clozapine was developed here in Switzerland by the Wander company under Professor Stille, a pharmacologist working on the dibenzodiazepi-nes; it was from this line of development that dibenzepine and clozapine came. It is interesting to note that it was a very small group of pharmacol-ogists, doing excellent work, who produced the important drugs. Today we have big institutions, which are no more productive than the small labs they had at that time. Clozapine was then tested in open trials. One of the main investigators was Engelmeier in Germany. You will have heard of the Fünfer Ring from Professor Hippius. The Fünfer Ring consisted of five German investigators: Bente, Engelmeyer, Heinrich, Hippius and Schmidt, from five different universities, who were the real pioneers on the continent of the methodology of antipsychotic drug assessment. They developed a symptom checklist. In Switzerland we were especially interested in depression: our five university hospitals were linked together a little later. We developed a checklist, or rather a rating scale, for depression and hypomania. The German and Swiss groups then joined and together developed the AMD and AMDP systems for Methodology and Documentation in Psychiatry.

By the time clozapine came to be tested, the 10 of us were already cooperating and we were later joined by Peter Berner from Vienna. Clozapine was tested in open trials in all the centres and incidentally found to be efficacious in treating insomnia. This was a very important finding. Clozapine worked for the insomnia of barbiturate-dependent persons – barbiturates could be replaced by clozapine in very small doses. Clozapine was available in 10 mg tablets and you would administer 5–10 mg only.

The main theme, of course, was clozapine's sedative and antipsychotic effect, which was quite obviously present. We published an open study in 1971, of which I was the first author – only because the names were listed alphabetically. Then we in Zurich produced the first double-blind study comparing clozapine to levomepromazine, which we chose because of its sedative effect. We wanted to have a drug more or less equally sedative and with low extrapyramidal side-effects. Clozapine's efficacy was clear right from the start. Its reinvention in America for the treatment of chronic schizophrenia with negative symptoms had great commercial and scientific impact.

But clozapine was recognized from the outset as being an important drug, even though we had a lot of trouble with it. The first problem was proving efficacy. We had a few double-blind studies and two or three open studies when Wander was taken over by Sandoz. A big meeting on clozapine was organized in Bern; Sandoz completely rejected that it could be an antipsychotic, especially the people from Canada, America and other English-speaking countries. They wrote it off as poorly investigated, having only side effects and no efficacy. Then the agranulocytosis risk appeared in Finland with deaths of patients. All the cases were traced and carefully examined by Dr Amberg, the internist at Wander, and clozapine was withdrawn from the market in most countries. It was not withdrawn completely here in Switzerland. It continued to be available, because it was known to be very efficacious not only by those who had investigated the drug but also by all the hospital clinicians with patients being treated with it. We had so many chronically schizophrenic patients who had shown significant improvement on clozapine that we put pressure on the company to carry on producing it. Dozens of individual letters were sent by the heads of the hospitals and others to the directors of the company – arguing that it was unethical to stop production. The company wanted to kill the drug off, but it was maintained because of our opposition.

In a second stage, clozapine was reintroduced in all countries. It was not possible for psychiatrists to stop all clozapine treatment when patients were discharged and so it gradually returned as a post-discharge treatment. But the person really responsible for introducing clozapine into the United States was Nathan S. Kline. Whenever he visited me in Zurich he would enquire about new drugs; I mentioned clozapine or HF1854, which was the investigational number. I recommended him to try it and gave him some, which he took back to the United States where he prescribed it to his patients. When he was no longer able to get clozapine from the company, he sent patients to me; so I started to treat American patients decades ago when clozapine was in its early stage of development. Nathan S. Kline was the first person in the United States to recognie clozapine's value. But then he was always ready to try out new things.

Tell me about Kline.

Nathan S. Kline was an extremely dynamic man and a very good friend. I got to know him on one of his visits in Zurich. The range of his activities was very broad. You may have heard of the admirable work he did for immigrants for example; he supported 150 or more immigrants in the United States, providing them with work or financial support. That was just one one of his merits. Another exceptional thing was his activity founding hospitals abroad: one in Liberia, one in Haiti and another in the Far East, I believe. He raised the money from the drug companies not only for hospital building but also for the supply of the drug treatment and for staff training in Canada or the United States as well. I find that quite admirable; it shows just how energetic he was that he could combine all this with being Director of Research at Rockland State Hospital.

He was, to my knowledge, the first psychiatrist to build up a large databank on hospital patients and their treatment. He did this with Eugene Laska, who is still one of the leading mathematicians in the field. They had a large computer centre funded by the money Nathan Kline had raised. He was extremely active in the field of computerizing psychiatry; he gave us all his computer programs, programs which had cost over a million dollars to develop. He was a very generous man. He was also very active as a practitioner. He not only did research at Rocklands, he also had a large drug practice. He had an initial long interview with his patients, which was frequently video-taped. After that the patients were seen by his assistants, and he saw them again if there were any problems.

But above all he was a man with a special nose for new things. He had enormous enthusiasm and was able to recognize what was important and new. His interests within psychiatry were very broad, and that's one of the reasons why he came to be such a pioneer in the field of psychotropic drugs. He was one of the very first in the world to use iproniazid, which is proof of his flair and interest. He was also an extremely trustworthy friend. He was very active, a bit hypomanic even and never needed much sleep. At 7 o'clock in the morning he would already be knocking at his patients' doors in order to visit them; after that he would drive to the hospital for his research and in the evening he would see more patients. He was a highly motivated doctor, there's no doubt about that. That's Nathan Kline as I knew him.

You said that he was one of the first to collect a large database of patients but you've also gone down this route with a view to tackling some of the myths that have been around psychiatry. One of the first myths that I heard you talking about was at the BAP guest lecture in 1987, when you suggested that there is a common belief that antidepressants can cause a switch into mania but that there is no evidence that this is the case.

Well, I got into data processing very early. I had always been interested in statistics. In 1959 Bleuler gave me a research position for a year and a half, which was sponsored by Geigy in order to test imipramine. I started a large study covering 200 patients, (150 inpatients and 50 outpatients), all of whom I treated myself. For more than 18 months I did nothing but treat depressive patients, which is quite an experience. I nearly became depressed myself. All the patients were drug-naive, at least in present-day terms, although some had been treated with opium, amphetamines or barbiturates.

This study brought me into close contact with Geigy, where Peter Weis was in charge of documentation and statistics. Peter Weis was a chemist but had the task of computerizing the data. At that time only the big banks and big drug companies had computers. The university didn't have one yet. I had the data punched in and computed in Basel by Peter Weis and in 1961 I published a larger analysis on imipramine dealing with predictors of response.

I then got involved in computerizing the AMP, which was more or less a consequence of receiving the computer programs from Nathan Kline. The big push for data processing in psychiatry at the time came mainly came from psychopharmacology – statistical analyses, which required computers.

As to the myths of psychiatry, I don't know. The hypomania issue is certainly one of them. We are autistic in Eugen Bleuler's meaning of the word: we are full of wishful thinking; if we do something and something happens we are always tempted to think that we were the cause of what may in fact be just a chance phenomenon. So if you treat a patient and he gets better, it's a temptation to believe it is because of our treatment, while we know perfectly well that we have to control for the spontaneous course of the disorder, for the placebo effect and so on. This also applies to the switch to hypomania, which for a while was even taken as an indicator of a drug's antidepressant activity. It was maintained that if a drug didn't cause a switch, it wouldn't be a good antidepressant.

I was very sceptical about that from the outset because of other studies I had done on the natural course of the disorder with representative samples, where I had seen the switch occur very frequently without treatment. I had also seen such switches in patients on imipramine, but when I investigated their previous histories, I found that the majority were bipolar patients (Angst, 1965). I therefore carried out retrospective studies going back to the beginning of the century, collecting hundreds of case histories from hospital records, prior to and after the introduction of psychotropics and ECT, in order to see if the switch rates had changed at all over those years. And they hadn't (Angst, 1987; 1992).

W. Bunney's extensive 1978 review of multiple studies on the switch concluded that it was drug-induced; but of course if you have an overall switch rate of 7–8%, it consists of uni- and bipolar cases taken together; however, if you split them, you find that a very low percentage of the unipolar cases and a very high percentage of the bipolar cases subsequently switch from a depressive episode into hypomania or mania. The main factor then in the studies he reviewed is the ratio of unipolar to bipolar patients, for which there was no control. Ideally, the existence of drug-induced hypomania should be shown by means of placebo-controlled studies; however, I know of no studies which have established it by this method. Switching is also a rare event compared to other side effects, which makes it difficult to obtain reliable rates; this is probably a subject for meta-analysis. The problem is that even today there are methodological shortcomings in measuring the switch to hypomania. It's not on the rating scales usually applied for drug evaluation. Our ratings are one-sided – depression-rating scales measure only depression – and the spontaneous reports are, of course, not very reliable. I wouldn't rule out the possibility of a switch occurring. There may be a small percentage of cases which switch on certain drugs, amphetamine or whatever, but I simply do not believe that the majority of switches are drug induced.

So it's not inconceivable then that the antidepressants may also be antimanic in that after all ECT is both antidepressant and antimanic.

Well, that is the other problem which is raised by this question. There are the studies on imipramine carried out by Akimoto (1962) in Japan. He used up to 400 mg of imipramine in the treatment of mania and reported successes and sedative effects, which is very interesting.

We've completely lost sight of this possibility – partly I suspect because the catecholamine hypothesis came along and very simplistically said that there is a lowering of amines in depression and therefore there must be high amines in mania and, ipso facto, any drug which increases amines couldn't be used in the treatment for mania.

This question is dealt with in the monograph on imipramine which I wrote in 1970 with Theobald and others from Geigy. That monograph summarizes over 4000 references, including something on the drug treatment of mania. Akimoto's success in treating mania with drugs was impressive and it hasn't been disproved. Such high doses of imipramine have been discredited mainly because of side effects, such as epileptic seizures.

One of the other myths that you've been interested in more recently is the target symptom myth.

The target symptom concept was introduced by Freyhan in 1960, who was at St. Elizabeth's Hospital in Washington DC. His paper on target symptoms was based on open trials with imipramine mainly. Of course, the majority of depressives are retarded, not agitated, and the general impression was that imipramine worked better in retarded cases than in agitated ones. Agitated patients are very difficult to treat anyhow; they respond well to ECT. So the concept of target symptoms was formulated solely on clinical grounds. Randomized trials were lacking, and it was more of a clinical intuition that a sedative drug should be given to an agitated, and non-sedative to a non-agitated, form of depression. This was the basis of Kielholz's idea of three components of the effects of antidepressants, activating, mood-improving and sedative effects. He classified antidepressant drugs accordingly. I don't believe in these three components. There is no doubt that drugs can show more activation or sedation from an experimental point of view, but that does not provide evidence for a differential indication of drugs, answering the question which drug is more suitable for which type of patient.

Paul Kielholz's recommendation now belongs to common-sense psychiatry and has spread world-wide. In my opinion, though, many of these ideas have not been soundly proved by empirical data.

What do you mean by that?

The common sense view is that an agitated depressive will respond better to a sedative antidepressant like amitriptyline than to a non-sedative drug like moclobemide and vice versa for a non-agitated depressive. But this is simply not proven. A meta-analysis we carried out comparing sedative antidepressants and moclobemide clearly showed that there was no difference in efficacy between patients with low or high agitation.

I'm not convinced about this whole matter of selective clinical profiles for antidepressants. An exception may be amphetamine. I have treated many depressives with amphetamines, as have others like Nathan S. Kline, Donald F. Klein and others. In the early 1950s opium and amphetamine were the main drugs used to treat depression.

The drug available on the market was pure dexamphetamine and a combination with a barbiturate in order to have a sedative effect. Some of us still use amphetamine pure or in combination with a standard antidepressant in refractory depression. Over the years I have certainly seen many patients who do not just show activation under amphetamine but also mood change, a clear elevation or improvement in mood, which points to a true antidepressant effect as well.

Anyway, we now know that all the standard and modern antidepressants have roughly similar efficacy; there is little evidence of a differential activity profile in the subgroups of depression; they all respond to the same extent. Indeed, it is the syndrome of depression across a whole range of disorders and symptoms which seems to respond, while within the depressive syndrome there is no clear evidence of substantial differences between drugs. I therefore think the target symptom concept is a myth. It may be better to apply non-sedative antidepressants; this has been shown by the findings of Ian Hindmarch on the unfavourable effects of standard sedative and anticholinergic antidepressants on cognition, learning, driving and memory. I think it is important to have non-sedative drugs and to use them. Today's SSRIs or RIMAs have great advantages over the standard antidepressants.

Given that the target symptom approach falls down and given also that the target neurotransmitter approach has fallen down, people like Herman van Praag have gone back to an Adolf Meyer type language, it's all just reaction formation. Do you take this kind of approach?

Herman van Praag and Leijnse developed the theory of a functional pathology in 1965, which hasn't so far been disproved. What is clear today is that all transmitter systems are interrelated, which doesn't lend credence to the simplistic views of the action of drugs or of the relationship between personality types and transmitters proposed by some. It may be correct to think along the lines suggested by Van Praag in a more dynamic sense, based on syndromes which cut across psychiatric classification.

Psychopharmacology stimulated a syndromal approach very early on. It has always been thought that the drugs work on core syndromes and not on disorders. This idea is now better founded. It makes little sense to stick to a rigid, static system of classification but might be more promising to look for general functional syndromes of behaviour or mood regulation. In these terms, I think I would to some extent agree with Herman van Praag.

The third group of myths you've taken on to some extent is one you've taken on through your involvement in the development of moclobemide. The MAOIs as a group of drugs have been more subject to myths than any other group of psychiatric drugs.

I was involved in research on iproniazid and isoniazid in 1956 before they were used in psychiatry. I carried out a trial on iproniazid and isoniazid in multiple sclerosis, which is published in the *Swiss Medical Journal*. At that time, these drugs were used in the treatment of tuberculosis. A paper from Vienna reported Gram-negative bacteria in the CSF of multiple sclerosis patients, suggesting that it was a special subtype of tuberculosis and that it should be treated as such, which is what we did – but without any effect. Without any therapeutic effect, that is, but we did see a lot of side effects, which is the point of the episode. Iproniazid turned out to produce peripheral blood changes. We found extensive erythrocyte destruction. I made a lot of bone marrow punctures and looked at the findings together with a very good haematologist colleague; they were quite clearly a side effect of iproniazid.

All this was before iproniazid was introduced into psychiatry. After the first symposium on iproniazid in Zurich at which the Roche Company presented its data, Bleuler asked me whether we should introduce it. I advised against, because it was toxic. My scepticism was also based on the literature, which showed that it can create confusional states. Although we did use iproniazid to a minor extent, it was never really a major antidepressant drug and it wasn't a great success on the Swiss market. Subsequent drugs like parnate, tranylcypromine or phenelzine never broke through as antidepressants either.

The fact that the MAOIs had a restricted indication, being targeted at the syndrome of atypical depression, didn't make them great drugs. If they are only suitable for a subgroup of patients – and an ill-defined one at that – one may well ask why they should be used at all. When I did use these drugs it was mainly in combination with tricyclic antidpressants in treating therapy-resistant cases.

I remained interested in the MAOIs because of reports from England and America. I ordered phenelzine and tranylcypromine from abroad for use in treating depression, but the results were never very impressive or were insufficient to offset the dietary and other problems such as inter-action with other drugs. So the MAOIs remained second or third choice drugs. In the 1980s the advent of the new reversible MAO-A inhibitor (RIMA) moclobemide, gave us a fresh opportunity in the field of MAO inhibition.

Looking at the MAOI story though the MRC trial which suggested that they weren't effective, was probably a poorly done trial, with too low a dose of phenelzine; the liver problems that they caused may have been as much caused by co-prescription with the barbiturates – anyway, you don't find these problems now – and then the famous cheese effect, even in the case of the older MAOIs, seems to have been something of a myth, in that it's very hard now actually to prove that there were ever many people who had a serious problem with the cheese effect other than those who were on tranylcypromine. But for whatever reason, this group of drugs got branded and it's very very hard now for . . .

Yes, in 1965, I was at the Maudsley for a couple of months under Michael Shepherd where I did a retrospective record study by analogy with the MRC trial. Erwin Varga and I went over more than 800 hundred records documenting the treatment results of phenelzine, imipramine and ECT. We confirmed the results of the MRC trial: phenelzine did not perform well compared with imipramine. ECT was the most effective. It is not clear what the poor response to phenelzine really means, given what we now know about moclobemide. The MAOIs should work, at least in adequate doses. It was probably a major error to recommend their use mainly for atypical depression.

Well, was the idea that it was specific for particular kinds of depression more a marketing ploy rather than anything based on scientific evidence?

My view is that we simply didn't have good clinical studies on the classical MAOIs, and the drug companies were not sophisticated enough at that time to attempt any really systematic investigation of them. The MAO inhibitors have never been investigated across all indications to anything like the extent we see for new drugs today. That's my opinion at least.

On that point, it seems likely that there's only going to possibly be one or two more RIMAs introduced into the market and even these compounds are ones that entered development some time ago, so in a sense they are part of an older generation of compounds. Is the golden age of psychopharmacology drawing to a close?

I don't share this opinion. Let's start with the antidepressants since we're on the subject. A ceiling has been certainly reached as regards side effects. The new drugs have so few side effects that they barely differ from placebo; there's not much further one can go. The ceiling may have been reached on tolerability, but there's a long way to go to optimal efficacy. There, too, we certainly currently have a ceiling effect, in that all anti-depressants have the same limited, modest efficacy. We still don't have a truly powerful antidepressant. The potential for better drugs is vast. Good antidepressants, in my view, would be drugs which, like good hypnotics or good analgesics, worked within a few days, if not hours and had higher success rates than 50 to 65%. However, it's my hypothesis that if a new drug really acted faster, it would probably also be stronger; with a higher response rate. The companies will have to look for quicker onset of action and will hopefully focus on non-sedative, stimulant drugs. They won't return to amphetamine but to similar substances.

In contrast to antidepressants, tolerability is still the main problem for antipsychotic drugs. On the other hand, their onset of action is rapid and their effect is more reliable, improving the positive symptoms considerably. But these drugs do not generally cure the condition, which means that there is room for improving action as well as tolerability. The development of receptor sub-typing is likely to play an important role. I wouldn't rule out improvement on both tolerability and efficacy by much higher specific and local action of the drugs in the CNS. So far, experience at least shows that more selective action does not reduce a drug's efficacy. There is no proof, for instance, that the serotonin-specific reuptake inhibitors are any less active than the tricyclics. There may be some differential indications, although that's not really proved in my view.

But in the case of the antipsychotics, arguably the most potent drug is clozapine, which is as non-specific as you can get, and the least potent are the highly selective D-2 blockers.

Yes, but even if that is the case, it doesn't exclude the development of more specific, less toxic and better-tolerated drugs. I think we are still in the early stages of development and I wouldn't be too pessimistic. The whole field of receptor sub-typing seems to be very promising for psychiatry from a dynamic point of view; and I think it could revolutionize psychopathology and pathogenetic theories, cutting right across all sorts of behavioural syndromes. There is some evidence at least for the assumption that certain regulatory systems cut across functional behavioural systems. So I repeat we shouldn't be too pessimistic, as was the case for benzodiazepines, where some drug companies, wrongly to my mind, decided to withdraw or scale back their interest.

The benzodiazepines provide a good example of how the whole issue of partial agonist or partial antagonist hasn't been sufficiently explored. For instance, we had access to oxaprotiline, developed by Roche, a drug which was a partial agonist but behaved clinically like an antipsychotic. Now, if we had benzodiazepine-type antipsychotic drugs, avoiding all the extrapyramidal problems, it would be just great. So, there is some potential left for new compounds with new pharmacological principles.

But aren't we in a climate where it's harder and harder for a company to recoup their costs. The pharmaco-economic prospects facing companies wanting to launch psychotropic drugs that do not differ radically from what has gone before are not good.

Yes, that is a enormous brake. Development has certainly been slowed down by the registration and safety demands and costs, for example. I think this has had a damaging effect of the strategies of the companies, making them over-anxious and unwilling to take risks. Risk-taking behaviour by individuals in the companies is not rewarded, and there's no doubt that to develop a drug has become a major financial risk. It's not that there is no potential. It's rather that society has an exaggerated need for ever more security.

Why do you think we've got so neurotic about drug development?

Well, it's a combination of factors. There is a hostile attitude against everything which is chemical – even though nature is chemical. This interreacts with the whole Green movement, which favours an alternative, more natural way of living and food intake, avoiding all chemicals, which are defined as poisons. Then there's the distrust of science, scientific thinking and scientific proof, which stems from the 1968 movement, and inevitably results in an irrational bias against scientific methods in proving efficacy. In Switzerland at the moment natural healing has a large following, with all sorts of unproven medication and natural products selling well. Medical science has partially lost its prestige in society, with more distrust than trust in scientific methods and overconfidence in all homoeopathic products.

It's really odd that there should have been such a change in so short a period of time. When the drugs were introduced first there was the idea that nature, and particularly disease, was bad, or at least potentially hostile, and they had to be contained by man. Now we've gone to the opposite extreme. Nature is good. Man is the fly in the ointment. Where does that change in thinking come from?

To my mind it stems from the 1968 movement, which was romantic, mystic and irrational. That is why Jung's psychology, with its theory of archetypes and stress on emotional development, or the writings of Herman Hesse, who was treated by a Jungian analyst, had a special appeal. All the mystic experiences of the LSD movement to change what they called consciousness were irrational in a way. This anti-rational movement is still very much alive and partly explains the opposition to drug treatment, which is thought to be inhuman and merely chemical, as opposed to human and more emotional types of treatment.

Another factor is the belief that human beings are being increasingly poisoned by the environment. No one would deny that there is environmental change and pollution, but current concerns are that our present life style and civilization are far away from nature and must therefore be unhealthy. So we have this polarization: on the one side advocacy of a return to nature, and drug treatment is one of the demons on the other side.

Yet another aspect in the rising costs of developing drugs, as I mentioned earlier, is an exaggerated demand for security. Switzerland is a good example. Increased wealth brings over-insurance. People would like to avoid having to take risks in their lives – up to death. As regards drug treatment, people want it to be safer than it can possibly be.

Let me re-introduce the question of psychotherapy here because psychotherapy is often put forward as being much safer than drug treatment. You began as a psychotherapist and recently, at least, there've been some claims that treatments like cognitive therapy and interpersonal therapy are useful for depression – although I know you are somewhat sceptical about claims for the efficacy of psychotherapy in depression. Do you think the vogue for therapies links up to this question of risk?

I was interested in both interpersonal psychotherapy – IPT – which was created by Myrna Weissman and Gerry Klerman and in cognitive therapy – CT – founded by Aaron Beck. I looked carefully at this development but am not entirely convinced that the evidence for the efficacy of these techniques would meet the requirements for registration as new treatments if the same standards were applied as for drug treatment today. There are not enough well-controlled studies proving psychotherapy's efficacy against placebo, controlling for severity of depression. For instance, the evidence from Irene Elkin's NIMH study – the biggest carried out in the field with about 400 patients – a very well-designed study using well-trained therapists, is not convincing as to efficacy. On conventional measurements, at least, such as the Hamilton Rating Scale, neither CT or IPT was any different from placebo over eight weeks.

In 1989 I organized a workshop in Zurich, at which Aaron Beck represented CT and Bruce Rounsaville IPT. The results of the NIMH study of Elkin *et al.* which were presented at the workshop showed no difference in efficacy between placebo and cognitive therapy on the Hamilton Depression Scale. Aaron Beck was disappointed and angry and maintained that the therapists had not been well trained, but he was contradicted by Brian Shaw from Canada, who had trained the therapists for the project. Moreover, Aaron Beck himself had been a consultant for the whole project. I therefore concluded that CT must be very demanding to teach and to learn, which would tend to favour the application of IPT, which has been shown to be at least as efficacious as CT.

So the big studies on the psychotherapy of depression are not convincing, and data analysis has shown drugs to be clearly superior in severe depression. Psychotherapy is frequently recommended in the treatment of minor depression, which is to ignore the fact that there is a lot of evidence that in minor depression it is not possible to prove efficacy either with drugs or psychotherapy. But despite the lack of definite data on the psychotherapy's efficacy, it should always be used. I would, though, recommend learning IPT as a first technique, because it is easier to learn and it gives the patient the necessary information about his disorder. It underlines the social roles and quality of life of the depressed patient and highlights important aspects of depression that lie outside clinical features identified by the rating scales.

Medicine's neglect of these aspects has damaged its reputation. This whole area of a patient's social roles, support and networks is extremely important, not only for depression, but for all disorders. So I am very much in favour of psychotherapy combined with drug treatment but would never advocate replacing drugs in the treatment of moderately or severely depressed patients by psychotherapy alone.

But there's another point I'd like to make. I am now predominantly an epidemiologist and therefore interested in the pharmaco-epidemiology of fluoxetine. The wide use of this drug is a very interesting phenomenon. I would say that there is a big natural experiment in progress, one which I'd be very cautious about judging. I would tend to the view that there's no reason why people should not take an SSRI if they get better. If they resort to cigarettes or alcohol for, example, why should they not take a drug which is less toxic than nicotine or alcohol?

From an epidemiological point of view, there's a high prevalence of mild depressive, sub-threshold syndromes; many people are mildly pessimistic, depressive, obsessional or hypochondriacal throughout their life time. We know from the lithium data that effective prophylaxis can decrease obsessionality. This may also be true for the SSRIs. A person taking an SSRI may have the impression that a character trait is changing, for example, that depressive traits, pessimism, joylessness or chronic fatigue, are diminishing. If these symptoms have been chronic, the subject may consider them as part of his personality. But there are no grounds for assuming that personality disorders are essentially different from psychiatric disorders. In some cases I would say they belong to the same spectrum; for example, a person with a cyclothymic personality belongs to the bipolar spectrum and a depressive personality belongs to the depressive spectrum, in my view. There is good reason to assume that drugs will act on personality disorders if they belong to the target spectrum. We know that, across a certain spectrum, drugs are unspecifically efficacious.

So I would say that it's perfectly possible that many more subjects in the population could benefit from such a drug. And the number is far higher than you would think. New epidemiological studies show that depression as such is much more prevalent in the population than previously thought. There's extensive sub-threshold morbidity, which has been shown to be socially relevant. So I repeat I would be very cautious about judging the widespread use of SSRIs. How to handle such a possibility is a political, social or ethical question. I am not an advocate of flooding the population with antidepressants, but the whole field needs careful research, a scientific approach rather than just opinion.

Let me pick up on some epidemiological issues. While you've been here, Zurich has been a centre for epidemiology. Now one of the things that's come out of this is the idea of recurrent brief depression. Do you want to comment on how that came about?

The concept of recurrent brief depression was a by-product of the methodology we were using. When I started the studies, I hunted around for instruments for assessing morbidity in normal populations; the PSE was the only structured interview available, but it was not really suitable for that purpose. The PSE was designed primarily as an interview for psychiatric patients suffering from schizophrenia and severe affective disorders. Whereas we wanted to cover the whole field of functional somatic syndromes, together with psychological syndromes, including for instance gastric functional complaints, headaches and insomnia. So we created the SPIKE interview, which is comprehensive and picks up milder symptoms and syndromes. Applying the SPIKE interview, we assessed systematically the number, length and frequency of symptoms, and it emerged that brief spells of depression are frequent among treated depressives who do not meet the diagnostic criteria of DSM. The question was then: what frequency was needed for case definition and how that could be validated; we then came up with the concept of recurrent brief depression.

Our study contained other groups of non-recurrent and less recurrent brief depression, but these were just not as valid and would have raised the prevalence of affective disorders in the population to a percentage that would have been meaningless. So, we settled on recurrent brief depression. But that was not all. We found brief spells, of a few days, in hypomania, neurasthenia, anxiety and insomnia. There is, in fact, epidemiological data from England showing that in many cases the consumption of hypnotics is not chronic but occurs in brief spells, which is linked with brief insomnia. Fatigue, too, can occur in brief spells. The same is true for hypomania, something which I consider to be quite important clinically, because it means that such subjects belong to the bipolar spectrum. But these brief spells are simply not investigated or considered. So recurrent brief depression is just one brief psychiatric syndrome we have described.

Is recurrent brief depression distinct from the kind of brief depressive episodes that go with borderline personality?

Well, there is no specific research on that. Two other groups, those of Montgomery and Staner, have been involved in the area of personality disorders. Stuart Montgomery started with a group of repeated suicide attempters, to whom he gave flupenthixol and several SSRIs as a long term medication; he couldn't see much change against the measures he had used. Of course, from a phenomenological point of view, a group of frequent suicide attempters is bound to include many personality disorders. This may be true for about 80% of suicide attempters. Therefore, such a group cannnot be representative of recurrent brief depression and indeed Montgomery didn't define them as recurrent brief depressives at the beginning of his trials.

Staner, from the Mendlewicz group, studied intermittent depression and assessed personality diagnoses. They found a high rate of recurrent brief depression. They also showed that about 14% of major depressives received a diagnosis of a personality disorder in contrast to about 4% in the group of recurrent brief depressives. This finding does not suggest that recurrent brief depression can be explained by personality disorders. Those are the only data on personality disorders currently available. A study on personality disorders is being conducted in Zurich by Johann Walter Meyer, sponsored by the Swiss Science Foundation, with interviews of patients whom we had earlier diagnosed as suffering from recurrent brief depression or major depression. This will be the first epidemiological study to assess both recurrent brief depression and personality disorders. Although it involves a sample of males only, it will probably answer the question of the overlap between the two.

If we take a group who have recurrent brief episodes who don't have a borderline personality, any ideas what mechanisms could be causing recurrent brief syndromes, whether depressive or whatever?

I think it is an endogenous mechanism. These subjects are rapid cyclers, with brief spells, which are difficult to treat. If you ask them as we did in our interviews about life events, using standard instruments, they don't report the occurrence of life events in connection with these repeated brief episodes. Someone is more likely to make associations when he has had one or two major depressive episodes; the more you have, the fewer precipitating events you can find. The fact that fewer and less intense events are involved over time may also be an effect of kindling. The threshold for manifestation or the threshold for sensitivity to stimuli may change. This is the view of Robert Post, whose kindling theory may also be applicable to recurrent brief depression.

I have also looked at all the case histories of RBD subjects and their personalities and they are not very deviant from the norm. Many of them are living under considerable stress but performing quite well in life, in other words, many are quite strong, stable individuals, not borderline subjects at all.

Let me raise the other issue which comes out of the Zurich epidemiology work, which is that contrary to prevailing views that depression is much commoner in women than men, if you go out into the community, as you have done, you find that there's an almost equal prevalence . . .

Well, the sex ratio depends very much on co-morbidity. The analysis of pure recurrent brief depression shows that the prevalence is almost equal – close to 1.1 or 1.2. In the Zurich study we found this also applied to major depression if you exclude the co-morbid cases. On the other hand, taking double depressions, there is a several-fold preponderance of females. So the more complicated and severe the case is, the more common it is among the female groups. I don't know what this means. The hypothesis of Susan Nolen (1987), an American psychologist, is that the sexes have different coping strategies. It would appear that females ruminate, blame themselves and try to find subjective reasons for their depression much more than males do. Males would be more likely to act out, go out and try to forget, drink, or try to overcome their depression through sport. This male strategy might be better. The females may get trapped in a vicious circle, which intensifies the severity of episodes and increases their vulnerability to depression over the years. So a psychosocial effect may be involved. Another possible reason is hormonal. Androgens influence aggression and may also determine male coping strategies. I do not think that the explanation for the sex ratio is to be found in the X-chromosome, something which I advanced in 1966 in my monograph but which I now consider to be too simple.

We lack a European forum. We've got ECNP and AEP but do they actually provide what we need in Europe? Compared to the Americans, who are so organized.

Yes, the CINP has changed and declined since becoming a huge world congress. It has too many parallel sessions and has lost its coherence. Earlier meetings always ended with all the symposia Chairmen presenting a synthesis of their results in a plenary session; this gave an extraordinary overview of the whole field. This practice has been abandoned and forgotten. At a meeting nowadays you are confronted with dozens of parallel sessions and time-consuming choices between them.

The balance of ACNP has changed: as its clinical element has declined so has its interest to clinicians. While it may have gained scientifically, I don't think it fulfils its former role of bringing together basic science researchers and clinical scientists. I think the area of clinical research has been grossly neglected. I find that the development of ECNP, embracing clinical and experimental research, is currently more promising. Over the past few meetings it has developed well and has maintained a clinical course. This is interesting in view of the foundation in the States of an American Society for Clinical Psychopharmacology by way of reaction to the changes in ACNP.

As you say, the area of clinical trials needs development. We've had something of a hiatus since the 1960s. It seems to be only recently with the European Consensus Conferences on Methodology that there is any movement returning to the field.

Yes, little has been happening because the drug companies' main interest is in meeting the FDA requirements, and new methods are a lower priority. This is why we launched in Zurich the European Consensus Conferences on the methodology of clinical trials. In 1994 in the context of the ECNP Conference in Jerusalem, a full-day methodological meeting was organized by Stuart Montgomery attended by Paul Leber from the FDA and representatives of most of the drug companies. It was quite obvious that new methodological developments will be of great future interest. One example is the development of new criteria for the onset of action of drugs.

Another neglected area is self-assessment: for instance, daily self-assessment by the patient. A new rating scale has been developed by John Rush, the IDS, a depression inventory of 28 items, existing in two versions, for self and observer ratings; the correlation coefficient between them is 0.95. If that is true, one could replace observer ratings for ambulatory patients by daily self-ratings and determine more precisely the onset of improvement. I would also recommend regular application of a global self-assessment of depression on the line of school marking systems. In Switzerland for example school marks range from 1 to 6 and I have started to apply such a scale in the daily assessment of depression. Because they feel immediately at home with such a measure, patients are able to define their ratings very precisely, right down to decimal points. The advantages of a familiar scale over an invented and artificial one are obvious. On the whole, the methodology of drug trials is a neglected area in psychopharmacology and deserves far greater attention.

Select bibliography

Angst, J. and Theobald, W. (1970) *Tofranil*. Verlag Stampfli & Cie, Berne.
Angst, J. (1987) The switch from depression to mania or from mania to depression. *Journal of Psychopharmacology*, **1,** 13–19.

13 George Beaumont

The place of clomipramine in psychopharmacology

Start from the start.

My career has been very varied. In the very early days I did some psychiatry. I think it was either my fourth or fifth job when I was a resident in Howard Kitching's Unit. At the time he was well known in Manchester. But I really began by wanting to become an obstetrician and gynaecologist. I went quite a long way along that path but then became disenchanted because some of my colleagues, who were then senior registrars, were not getting consultant appointments until their early 1940s. It seemed as though there was going to be a long wait so I decided to change course. With the benefit of hindsight it was a mistake because the situation began to improve shortly afterwards – but I wasn't to know that.

So, I gave up obstetrics and gynaecology and decided to become a GP. I wanted to broaden my experience so I took a psychiatric job and also worked for a while in paediatrics. I entered general practice in Stockport in 1960 and soon developed quite an interest in psychiatry.

However, as time went by the workload steadily increased, there were some problems with partners and I became very disillusioned. One Saturday, while I was on duty, I was reading the BMJ over lunch and in it I saw that Geigy Pharmaceuticals were advertising for a medical adviser. Really just a 'flyer'. I applied and to my surprise I was offered an interview. It was a complicated time in my life, too, because my wife had just had our first daughter and I was trying to organize things at home as well as sort out my future. However, to cut a long story short I was offered a job.

I think that what interested Geigy was not only what I had done medically but also that when I was a medical student I had been President of the Union. I had done a lot of committee work, as well as being heavily involved in politics. I think they were intrigued by this combination of medical training and experience in administration and public life.

Based on an interview previously published in Beaumont, G. and Healy, D. (1993) The place of chlomipramine in the history of psychopharmacology. *Journal of Psychopharmacology*, **7**, 378–88. Reproduced with permission from the *Journal of Psychopharmacology*.

There were, in fact, two jobs available, one in rheumatology and one in psychiatry. I could pick whichever I liked. My reasoning was – since I had never done any rheumatology but once did a job in psychiatry, I ought to take the psychiatric post.

In those days, the industry was rather 'primitive'. There had been little development in regulatory affairs and there were no formal registration procedures for drugs. It was all very simple. When I arrived at Geigy I was somewhat astonished. I was given an office and then asked my boss, Dick Gosling, what am I supposed to do. His answer was very simple – 'we would like you to look after some of the old psychotropics and you can evaluate a new one we have called clomipramine and see what you make of it'. So with that limited brief I had to sort myself out and learn about what we now call pharmaceutical medicine.

Clinical trials were relatively simple in those days. A patient entered an antidepressant trial simply if a physician 'thought he was suitable for treatment with an antidepressant drug'. This was the only criterion used to select trial subjects.

So we started a series of studies with clomipramine. I don't remember exactly when it was that I began to suspect that there was something different about clomipramine compared with the other then available antidepressants. There were few signs in the literature that there was something special about this compound. To be truthful I think that the first person to recognize that clomipramine might have some other interesting properties was a Frenchman called Guyotat. He made a passing reference to its use in a review of a series of patients treated in an uncontrolled study. However, it was a discovery that Professor Lopez–Ibor was running in a Unit in Madrid in which clomipramine infusions were administered to patients with a variety of psychiatric disorders that really stimulated my interest. In those days there was a certain popularity for administering antidepressants by infusion.

I thought it was the only one that was actually produced as an infusion?

It may have been the first, I am not sure, but subsequently, there were others. Whether there was really a sensible rationale for infusion rather than oral use, I don't think we knew. In the first instance we felt it was something just worth trying. However, I did eventually come to the opinion that there was a rationale for intravenous use. This was based on observations of treated patients. Clomipramine is highly sedative when given intravenously but not when given orally. If you went to any of the hospitals which had established an intravenous infusion unit, you could see all the patients fast asleep. I suspect this is something to do with first-pass metabolism. When infused, not all the drug is metabolized, as it is following oral administration, and some reaches the cerebral circulation in its unchanged form.

As far as Lopez-Ibor's use of clomipramine was concerned, I was particularly impressed by the success claimed in obsessive – compulsive disorder. It struck me that maybe this was something which made clomipramine different from other antidepressants. This was probably a marketing view rather than a medical one. I was looking for a niche for the compound and I thought 'well nobody else has used antidepressants in OCD'. At that time I had no idea how common OCD was but it seemed a possibility.

I had already made contact with a number of psychiatrists in the UK and they were using clomipramine. I suggested that they might try using it in obsessive – compulsive disorders. Their reaction was favourable since it was acknowledged that it was a difficult condition to treat and resistant to any drugs available at the time. Anything, they thought, that worked would be a tremendous therapeutic advantage. I arranged for four or five of them to visit Madrid. I had been in touch with Professor Lopez-Ibor and asked if we could visit his hospital. He made us very welcome, entertained us and told us about his work with clomipramine. We were all excited by what we heard.

When we came home we established a number of uncontrolled studies looking at the use of clomipramine, given either by infusion or orally, to patients with OCD. Straight away we encountered difficulties. We had no means of accurately measuring the effect of the drug. There was no generally accepted rating scale for OCD. A literature search led us to the Leyton Obsessional Inventory and we used that for some projects. We also 'invented' a scale of our own. It was rough and ready by today's standards, but, importantly, measured features such as avoidance, resistance and interference. The end results were encouraging. Patients seemed to be improving – of course there was no placebo control.

Around this time we went to Canada for a joint meeting on 'The Management of Obsessional and Phobic Disorders'. Some Canadian psychiatrists had already become interested in what we were doing. This was subsequently reflected in the fact that clomipramine was licensed quite early in Canada, whereas great difficulties were experienced in the United States.

I think the next important milestone was reached when Isaac Marks became interested. He ran an important study but he was very reluctant to deprive any patient of what he considered were the benefits of behaviour therapy. This made it very difficult to establish proper controls. However, some positive results were obtained. Subsequently Isaac Marks suggested that only patients who were also depressed obtained benefit from clomipramine. I don't accept this view because the protocol was designed to specifically exclude significantly depressed patients. These so-called depressives who benefited were only showing scores of less than 14 on the HDRS and I don't believe this indicates 'significant depression'. Nevertheless Marks concluded that the drug was no better than placebo in relieving symptoms of OCD, that it was no different to any other antidepressant and that behaviour therapy was the treatment of choice.

Stuart Montgomery questioned these conclusions and suggested that we ought to perform a placebo-controlled study in which the issue was not complicated by the offer of behaviour therapy. Montgomery, therefore, performed the first definitive placebo-controlled study which established that clomipramine was effective in the management of obsessive – compulsive disorder.

It was about this time that I left Geigy pharmaceuticals as it was then. My reasons for leaving were essentially personal. When I joined the Geigy company, the medical department was based in Manchester and subsequently in Macclesfield. When the merger between Geigy and Ciba took place the department was relocated in Horsham. At that time I had children who had reached crucial stages of their education and both my wife and I had widowed dependant mothers who were growing old and needed our attention. We had a family meeting at which it was decided that although I had been offered an important post in the new department, there was no way that we could leave the Cheshire area. I therefore left Ciba–Geigy and with some relucance returned to part-time general practice, setting myself up at the same time as a freelance medical adviser. With one of my new GP practices I also established a contract research organization.

There are a couple of features of the Geigy experience which ought to be mentioned. At the same time that we were investigating the use of clomipramine in OCD we were also looking at its use in phobic disorders, especially agoraphobia and social phobias. At that time the concept of panic disorders had not become well established but looking back I think that panic was a feature of phobic disorders that interested us.

I mentioned that after I left Ciba–Geigy I was involved in the establishment of a contract research organization. The company was mainly concerned with trials in primary care. We recruited and trained GP investigators. Although we worked in a variety of clinical areas we tended to specialize in the evaluation of psychotropic agents. I had already been involved in the development of general practitioner research whilst at Geigy. I had set up a General Practitioner Research Group and used it extensively for antidepressant studies. I recognized early on that there was a great difficulty in finding suitable or adequate numbers of patients in psychiatric clinics. One really had to go out into the community and use well-trained GPs to look for patients with depression, phobias, agoraphobia and so on.

Just to chase the Ciba-Geigy end of OCD a wee bit further, how much does the industry create the market? Since Anafranil of course we've had the major surveys in the States which have shown that upwards of four million people in the States have OCD and by inference somewhere like 1 million people in the UK must also have OCD. These surveys have been sponsored by Ciba-Geigy, so to some extent we've got a situation where Ciba are now creating the market. Any comments?

Yes. I think that to some extent the industry can create a market. If you look back at the history of clomipramine, the idea of using it in OCD started in the Medical Department of Geigy UK but I have to admit that I did have the possibility of a marketing advantage in mind. When you are faced with a wide range of drugs, like antidepressants, you are trying to find something which makes your drug of a special interest to investigators and subsequently prescribers. As soon as I realized that there might be something which set clomipramine apart from the other anti-depressants, I vigorously pursued it.

Of course as soon as I started to get some favourable results, my marketing colleagues became extremely interested and anxious to pursue the indication. But I have to say that initially the interest only seemed to be in the UK. We got little encouragement from our European colleagues. They came into the project later in the day. I don't think that at first they realized the potential.

The big opportunity, which would not arise now, came when it was time to licence the drug. There is another strand to this story which is what happened to the licensing of drugs. When the evaluation of clomipramine started we are talking about the days even before the establishment of the Dunlop Committee. Eventually the CSM was set up and the Medicines Act came into force. But in those days companies did not have registration or regulatory affairs departments. As far as clomipramine was concerned I literally had to write every word of the submision. I did nothing for three months but sit in my office and write it starting with basic chemistry and working my way through to the clinical results. In addition to the documentation in support of the depression indication I also included the results of our OCD studies. We were very fortunate because the indication was approved right from the early days. It would, I think, have been much more difficult now. But, of course, the result was that clomipramine was the only antidepressant approved for the treatment of OCD.

At the beginning I don't think we realized that all this had anything to do with the 5-HT story. But when we realized that there was an effect in OCD and maybe in social phobias and agoraphobia, we asked ourselves what is different about this drug. When we looked at the profile we realized that although by no means selective, clomipramine was the most powerful inhibitor of the reuptake of 5HT then available. The situation was complicated by the fact that clomipramine is metabolized to desmethyl-clomipramine, an inhibitor of noradrenaline reuptake. We began therefore to wonder whether the use of intravenous clomipramine, and particularly the success claimed by Lopez-Ibor, fitted the 5-HT story.

Just one last point: did Arvid Carllson interface with you at any point or did he get his ideas about 5-HT independently?

He did not interface with us. He may well have interfaced in Europe, I don't know, but there was no direct link with us at that time. Later on when we began to think in terms of 5-HT, people looked at the more selective 5-HT reuptake inhibitors and asked whether the anti–OCD effect was a property common to all of them. They do appear to have this but clomipramine remains the 'gold standard' to which everyone must aspire. I believe that in some countries, such as France, you must show that a drug is as effective as or more so than clomipramine before you can have it licenced for the treatment of OCD.

How does it feel to have been associated with one of the most significant psychopharmacology stories?

It has been quite a thrill. I would not claim that we started it. It was started by people like Lopez-Ibor but I think we pursued it more energetically than others. What then began to happen was an old familiar story. Everyone at that time thought that OCD was an unusual, bizarre and rare condition but as soon as you have a treatment for a condition you discover that it is more common than everybody supposed it to be. What is so exciting now is that there is a lot of epidemiological work emerging which indicates that OCD is a relatively common condition – a condition also which may be co-morbid with depression.

After I left Ciba-Geigy the company seemed to lose interest in psychopharmacology. There was a hiatus when very little seemed to happen. Now they have brofaromine but even that seems to have been allowed to fall behind the competition. I think this loss of interest to some extent extended to carbamazepine, especially to its wider potential uses.

I was slightly involved with carbamezapine at one stage when I was leading the psychopharmacology team. Of course the success of carbamezapine was due to the work of Alan Galbraith but his main interest was in epilepsy. I started to pick up the suggestion that it did have some applications in the prophylaxis of bipolar disorder but this was not given a high priority by the company at that time. Now of course it has been developed for that indication, especially internationally. To some extent however I feel that Ciba-Geigy opted out of psychopharmacology.

Why do companies do that. Why do they opt out of what is potentially a huge market?

I find it difficult to understand but I suppose they had important products in other areas of medicine – like rheumatology and cardiology – which they wanted to exploit and which therefore deserved more interest and attention.

I tend to feel that companies often perceive these areas as 'real medicine'. I believe that the problem we have with psychiatry even pervades the industry, in that peopole do not consider psychiatry a worthwhile area to work in compared with, for example, the treatment of hypertension and ulcers. These conditions constitute proper medicine whereas psychiatric disorders do not. So companies get more excited about antirheumatics, antihypertensives and so on than about antidepressants. I think this is why Ciba–Geigy lost its way in psychiatry.

You have had an initiating role in another area of psychopharmacology, namely the psychopharmacology of sex. With recent reports that up to one third of younger men have premature ejaculation problems, something that 5-HT reuptake inhibitors may help significantly, this seems an area that is set to grow. Could I get you to tell me how all that came about?

There were two chance findings that started it. The first was at Winwick Hospital in Warrington where there was a clomipramine infusion unit. I used to visit the hospital regularly to follow the progress of a trial. I went into the unit one day and talked to some of the patients. One of them, a bright guy and in fact a research chemist, was being treated for depression. I asked him what he thought about clomipramine and in particular whether he had experienced any side effects. 'It does funny things to your sex life' he replied. I asked him to explain. ' I come here for five days and go home for the weekends' he said, 'when I was beginning to feel better and more interested in sex I found that when I had intercourse with my wife I could not ejaculate. I suspected it might have something to do with the treatment. I did not want to stop taking clomipramine altogether (he took capsules at weekends) for fear of slipping back but what I found was that if I fiddled with the dose I could control the way I ejaculated. I could slow it down or stop it altogether'.

I was intrigued with this finding so I contacted Ray Goodman, a sexologist working in Manchester. He too was interested in the observation. Since Ray was running a clinic for the treatment of sexual disorders I suggested he might do a trial of clomipramine in premature ejaculation. He agreed to perform an open study. When I looked at the records of patients in other studies I realized that fairly big doses of clomipramine caused men to have failure of ejaculation altogether and I suspected that even higher doses caused failure of erection. So I wondered what the effect on premature ejaculation was of low doses and whether one could 'titrate' the dose to produce the desired effect. So we used small doses in Ray Goodman's trial and found as little as 5 mg or 10 mg would have the desired effect.

The results aroused considerable interest. The trial also showed that it was not necessary to take clomipramine all the time. It could be taken in a single dose about four hours before intercourse. Of course this kind of treatment does introduce an element of planning into sexual relationships – spontaneity is rather destroyed.

About the same time was the second chance finding. In those days we used to receive what were called case report supplements. What happened was that if one of the representatives called to see a doctor and he or she reported something untoward, this was written on the form. All of them came into the office. One of the jobs of the then multi–purpose medical adviser was to answer all these queries. When I came in in the morning there would be a pile of reports on my desk and I would write to all the doctors concerned. One day I picked up a report from a GP working near Peterborough. He had said to our representative 'you know that women who take clomipramine can't have an orgasm'. I thought this was a very interesting observation for it fitted in with our findings about ejaculation. I went to see the GP who gave me a very good description of a female patient who had been put on clomipramine and who complained bitterly that she was unable to achieve orgasm. When she stopped the drug she was orgasmic again. So we started to enquire more into this area and examine some of our trial reports and found that not only did males report interference with ejaculation and even interference with erection at high doses, but females were sometimes anorgasmic.

It is interesting again, with the benefit of hindsight, to see what is happening now with the new 5–HT reuptake inhibitors. There are similar reports of these drugs interfering with ejaculation and sometimes with orgasm.

We have never really got to grips with sorting out the psychopharmaoclogy of this – was the effect peripheral or central? It is something I would like to have done but there was a certain amount of opposition from the company at that time. In fact I got into trouble with the Managing Director after presenting the findings for the first time at a conference in the Channel Islands. I didn't know the press were present – in fact I don't think they were – someone must have leaked the story – but when I walked into the office on the Monday morning following the conference, the MD came into my office, infuriated, and slapped down a copy of one of the tabloids on my desk. 'What the hell's all this about George?' There in the paper was the claim that a new wonder drug improves your sex life.

The company was somewhat Calvinistic in its philosophy and I was told 'lay off this subject – we don't want this kind of publicity'. So I never really pursued it energetically, although I have always retained my interest in the sexual effects of drugs. I ought to mention that after the initial reports we were involved with a number of people, including Barry Everitt, who were looking at what you might call the psychopharmacology/anatomy of these effects. But as I say we did not pursue it as energetically as we should have.

The idea that the pharmaceutical industry might develop drugs for sexual disorders was something quite unheard of in those days. It is interesting to see that now there are people coming from pharmaceutical companies, as they did at the BAP meeting in Cambridge, saying 'here's a great area of opportunity'. It has always been one of those neglected areas despite the fact that sexual problems/are very common.

With all the publicity on drug treatment of OCD in the US these days does it ever seem like they are reinventing the wheel?

Yes. In the 1970s I made several trips to the United States with the Geigy team who were appearing before the FDA in an attempt to register clomipramine. Many obstacles were put in our way, mainly in relation to toxicology, and it became very obvious that clomipramine would not get a licence in the USA for depression despite its acceptance and popularity elsewhere in the world. Eventually we gave up.

Clearly there was a demand in the States for clomipramine at that time, especially for the treatment of OCD. I think some was brought in from Canada where it was approved. Sometimes parents and relatives would come to the UK to try and obtain clomipramine. I would be sitting in my office and the telephone would ring from a London Hotel. The caller for example, would say 'I have brought my wife over from the States, she has terrible obsessions, can you supply me with some Anafranil?'

Gradually, interest in the States grew (there were always a few enthusiasts) and although there was reluctance to accept our original claims, eventually they had to. Recently clomipramine has been licensed in the US for OCD. Now, of course, there is a flood of publications and booklets from Ciba-Geigy. Much of what is being said was described in the UK 20 years ago. I must admit I am mildly amused for it does seem like the Americans are reinventing the wheel.

Could the OCD story have happened if it were all starting off now?

I have great doubts whether it would happen now. You have to refer back to the regulatory situation as it was in those days. Then it was possible, as I used to say, to play hunches. I used to like the phrase 'flying a kite'. I would go to my boss and say 'how about flying a kite on this one. It looks as there may just possibly be something in it'. You have to remember that serendipity played a major role in the discovery of many medical treatments not least in psychiatry. The discoveries of both the tricyclics and the monoamine oxidase inhibitors in depression were purely serendipitous.

In the early days there was not the strict regulation that there is now. Now, without a CTX at least, my boss would not be able to allow me to play my hunches. So you have to prepare a substantial dossier before you can 'just try something' and the company would probably think it was not worth the expense.

I wonder whether companies would play hunches now. They have to go for the 'big chance' and I suppose that in psychiatry the big chance would be depression. The attitude would be that depression is a multi-million pound market and we want our share of it – we can't be 'playing around at the fringes with strange conditions like OCD and phobias'. So I wonder whether if history were to repeat itself the same thing would have happened now.

You've also had a role in setting up the Diploma in Pharmaceutical Medicine.

When I joined the industry in 1966, it was becoming respectable to be a pharmaceutical company medical adviser. But if you look back at the history of doctors in the industry in years gone by they did not have a good reputation. It was a standing joke that the industry was the place for doctors who had been struck off and abortionists. It was the only place where they could work. I'm sure it was not as bad as that but that was the joke.

Those of us who worked in the industry felt increasingly that pharmaceutical medicine should be a speciality in its own right. There were developments, both in the UK and in Europe with regards to accreditation and specialized registration. I, and others, became concerned about how the doctor in the pharmaceutical industry might fit into any new framework. Was he or she in danger of becoming a second- class citizen?

At one time you could move about easily in medicine. You could move out of practice into industry then back into practice either general or hospital. As the years have gone by this mobility has become increasingly restricted. You have to do it the right way following the approved training courses. So it became obvious that it was necessary to establish some kind of status for doctors who worked in the pharmaceutical industry.

At that time most of us were members of the Association for Medical Advisers in the Pharmaceutical Industry – AMAPI for short. I have had various offices in the association including that of Chairman. Some of us in AMAPI started to think what we could do to improve our professional situation. We consulted various learned bodies including the three Royal Colleges of Physicians of London, Edinburgh and Glasgow. They said they could do nothing until we could establish that there could be a proper course of training that could lead to a professional qualification. We had to show that pharmaceutical medicine was a subject that could be taught and that pharmaceutical physicians could be trained.

I was serving on the AMAPI Committee at the time and I was given the task of setting up the first training course in pharmaceutical medicine. It was run on a modular basis over a year. Having done this the Colleges then accepted the principle that pharmaceutical medicine could be taught and the three Colleges of Physicians agreed jointly to grant a diploma in Pharmaceutical Medicine. The examination came under the aegis of the Edinburgh College and was held there.

The problems that AMAPI then faced was that, by its nature, it was not a training organisztion. The course needed to be embraced by some academic institution. We thought that ultimately the diploma would lead to specialist registration. That hasn't actually happened. However, pharmaceutical medicine has now moved farther with the establishment of a faculty. Shortly we will have an examination for membership of this faculty of pharmaceutical medicine of the RCP which will be on the same level as the MRCP, FRCS, MRCPsych or similar professional qualifications

But returning to the 1970s, I and my colleagues tried to interest academic institutions in taking over our course. We found considerable reluctance and we were in a 'catch 22' situation – if no one could be trained there would be no one for the Royal Colleges to examine. To cut a long story short I eventually persuaded the Welsh School of Pharmacy in Cardiff to take over the course. Since then the Diploma in Pharmaceutical Medicine has become well established.

Cardiff has since also established a course for a Diploma in Clinical Science for clinical research executives or associates who are scientifically but not medically qualified. A course for a qualification in Regulatory Affairs has also been established. I was to some extent involved in the Diploma in Clinical Science and was the first external examiner.

There is, of course, a problem for non-medically qualified scientists working in the medical departments of the pharmaceutical industry. What is their career structure? They cannot become a medical director because by definition a medical director has to be medically qualified – but that's another story which has created problems even with the BAP.

Do you want to carry on with that?

It's an old story really. The pharmaceutical industry was not developed by doctors. In the first place it was developed by chemists and pharmacists. It was not until we started to be concerned about the safety of medicines that doctors were needed in the industry. So in the days when I entered it, doctors were a relatively new phenomenon. One immediate problem was financial as much as anything. The industry found it had to have physicians because the world was changing but the chemists and pharmacists, very bright people, were very reluctant to accept this. Moreover, salt was rubbed into the wound because the industry had to pay the sort of salary that a physician could earn as a hospital consultant or general practitioner, in order to attract the right people and such a salary would be in excess of what the pharmacists and chemists could demand. So you had a situation where you had people who were better informed and had been more involved in the drug development process having to accept 'upstarts' from the medical profession who know less but earned much more. It was a difficult situation at that time.

It was not, of course, quite the same as the CRA, Clinical Research Assistant, situation which in a sense has come about for the opposite reasons. The industry has found that because physicians are so expensive, it can pursue research by employing people with other scientific qualifications, who are not as expensive as physicians. The problem for the CRA, however, is the lack of a career structure. It is not really possible to get to the top of a medical department if you are not medically qualified. To progress you need to move into marketing or product management otherwise you are in limbo.

CRAs have tried very hard to improve the situation. They have established their own professional organization and they have their diploma but I still feel that they have an identity crisis.

Can we pick up your role in the BAP story?

Those of us who worked in the industry had been meeting with physicians from hospital practice and academia regularly. In my case it was with psychiatrists. But apart from the old RMPA meetings there was no forum where we could all get together. When we did meet it was purely on a clinical trial level. There was a need for a more general exchange of ideas.

Who in particular would you meet?

One would immediately think about people like Alec Coppen and Max Hamilton. We wanted a forum where, as I have said, we could meet not in the context of 'you're being paid for a clinical trial' but in a much freer atmosphere where we could exchange ideas.

I think several people had thought about setting up some sort of association about the same time. That was not really surprising because we all 'chatted' to each other at conferences, at the bar or over dinner. So the same thought would be going through several people's minds.

I thought that Trevor Silverstone and I were the first to think about it. We were attending a meeting of the ECDEU in New Orleans. We had dinner together at Antons and breakfast at Brennans. I don't remember whether it was at dinner or breakfast but at some stage we said why don't we set up an organization in which industry and clinicians can get together. So we returned from New Orleans full of enthusiasm only to find that we had been pre-empted by David Wheatley, Syndey Brandon and Anthony Hordern – all people who I knew well and with whom I had worked in various ways. So I suppose they were the people who really started it. They were the people who wrote the famous letter which started the ball rolling.

Eventually a group of about 20 of us got together in the RSM to set up the organization. Of course David Wheatley was involved as was Anthony Hordern, who was then working at Kings, as well as Sydney Brandon, Alec Coppen, Max Hamilton and so on. From the industry there was an important person, who doesn't get mentioned nowadays – that's Gerry Daniel. Gerry worked for Squibb and was very interested in schizophrenia. In the first instance it was industry physicians and clinicians who met and I suppose this was at the root of some of the suspicion that other people had for what we were doing.

We had no bad intentions – it was just the way it happened. Initially there were several sources of criticism. For example, some people thought we should have set up a body associated with CINP and Philip Bradley. At first he was very much opposed to what we were doing although eventually he joined us.

I was elected to the first council and took the post of meetings' secretary. I had the task of organizing the first BAP meeting. I am ashamed to say that the result was disastrous. I managed to attract about 25 people to the first symposium at the RSM. When I look at the success of the BAP meeting in Cambridge now I realize how paltry those early efforts were. David Wheatley took over from me and did much better. Eventually the meetings became quite well attended.

I suppose that the first really big meeting was the fateful one in the Channel Islands which created so many subsequent problems. It was something of a watershed really. Perhaps because the impetus in planning the meeting had come from people on the industry side, like Gerry Daniel and myself, our idea was to put on a really superb event, which I supposed we modelled on the kind of meeting the industry would organize. In fact I was very much responsible for the selection of the venue. I had already organized many meetings in Guernsey. So I introduced the BAP to a professional meetings organizer who I knew. He suggested a new hotel in St Pierre Port called St Pierre Park which had excellent conference facilities. We thought it was a wonderful idea – we would have everyone together in the lovely island of Guernsey. Little did we realize what would happen. In a sense that was really when 'the bubble burst' as far as the non-industry, non-clinician side of the organization was concerned.

The views seemed to be that this was just a 'bun fight' for wealthy clinicians and pharmaceutical company personnel and that the rest of the members could not afford this kind of thing. I think that many of them felt that unless there were changes in the organization they could not continue to support it. And a number boycotted the meeting. There has never been a meeting like it since. Inevitably we had to move to the frugality of student rooms and university venues.

Of course I was not meetings' secretary at the time but because I was involved in the choice of venue, I have to accept some of the blame.

Going back in time I played another role in the association. It needed a constitution. I had been involved in constitutional affairs as a student politician and, as President of the Union at Manchester, had been involved in revising its constitution. I brought it along as a model to a meeting and Max Hamilton who was then Chairman, said 'seeing as you know so much about constitutions you had better write one for the BAP'. So in collaboration with Max I produced the first constitution. Although it has been modified since I think it is still basically the one that we wrote.

It appears to be the outline on which the ECNP constitution was also built. What were the contents of the early meetings, what were the issues, programmes?

One of the earliest which I set in motion was on the sexual effects of drugs. The proceedings were published as a monograph which I think is still around. This choice reflected my early interest in the subject. As I said I did not make much progress with the company so I suggested that it might be an area the BAP would consider. The meeting was held at Queen Charlotte's Maternity Hospital in London.

Other meetings were on subjects like the measurement of depression. I remember that one of the first meetings I organized was on the teratological effects of psychotropic agents. I was interested in the subject particularly of drug effects in pregnancy and lactation. The meeting was held at the RSM and I recruited some good speakers but there were only about 25 people in the audience. I was very disappointed. Strange how this has since become an important issue but few psychiatrists or psychopharmacologists seemed to be very interested in it then.

What about the BAP council meetings during the early days? What were they like, what were the interactions like, what were the issues?

In the early days they were very friendly. Most of those on council were either academic clinical psychiatrists or people from industry. But gradually others, like Paul Spencer from UWIST, became involved. Most of the problems that we had arose outside the council. We thought we were doing a decent job and there was a good group all of whom got on very well together. The flack was all coming from outside – from bodies like the Institute of Psychiatry.

Tell me about the Institute of Psychiatry – the Maudsley

Well, I don't think I really understood why they seemed to take exception to what we were doing. I suppose that in a way I felt they were adopting something of a holier-than-thou attitude. Firstly, I suspect that they were extremely wary of any kind of relationship between psychiatry and the pharmaceutical industry. Secondly, I think they felt that we were setting certain standards that we were not entitled to.

One of the biggest problems of all was the name. Nobody could think of a satisfactory name for the association. Initially the name 'British Academy of Psychopharmacology' was suggested. With the benefit of hindsight this was foolish since by calling it an academy, we seemed be establishing 'academic' standards. Perhaps that was what caused the Institute of Psychiatry to object. I suppose people thought of the title academy because there were bodies in the world that took the title 'college' – the ACNP and the CINP, for example. You might ask what right has the CINP to call itself a college – it's really just a group of people who get together and formed an organization.

So I think the name had a lot to do with the problem. Malcolm Lader for example objected to what we were doing and so did Philip Bradley. There were also objections from non-medically qualified psychopharmacologists who said the BAP was no more than a marriage between the marketing orientated arm of industry and clinical psychiatrists who would earn fees by performing clinical trials.

It took a long time to overcome these prejudices. Eventually we did, although Tim Crow never accepted us.

The other view that was actually put forward by Tim Crow was that if clinical people were going to do proper science they should be in the appropriate scientific organizations such as the British Pharmacological Society; what do you think of that?

It is all very well to say that but if you go back to where we started the rationale had a lot to do with clinical trials. Psychopharmacology needs well-executed clinical trials. We cannot make any progress in terms of applying the principles of psychopharmacology unless we subject products and ideas to proper clinical trials. By the nature of things most clinical trials were set up by the industry. The industry's standards were sometimes open to criticism so we wanted to involve clinicians in a dialogue in order to help improve our standards. On the other hand clinicians would not do many clinical trials without our help. As I have already said, we wanted to create a forum in which interactions could take place. It is all very well saying you should join the right society. What society should people who worked in industry have joined if they wanted to achieve these aims? The comment about joining the right society is nonsense really. There was a need for a forum in which the relationship between the people who produced the compounds and those who assessed them clinically could be developed.

You've had an interest in eating disorders also?

My original interest in anorexia really stemmed from observations that clomipramine could cause weight gain irrespective of any change in appetite. We received a number of anecdotal reports that anorexics benefited from clomipramine. The thought we had was that you might be able to institute drug therapy initially and then provide psychotherapy. The issue became somewhat contentious because although some clinicians were using clomipramine others were against the idea of using any kind of drug in a disorder which they considered to be essentially 'psychological' . I did have some contact with Arthur Crisp but we never really pursued the subject. It fascinates me now to see that manufacturers of SSRIs, whilst not claiming success in anorexia, are doing so in bulimia. But of course bulimia didn't exist at that time. Russell introduced the idea some time later. Nevertheless, I did feel that the eating disorders was an area of psychiatry I would like to have explored more. I think recent experience supports the possibility that there may be important relations with 5-HT.

As well as the eating disorders, you've had an interest in sleep?

I suppose that my interest in sleep began in a very routine way. Whenever you are investigating a psychotropic drug there is a standard package of investigations which needs to be done. This will include studies on the effect of the drug on sleep.

As far as clomipramine was concerned there were a few important spin offs of this approach. We found that with TCAs, especially clomipramine, there was suppression of REM sleep after the first dose. This observation leads one to ask why is it that the drug has a dramatic effect in the brain following the first dose and yet it does not significantly alleviate depression for several weeks. Clearly the drug has entered the brain, and is acting immediately – so what is the explanation?

One thing we did believe, then, was that REM suppression and anti-depressant activity were in some way related. Some people still hold this view. Of course there is a shift in the patterns of sleep in depression. However, at that time it had not been suggesed that REM latency might be a marker for depression. Although we had a lot of ideas I don't think we pursued them as vigorously as we might have done.

One thing, however, that we did pursue fairly actively with David Parkes, was the possibility that a compound like clomipramine, being such a potent suppressor of REM sleep, might be useful in the management of narcolepsy. The outcome of the trials performed is now reflected in the conventional wisdom that although clomipramine has little effect on narcolepsy itself it is a valuable drug for the management of cataplexy. I think that clomipramine is still the first line treatment for this condition.

Another area of interest which we have not so far mentioned was the management of pain. Again this originated from anecdotal reports that the addition of antidepressants to an analgesic regime was of value especially in some chronic pain conditions. I set up a research project, mainly centred in UWIST, and a whole series of papers resulted from this. The group in Cardiff were already interested in opiate receptors.

I think that what emerged was the concept that pain and depression are probably rather similar processes. Depression is, if you like, a kind of mental pain. I think that there is some evidence for a common mechanism. I don't think that it is just a question of low pain thresholds in depression which revert to normal when the depression is treated with an anti-depressant. There is some other property of antidepressants that is associated with the relief of pain. We published a number of papers on this subject and I organized several conferences on pain and its management.

It is very interesting to see that clomipramine is still considered to be an important compound even though it has not been energetically pro-moted since the late 1970s. I think the psychiatric community has recognized that it is a drug that has important qualities. For example, it has become the 'gold standard' in OCD and in the area of resistant depression it is still one of the most favoured drugs for inclusion in 'cocktails'. I think it has been recognized that there is something rather special about clomipramine. Even though rather neglected by Ciba-Geigy in the UK for 13 years it is, interestingly, still a market leader in some countries.

Let me switch completely to the issue you raised earlier about GP trials and also the role of GP's in the development of psychopharmacology and the BAP.

We identified the need for general practitioner trials a long time ago and it was for this reason that, when I was working with Geigy Pharmaceuticals, I established a general practitioner clinical research group. I needed relatively large cohorts of patients for some of our clinical trials. It was clear that these were not to be found in psychiatric practice. Even if they existed at all recruitment would take a long time and there were considerable marketing pressures to get things done quickly.

We knew from the results of epidemiological surveys in general practice that, for example, there was a large number of depressed patients many of whom were not being treated. Perhaps we were somewhat ahead of our time when in the late 1960s and early 1970s we decided to recruit GPs, train them how to recognize and rate depression and then use them as investigators. I think we were among the first groups to use video film of patients for training purposes and organize inter-rater reliability exercises.

You can draw a more recent parallel when you consider developments with the new anxiolytic agents. If you want to perform trials in generalized anxiety disorder (GAD) and go to psychiatrists in search of suitable patients they cannot find them. The only place that you will find subjects who fulfil the criteria for GAD are in general practice so you have to accept the same policy that we adopted for depression.

The GAD situation raises a more general issue. At different times the availability of certain types of patients is at a premium. When the beta-blockers and subsequently the calcium channel blockers were being developed, a 'virgin' hypertensive patient was 'worth his or her weight in gold' because every company wanted to put them into clinical trials. This has recently been the case with GAD and in consequence very large fees have been paid to clinical trialists. I must say that I find it just a little disturbing when patients like this in general practice are worth so much.

Certainly I feel that research in general practice has contributed considerably to clinical psychopharmacology. Some of us who were involved in this development were also prime movers in establishing the BAP. I firmly believe that drugs need to be tested in the environment in which they are ultimately to be used. Somehow I feel that the BAP has rather lost its way in respect of this aspect of psychopharmacology.

Should phase II work be happening in general practice?

There are two ways of looking at the question. You could argue that patients in general practice are not particularly 'clinically' depressed. They are really people with stress related problems and depressive symptoms who are likely to recover spontaneously and therefore do not make good clinical trial subjects. Alternatively, you could argue that the patients who psychiatrists see are not representative of the universe of depressed patients. They may be non-responders who have had considerable previous exposure to psychotropic agents or their depressions may be complicated by social and personality problems.

I think that if we really believe in the DSM-IIIR approach to major depressive disorder and dysthymia and if we train our investigators properly, large cohorts of patients can be identified in general practice who fulfil the diagnostic criteria. I certainly believe that it will be easier to find them there than in psychiatric practice. By the same token you are not going to be looking for bipolar disorder in general practice – you will only find that in psychiatric practice.

This means that it is entirely justifiable to consider performing phase II studies (late phase II at least) in primary care settings. In a sense this brings me back to my comments about psychopharmacology. Psychopharmacology is not just an ivory tower exercise – important though that may be. If we want to know how drugs behave we will need to know how they are used and with what effect. This then takes us beyond the conventional clinical trial. We have all had the experience of trying to extrapolate the results of clinical trials to everyday practice only to find that some of the optimism expressed was unfounded.

In terms of who actually makes the contributions to psychopharmacology who do you think it is; do you think it is the marketing people or is it the people who 'see' the molecules, the chemists.

The truthful answer has to be that they all do. Looking at the question historically I think that it would be fair to say that in the early days scientists made little contribution to the development of psychotropic agents. Clinical observation was more important. Two of the most important advances – the discovery of the MAOIs and the tricyclics – were entirely due to serendipity.

Following the clinical observation that these substances relieved depression, the scientists looked at their actions discovering for example that tricyclics inhibited the reuptake of noradrenaline or 5-HT. To assume, however, that these observations explain what is happening in depression is a rather large jump. The two may be totally unrelated. I suppose that when you see how nowadays scientists can 'construct' compounds that 'fit' receptors there is a lot more 'science' about than there used to be. Nevertheless, we have to be very humble and remember that some very

recently introduced psychotropics owed their discovery to a large element
of serendipity.

It is not just clinical observation or science, however, that determine
whether drugs succeed or not – political, economic and commercial
factors all play a part. We should not lose sight either of what might be
called cultural considerations. Diseases are not universal – they exist in
some cultures and countries but are unheard of in others. I well remember
when I worked in the industry being asked to organize a clinical trial
programme on psychovegetative dystonia. I was told that it was a very
common condition (in fact in one European country it was the common-
est reason for sickness certification). I never really found out what it was,
never mind showing the effectiveness of drug treatment. One of the great
imponderables about marketing drugs is why drugs succeed in one country
yet totally fail in others despite trials being done in the same indications,
using the same protocols and employing 'the same rating scales'. There
are many examples of one country's 'best seller' being a non entity in
others, such as viloxazine in South America and maprotiline in France.

Is part of the problem that we have had no really new drugs since the mid-1960s?
  You could say since the late 1950s.

Yes, I think it is. We have made great strides in reducing side effects and
toxicity but as far as clinical efficacy is concerned we have really made
very little progress.

*What about the question of risks and benefits. Are we going to end up with no
clinical work at all?*

This issue worries me very much. The relationship between risk and
benefit has changed dramatically and I suspect that the pendulum has
swung too far in the wrong direction. I accept that one of the principles
of medicine is 'first do no harm'. But we are in danger of reaching a
situation where in trying to avoid doing any harm we do not do any
good either. Risks that were once acceptable are now unacceptable.
Everyone – patients, doctors and particularly lawyers – have to accept
that there is an element of risk in every medical procedure. When I am
asked this question I always recount one of my early experiences as a
house officer when I saw a young, healthy 21 year old die from swallowing
an aspirin. It sounds ridiculous – he had a headache, swallowed an aspirin,
had a gastric bleed and no-one could stop it.

It seems now that we are reaching a situation where no risk, however
slight, can be accepted. Medicine is becoming increasingly defensive.
Drug evaluation is particularly vulnerable. Because of such problems as
indemnity, insurance and the use of placebos we could find that it is
virtually impossible to perform clinical trials. I think we shall never again
be in a position to 'play hunches' like we used to do.

14 Donald Klein

Reaction patterns psychotropic drugs and the discovery of panic disorder

My first encounter with your work was when I was in Cambridge, in 1986. I became aware of it through Martin Roth's involvement in the Upjohn trial of alprazolam in panic disorder. Even then, in the UK, most clinicians weren't prepared to accept that panic disorder was a real entity. Your name was there as the person who created the concept. Now I am hopeful that this book will get beyond the psychiatric profession and out on the streets and panic disorder is interesting here in that it's come from nowhere to being one of the concepts that everybody, even the person on the street, knows about now.

The next time your name came into the frame was talking to a colleague from New Zealand, Peter Joyce, about an idea I had which is that tricyclic anti-depressants are potentially as antimanic as they are antidepressant. He said 'ah ha, one person who has really tested this way back in the 1960s was Donald Klein who when people came into hospital randomly allocated them to antidepressants, antipsychotics or whatever, regardless of the diagnosis and it looked like people with mania didn't do well with antidepressants'. Do you want to pick up on either of those two points?

I think maybe I ought to start out with going to Hillside. Back in 1959, I was working in a research department at the Creedmoor State Hospital. I had gotten interested in psychopharmacology from the time I had spent in Lexington during the early 1950s but I was initially interested in being an analyst. In those days, it was really the only game in town if you were interested in doing something intellectual in psychiatry. I had actually started in the New York Psychoanalytic in 1957 and in 1959 a job opened up at Hillside and I went to work for Max Fink.

Max Fink was a neurologist and psychiatrist and he ran the Department of Experimental Psychiatry there. He was a diagnostic nihilist and at that time that was not a stupid thing to be because there were extensive studies carried on during the 1950s by psychologists showing that psychiatrists had no inter—rater reliability whatsoever. They could barely tell psychosis from non-psychosis and that was about it. So Max's attitude was that it was foolish to think in terms of diagnosis. I was perfectly willing to go along with that at the time. Now the way Hillside ran, it was essentially a long-term psychoanalytic hospital. The average length of stay was 10 months to a year. Two hundred beds and they all got intensive psychotherapy. The deal that Max and I were able to work out with Lew Robbins, the Head of the Hospital, was that I would be the only person in the hospital who could write orders for medication.

Now I'd write anybody's orders. The way this worked was, if they wanted to medicate a patient, which meant that psychotherapy had failed and the patient was in the hospital for eight months already and they were getting concerned about getting them out, they would have to call me before the patients were put on medication, which would give me the opportunity to ask why they wanted to put the patient on medication. Then I would see the patient and speak to the ward staff. I would write whatever order they wanted and then I would see them weekly and talk to the ward staff and talk to the therapist. And every time they wanted to change the dose, they had to tell me and I would write it.

It was the best learning experience I ever had. Because what it did was it gave me a tremendous opportunity to see how other people handle patients. They'd do all sort of things I would never have done, sometimes right, sometimes wrong and also to get a real idea of the sociology of prescription in the psychodynamic framework. So, for instance, you'd have the following sort of story, they'd call me and say 'look I want Mrs Jones on thorazine 200 mg' and I'd say 'why' and they'd say 'well, she's schizophrenic' and I'd say 'yeh, but she's been here how long, 10 months, and she's been schizophrenic all along why do you want to give it now?' They'd say 'well, she hasn't responded to the therapy and we think that it's probably a good idea'. When you'd talk to the patient about it, the patient would say its okay by me but it means the doctor has given up on me. When you'd talk to the ward staff about it and they'd say, 'she kicked a maid last week and we're not going to put up with that'.

Anyway, it was tremendous. At the time everyone was called schizophrenic, nobody was thinking diagnostically. To think in terms of systematic descriptive diagnosis was a sure mark of a superficial mind because everybody knew that that was just the symptomatic manifestations of the internal conflicts which is where the real action was. So people got treated quite randomly and so my first couple of papers were on a hundred patients treated with thorazine and a hundred patients treated with imipramine. What I did was to isolate different reaction patterns. They were published in the *American Journal* and *Archives* back around 1962.

Now in that very first paper on imipramine I noted there were a group of patients who had periodic, I guess at the time they were called anxiety attacks, who got better on imipramine and that was very startling. It was a good clinical observation, if I say so myself. Now Frank Ayd did a paper in which he talked about the effects of imipramine on neurotic patients.

Another guy named Doug Goldman, who is dead now, had also written a paper on imipramine and neurotic patients. But neither of them actually singled out panic attack as being the key variable that was changing with imipramine.

Now how I first noticed it was that some doc called me up and said that he had a patient who was schizophrenic and they tried thorazine on him and he'd gotten worse and would I see him. Which I did. And this fellow was hideously anxious, extremely dependent, extremely demanding but he wasn't delusional and he wasn't hallucinated and he didn't have thought disorder and he didn't have any restriction of affect. He was so impaired in his functioning they had concluded that he was schizophrenic. Thorazine made it substantially worse which it does regularly when a patient has panic disorder.

Going over the thing, it turned out that he had these periodic panic attacks or anxiety attacks – later I called them panic attacks. So I talked to the residents about that and said 'I don't know what to do with this guy but I've been working with this new drug, imipramine, and it seems to have some funny anxiolytic effects when you give it to agitated depression and who knows maybe it will work here'. So essentially we had a patient we didn't know what to do with and also we had a drug and we were unsure what it did so we mixed them together. It was pure empiricism. And so after each week we'd see the patient and he'd say 'this drug is terrible and it's not helping me, I am getting worse, when are you guys going to help me?'. And we'd up the dose and say 'see you in a week'. After about the third or fourth week, the patient was still complaining bitterly, very anxious, 'it's terrible, I can't go around the grounds by myself'. The psychotherapist said that this drug was a waste of time and the psychotherapy supervisor said it was a waste of time but one of the nurses said to me 'he's better'.

I said 'well how do you know he's better?' I asked several nurses and they all agreed but they didn't know why he was better and finally one good clinical observer said that 'well you know he's been in 10 months and 4 times a day for the past 10 months he has been running to the nursing station saying he was dying. And we'd hold his hand and say no, there's nothing wrong with you it's just this terrible anxiety, the doctors have checked your heart out, you're not going to die and 20 minutes later he'd wander away and 2 or 3 hours later he'd be back and he hasn't done that for the past week'. So I went to the patient and said 'I understand you're feeling better' and he said 'who told you that? What a ridiculous idea'. And I said 'well, one of the nurses told me that'. He said 'well, what do they know'. And I said 'well, isn't it true that you've been running to the nursing station daily for 10 months now' and he said 'absolutely'. I said 'and you haven't done that for the past week'. And it stunned him. He had no idea he had changed his behaviour and he said 'well that's right'. So I said 'how come'? And he said 'um, I guess I've learned they can't do anything for me' and I said 'you've been here 10 months and this week you learned that they can't do anything for you'. He said 'well you've got to learn sometime'. The guy's a premature behaviour therapist.

Now of course what happened, which became plain with a series of patients, is that it was the panic attack; that was the proximal stimulus that led him to run to the nursing station. When you panic you reach out for help. And that's what he did. And then when the panic stopped, he wasn't running to the nursing station but he was still terribly anxious. He still wouldn't go around the grounds by himself, somebody had to walk with him. What struck me was that we have to distinguish the panic attack from the state of chronic anticipatory anxiety – they are just not the same thing. And that for us to continue calling it an anxiety attack in the context of chronic anxiety is exactly wrong so that's why I came up with the neologism.

Where did you get the actual term from?

I don't know. It came out of the blue somewhere. If you look in Joan Rivière's old translation of Freud, which I had read because I was in analytic training; in the Standard Edition they use the term 'anxiety attack'; in Joan Rivière's edition they are called 'panic attacks'. And that was the edition I knew, so I may have picked it up from there.

There are always people who like to trace things back and they say, well, you can see the concept in the old German literature.

Oh, yes, you can. Freud in 1895 described it beautifully. In his 1895 paper on detaching the syndrome of anxiety neurosis from neurasthenia, he points out quite clearly that people who have agoraphobia remember the onset of the agoraphobia with the occurrence of an anxiety attack. That is the second thing I noticed – going back to the patients. Once I started focusing on the attack, it occurred first, and the phobia came second. Then I thought of it as a three-layer cake – the panic attacks began an anticipatory anxiety and then you avoid the situations in which if you got a panic attack there, help couldn't get to you and that's what is called agoraphobia.

So I saw that as a nice sequence. And Freud says that. And Freud also describes in a number of case histories something which has just recently struck me as being the key issue in panic attacks, which is the extreme feeling of suffocation, the very marked respiratory distress that occurs in the panic attack and that's actually why for a short period of time Freud accepted Rank's birth trauma theory. He accepted this because what was the birth trauma – the birth trauma involved the cutting off of respiration and that's what Freud said very clearly. That's the trauma– the feeling of suffocation. Any way he gave it up very quickly. It was a rather transient idea of his. And long before Freud, Westphal described anxiety attacks and if you talk to Pierre Pichot he tells me that some Frenchman described *angoisse paroxysme* back in 1830.

So, it's not like it's a new observation. What's new is that I put it together a different way. I think what's new also is that it's not anxiety and nowadays I'm saying it's not even fear and that is because you have no hypothalmic – pituitary – adrenal activation in a panic attack, neither during a clinical panic attack or during a provoked panic attack.

So, what is it?

I think it's a suffocation false alarm. I think that people think they are suffocating and I've got a lot of circumstantial evidence for it.

Are there two entities that may at times look the same: one which involves the respiratory symptoms and hyperventilation and one which doesn't?

It's hard to say. The English psychiatrists, Brandon and Briggs, published a reanalysis of the Upjohn study in the *British Journal of Psychiatry*, in which they had imipramine versus alprazolam versus placebo. What they did, which had nothing to do with my work at all, was they cluster-analysed the symptomatology of the patients and how they described their panic attacks. It turned out that 70% of the patients had respiratory symptomatology and about 30% didn't. When you lay it out, if you look at the whole group, imipramine and alprazolam are the same but in the patients with respiratory symptomatology imipramine is better than alprazolam and for the patients without respiratory symptomatology alprazolam is better than imipramine.

Well, that's interesting; that sounds like we have two different processes. One panic disorder with respiratory symptomatology, another panic disorder without respiratory symptomatology. But one of the problems there is that it could be a misdiagnosis. Jerry Rosenbaum also re-did the Upjohn study. So I called him up and I said 'look, you guys have a chance to replicate what Briggs did', because one analysis, you know, you don't quite believe. They couldn't replicate it and the reason they couldn't replicate it was that well over 90% of their patients had respiratory symptomatology. So, what had happened to the 30% in the Upjohn study? Now I know social anxiety is frequently misdiagnosed as panic disorder so the possibility may be that they had a lot of social phobics in that study, who imipramine does nothing for, but alprazolam is a good drug.

Can I pick up on one more thing. One of the things that happened with the coining of panic disorder was that the old idea of hyperventilation syndrome, which was common for 10 years, at least in the UK– everybody was talking about hyperventilation syndrome and of course the treatment is to breathe into a plastic bag or whatever. Is there some interface between this and panic attacks then?

Yes, I understand but a panic attack takes four minutes; by the time you've got that paper bag up there you've got occupational therapy. You're giving the person something to do until the panic attack has gone away. There's a guy named Van den Hout, a Dutch psychologist, who's done a controlled study of rebreathing and there's nothing. The hyperventilation types claim that it's acute respiratory alkalosis that provokes a panic attack but Jack Gorman and I have found that's just wrong.

We noticed that during our lactate-induced panic attacks the patients did hyperventilate and we said well we really ought to address the issue of hyperventilation. So we thought for a while how can we get people to hyperventilate and not get a respiratory alkalosis. I forget who had this idea but somebody came up with the idea that if you hyperventilate in 5% carbon dioxide, you're in dynamic equilibrium because there's 5% carbon dioxide in the lungs. So you're blowing out as much as you're breathing in and you can't get an acute respiratory alkalosis under those circumstances. So we said great and the study we did was we had a new computerized plethysmograph, for measuring every breath, and we either put them in room air to hyperventilation or hyperventilation in 5% carbon dioxide. The theory going in was they would panic with ordinary hyperventilation and they wouldn't panic with carbon dioxide.

It was exactly the opposite. And we got no panics with hyperventilation and that's been now replicated by five other people. What happens when people with panic attacks hyperventilate is that they don't like it, they feel dizzy, they feel depersonalized but they don't panic. In carbon dioxide they panic like crazy. This is what got us to thinking along the lines about the suffocation alarm.

Basically if you look at the challenge studies, Pitts came out during the 1960s with the finding that intravenous lactate produced panic attacks in patients with panic disorder and nothing else. And he was instantly attacked on the same ground as David Clarke is talking about, that it's simply psychological. The person, they get symptoms, it reminds them of a panic, it frightens them, they get emotional, and they spiral into a panic attack. Pitt's answer to that was that he gave the patients EDTA, a powerful calcium chelating agent; it threw them smack into tetany but they didn't panic. So the idea that they are just responding to a non-specific stress and they produce this syndrome is silly but that hasn't stopped it. Since then it has been shown that insulin doesn't cause panic and physostigmine doesn't cause panic and 5-HT-P doesn't cause panic and all sorts of weird things that you give to people.

Don't cause panic. But the cognitive therapists would say well, okay, but cognitive therapy works.

No better than simple non-directive support as Shear showed. There's nothing specific about it – there are four different studies showing that when you compare cognitive therapy against an acceptable credible therapy the other therapy always works as well. So, I think that they both work is possible. Even then there has only been a single one, comparing cognitive therapy against medication against placebo in a sample where the medication is shown to be better than placebo. Black, in the *Archives*, showed fluvoxamine was much better than placebo but CT was barely better. David Barlow tried that but medication was no better than placebo in that trial. That's the story. Jack Gorman is doing the study now – the one that I've just described – and when that comes out we'll know something, but up to this point it's all fluff. Both the specificity is fluff and the actual demonstration of efficacy is fluff.

Can I ask you, this whole area has created – well wars is the word that comes to mind – the series of articles in the British Journal of Psychiatry *where Isaac Marks and others attacked the Upjohn work; there isn't anything else quite like it in the psychiatric literature. Passions seem to get aroused on this one. How do you account for it?*

I think it's Isaac. I've known Isaac since the early 1960s. Isaac is an extremely smart man and his first book on 'Fears and Phobias' was a wonderful book. It was just terrific but he missed the boat. I told Isaac back in 1963, 'you know, isn't it strange imipramine blocks panic attacks' and he just scoffed at it. I told the same thing to Martin Roth. He tried imipramine on some of these people and said 'it's just poison'. I can believe that because there are people who are hypersensitive and apparently he had some bad luck. But Roth converted later and took part in the Upjohn study, whereas Isaac has been relentless in his attempt to downgrade the importance of panic attacks. He had the opportunity to run with this idea but he didn't. He did a study on imipramine in panic disorder and found nothing. When Al Raskin re-analysed his data, he found a big finding Isaac had missed.

I didn't know that one. No. Is it broader than just panic disorder. Is it antidrug treatment because he had the same gripe with the use of 5-HT reuptake inhibitors and OCD. With clomimipramine in particular.

Well sure, I think Isaac has converted into a learning theorist. I don't know if you've seen these articles by me and my daughter, Hilary Klein, that appeared in a book that Peter Tyrer edited for the British Association for Psychopharmacology. There's two chapters in which we say yes there's an argument and let's handle this argument and list 27 arguments about panic attacks according to Marks and refute every one of them.

How important do you think the coincidence of interests with Upjohn was in helping get panic disorder on the map?

It was already on the map. I'll tell you how panic disorder got on the map. I was writing articles on panic disorder and I had got about four good studies, well controlled, showing that imipramine worked. And also Pitts had done his work on lactate and they got a lot of play. I think one of the major reasons the impact wasn't bigger was that I was working at

Hillside Hospital, which is a small non-academic hospital. I had no university appointment. But then, somewhere around 1978/79, Ballenger and Sheehan published a paper out of Harvard, where they were both residents at the time, saying well, we've decided to check Klein out and he's right – we did a double-blind placebo-controlled trial and by God it's true. That's what happened. I don't blame people for not paying more heed before because it's nice to have an independent replication. It was the first time there was a replication and in Harvard of all places.

If it comes from Harvard it has to be true!

Has to be true. That's what did it. So when the DSM-III came along I was on the Task Force and Bob Spitzer, who was the chairman of the committee, was fierce about getting panic disorder into the thing.

Why was he so keen?

He had had some personal clinical experience and thought it made sense. And that the data was good. The data was actually better than it was for many other things and at the time.

Could it have been, he was keen to sort out the whole neurosis concept and in a sense to do away with it. Was this the Trojan horse. Did he see one of the ways to . . .

No, obviously I've been doing some thinking on this. Bob said to get into DSM-III you have to have inclusion criteria and exclusion criteria and the concept of neurosis is basically a concept based on exclusion criteria only. What a neurosis means is a person who is not psychotic, but there's no body of inclusion criteria. There is nothing in common between all the various things that are called neuroses in terms of inclusion criteria. That's the reason that they got rid of neurosis. It just didn't make any sense in terms of an organizing principle.

The only sense it made was if you adhered to a particular etiological theory and we weren't having any of that. That caused a tremendous amount of political fights. I don't think that panic disorder was particularly brought in with regard to neurosis. I think it was just that Bob and the Task Force thought it was a good idea. One of the things that is funny is that we had an argument then about agoraphobia without panic disorder and I said that panic disorder was the necessary but not sufficient precursor of agoraphobia. So is stand alone agoraphobia a real thing? I said probably not. Bob said shall we take it out but I said leave it in and we'll see how often it gets used. Clinically it's never used. But epidemiologically it turns out that ECA studies and the study done by Wittchen and Angst in Europe found that there is three times as much agoraphobia without panic disorder as there is of agoraphobia with panic disorder. That was used by Wittchen and by Marks as evidence that basically the relationship between panic disorder and agoraphobia is fallacious.

I never quite understood it. I looked at the criteria for agoraphobia and the criteria for agoraphobia are one out of six fears, one of them being afraid of being in a crowd. So finally Myrna Weissman did a clinical review and she got about 23 patients who in the ECA study had come out with agoraphobia without panic disorder and found that 22 of them didn't have agoraphobia. They all had simple phobias. They weren't massively restricted with regard to travel. Anyway, what happened was that the epidemiological criteria were such that a lot of people who were diagnosed as having agoraphobia just didn't have it.

One of the other things she did with all data of course was to flag up a link between panic and suicide.

That's a very controversial point. I think in the context of depression that panic is an exacerbator and that may well drive a person to suicide but that pure panic disorder is a increased risk for suicide, I rather doubt. But she said it did.

Lepine in France didn't find it and we went back in our records and we didn't find it. Let me tell you what we did find. In the ECA they register whether the person has suicide attempts and whether they have panic disorder but there is no timing, you didn't know which came first. In our family study, we have exact records. We found out that in pure panic disorder the increase in suicide attempts was there, except that we had a 7% rate of suicide attempts anteceding pure panic disorder. It occurred during adolescence and separation – anxious people are very prone to suicide attempts, with their displays of 'you've got to help me'.

The fact that panic disoders and mood disorders both respond to the same drugs, does that point to a link between the two or not?

No, not all of them work. First of all our best antidepressant is ECT and ECT did not work on panic disorder, it makes it worse. Maprotiline does not work for panic disorder, bupropion does not work for panic disorder, so it is not all antidepressants. Nonetheless it does seem funny and the incidence of depression in people with dyed-in-the-wool panic disorder is sky high. Now, Myrna has just published a paper in the *Archives* in which she did a nice family study in which she says that they sort independently, so that they are not really related to each other. The fact that they happen to be together is just an accident. We did our own family study and we've got some indications that that's not true – there are people with panic and depressions that run together in families. It's actually significant on one test so it's there but it's not tremendous. So I think that's an unresolved question. It comes to just what the relationship is then.

But certainly, in terms of the common role of antidepressants, that's not correct. And of course the high potency benzodiazepines work on panic but don't do much for depression.

Let me hop for a second. As regards depression you outlined the concept of endogenomorphic depression and argued that anhedonia is a key issue for people with mood disorders. Do you want to run through that? Listening to Prozac has popularized some of these ideas.

Well, yes, that was essentially derived from my inpatient experience in Hillside and you would see people who were just basket cases. We saw hundreds of guys with melancholia which you just don't see anymore. These people were profoundly changed: nothing made them feel good, nothing. Food tastes like cardboard, sex was nothing, and when their family came to see them they couldn't, didn't, care less. And then we'd give them imipramine and three or four weeks later the veil dropped and all of a sudden we had this whole new human being. On the other hand there were patients who had many depressive complaints and you'd give them imipramine and nothing much happened. But we had them in the hospital and I'd see these patients after they came in and I'd interview them and they'd tell me life was terrible, nothing moves them, they can't get any pleasure out of life and I'd see them 20 minutes later laughing it up in the corridor. Now those were the people who imipramine didn't help.

So it came to me that the difference seemed to be the ability to respond to pleasure and that's what led me to the endogenomorphic idea. I think on the whole for severe depressions, moderately severe depressions, there's a useful distinction. I also now make the distinction that I don't think I'd made in that article between consummatory pleasure and appetitive pleasure. Essentially this comes down to is that I think there are two sorts of pleasure. Freud said that pleasure was a reduction in tension. And he obviously had orgasm in mind or being satiated with food. But as he himself says somewhere, it seems hard to deal with fore-pleasure on that basis; a very pleasurable period with rising excitement. What he says well links in with the descrescendo, the orgasm, but that's not very satisfactory as a theory. There are people who do rock climbing, and they go jogging, all these things give you pleasure.

The ethologists a long time ago made the distinction between appetitive activities and consummatory actitives. Consummatory activities were largely highly stereotyped, species-specific devices for either self-preservation or procreation and appetitive activities were everything that got you in a position for doing consummatory activities and it struck me that there are two different sorts of pleasure there. In a sense you might say it's the pleasure of the hunt and the pleasure of the feast. They are not the same thing.

Looking at the severe patients it struck me that their pleasure of the feast and hunt were both shot. But that the patients who respond to MAO inhibitors as compared with patients who respond to tricyclics, their consummatory pleasures are intact but their appetitive pleasures were distinctly not there. Normally when you anticipate having a good time, you are already having a good time. You've already got a glow of pleasure in anticipation. They didn't have that. And you know you might say to someone 'let's go to a party' and they say 'parties are a bore' and you would say 'that's funny I saw you at a party a couple of weeks ago and you seemed to have a good time' and they'd say 'no, no, I didn't really have a good time' but you drag them to the party and they do have a good time. In anticipation it's a bore, it's unrewarding but in the actual consummatory activity, it's not bad.

Now, although I think that's held up pretty well, there is one fly in the ointment. Recently Fred Quitkin, who's worked with me for 30 years now, a very good guy, did a study where he took 500 patients and did this comparative study on imipramine versus phenelzine versus placebo. They had to have emotional reactivity, and they had two out of four, what we call atypical signs, which are basically overeating, oversleeping, rejection sensitivity and a sense of tremendous fatigue. When we took people into that trial, people showed up with only one of the four. So we figured well, why waste it; we will put them in and handle them separately. Then people started showing up and they had 0 out of the 4, but they did have depressive complaints with a reactive mood and they did not have endogenous signs. So, we took them too. We only had a small sample, about 60 I think. Amazingly, they responded both to imipramine and phenelzine. Whereas if they had any one of those four signs, imipramine was barely better than placebo and phenelzine was much better than placebo.

So I don't know, it's conceivable I'm wrong. Consummatory anhedonia may be an aspect of severity. It may well be that what I am calling the atypical signs are actually signs of a particular kind of disturbed physiology, which is like in amphetamine withdrawal. If you take somebody, anybody, and you give them 30 mg of dextroamphetamine a day for a month and halt it you can produce someone who is over-eating, oversleeping, sensitive to rejection and completely fatigued too but I don't think that's a complete answer.

Mention of Fred Quitkin brings to mind the idea that it should be possible to work out what a drug does from the pattern of responses to it.

Fred and I worked on that for quite a while and Fred grabbed the ball and carried it. The logical analysis of drug effects has taken second place. We just did a Markov analysis with Don Ross, who's our statistician. Now a Markov analysis is like this: in the simplest situation, you've got two states. You're either okay or you're not okay. You measure everybody every week and ask them whether they're okay or not-okay. Now you end up with four transition probabilities. You can either go okay-okay, or okay-not-okay or not-okay-okay or not-okay-not-okay. So you have a matrix of transition probablities between each week. There are statistical tests for analysing whether that matrix is constant over time or changing over time. And if it is changing over time, when does it change over time?

Well, it turns out in our analyses that for placebo it's a constant matrix; there is nothing that's happening obviously, it's all noise from week to week. Whereas with both imipramine and phenelzine there are marked discontinuities. That is a crucial issue for drug development. In phase II drugs, they don't have placebo. Now most drug houses look at people when they come in and people when they go out and they say 'oh, look, 50% of them get better, it seems like the drug is working'. But when you apply Quitkin's pattern analysis or this Markov analysis you can ask are they really getting better in the way that looks like an antidepressant response for instance.

Well, why has the industry not picked this up because it seems to me that we need to get out of the rigid placebo-controlled double-blind randomized control trial.

Well, I think the industry are very conservative. Secondly they've got the FDA on their back and the FDA and Paul Leber doesn't think badly of our work but nonetheless he could have a lot of second thoughts about accepting a study on those grounds. My belief actually is that it would be good for the industry in Phase II but in Phase III you're probably stuck with pretty much the usual thing.

Can I bring up a further issue, which sort of plays into this one, which is that you've been talking about clinical entities, the clinical needs of trials and trial design, etc. I'm aware that within ACNP there's been a feeling for some time among the clinical people within it that ACNP is going the wrong way. It's going too much down the road of becoming a Neurosciences Society.

I said that back in 1980 when I was President of the ACNP. The ACNP was founded by clinicians – Frank Ayd, Heinz Lehmann, Nate Kline and others. It was bankrolled by the drug industry on that basis. First of all, they immediately set themselves up as a limited society – they were only going to have a certain number of members and they said they were only taking the best. The fact of the matter is that it's far easier to demonstrate your scientific skills in non-clinical areas. You can do very highly technical work on rats and you can study the physiology, the brain chemistry and you can do wonderful things so that when you start comparing the CVs, the bibliographies, of people who are doing clinical work with people who are doing preclinical work by any usual test the preclinical people were outstanding and the clinical people were finding out if this drug worked and if that drug worked.

Which looks much more . . .

Which looks much more pedestrian and uninteresting. Also the whole ideology is that the basic science provides the ground work for the proper understanding of clinical science. That's the way people think. It doesn't mean that they are right. They really hadn't got together close enough yet so they still have two pretty independent tracks.

What happened essentially was that I did an analysis of the membership of the ACNP back in 1980 which showed that the number of clinical people working with whole human beings in clinical settings was steadily dropping and that the number of non-clinical scientists was steadily rising and that we were on our way to being a neurosciences organization. The charm of the ACNP was the attempt to integrate the two – you wanted the non-clinical scientists and clinical scientists in the hope that maybe you would strike a spark somewhere. What was happening was the ACNP panels were becoming more and more 5-HT-14 receptor orientated and what that means to the rat – with no attempt even to get at clinical relevance.

There was one session at ACNP, where there was about one clinical panel only in the whole meeting and no attempt by any panel to take this into account. So I said enough is enough. The ACNP programme committee is trying to respond to that and more credit to them. I think that that's good. In the meantime, they don't have a serious commitment to the whole idea of educating practitioners and I think this is necessary because a number of studies now have shown that most practitioners are doing poorly. The RAND study, for instance, by Ken Wells in which he essentially tracked depressives through the primary care system. The vast majority of them never got diagnosed. And once diagnosed never got treated.

You did more though than just say to ACNP enough is enough. You went and formed your own society. Tell me about that.

Actions speak louder than words, that's all. It's interesting what happened actually. Paul Wender and I had been friends for many years. Paul's a terrific, guy who has done remarkable work in at least two areas, one being childhood minimal brain dysfunction and attentional deficit disorder. He is the leading figure showing that attentional deficit disorder persists into adolescence and beyond. And the second was his work with Seymour Kety on the adoption studies in Denmark. Now Paul and I had gotten friendly and we wrote a book back in 1981 on *Mind, Mood and Medicine* (Klein and Wender, 1981) and somewhere along the line we decided depression had been treated badly and we formed an organization called the 'National Foundation for Depressive Illness', which was a non-profit corporation – which did not do very well. We had difficulty raising money. Senator Hatch had a man on his staff who was really depressed, and Paul's treatment of him opened Hatch's eyes. He said 'my God, this stuff's real'. And he asked 'is there anything I can do for you' and we said 'you can raise some money for us'. So he joined with Senators Kennedy,

Metzenbaum and Kassenbaum and helped us throw a fund—raising benefit.

Now our funds were going steadily downhill. We had that one big bolus of money but amazingly we had been unable to really capitalize on that. At the time that we were getting fed up with the narrow focus of ACNP, we decided one reasonable use of NAFDI money would be to bankroll this other organization and help depressives out by increasing the education of practitioners. So essentially the ASCP was sort of godchild of NAFDI. It has a separate board, completely independent and we've got a set of by-laws and so on, except that Peter Ross, who's our administrator for NAFDI, is also the administrator for ASCP. And I guess it will stay that way for a while. So that's the reason we were able to get this organization off the ground because we had some backup.

Will the industry move over do you think?

They haven't. That was one of the major concerns of the ACNP that we would end up cutting off their pipeline.

What would happen do you suppose if the industry did begin to move over?

Beats me. I presume what would happen is the ACNP would develop more clinical interests.

Or else they'd put a contract out on you!

There was a fair amount of hard feeling over that, but they recognize that we are not simply out to get the ACNP. We've got two Presidents of the ACNP on our board, myself and George Simpson. And they can recognize that they have got to change.

I think we're faced with just the same problem with the BAP at the moment. BAP, like ACNP, was begun by clinical people who brought basic scientists in and in recent years has begun to move down the road of becoming a neurosciences group.

I don't think you have ever been a closed limited membership organization. That makes a big difference because if you only take 10 people a year and you've got 75 applications, you go for the fat CVs.

One of the other problems is that the basic sciences are very much a case of doing crosswords as it were. Sort of problem solving. You pick the problems that you can solve at any particular time. Clinically though it isn't the same. People who work in the clinical field really don't have a choice about what problems they can tackle or not. They are faced with things that may or may not be solved by them and hence you get . . .

Do you know the joke about the drunk and the lamp-post? There's this drunk wandering around the street and the cop comes along and says 'what are you doing' he said 'my keys, I dropped my keys', and the cop says 'oh you've dropped them by the lamp-post here'. 'No' he said 'I dropped them down there somewhere'. So the cop said 'well why are you looking down here' and he said 'well here's where I can see things'.

So you're saying that basic science people are working around the lamp-post.

I respect basic scientists and was a basic scientist myself briefly. I was a chemist. But there is still an enormous gap between basic science and clinical relevance.

On that point, let me take you back and ask you why you went into medicine at all. What your career path was into medicine?

It's easy actually. I was 15 when I went to College . . . stumbled on Freud. And he was talking about all the things that interested me. Sex and girls. I was always a sceptic. I never bought it. I said it's very interesting. So I got the idea of becoming a research psychoanalyst. That there would be some way of testing these ideas out and then it turned out to be a psychoanalyst you had to be an MD so I went to medical school.

Did you at any point think about changing on your way through medical school?

Well, from my psychiatry courses I nearly did. They nearly made a haematologist out of me. The psychiatry courses were terrible. Terrible. We had one guy who would read to us from a book. And finally we delegated some people to go and talk to him, and said 'we all know how to read'. And he said 'this was our resistance against understanding the real truth'. So that was terrible. I had a good friend, a fellow named Norman Kretchmer, who was in my class, who already had a PhD in biochemistry. He had his own lab and I worked through College as his lab tech. So I got involved with basic science. It was a lot of fun. We built our own chromatography apparatus. But I maintained my interest in psychoanalysis.

I really did like Medical School and I liked medicine, I liked the whole thing about physiology. Then when I got out of Medical School, I went into the public health service. The US Public Health Service Marine Hospital. That was largely because the Korean War was on and I didn't want to go to Korea and if you were in the Public Health Service, the draft was not enforced. Essentially I was with the coastguard medical officers. I anticipated finishing my internship and then I would spend two years on an Indian reservation and that was okay. Better than Korea. In fact I got fired. At the end of my internship about 30 days before it ended, Eisenhower abruptly reduced the force in the public health service and they dropped out the bottom half of the entire class and I was out of a job and vulnerable for the draft.

So I went scurrying around and I landed as a first-year resident at Creedmoor State Hospital. At the time we had no medication, this was

1953, we had 6000 patients and I walked in and said to the head of the male admitting services 'Dr Klein reporting for duty sir'. He said 'yes Klein, here's this little book which is going to teach you how to do a mental status. You'll be admitting 20 patients a week and there are 300 patients to take care of'.

That was the extent of my psychiatric education. That was all I got and it was okay because I enjoyed being on my own then. I was being thrown into a snake pit. It was just terrific. I saw so many strange things. People were really untreated and they were completely out of it. At that time I began to get a little doubtful about psychoanalysis. It was very difficult to see how it applied to these people. I was getting noises from the Draft Board, so I called the public health service again and said 'look I've got a whole year of psychiatric education now, is there a place for me?'. And they said 'yes as a matter of fact we have a place for you down at Lexington, Kentucky in the Narcotics Hospital'.

So I went down there. When I got there they said 'who are you?' and I said 'Dr Klein' and they said 'never heard of you'. It turned out my papers had fallen behind the files somewhere and I was really supposed to be in Anchorage, Alaska. Lexington was wonderful. It was a 1000-bed prison. It had 700 prisoners and 300 volunteers at any one time – women and men. I had zero experience with drug addiction so they put me in charge of the women's unit and in charge of withdrawal. I had to learn fast. It was the most interesting experience.

At the time, they had the best human research set up in the world. Abe Wikler and Harris Isbell ran the Addiction Research Center. Abe came out with probably the very first text on psychopharmacology. It's called *The Relationship of Pharmacology to Psychiatry*. It came out in 1955.

Pretty early.

Too early because he missed the antidepressants and he just had one reference of chlorpromazine so the book died. It's one of the great books. Wikler was one of the smartest men I have ever met. He was really something. And so in Lexington I got exposed to the first trials on LSD, reserpine and on chlorpromazine.

Tell me about all this.

I was running the withdrawal ward and Abe came over to me and says we've got this new drug, its called chlorpromazine and we think it may be like morphine – it's safe enough. I said 'why do you say it's like morphine' and he said 'well, when people take it, they get sort of quiet, they go on the nod, but they are not asleep and they are not ataxic and their pupils get small' (which was not true). So they had this ward with prisoners and volunteers and they gave this guy a shot of chlorpromazine and asked him an hour later 'how is it' and he said 'doc, I don't know what that shit is, but it will never sell'.

And he was right!

He was right. It's never sold on the street. But it was a wonderful ward. One day a foundation grant showed up for work on LSD, you know it was Korean War times and there was tremendous interest in brain-washing. They had these pilots who had been shot down in Korea, who were appearing on TV saying 'I'm a tool of Western Fascists and they made me do this and every right-thinking person will curse America'. Everyone was saying how could one of our pilots do this. It's very easy: put a gun to someone's head and they'll say anything. But people got more concerned about brain washing and about strange drugs being used. LSD had just been described by Hoffman and Stoll in about 1953 and do you remember how that happened?

Yes. It's curious though, Hoffman took the stuff around 1948 but as you say it was round 1953/54 before I've seen anything in print.

Right. Well Stoll was the psychiatrist who wrote up Hoffman's experiences. He wrote this wonderful paper on LSD. And Stoll came to Lexington to tell us about it and they opened this foundation and gave us money. We found out about 10 years later that it was CIA money. The CIA had set up research studies on LSD all around the country and their interests were basically technical – with whether you could use the stuff in war or for espionage and brain washing.

It was my job to select subjects for the LSD experiments. Our criteria were quite clear; they had to be hopeless cases, antisocial psychopaths who had at least two five-year sentences, or drug addicts for twenty years and the chance that they would be rehabilitated was zero. And they were happy to volunteer – everyone volunteered. And so we had the opportunity of watching LSD being used. What was funny was that it was done very antiseptically. People were put in litte cubicles on a bed, filling out a questionnaire and there were none of these revelatory experiences.

No, that seems to be the group phenomenon of it, doesn't it?

Yeh, you have to do a lot of introductory work to get a transcendent experience, which is an entirely strange thing. You'd walk in and say 'how are you doing', and they'd say 'fine', 'anything unusual happen?' 'no, you just turned green and the walls turned yellow'. So strange things happened but there was no big revelation. LSD seems to be an amplifer. Then chlorpromazine came in and they did a double-blind placebo-controlled chlorpromazine trial and a double-blind placebo-controlled reserpine trial on my ward.

These were not my studies, I was in the last six months of the two years I was in Lexington. They moved me over in charge of a World War I Veterans' ward. These people had been psychotic for 30 years. They were out of it completely. We gave some of them chlorpromazine and I remember a guy who hadn't said anything for 30 years comes over to me after a few weeks and said 'Doc, when am I getting out of here?'. It was Rip van Winkle. He had remembered nothing. The last thing he remembered was in 1916 going over the trenches. That was an honest to God miracle. The whole idea of chlorpromazine just making people quiet, you know, it's so silly. So, I was involved in facilitating these two studies. Essentially, reserpine wasn't very good but chlorpromazine was great.

Tell me about reserpine. Had Kline done his trial prior to this or was this a trial that he was also involved with?

I think this was contemporary with Nate Kline's trials. There was some guy in India, who had done some reasonably good work with reserpine and there was a lot of interest as to whether reserpine and chlorpromazine acted differently in treatment or whether they were affecting people differently. In my opinion reserpine was just an inferior drug to chlorpromazine. It didn't work very well. It slogged people. On chlorpromazine many people who were withdrawn and almost mute actually woke them up. That never happened with reserpine. But I think reserpine has actually been insufficiently studied.

So after Lexington?

After Lexington I went back to Creedmoor and I got involved in research at the Creedmoor Institute of Psychobiologic Studies. It was an outfit run by Arthur Sackler. Arthur was an amazing man. If you go down the mall in Washington you see the Sackler Museum. That's him. And he's got a wing on the Metropolitan and he's got a Sackler Museum in Peking. I don't know where he got all his money from but he apparently got into medical advertising, when medical advertising was just starting post–World War II and he just cleaned up. He was a biological psychiatrist at a time there weren't any biological psychiatrists. He had two brothers. And he ran the Creedmoor Institute of Psychobiologic Studies and I was sort of kibitzer over there during my first year residency.

They had a theory histamine was the problem in schizophrenia and he would give patients histamine. At the time we were using sub-coma insulin on our acute admission ward. You give people small doses of insulin and they sweat and they lie in bed and they gain some weight. I doubt it did much for them but its a pretty good sedative. I convinced them to use this histamine biochemotherapy so we took one ward and we gave people insulin and another ward had histamine biochemotherapy. We never got to randomization or blinding but the people who had histamine biochemotherapy did badly. And that was the end of that study.

When I finished my residency, I went to the Creedmoor to work full time. Somewhere along the line they had a study on autism where there were several analysts who were convinced that autism was caused by the family. They had six families in treatment, the mother was in treatment, the father was in treatment, the child in treatment and the dog was in treatment. They got nowhere for a year. That was interesting. I was taking care of two autistic identical twins, who walked around on their toes, slapping their chest with their hands. I said to the chief analyst 'their mother did that?' That programme was cancelled and we were shifted to geriatrics.

So we did a study on dicumarol in cerebral arteriosclerosis – a proper placebo-controlled study. And essentially we found that they lived longer but it didn't help them mentally. That got published. It was my very first paper. Then we did a study on mepazine, which is a phenothiazine that is distinguished for being the only phenothiazine that just doesn't work. It came with glowing reviews. To our surprise it didn't help and it was eventually taken off the market. It made a very good active placebo.

Then the opportunity came to go to Hillside. I was in analysis, since 1957. My job in Creedmoor was frankly a sinecure and I was busy being analysed. I kept telling my analyst that I was interested in doing something more systematic and interesting in the way of human experimentation, which he told me was my sadism. We just had to work that through. I went to Hillside. Max Fink was there and he was really a dynamo. Extremely sceptical. He kicked me into high gear. From leading a fairly leisurely life at Creedmoor, I started working very hard and that was fine. I lasted in analysis for a couple more years. I told my first analyst that we are not getting anywhere and he agreed very happily so they gave me another analyst who was a complete idiot. I lasted about five months with him.

After our initial couple years' experience of imipramine and phenothiazines, Max and I did this random trial. Everybody, no matter what they had, got randomized either to placebo, imipramine and chlorpromazine. We used big doses. We used 300 mg of imipramine, 1200 mg of chlorpromazine and we did it on 150 patients. Max left to become the Director of the Missouri Institute of Psychiatry and I continued there and I did the whole study again. So we did actually 300 patients. I think it was the largest, randomized placebo-controlled study that had ever been done in one place. We published a series of articles on that trial, in which we showed a lot of things that have been forgotten, like chlorpromazine is an excellent antidepressant, which doesn't fit with any of the current theories.

Are the current theories marketing driven?

Yeh. And even the simple theory that Schildkraut came up with about noradrenaline deficit in depression and excess in mania didn't fit chlorpromazine.

So how come our theories went the way they did in the face of this kind of trial? People just don't reference your trial.

Contradictory facts never sink a theory. It's a better theory that sinks a theory. These theories were obviously no good but there weren't any better theories around. They account for 40% of the facts. They didn't account for 60% of the facts but we had no other theory that would even account for 40% of the facts. So that's the reason the theory survived.

Do we have one yet? It seems to me we're in a vacuum. People don't believe the amine theory yet the industry still builds drugs as though amines are what it's all about.

I think that when you look back over what we've learned in the past 30 odd years about drugs and psychiatric illness, there are two things that seem to me to be completely outstanding. One is that the major psychotropic drugs don't affect normal human beings.

Well, chlorpromazine affects normal human beings – it gives you parkinson's, it demotivates you and, okay, right, it won't show up on cognitive function tests but that's because we don't have good cognitive function tests.

That's not necessarily relevant to its antipsychotic activity. My understanding of antipsychotics is that they wake people up.

Well, certainly they can bring you out of things that you are absorbed in. They bring you back. Sure.

So that's a little hard to reconcile with what you're saying. There are other phenothiazine like drugs that are not antipsychotic that all do exactly that – phenergan for one – people are quiet on that, they are unmotivated, but that's not antipsychotic at all. So, I think it's probably a parallel but not the central effect. Imipramine doesn't do anything to normals.

My major point is that I think there are two different sorts of drugs. There are drugs that are rheostat drugs, that is what they do essentially is they alter your level, like an antacid: that is, if you have hyperacidity we can make you have normal acid; if you've normal acid we can make you subnormal. And then there are other drugs that are essentially like aspirin and the psychotropics are more like aspirin. If you've got a fever aspirin will bring it down to normal but if you've got a normal temperature it won't make it go lower. So its fixing a derangement and that's what I think these drugs are doing, fixing a derangement.

What's striking about chlorpromazine, for instance, in manic depression is that it will make the mania better but it will also make depression better. That sounds to me like if you had a thermostat that was insensitive. If we were to plug the sensor in backwards, you would turn negative feedback into positive feedback. So what you've got to do is fix the detector; I think that's a useful analogy.

One thing we've learned is that there seems to be normalizing drugs, which speaks for a cybernetic circuit pathology. The other thing is that psychopathology is largely genetic. At present we lack an understanding of the functional circuitry of the brain. Things like receptors are just the very peripheral edge of the thing – all these wonderful things they talk about happening at receptors, happen 10 seconds after you give the drug.

Yes, I agree totally.

So why does it take six weeks to get better? I'd say and have been saying for years is that the right way to go is behavioural genetics. We should breed animals for pathology. And they have actually done that to some extent, they have some anxious strains of rats. But I think you can breed for separation anxiety. I think we can breed for anhedonia. And that would be far more interesting. I have never been able to sell that to anyone, I can't sell it to the pharmaceutical houses or to NIMH.

Look at Eric Kandel, basically what's so bright about Eric is that he has a functional analysis strategy. He takes the simple organism and takes a simple function like siphon retraction and then he works out the circuitry, so he has a greater understanding of what happens when you do this and do that. But most of the stuff that's going on in receptorology is not related to a functional context. So no matter what you find it remains a mystery.

That's what actually got me so interested and excited in my recent stuff on respiration because with that I've got a functional context, which is the idea of a suffocation false alarm.

Can you flesh that out?

Well, I've got a general framework which is that many diseases are malfunctions of evolved functions. Now since carbon dioxide and lactate increments can cause panic in panic patients, you have to ask what causes this naturally and both are caused by hypoxia. Carbon dioxide goes up when you're not having enough oxygen and lactate goes up from pyruvate, again when you're not getting enough oxygen, so they are actually two physiological signals that you may be in potentially suffocating circumstances. Taking a functional viewpoint, I got the idea that panic disorder people have a hypersensitive suffocation alarm.

So I started to read the literature. The flip side of this is that some people ought to have hyposensitive suffocation alarm systems and I found them; these kids with Ondine's Curse. These kids are born, apparently healthy; they put them to sleep in the crib, they go to sleep and they die. This isn't sudden infant death though because if you catch them when they are just turning blue and you wake them up they start to breathe again. They then go back to sleep and they stop breathing again. And you wake them up and they start breathing. They only discovered this 20 years ago.

Ought it to be more common, given that panic disorder is so common?

Well, look at the flip side . . . panic disorder doesn't kill you and so if it gets evolutionarily weeded out that's difficult. Anyway, they are now able to keep these kids alive with phrenic driving. They go to sleep at night and they have a radio–frequency broadcaster that zaps them every five seconds, so their diaphragm contracts and they're all right. They now have a group of these kids, who are in their teens. There's a woman named Debra Weese-Mayer, who's a paediatric pulmonologist out in Chicago, who I was lucky enough to hook up with. She has the biggest collection of these kids and what's really interesting about them is that they don't have any suffocation reflex at all. They don't know what it is to suffocate. You put them in pure carbon dioxide and it doesn't stimulate them; they turn blue quite happily.

Now the idea of a suffocation alarm signal, sounds like an unwarranted reification, doesn't it? You've got 3000 different things going on in your body that depend upon a flow of oxygen. The oxygen gets cut off, everything goes to hell. With the suffocation alarm centre cut off everything should be signalling that things are going wrong but it doesn't work that way in these kids. Furthermore imipramine, I argue, downregulates the suffocation alarm signals and that's why it works. So what should these kids get from it – they've got barely enough suffocation alarm signals to begin with? – They stop breathing.

Do they?

In some ways they have panic disorder inside out. There's some quite interesting stuff there. Megacolon is one per 5000 births but a third of these kids gets megacolon. Now megacolon is a segmental absence of nerves of the myenteric plexus in the gut which happens to have a high concentration of serotonergic neurones. So they've got an absence of serotonergic neurones peripherally, what about centrally?

Another thing about panic disorder is that half the people who have it have a history of separation anxiety. And how do you fit that together with suffocation? It struck me that it might have something to do with endorphins because endorphins downregulate carbon dioxide sensitivity and also downregulate separation anxiety. So, perhaps we have some sort of endorphinergic deficit. Which made me wonder just how anxious are all these kids with Ondine's Curse. You know the highest epidemiological risk factor for anxiety is chronic illness and these kids go to bed every night liable to die that night. If the machine malfunctions, they would die. Many of them have had tracheotomies, they get lugged into the hospital. Their parents are frequently so anxious about them they stay up with them all night, every night. They get dragged into hospital for a week in a year and they get probed. They know they've got this thing that isn't going to go away. Should that be an anxious kid?

Should be.

By any of the usual standards. I said if they are really panic disorder inside out, maybe they're not anxious. So we did a study with Daniel Pine. They are not anxious, which is remarkable. But the thing that recently has me the happiest, because if this works out I will be very surprised and pleased, is, one of the aspects of the suffocation alarm theory is that any suffocating circumstances should be panicogenic. And in fact this is largely true. People trapped in a mine go nuts. However, the one thing that bothered me was carbon monoxide because carbon monoxide asphyxiates you but you don't panic. You just go off nicely and that was extremely irritating. And . . .

Has Sol Snyder solved that for you?

He has. I commented on where the suffocation alarm system is in the brain. I said I'm not sure it's in the brain, maybe it's in the carotid body. The carotid bodies are actually measuring the oxygen and carbon dioxide and relaying it on to the brain so the sensor could be there. Now Sol has shown not only is carbon monoxide a neurotransmitter, it is the neurotransmitter in the carotid body. What does it do in the carotid body. It turns the carotid body off. So maybe the reason you don't panic is that you get the carbon monoxide and it knocks out your alarm system. If that's right, carbon monoxide should be an antipanic agent and should block the carbon dioxide effect. That's a study we're doing.

Who've hit you as the key people of the last 30 years?

Wikler, Fink, Sol Snyder, of course. I naturally think of people I know, who actually trained with me like John Kane, Fred Quitkin, Arthur Rifkin, Jack Gorman and Mike Liebowitz. Leo Hollister did excellent work, Gerry Klerman, Jon Cole was a real leader. He is an extraordinarily erudite, funny man.

What about this book Listening to Prozac. *It seems to me that this, for the first time 30 years later, is where the impact of the psychotropic drugs has begun to reach down to street level in the US. Now you're cited widely in the book as being a . . .*

Peter Kramer and I have been corresponding over the years. I always like the way he writes but I think the reason Peter's book is so popular is because it makes an appeal to wishful thinking. Why was psychoanalysis so popular? It appealed to the belief that you would be a whole new human being and that you would be not just taking care of a few lousy symptoms. It was going to change you radically. And that was tremendously appealing to people. Everybody wants to be saved or cured.

Now, when people talk about medication, they ask 'does it cure?'. And I say it's not going to cure you; if you stop the medication you may very well have a relapse. It's not a radical cure, it's a symptomatic management and it does pretty good but that's all it is. That doesn't stand up in competition with the psychoanalytic goal. Well, Peter comes along and says Prozac is going to make a new person out of you and all of a sudden it's all over the papers. He's appealing to the same level of wishful thinking and that's why it's so popular. The medications have not become popular because they work. They have suddenly become popular on the basis of the same sort of curative promise.

Select bibliography

Klein, D.F. and Fink, M. (1962) Psychiatric reaction patterns to imipramine. *American J. Psychiatry*, **24 119,** 432–38.

Klein, D.F. and Fink, M. (1962) Behavioural reaction patterns with phenothiazines. *Archives of General Psychiatry*, **24 7,** 449–59.

Klein, D.F. (1972) Endogenomorphic depression: a conceptual and terminological revision. *Archives of General Psychiatry*, **24 31,** 447–51.

Klein, D.F. and Klein, H.M. (1989) The definition and psychopharmacology of spontaneous panic and phobia and The nosology, genetics and theory of spontaneous panics and phobia, in *Psychopharmacology of Anxiety*(P.J. Tyrer, ed.). Oxford University Press, New York, pp. 135–62; 163–95.

Klein, D.F. (1993) False suffocation alarms, spontaneous panics and related conditions: An integrative hypothesis. *Archives of General Psychiatry*, **24 50,** 306–17.

Wender, D.H. and Klein, D.F. (1981) *Mind, Mood and Medicine: a Guide to the New Biopsychiatry*, Farrar, Strauss and Giroux, New York.

15 Herman van Praag

Psychiatry and the march of folly?

A number of people I've interviewed mentioned the trouble you had in Holland during the 1960s when it was not fashionable – almost not possible – to be a biological psychiatrist. Do you want to tell me something about it?

To clarify that I need to bring up some historical data. I started my residency in psychiatry in the late 1950s. I had always been interested in research. I did research in Neurology as a student at the University of Leyden and later in the army, and then I started training in psychiatry as a future neurologist. At that time, in Holland, you had to do one and a half years in the 'sister' discipline. I started out with psychiatry. I had left the army on 30 March and I started on 1 April 1958 – at the very time that the first MAO inhibitor and the first tricylcic was introduced. Well, the first monoamine inhibitors were immediately fascinating to use because they exerted antidepressant effects and it was already known that they had an effect on monoamines. So from that time on, I was captivated, amongst other things, by the question whether there is any relation between antidepressant action and changes in brain monoamine function and metabolism, and whether there is anything amiss with brain monoamines in depressives responsive to those antidepressants.

So I started to work from the very first day of my residency with Bart Leynse who was a biochemist. At first he was somewhat hesitant. In the 1950s, for a biochemist to work together with a psychiatrist! Could it harm your reputation . . . but in the end he accepted and then I worked on that topic and I wrote a thesis – a combined psychiatric/biochemical/pharmacological discourse – about the significance of MAO inhibition as a therapeutic principle in depression.

I defended my thesis in 1962. I finished my residency in 1963 and subsequently I worked for three years in Rotterdam as Chef de Clinique (clinical director) of the Psychiatric University Clinic. In 1965 I was invited to come to Groningen to start a Department of Biological Psychiatry. How come? That was the single idea of someone who was to become a very important man in my life, Dr Dijkhuis. Sitting on the board of a University, at that time, was a more or less honorary position, but there was always one professional and full-time board member and in the 1960s that full-time board member happened to be a former general practitioner, Dr Dijkhuis. He had read my thesis and in one way or another he felt that the question of the link between brain and behaviour was novel and important.

So he asked me to come to Groningen and I got all the money I requested to set up a Department of Biological Psychiatry. At that time that was an enormous amount to invest in Psychiatry – I needed facilities for pharmacology, biochemistry, animal behaviour and neurophysiology and a clinical research unit. I accepted the position. I remember very well I discussed it thoroughly with my wife. It was the mid 1960s, the heyday of psychoanalysis, of psychodynamic thinking. Assuming the official role of Head of a Department of Biological Psychiatry, the first of its kind in Europe, in that era would mark me for ever as Mr Biological Psychiatry, an idea I didn't like. I feel too that I am a full-blown, all-round psychiatrist. I like biological psychiatry, but I'm more than that concept implies. Yet the challenge appealed to me and I went.

My presentiment came true. I was pinpointed and earmarked as Mr Biological Psychiatry in Holland. At the end of the 1960s, a social revolution took place – in America it was politically orientated with the Vietnam War as a focus, but in countries like Germany and Italy and Holland, it was a anti-establishment movement – and biological psychiatry became a focus of the revolutionaries. Biological psychiatry was reactionary, was conservative, was anti-human, it was everything bad, politically, medically, therapeutically. And so antipsychiatry developed. There exist no psychiatric diseases, according to the most extreme protagonists; there is just labelling by a society that doesn't accept unusual behaviour.

Antipsychiatry became more and more influential and biological psychiatry more and more unacceptable and I was Mr. Biological Psychiatry. In 1977, I went from Groningen to Utrecht, in the heyday of antipsychiatry, and antibiological psychiatry. Groningen is located more eccentric than Utrecht and was less extreme, and so biological psychiatry had been more or less accepted. The most extreme revolutionaries were located on the Western coast – in Amsterdam and Utrecht. The Psychiatric University Clinic, after my arrival, became a focus of political turmoil and my very presence there became highly politicized. Frequently there was trouble in terms of disturbed symposia, disturbed lectures, protests against biological research, street riots against electroshock treatment, even physical threats.

I've heard from people like Alec Coppen that when they went over to talk to meetings in Holland, they found that there were demonstrators outside the lecture theatres.

Oh yes, we had police there. It reminded me of the 1920s and 1930s, of the clashes in Germany between the communists and the fascists. That time too, there existed a highly politicized environment that incorporated all kinds of extraneous domains. What has biological psychiatry to do with conservatism, reactionary convictions? – but all of a sudden it was, within medicine, the symbol of everything that at the time was unacceptable. Psychiatry it was claimed had nothing to do with the brain. It had even little to do, according to some antipsychiatrists, with inner psychological workings. They were also, but not so vehemently, against psychodynamics. It was all caused by social factors, maybe by relational factors but in particular by social ills. So, those were stirring, but interesting, times.

Did it ever get to the stage of being actually worrying to you or your wife in terms of serious threats to your personal safety?

Yes indeed, including the children. There were times when we had to have police protection. My family, more than I, suffered in consequence of that. I, to an extent, was concerned, but on the other hand I flourished; I am at my best, I think, when I have a cause in mind, which I can defend and fight for and I felt the biological approach had a lot to offer to psychiatry, that it was a cause worth fighting for – scientifically and clinically – in terms of providing novel treatments to psychiatric patients. I felt I did progressive, not conservative, things, since I was working for the betterment of diagnosis and treatment. That is not reactionary. Rather it is a progressive attitude and I liked to defend it. So it never occurred to me to resign. If you ask me: were you perfectly happy with the situation? I would say: no, but I didn't suffer. Also, something which was very important to me, was that the Dean, the President of the Hospital, the Faculty, and the staff of the Department, were always behind me, both in Groningen and Utrecht. They always thought the work was important. No-one in the University or the Hospital or the Department ever tried to belittle or discourage me or say: 'van Praag, maybe you should shrink your activities a little bit, keep it more in the background'.

Why do you think it happened? You've mentioned the whole 1968 period but one of the other things I've heard you mention before is that there is a certain Calvinism within Holland. Do you want to elaborate on that?

Indeed, that trend exists. Even among the revolutionaries. Holland is in nature still a very Calvinistic country. The churches are empty, but yet it is a nation which has a strong Calvinistic mentality, in that principles are highly important; you can not and should not compromise on principles; the right thing to do is: implement your principle, whatever it costs. There is little tendency to relativize; to reason. Yes, there are principles, but there's also a practice, real life, and maybe we should discuss whether the principle should and can be fully implemented. That religious fervour inspired the antipsychiatric movement. Likewise, it dictated the idea that the spiritual is a domain independent from the physical and that the former domain is of a higher order and of greater value than the physical.

The idea also that something in the human psychological existence is immortal, independent from the body, from the brain; that there is something incorporeal that survives death. That belief system was being questioned, in the opinion of my opponents, by my work.

I replied, that there can be no behaviour, no experience, without corresponding cerebral underpinnings. But the very idea that by ECT, by use of a machine or a drug, you can change the mood of a guilt-ridden melancholic patient, ran counter to ingrained ideas of Christianity and particularly of Calvinism. I think, though I can't prove it, that an element of that philosophy gave antipsychiatry its fervour. The unwillingness to accept that the psychological realm, though of course different from the physical, can actually be influenced by physical means, that you can study the physical underpinnings of whatever psychological process, was anathema to antipsychiatrists. Listen, I'm not a theologian; if you believe that there is something in the human existence that is immortal, by all means, think so, I do not deny it. But it is not the object of my studies. That's a subject for theology. I study phenomena which I consider to be dependent on a functioning brain. If there's more, it belongs to another discipline.

So the late 1960s and the 1970s represented a highly politicized era, that was highly revolutionary and antibourgeois. Any type of establishment, anything that was believed in by fathers and mothers, was rejected. Biological psychiatry, moreover, had to struggle against the combined force of religious convictions regarding the immortal soul and the firmly Calvinistic inclination to adhere to (antipsychiatric) principles, even if they turn out to be unpractical, not useful or even wrong.

To the point now that ECT is still very difficult to use in Holland, isn't it?

Yes. I find it almost unbelievable. Almost the first phone call I had when I came back to Holland two years ago, was the request to sit on a Committee to judge ECT. I said: 'has nothing changed in all of these years?' and they said 'well you know the parliament has asked questions'. I said: 'what questions – let them read. ECT is not a panacea but there is enough data to show them that it's a legitimate method within certain diagnostic borders'. Gradually, however, the resistance is easing up. When I was in Utrecht, we were the only department in Holland practising ECT. I contended: that is unacceptable – you prevent a treatment that has been shown to be effective for a substantial number of patients and for what reasons? You call it ethical reasons but you're talking about your private ethics, not the patient's interests. Nowadays ECT is permitted, but only in certain centres, with all kinds of protective measures. I am not against protective measures, but if you have a therapeutic method available only in a few centres, you can be sure that many patients will not be treated. Distance is a therapeutic handicap.

I can give you another example of unethical political influence in psychiatry. For years in Holland there was no MAO inhibitor available. Even though there was clear evidence that MAO inhibitors can be efficacious in major depression and in atypical depression. Many didn't 'believe' in them, but in fact not to have those drugs available was unethical.

Remarkable, isn't it?. And this is despite the fact that there are two large pharmaceutical companies within Holland. One would have thought that the industry could do something more to . . .

But the industry, in the 1970s, and 1980s, was very much in that same boat – it was considered devilish. The industries make money, make big money out of drugs and they were in the eyes of many, as much detestable as biological psychiatry was. They failed to have a counterbalancing effect.

Frankly, to be looked at with suspicion is not a prerogative of biological psychiatry. The notion that people have to be protected against psychiatry is by to means rare. Recently, in Holland a new law was passed, that makes it extremely hard, much harder even than ever before, to admit psychiatric patients. Again – whose interests are we serving this way – certainly not those of the patients. It is as if psychiatrists are dangerous: Pied Pipers of Hamelin, who tend to admit people against their will, and against their best interests. It took 10 years to prepare the law and now it's implemented. I think this is terrible; absolutely terrible that you cannot admit patients who are floridly psychotic but not genuinely dangerous. Is this ethics? This is anti-ethics, ethics upside down.

Let me hop for a second – you left Utrecht and went to the US but before I pick up on that I want to pick up on the fact that you came back from the US to Maastricht to unify the Department. Now why was unification necessary? It seems an extraordinary need.

Sure, but it had a direct relation to what we just discussed. Maastricht is Holland's youngest University. It is 20 years old and the department of psychiatry started from the beginning as a tripartite organization. That was still true when I came two years ago – there were three independent Departments of Psychiatry. One was called Social Psychiatry; the second Clinical Psychiatry, that's hospital psychiatry; the third Psychobiology and Neuropsychology. Independent Chairs, independent budgets. The university felt perhaps it would be a better idea to unify it.

I know it sounds a bit pathetic, but our profession is truly dear to my heart, so I thought unification was a very good cause. In addition, I have always liked management, apart from teaching and research. In New York, I performed a similar but much larger unification job. I had experienced how interesting this kind of scientific management can be and so I liked the idea. I had a secondary reason, which was to be near my children and grandchildren. Finally, after almost 11 years in New York, I was restless enough to say well let's climb one more mountain. A possible hidden motive was the wish to obscure the inevitable ageing process. I liked the idea of starting again and feeling younger than I really am.

You went from Utrecht to Einstein. Can I ask you how that came about – did you go partly because things were so hot in Utrecht?

I know that some people thought so, but no that was not the case. I liked my job in Utrecht. It included sometimes fierce fighting but it was for a good cause and, as I said, the Department and the Faculty and the Hospital were behind me, unconditionally. No, I was called, completely unexpectedly one day, by the Dean of the Albert Einstein College of Medicine, Ephraim Friedman. The chairman of the search committee was Dom Purpura, the brain researcher – later he became the Dean. They called me and also the late Nate Kline. I knew him very well. They asked me would I be interested in coming to Einstein as Chairman with two special commissions. First of all, to unify psychiatry at Einstein and Montefiori and their affiliated hospitals and secondly to boost research. The last Chairman had been Ed Sachar, and with his appointment, the Dean had tried to open the doors to research. For a long time the Einstein department had been highly psychoanalytic. Ed Sachar, however, left Einstein after less than two years to go to Columbia; an interim chair, Wagner Bridger, was appointed and subsequently they asked me. Well, I hadn't given it any thought. I had been many times to America but my wife was not so interested. The dean said come, look for yourself and let your wife join you and so we came. I found it, first of all, interesting from the management point of view, which at that time was not very much the responsibility of departmental chairmen in Holland. The American experience looked fascinating, to my wife as well. Also I felt a bit flattered at being invited to come to Einstein. So, after some negotiations, I went.

What kind of situation did you find there. Was it still analytically controlled?

In many ways, yes; though Einstein more so than Montefiore. I had to unify those departments and I must say I was happy that the former Chairs, the acting Chair in Einstein and the regular Chair at Montefiori, had already left. It would have been very difficult to work together. There was nothing about the unification in writing. In the more or less typical, classical American way, they said: 'van Praag you have accepted, we are very interested in the outcome, but you do it any way you want'. That's still one of the most inspiring aspects of the American society. Confidence in and high regard for initiative and improvisation. Just do it; you know, you're not governed by 3000 or so rules like in Holland – do it.

So there were two Academic Psychiatric Departments each with their own affiliated hospitals. I tried to achieve a number of things. First of all the unification. What they had in mind was academic unification – combining the research, training and teaching. But I felt that it was a unique chance to bring about a clinical commonwealth as well. The two institutions and their affiliated hospitals together covered a large segment, 80%, of mental health delivery in the Bronx, a borough of 1.3 million people, so I felt that the Department could become a true comprehensive network of facilities.

The Dean once said to me, 'van Praag you work so hard also in the clinical domain, but it's not necessary'. I replied: 'But I like it, it's an interesting experiment to have an Academic Department so much involved in management of day-to-day clinical activity; having the chance to demonstrate that we are not living in ivory towers but down to earth; contributing to better organization and innovation in mental health delivery'. So that was one task – unification, academically and clinically. I promoted research. I recruited a considerable number of research-orientated people, not only in biology. For instance: when I arrived the payroll mentioned one half-time behaviour therapist. We were responsible for more than one million people, among whom were many chronic patients, and there was one half-time behaviourist! That I felt to be absolutely unacceptable.

I've tried to implement what I have always preached: a harmonious development of psychiatry, with balanced attention for biological, psychological and social determinants of abnormal behaviour and for the corresponding treatment methods. Yes, I do believe in psychological interventions. There is little proof for the efficiency of psychodynamic psychotherapy but for cognitive and behavioural approaches there is. It would a priori be silly to doubt that you can change behaviour by learning; normal behaviour changes – why then not abnormal behaviour? Psychodynamic psychotherapy, I'm willing to give the benefit of the doubt. It is hard to believe that one can understand present behaviour without taking the past into account. If that is so, the assumption that one can lighten the present, by clarifying the past, seems reasonable. So, I tried to build up a multidimensional, research-orientated department. I also established a stronghold in the biological sciences; there existed one basic lab when I came and there were five when I left. Certainly there were still many things to be desired, but the basic model of an academic psychiatric department had been built up, at least the model I prefer.

I regret the tendency to make psychiatry monodimensional, whatever that dimension might be: psychoanalytic, social or biological. You know, the idea that schizophrenia is a brain disease, that is a terrible simplification, originating in the 19th century, but presently revitalized. Of course, it is a brain disease, but it is much more than that. There are many more variables involved. The brain dysfunctions do not drop from the skies. They are a product of a host of noxious variables that can be psychological, relational and environmental in nature. This applies to the entire field of abnormal behaviour; to deny that would be unscientific, even if presently 'politically correct'. Tunnel vision is not to the benefit of our patients and not to the benefit of our profession as a science.

So I have been viewed in Holland as a *pur sang* biological psychiatrist, but in fact, I am and have always been a generalist. My first inaugural lecture (1968) was entitled 'The Complementary Relation between Biological and Psychodynamic Psychiatry'. Its broad basis is what determines the charm, the importance, of the profession. It is a three-dimensional structure and our professional identity is in keeping. We are no more than amateur psychologists, amateur sociologists, amateur neurobiologists but we are not amateurs when it comes to bridging these divides. Synthesizers, that's what we are and should remain.

Let me switch to a few of your ideas about what we've learnt from the use of drugs and research on drugs. From the start you've been associated with two ideas – the 5-HT hypothesis and a dimensional approach towards things. You can pick up either of these. Alec Coppen says that the 5-HT idea was a North Sea idea between yourself, himself and Ashcroft up in Aberdeen.

Yes, I could agree with that. But I have been more than that; I have been a monoamine man. I have worked in Groningen with Jacob Korf in monoamines, not only with serotonin. Serotonin was neglected in America, where gradually it was only catecholamines that counted. But Korf and I, we always have tried to study, for instance in the CSF, both serotonin, noradrenaline and dopamine metabolism. I have worked together with neurologists in Parkinson's disease as well as with psychiatrists in depression to investigate what monoamines steer. Serotonin was only one of the variables we were interested in. In the USA, for many years it was all catecholamines; so the few people that remained true to serotonin, became the 'serotonin-people'. Yes, we were, but we had more irons in the fire.

Now the dimensional ideas. From the beginning I had difficulties with nosology. One of my teachers, Rümke, was a convinced nosologist but I didn't see the light. I saw so many patients of which I felt 'yes, they are depressed; yes, they are psychotic, but to claim that they fulfil strict criteria for any particular diagnosis, no'. In depression you see so many anxious people; people with panic disorder, with obsessions and so I . . .

But you introduced the notion of vital depression in the 1960s. You were one of the people associated with trying to pick out a form of depression that might respond to drug treatment.

Yes indeed, very early on, in the late 1950s, we tried to operationalize the various forms of depression: vital depression, personal depression and mixed forms. Those are, however, strictly syndromal concepts without any further nosological connotations. If you want to study, for instance, vital depression, we reasoned, you have to define the concept. You have to describe in detail what you're dealing with. The term endogenous I didn't like because it was so much linked to absence of precipitating events and to heredity. We reasoned we need terms that, etiologically, are totally neutral, that are purely symptomatological and descriptive, without any connotation as to severity, duration, or causation. Moreover, we developed, and we were the first to do so, a structured, standardized interview for the diagnosis of vital depression. Okay, of course, nothing as elaborate as the present day's standardized interviews, but it was the first of its kind. The Hamilton had just been published. But the Hamilton is . . .

Just a checklist . . .

A checklist, yes, and we wanted to study and compare the various syndromal depression types. What are antidepressants doing in which syndromal type of depression; are monoamine systems disturbed in certain syndromal types of depression? So it was necessary to operationalize types of depression and to develop an instrument to assess those. All that, by the way, was, of course, anathema to the at that time ruling class of psychoanalytic psychiatrists. Operationalization of diagnoses and standardization of interviews was robotic; it was, as one said to me, destroying the very fabric of psychiatry. This approach was hardly acceptable in the 1950s and 1960s.

We focused our studies on a well-defined and assessable syndrome, that is, the syndrome of vital depression, so that it would be as clear as possible what we were talking about. We studied 'pure' cases, but at the same time it was clear that relatively few patients were 'pure', that many showed also features of other syndromes. So in order to be able to give a precise diagnostic evaluation of a certain patient, a strategy additional to precise syndrome definition had to be pursued, one I have designated as 'functional psychopathology'.

We reasoned as follows. The basic units of disease in psychiatry are the psychological dysfunctions, such as deviations in mood-, anxiety- and aggression-regulation; motoricity; level of initiative; perception; cognition; memory; concentration, and many others. Hence, to obtain a clear picture of what in a given patient is dysfunctioning and what is still normally functioning, one has to dissect the psychopathological syndrome(s) into its component parts, that is, the psychological dysfunctions. They should be assessed and measured, and if no adequate psychometric instruments are available, those should be developed. In this way a, what you might call 'psychiatric physiology' will be developed, elevating psychopathology to a truly scientific level. Diagnosing in psychiatry, I maintained, is a three-tier process: the disorder should be established, the syndrome characterized and finally the functional composition of the syndrome(s) determined.

I consider myself as a nosological sceptic. The third diagnostic tier is closest to my heart. I realize, however, that we need a common, simple language to communicate. The disease-based-system meets these terms, though it is a primitive and imprecise language. I do not want to do away with categories, I want to have the system functionally complemented. For my teacher, Rümke, convinced nosologist as he was, those ideas were anathema, but he was a great man and tolerated dissident residents.

In the review you wrote of my book *Make Believes in Psychiatry* (Van Praag, 1993), you mentioned that it seems I have prophesized several developments in psychiatry already in the 1950s and 1960s. The remark was ironically meant, I think, but in all modesty, it can be said that many ideas I have professed during my academic life, occurred to me at an early stage in my career. It sounds pedantic, but I cannot help it.

How much does the dimensional approach that you've taken, where you've been interested in concepts like irritability, how much does that link or otherwise to Fritz Freyhan's ideas of target symptoms?

Not the same. People always raise this issue. One example, I don't study acoustic hallucinations. Marius Romme in my Department in Maastricht has done interesting studies with people who hear voices but who are not psychotic. What I'm interested in is not in hearing voices as such but in the underlying psychological, i.e. perceptual disturbances. That is what functional psychopathology is all about. It is not the symptom as it is being characterized by the doctor or formulated by the patient but the underlying neuropsychological disturbances that are being studied and related to neurobiology. Symptoms are not what I have in mind. It's really a psychiatric physiology I hope to establish. The term dimensional, in fact, is not adequate. I don't follow so much a dimensional approach, but rather a functional approach.

Well, now could I ask you how that links then to the work of Eysenck during the late 1950s and early 1960s because he had this idea that people fall on different points of a set of physiological dimensions and that people could be picked out by drug challenge tests. Arguably it would be awfully useful if we were to do that nowadays, because so as far as I know the work is still valid.

No doubt. I am not a connoisseur of Eysenck's work, but what I am unhappy with is the small number of dimensions he uses – for example, introversion – extraversion. Dichotomies make me uneasy. It's too simple to divide people into two groups even if you link them dimensionally. Eysenck is a dimensionalist but his system is too meagre. Defining personality or psychopathology on too few dimensions means an unacceptable simplification of mental pathology. This doesn't detract from the fact that Eysenck's system is still a useful starting point.

One of the problems though for the Eysenck work appeared to be that the models worked beautifully while we only had stimulants and sedatives, but once we began to get the tricyclic antidepressants which were neither stimulant nor sedative they didn't fit into the framework.

But what is the framework? Again, it is too much a reductionistic hat rack. In the psychological apparatus, there is an innumerable number of functional abilities and the dimensions, or better still the dysfunctions, to be distinguished, should reflect the complexity of the psyche. The human mind is much too rich for simple dichotomies such as: extraversion/introversion, or type A/type B personalities. Once more, functional psychopathology I define as the product of systematic dissection of psychopathological syndromes in their component parts, that is, the psychological dysfunctions, and of a personality structure in the component personality traits and subsequent measurement of dysfunctions and traits in a, hopefully, sophisticated way. Each psychological (dys-) function and each personality trait can be taken as a dimension that reaches from zero to maximally present.

If we, eventually, hope to understand brain and behaviour relationships, the functional approach is, I think, the way to go. I find it hard to believe that one day we will have unravelled the biology of, for instance, type A-behaviour or of the concept of extraversion or find specific drugs to influence them. They are too broad. I find it much more likely that one day that will be the case for behavioural components like increased aggressiveness, impulsivity, lability of mood, to give only a few examples.

You have introduced in your book, the idea of a stem and branch − that it's maybe worth chasing 5-HT the whole way through a range of behaviours. Do you want to comment on that?

Yes and no. Chasing 5-HT through a range of behaviours, but searching for relations between 5-HT and components of those behaviours. The same is useful for noradrenaline and dopamine. In fact in a paper in 1975 we reported that the dopamine disturbance found in Parkinson's disease, that is, lowering of CSF HVA, is not restricted to that disease, but is also found in retarded depression and in inert psychotics. Apparently, we postulated, it relates to lack of initiative rather than to a particular diagnosis. Serotonin disturbances in the brain, we have hypothesized, are related to instability of aggression and anxiety regulation, and noradrenergic dysfunctions to hedonic disturbances. Biological dysfunctions in psychiatric disorders seem, thus, to correlate with psychological dysfunctions across diagnoses, rather than to categorical constructs.

Another example demonstrated by Renee Kahn and myself is that the augmented cortisol response to MCPP found in panic disorder turned out to be very strongly correlated with pre-test anxiety, rather than with panic disorder. Apparently it is not specific for panic disorder, it is rather related to anxiety, irrespective of diagnosis. I think there are many more examples to support this idea that brain dysfunctions correlate better with disturbed psychological domains than with the present day's categorical diagnostic constructs.

Let me chase this a bit further − what you seem to be saying is that there's a close link between brain function and personality. If so what do you make of the public health experiment going on at the moment with so many Americans taking fluoxetine?

The medical profession is never helped by perceived miracle drugs. Miracle drugs are myths. On the other hand, the fluoxetine uproar is probably telling us something. Fluoxetine, and I think it holds for SSRIs in general, are not merely axis-I drugs, active in depression, in OCD, in panic disorder, but in addition they seem to influence personality traits, personality dysfunctions, like impulsivity, irritability and lability of mood. The SSRIs might be the first generation of drugs that, indeed, affect personality traits.

I have seen several patients in whom that seems to have happened. The spouse said, 'with fluoxetine my partner became a different person'. Why? Before, in the morning he or she was explosive; an unpleasant, irritable person, I had always to be very careful not to get into conflict and now he/she is very different, much more tolerant, much more mellow. The reason for that is, I think, not a miracle, but the fact that personality traits are being influenced. I hope and I think that the more specific we will be in impacting on particular neuronal systems, the better the prospect of developing drugs that will benefit certain personality disorders. There is a genetics of personality traits, there is a biology of personality traits, there will be a psychopharmacology of personality disorders/dysfunctions in the future.

One could even argue that we're likely to get to the genes of personality traits and the biology of personality traits quicker than we were getting to the genes or biology of schizophrenia.

Maybe. Personality biology would not be without danger. Who wants to have his personality 'mechanically' changed? Personality pharmacology should be handled with great care and caution. Beware of cosmetic personality psychopharmacology. On the other hand, there are personality traits that are harmful for an individual as well as for his surroundings. If well-controlled, there is room for pharmacological personality reconstruction. The emerging opportunities to interfere in personality structure, I think, could be an explanation for the remarkable upheaval fluoxetine has caused in the media.

There is a history here actually. I went back and read some of Kuhn's early case histories and he describes exactly the same kind of phenomena that are described in the book Listening to Prozac *− of people who are sexual perverts, getting an antidepressant and their sexual perversion going away. This history has been lost. Do we just go around the circle sometimes?*

Well, I didn't know that observation of Kuhn, but we have been focusing for so long mainly on axis-I diagnoses and failed to systematically study the effect of psychotropic drugs in pure personality disorders or in co-morbid personality disorder. Maybe there are more drugs than fluoxetine that have an impact on personality traits. Also, you have to take into account that the authorities prevent this kind of research – the drug is marketed for depression or anxiety or some other diagnosis and to use it in another diagnostic category is generally not permitted.

With DSM-III, the psychiatric profession in the US went biological. With this book Listening to Prozac *it's as though at street level they are going biological.*

You are right. I regret this monomania. Let me make you a compliment. It seems different in the UK. British psychiatry, over the years, has been much more eclectic, more level-headed, less theory-driven. In the States official psychiatry is presently biological. You don't get any important Chair without being a researcher, with a biological track record. Biology and drugs are now considered to be the major pillars of psychiatry, the successors of psychoanalysis; too much, I think, in that other realms are being neglected. Cavalier-like people say 'oh, psychotherapy, that is for social workers and psychologists'. I think that attitude is destructive for the profession. Psychotherapy and the underlying theories are an integral part of psychiatry. Training in psychiatry should include biological and psychological theories; mastering of at least two forms of psychotherapy, as well as being an expert in the use of psychotropic drugs. Biology is domineering American psychiatry; not at the grassroots though. If you interview new residents you note that most of them want to be trained in the psychotherapies. But for 'official psychiatry' it's biological research that truly counts. And so a drug like fluoxetine gets enormous attention. Partly for good reasons. Partly it is pure sensationalism: the drug shouldn't be all over the newspapers, on TV, etc. that's a kind of circus. Again, we have no miracle drugs – after such a period of elation, disappointment will follow, to the detriment of the profession.

All of these concepts like irritability and impulsivity and this way of thinking are in your book Make Believes in Psychiatry *which I think is one of the few serious books in this area that could reach out to the public. But you said to me on the way here that you were surprised that there it has caused so little fuss.*

Well, I had guessed that quite a number of people would strongly and publicly disagree with my views on diagnosis and diagnosing; also with the chapter on 'Make Believes' – discussing the, what I have called in another context, 'nosologomania', embracing as we do all kinds of new disease entities of dubious validity, such as multiple personality disorder, chronic fatigue syndrome and winter depression. I do not, of course, deny that depressions may occur preferentially in the winter. I do not deny that some people are very fatigued and I do not deny that certain people may have dramatic changes in personality, but I very much question on the basis of the prevailing data that these are discrete entities – diseases that you can study as such, that you can develop specific treatments for, that you can scrutinize for their epidemiology, biology and so on.

I regret that the book has not generated more discussion. One might disagree with my critique, but I flatter myself with the idea that my arguments are relevant and that the points I have raised are of considerable importance for the further development of psychiatric research, particularly for biological research.

One of the reasons that there may not have been much correspondence to date is that there's widespread support for these views in the profession.

That is a very positive view. But it is also possible that people strongly disagree but find it not so easy to object to my points of view and then it is easier to be silent. Because if the majority is working as they do . . .

If the Zeitgeist *is going the way you want . . . then why object?*

That's right. So far the *Zeitgeist* is not in favour of what I am trying to say. So the majority just ignores it. I hope that you are right and that the majority thinks that my ideas are not so bad, but I wonder whether it's right. So far my ideas about functional psychopathology, functional psychopharmacology, verticalization of psychiatric diagnosing, my view that the DSM provides diagnostic guidelines unsuitable to guide bological research; my rejection of the 'nosologomania', i.e. the unfettered numerical increase of psychiatric 'disorders', have received little support and, again, too little attention.

You know, at the APA some years ago I organized a symposium on the DSM classification system and its validity or invalidity for biological research. It was a good symposium but there were few key figures from the DSM establishment present and the turnout was only 50–60 people. That struck me. In my opening speech I raised the issue – how on earth could the turnout be so low. These questions touch the very roots of our research efforts. If you have no diagnostic system that is reliable and valid you can forget the whole thing. I mean, in that case you can only pretend to conduct science, but you can hardly expect that your research will yield anything useful and reproducible.

Clinically, for daily practice, a highly inaccurate diagnostic system is perhaps still acceptable, because our treatments are so far not very specific, but for research it is fatal. If the psychopathological phenomena one studies are not defined in detail, and diagnosed in valid constructs, there is no basis for research. So not to be there to discuss those issues, I thought, was regrettable.

It was an expression of a state of affairs in the States, in which the DSM, as a system, as a diagnostic philosophy, is the new holy cow. It is the successor of psychoanalysis. You cannot and should not question its fundamentals. You can discuss for hours whether the duration of disorder A should be four months, or five months, or six months, or whether you should add a symptom or subtract another in a given definition, but the very roots of the system, the premisses on which it is based, are not open for discussion anymore. That attitude is extremely detrimental for the profession and for psychiatric research in particular.

It is fair to say, that so far in spite of 35 years, 40 years of intensive biological research, there is no single biological variable with any diagnostic significance. That might tell us something about the diagnostic approach we have taken − it should lead to reflection. How on earth could it be that nothing of diagnostic significance has been forthcoming. Okay it could be the crudeness of the biology that is to blame, but another possibility is that the diagnostic system is inept − and that option should be taken seriously.

The change of culture from Europe to the US must have been awfully interesting because concepts like irritability and impulsivity are European concepts, indeed continental European concepts, that aren't found in the American or English literature. You also moved over with a background in Kraepelin and interest in psychopathology to a country that then had little interest in either nosology or psychopathology.

Well, it was just when I came that DSM-III was introduced. There was a lot of protest against the new DSM concept but it was already introduced as an official APA document. But you see, there is an interesting American quality that is flexibility, ability to quickly change direction. It was fascinating to see how a continent that for years had been under the spell of non-nosological ideas − no diagnosis at all − the psychodynamic points of view, rather dramatically and quickly changed to a quite conservative neo-nosological approach. It was amazing to observe that a society could change so easily. From 'no diagnosis at all', a DSM diagnosis based on structured interviewing, was now considered to be mandatory, at least in the research community. America became more Kraepelinean than Kraepelin was, so to say.

The dimensional approach − again, I rather call it the functional approach − has not been accepted. Psychiatric diseases are what we study. One has to explore the antecedents, the epidemiology, the biology and what not of discrete and separable diseases. Diagnoses are being made by counting symptoms, preferably those that are easily observable, and those that are easily agreed upon by direct questioning of the patient. In the process of nosologization of psychiatry, the need arose to objectify psychopathology to put a value only on that part of the spectrum of psychopathology that is clearly observable or that is clearly indicated by the patient − 'yes I'm depressed, yes I'm very anxious' − rather than on experiential phenomena. Some years ago, in the *British Journal of Psychiatry*, I discussed the importance of reconquering that subjective domain by experimental psychiatry.

So apart from the non-acceptance of the functional approach, the tendency to neglect the subjective elements of psychopathology is a second reason I have to complain about impoverishment of diagnosing in psychiatry.

But there had to be a DSM-III, didn't there?

Oh, yes. The first step was right. Even if it's based purely, or mainly, on expert opinion there had to be a standardized, operationalized classification system. But we should have left it at that: at the DSM-III; until all the proposed concepts had been thoroughly studied and validated or invalidated. There should have been no DSM-IIIR nor a DSM-IV, unless based on solid data. What does, for instance, a concept like 'dysthymia' mean. Is it valid? Is it distinguishable from major depression, from certain personality disorders, from generalized anxiety disorder, from adjustment disorder? Such validating research would have taken much time, much effort, much money, but it would have been the way to real progress. If I would have been the director of the NIMH, I said one day to Fred Goodwin, I would have invested most of the research monies in that type of study, not in biology. Again, without a detailed map of psychopathology, psychiatric research, particularly biological research, is easily led astray.

So when I came to the USA I experienced a change from a dislike of diagnosing, from a highly individualized way of describing and interpreting psychopathology, to a rigid nosological approach. The new psychiatry, however, is seemingly precise, but in fact we have introduced broad, heterogeneous diagnostic concepts, insufficiently validated and too much stripped of subjective paraphernalia.

You've said there is something of a nosological mania now.

Indeed, it is absurd. There has been an exponential increase in the number of diseases from DSM-II, to DSM-III, over DSM-IIIR to DSM-IV; the number tripled. What a nonsensical state of affairs. And then to think that you can study all of these entities, rather pseudoentities, as discrete diseases, as if they were things in their own right, each of them having their own aetiology, pathogenesis, course and treatment. You know it's the clothes of the emperor again, a world of make believes.

We're almost back to the situation with Esquirol describing all the monomanias in the 1840s.

Yes, mainly on the basis of a few symptoms one decides on the existence of and pushes for the recognition of a novel disease, a disease with its own particular course, biology, outcome and treatment. A research programme is initiated, grant proposals are being submitted, patients recognizing the symptoms organize into lobbies. Soon the fata morgana looks like an edifice. I ironize a bit, but the essence seems to me true. So, after so many years of research I am to an extent disappointed. There are beautiful new methodologies; approaches; new psychotropic drugs;

interesting biological data, such as the imbalance of the CRH/ACTH/ cortisol axis in several patient categories, but their diagnostic value – if your diagnostic orientation is nosological – is little.

From the functional point of view, however, things look different. There is increasing evidence that biological dysfunctions correlate much better with psychological dysfunctions than with either syndromes or the nosological entities we distinguish.

On that point there seems to me that there's a major split opening up in a lot of the organizations at the moment, like the BAP and ACNP and possibly even CINP, where there's an explosion of knowledge within the neurosciences so that we've got 5-HT-14 and D-35 receptors, but who knows what the clinical relevance of any of these things is. How do we hold the field together?

That is certainly something I see with trepidation. How many receptors can one study in humans – if you want to study the balance between serotonin receptors and their relation to dopamine and noradrenaline receptors, there are so far maybe 35 in total – that's almost undoable. That certainly is an embarrassing idea. Two points here: first, nobody has demonstrated yet that all these receptors are functionally active or that they are sufficiently different functionally to deserve a separate categorization. It could be that for the transmitter X the receptor A and B and C functionally form one cluster and D and E another cluster, so that you could reduce the number of receptors to be scrutinized. If that's not the case and that is the second point, the only way out is to shift our attention to post-receptor events. Those seem to be less heterogeneous.

Are you saying these get more molar again, almost more physiological again.

No, I mean to say that we have to broaden our horizon. For years now we have been focusing on transmission per se and on receptor function. The latter field becomes more complicated every year, at least from the point of view of clinical research. The avalanche of new receptors is overwhelming. Perhaps we should broaden our efforts to include postreceptor events, trying to study second and third messenger systems. Here the number of possibilities seems to be more limited.

In biology things will become ever more refined and detailed. That is not the case in psychopathology. Clinically we are still working with very crude and imprecise diagnostic concepts, and the terrible thing is, we do not seem to realize that. The DSM system is regarded as a kind of endpoint, not as a primitive beginning. Discussions on how to refine psychiatric diagnosing are hardly ever heard. The gap between the degree of sophistiction in biological and psychopathological analysis is widening rapidly. That is devastating for biological psychiatry. The irreproducibility of almost all genetic findings in psychiatry, for instance, is probable the consequence of diagnostic inaccuracy. We need new diagnostic concep-tualizations, to even try to follow the biological express train and to translate the fruits of the neurosciences into new methodologies that are diagnostically and therapeutically meaningful. In my book *Make Believes in Psychiatry* I have tried to generate an impulse to that end.

Earlier you hinted at the role of the pharmaceutical companies in playing down the personality issue. What role has the pharmaceutical industry – both in terms of wanting to produce drugs for a category that will give them a sufficient return on their investment and the insurance industry wanting to pay for treatments for which there are outcomes – how much have they, between them, brought about the current dominance of categorical points of view?

There is a strong reinforcement here. For insurance companies, for lawyers, for court authorities and the like categorical constructs, 'diseases', are easy to handle. One has a disease, that's it. The client is a schizophrenic, a depressive. But if you would say: 'listen, there exists a 'basin' that is called affective disorders, it's not a diagnosis, it's just a global indication (comparable to the pronouncement: the person suffers from an abdominal disorder) and actually, this particular patient belongs in this category, but again, it is not a diagnosis; he has however a psychopathological profile that we can describe in detail and measure, though we cannot give it a specific name yet': that's much too difficult for insurance companies, for lawyers, even for doctors. So the DSM lobby is strongly supported by practising psychiatrists, by insurance companies, by lawyers, who all find it a neat, easy and practical system to structure their practices on and to ground the payment system.

   Dimensional, or better: functional diagnosing is complicated and does not lead to easily transferable disease concepts, but it gives a much better picture of the clinical reality of a given patient.

You've reintroduced into the argument recently, ideas not heard since Adolf Meyer – the idea of reaction formations. Tell me about his role in your thinking.

The reaction formation I always felt is an extremely interesting and valuable concept. The idea that there are a finite number of psychological domains that can be disturbed by biological or psychological or social stressors but not in a preconfigured way. The phenomenology of the response in a given patient is very much dependent upon such things as the hardware of the brain, its present condition, on environmental circumstances, on personality structure and so what ultimately transpires in terms of behavioural and experiential changes varies very much from individual to individual and within an individual.

   The basic idea of reaction forms to me is that there is a noxious stimulus, biological or psychological in nature, perturbing certain brain systems, but to a different degree; dependent on such factors as I mentioned a moment ago. Consequently, a number of domains, psychological and physiological domains, are disturbed though to a degree that varies individually. Thus the composition of the ultimate syndrome cannot be other than very variable. The reaction form idea explains much better than the nosological premise, why so few patients fit the definition of a particular disorder, why there is so much so-called co-morbidity in psychiatry.

If I have to bet, if you ask me do you believe in nosological entities, the answer is no. Deep in my heart I think the disease concept in psychiatry is probably a fiction. The existence of a limited number of reaction forms seems to me more likely; for instance, the basin of the affective disorders, the basin of the psychotic disorders, the basin of the dementing disorders and a few others. The expression of these disorders in individual patients however is as variable as the shape of clouds in the sky. One recognizes the cloud, but its configuration varies unpredictably. Attempts to uncover the cause of a particular reaction form, of a particular diagnostic 'basin', would be idle. To understand its biology one has to study the biological underpinnings of the psychological dysfunctions that make up that particular reaction form.

That is my belief system; but of course I keep wide open the possibility that I am wrong and that one day we will indeed discover the cause, the biology of, say, schizophrenia or some other categorical, diagnostic construct. But frankly, in that case I would be a very surprised man.

Let me try to phrase this viewpoint in another way. Take an entity like schizophrenia, considered to be a discrete disorder. In fact, it is as heterogeneous a concept as one can think of. It is a group of disorders characterized by a great number of psychopathological phenomena – e.g. delusions, hallucinations, cognitive disturbances, etc., etc.– and the individual psychopathology varies widely. The degree of delusion, the degree of hallucination, the degree of inertia, the degree of cognitive disturbance is variable from patient to patient. The prognosis of schizophrenia is very uncertain. Some improve, some recover, some do not. The treatment response is also very variable. This state of affairs allows for no more than one statement, that is, that the group of schizophrenic disorders is a diagnostic basin with a wide variety of expression forms, some correlated with discernible brain dysfunction, others not and with very different outcome and prognosis.

Within that diagnostic basin of schizophrenia I could imagine the existence of a particular subform, which could be called a nosological entity because it is very tightly coupled to a very circumscribed brain dysfunction. This is possible. But in general, the reaction form idea appeals to me because it is of great heuristic value and my bet is that the view of psychiatry as a compilation of independent diseases will eventually turn out to be untenable.

But apart from who is right and who is wrong, I want to emphasize again how extraordinary insightful the functional approach to psychopathology will be. What does it mean to say 'he suffers from major depression'? It tells you little about symptom picture, about prognosis, about functional abilities, about treatment response, etc. If you could, on the other hand, provide an analysis of what psychological functions are disturbed in a given patient and to what degree, and which of them are still functioning within normal limits, the informative value of such a statement is much higher.

These data could and should guide psychological interventions and in the future, I hope, also psychopharmacology. You remember I have introduced and advocated the concept of functional psychopharmacology. It holds that psychopharmacology will move away from a nosological, towards a functional orientation, in which drugs will be prescribed not to treat the presumed 'disease' ,but the basic, the primary psychological dysfunctions underlying a given disorder; much like the cardiologists are doing. They do not treat myocardial infarction as such. They treat the resulting cardiac dysfunctions and that with a variety of drugs. That is goal-directed, dysfunction-orientated polypharmacy; that is the direction I see also psychopharmacology develop. But, no doubt the denosologis-ation of psychiatry will be difficult because psychiatrists cling to the disease concept.

What the profession really want is a few tumours, isn't it?

Actually the tumour metaphor makes a certain, though limited, sense. A tumour is not a discrete disease. It also is a 'basin' of a variety of disorders with a few common clinical characteristics, such as the dysfunctional multiplication of cells. For the rest, they differ in degree of malignancy, growth rate, prognosis, treatment response, pathogenesis, possibly etiology etc. So, indeed, a concept like tumour and a concept like schizophrenia share the qualities of being a 'diagnostic basin'. One can carry the analogy even one step further.

Apart from surgical interventions, tumours are nowadays treated with a variety of compounds slowing down cell division; those are in a way comparable to the present neuroleptic treatment of schizophrenia. The search however is for treatments geared towards elimination of the various catalysts of morbid cell growth. A comparable goal we pursue in schizo-phrenia research: to find and treat the neuronal processes underlying the key disturbances of a schizophrenic syndrome. I presume that those pro-cesses will not be the same in every schizophrenic patient, but that there will turn out to exist a variety of schizophenias, much the same as we probably deal with a variety of tumours.

Currently UK psychiatrists are caught on a hook. The government have set up targets for health gain and for psychiatry the target is to reduce the suicide rate from something like 15 per 10 000 to 10 per 10 000 by the year 2000, which seems impossible to many. You are one of the people who is most associated with suicide research and with the idea that it might be possible to predict the people who are likely to kill themselves. Do you want to tell me how you got into all that and how it evolved and where, if anywhere, you think it's gone.

How we got into this was as follows: from the beginning I had two research targets: schizophrenia and depression and from depression research we moved into anxiety research, simply because mood and anxiety disturbances are so highly intertwined. It was via depression research that we began to see the advantages of functional psychopathology or dimensional analysis for biological psychiatric research. We discovered that low CSF 5-HIAA in depression seems to be related to the anxiety component of depression. Serotonin disturbances occurred in other diagnoses with increased anxiety as well. In the 1970s, at a conference, we mentioned that. Then, the reply was: in that case the finding is just non-specific. That is a misconception, I answered. It is non- specific syndromally and nosologically, but specific on a functional level, coupled as it is to the state of heightened anxiety.

A second derivative of our depression research was a growing interest in the biology of suicide and later also of aggression, simply because both are common in depression and highly intercorrelated. We knew, at that time, of course a lot of social and psychological predictors of suicide but nothing on biological predictors, i.e. on brain dysfunctions increasing the risk of suicide in a situation of unbearable misery. It was a novel research line in the 1970s and it provoked an enormous resistance among antipsychiatrists. Suicide, they said, had absolutely nothing to do with biology, but everything with social conditions and perhaps a little bit with psychological make up. Anyhow, we initiated research into the biology of suicide, but Asberg *et al.* in Stockholm were ahead of us. They found, as you know, a correlation between low CSF 5-HIAA and suicidal behaviour. Later this correlation was also found in non-depressed suicide attempters.

I should like to add that the story of low 5-HIAA and suicide in a way is a shame for psychiatry. The relation between low CSF 5-HIAA and suicide was first published in 1976. You would have expected soon afterwards an avalanche of papers trying to confirm or refute this finding; even more so because Asberg *et al.* had found that the variable CSF 5-HIAA contains predictive information. Low values of that serotonin metabolite seemed to increase the risk of suicide in the year after the index admission. Nothing of the kind happened. Only one repeat study, concerning the predictive value of CSF 5-HIAA concentration for suicide has so far been published. If an internist had published a finding predictive of, for instance, tumor growth, many papers would have followed soon afterwards. In psychiatry: silence was characteristic. That is a clear sign how non-research orientated, how non-biological the profession still is. Psychiatrists do not seem to believe that biological findings might have practical significance. If the Asberg findings had been confirmed on a larger scale, measuring CSF 5-HIAA should be routine in the diagnosis of multiple suicide attempts. Done skilfully, the lumbar puncture is a minor intervention, well worth the potential information it could provide. Search for less invasive methods with the same informative value would of course be indicated.

Who were the key people who influenced you?

I have to answer you in an apparent haughty way. I have had no real guides, no tutors, at least not in biological psychiatry. When you are at the beginning of a new development, there are few people who can influence you. You have to create a domain for yourself, your own image, your own career, your own philosophy, your own methodology. That's not to say that there are no figures in the field that I do not greatly admire. For instance, in the States, a man like Kety. He's a most personable man, a man of great intellectual power and great scientific standing. He was crucial for the development and the acceptance of biological psychiatry in the medical field, because of his knowledge, because of his diplomacy, because of his eloquence and his ability to phrase things in the right way.

People like Biff Bunney, Fred Goodwin and Bernie Carroll were brothers-in-arms in the early days of biological psychiatry, when it was still psychiatry's stepchild. And there were quite a few more. Some of them went to NIMH and made it into a very important institution that has influenced the profession very much.

There were more warriors, though initially not many. In England, for instance, I think that Alec Coppen was a man who from the beginning became a symbol of the importance of biology for psychiatry. In Germany, Hippius was one of them. In Switzerland Kielholz was fighting on behalf of psychopharmacology. He was prominent in WHO circles and increased the respect for psychotropic drugs within the medical profession. He was not so much a great researcher but a statesman, a man who could really translate the importance of psychotropic drugs to the politicians and to the general public. Rafaelson has been important; he died too young. In the States, there was of course my old friend Ed Sachar and he too died too early. Those early years of biological psychiatry were fascinating. A bunch of bright young men fighting for the incorporation of biology in psychiatry.

Ole Rafaelson was another impressive figure professionally and physically. He was very much involved, both in lithium research and bipolar depression. Copenhagen had an excellent metabolic ward and in addition he also had statemen like qualities and expressed them well at the WHO, where he and I established a Biological Psychiatry Programme in the early 1970s, in an attempt to get that field on the psychiatric map.

He seemed to have a feel for the need to bring on young people as well. Some of these high powered men don't always have that. They try to kick away the ladder. But he seemed to want to bring people on.

You're right. And so he was important not only as a researcher but also as a politician, in the best sense of the world. He was a charming man, also. Good looking, strong, a Viking-like appearance; in many ways he was a very visible creature. I should have mentioned also, apart from many others, Delay and Deniker. In the early days, they were heavy weights on the biological psychiatric scene; the proud discoverers of the neuroleptics, and they were acknowledged as such. Mogens Schou I forgot to mention; he almost single handedly 'made' lithium. His professional life was shaped around that little ion. But let me stop here and just mention that many figures of importance were not mentioned.

Can I take you to some more personal issues. You've been in a concentration camp.

Yes, for almost three years. That was a crucial experience in my life. An experience of how low mankind can sink; of the ultimate failure of humanity, both of the perpetrators and those that failed to interfere. On the other hand, for me as a person, it has had, paradoxically, positive effects. The camp experience has made me, I feel, stronger, more mature, more hardened and more armoured against the vicissitudes of life.

But I rather like to mention another momentous episode of my life, that you did not touch upon. That is my visiting professorship in Jerusalem, in 1976–1977. I went from Rotterdam to Groningen and from Groningen to Jerusalem, for one year. I had been invited to become Chairman of Psychiatry at the Hebrew University in Jerusalem. I seriously considered the offer. I worked there for a year as a visiting professor as a trial period. In the end I didn't accept; mainly because of the language. I felt so clumsy, not being able to speak, to understand and to read the language. I thought, how on earth can I function here as a psychiatrist. Besides, my wife and children had not joined me because my oldest son was sitting for his matriculation. Facing linguistic difficulties alone, make them look even more insuperable.

So I didn't accept. If you ask me, are you happy with that decision, the answer is: not quite. Would I have been happier in Jerusalem than I have been in the USA and in Holland? Perhaps. I have been a Zionist all my life. Jerusalem meant a lot to me and it still does. I didn't mention it but one of my motivations to go to New York was the notion of New York as 'little Jerusalem'. Einstein is part of Yeshiva University, being the only Jewish University outside Israel. So New York was partly a substitution for Jerusalem. Emotionally, being a Jew, I feel now, so many years later, it would have made more sense to stay in Israel.

As I said, I've been a Zionist all my life, but in 1948 when the State of Israel was established I said: now you cease being a Zionist – either you go to Israel or you don't. If you don't, you are a supporter of the State, but not a Zionist. A Zionist is someone who goes. I never went for all kinds of reasons. I was in the Concentration camps during the War and when I came back I first wanted to finish secondary school. After that I said I first want to finish my medical study. After that I said before I go I first want to be a psychiatrist. After that the offer from Groningen came to establish a Department of Biological Psychiatry and I decided I first want to do that job. So it never came to anything really, despite a lot of deliberations. Partly, it had to do with the language but partly I wavered for self-serving reasons. I realized that if you spent two or three years learning the language, you haven't got the time to do research. So that was also a point. Perhaps Israel would have been even more satisfying than New York, because the country means a great deal to me.

Let me ask you something. Earlier in the interview, I was teetering on the brink of asking you a question I've asked one or two people, which is why has psychopharmacology been Jewish? Not completely but if you look at the names – Kety, Axelrod, Snyder, Kline, 4 of the 10 Presidents of the BAP and a lot of other eminent people. Why is this? Can you tell me?

Well, it is not so easy to say. First of all, psychiatry has been a Jewish profession for many many years. Certainly psychoanalysis is. Also, it is not uncommon to find, relatively speaking, many Jews in new fields, both in the sciences and in the arts. Are we more ambitious than other people? Perhaps. Intellectual and later also artistic achievements were felt to be important in Jewish circles. Another factor could be that we have been a discriminated minority for so long. In that position, the urge to demonstrate that you are good, that you are not as bad as the discriminators think you are, that actually you are better than them, might develop, and among the Jews it apparently did. Besides, the description 'People of the Book' is no slogan. For centuries, studying biblical books and commentaries was part and parcel of Jewish life. Not only of the Rabbi's, but of the common people as well. Nothing was taken for granted. Discussion, dialectics, weighing words and concepts is ingrained in the Jewish mind. Two thousand years of exile has thus been a thorough school of intellectual discipline.

The dialectical intercourse, the constant challenging of each other's ideas; that is for me the magnificent essence of Judaism. Few dogmas are acknowledged. There exists no *catechismus*. Every statement is open for discussion. It is the power of argument that finally counts. In no other religion do you find this – if you read the Talmud one Rabbi claims this , but is immediately challenged by another Rabbi, the latter by a third and so on. That scrutinizing orientation could have been inducive of moving into new fields, towards new horizons. So I think there are a number of reasons that Jews are attracted to the yet unknown, to domains still to be discovered. Psychopharmacology and the area of brain and behaviour is just an example.

I think it is an interesting point that here we have an Irishman asking a Jew this question. Brendan Behan, an Irish playright said that all nations have a history but the Jews and the Irish have a psychosis. The interesting thing for me is that, whereas the Jewish response to this, at least in the psychiatric area has been to try to explore the frontiers, the Irish response has been the opposite. Until quite recently we more or less denied that we had a national mental health problem, even when we had more beds occupied per head of the population than any other nation on earth has ever occupied. It seems extraordinary. That two people can actually respond so completely differently.

The Jewish people are Jewish, the Irish people are Roman Catholics. Catholics have never promoted the study of the Bible, whereas the Jews, particularly after the destruction of the Temple, became more and more obsessional about studying the Bible and text *exegeses*. That has been an extremely powerful tool to sharpen intelligence and to encourage voyages of discovery; constantly asking questions about what God meant, and argue about the different interpretations. Catholics discouraged study of the Bible by the common people. Jews in the majority, have been literate for thousands of years. That was not the case with many other people. Jewish Rabbi's, encouraged critical analysis of data. Intellectual curiosity is probably the reason that Jews so much like to explore frontiers.

What about the camps. Do you want to mention them?

What should I mention. I was there for almost three years. That was one of the reasons for that chapter in *Make Believes in Psychiatry*, on the children of holocaust survivors. The way I read the literature, is that it is completely unproven that holocaust survivors failed in the upbringing of their children. Even for the holocaust survivors themselves, it is unproven that a large percentage decompensated afterwards; were mentally crippled. I think it is a shame that such ideas were ventilated. It is typically a psychoanalytic point of view that after such a trauma, such an existential nightmare, one can not be able to live a normal life and one should be unable to raise one's children properly. The facts do not speak, the theory prevails. The theory demands that many people should have been crippled, so never mind what the facts tell. There is, however, very little good evidence for lasting holocaust-induced mental pathology in the survivors as a group. Completely disregarded is the evidence that, thank God, a large percentage of the few survivors have done quite well and were very well able to raise their children in a decent and reasonable way.

I finished that chapter by saying that soon, no single survivor will be around anymore to say just that. I added that in spite of all the horror, the notion that for some the camps have been an ego-strengthening rather than weakening experience should be seriously considered. In my case, I have a strong feeling that it changed me profoundly, but not for the worse. This might sound paradoxical. You could suggest that I survived because I was strong. But I don't think so. I believe the camps have made me more defensible, increased my fighting spirit; it also augmented my contendness with what life has to offer; it instilled a measure of material modesty. The expectations I have of my fellow citizens are also low. Probably also a result of war experiences. I like people, but I do not expect much of them; that lowers the risk of disappointment.

So, if you ask me did the war influence the rest of your life negatively, my answer is: I don't think so. The stereotypes about concentration camp survivors I thoroughly regret. It reminds me of the terrible things psychiatry did to the mothers of schizophrenics and the mothers and fathers of autistic children – you know, blaming the parents for the misery of their children. The idea that the holocaust survivors were so bad for their children and reponsible for personality deformations in the second generation, is based on a similar theory-driven callousness.

Until the World War II, German and middle European psychiatry was the world force. After World War II, it was UK and US psychiatry. Is that because so many Jewish and other intellectuals migrated from Germany and middle Europe. This seems to me to be an obvious explanation although not everyone I ask agrees with me.

There was an enormous brain drain from Germany since 1933, in physics, in medicine including psychiatry and in the belles-lettres. Many of them were Jews, many non-Jews, but for obvious reasons the Jews were, relative to their total number, in the majority. Many went to the USA. I think Germany suffered greatly and until this very day has never regained its pre-war position – in the arts, in literature and in the sciences. I think the Americans would say: in the 1930s we were graced with manna from heaven: a cohort of immigrants from Europe who enriched the country enormously.

So things have changed since you went into psychiatry first?

It was indeed a totally different profession when I started in the 1950s. It has developed, notwithstanding all the criticisms one might have, into a scientific discipline. When I started there were hardly any drugs. There was one form of psychotherapy – psychoanalysis – often watered-down psychoanalysis. Indeed, I didn't mention it, but I witnessed a second revolution in psychiatry: the development of other, non-analytical psychotherapeutic strategies such as behaviour therapy and cognitive therapy and furthermore the de-individualization of psychotherapy; the inclusion of more than one individual – group, family or spouse – in the therapeutic process. When I was a resident, it was a crime of sorts, while treating a particular patient, to involve his or her spouse or children or any other important other. Not even for diagnostic reasons. That was considered to be psychotherapeutic malpractice. I could never understand the reason why. I thought, people are living together; why isolate them in treatment? Family and group therapy for me were a refreshing revelation.

So in terms of diagnosing mental disorders, of biological treatment, of brain and behaviour research, of psychological interventions, of epidemiology, of genetics, there has been so much going on in the profession in the past 35 years. I feel fortunate to have lived in that particular period and proud and grateful to have been an active participant. The combination of being a teacher/clinician/researcher, moreover, offers satisfying compensation in the times when one's research is not going so well. Diagnosing and treating patients, teaching students and supervising residents are creative activities in their own right. We, clinical researchers, really enjoy the best of every aspect of academic life. And finally, permit me the platitude, research is important. If your daughter, your spouse, your father becomes psychiatrically ill, you thank God that there have been researchers, that there is development, progress, that there are pills, treatments and even preventative measures nowadays.

That's a very upbeat note on which to end but given all you had to say about DSM-III, I can't resist citing the quote at the start of your book Make Believes in Psychiatry *from Barbara Tuchman's* March of Folly *to the effect that a folly is something that is perceived to be counter-productive in its own time and not merely by hindsight, that alternative feasible courses of action should have been available and that the policy should be that of a group rather than just of an individual.*

Select bibliography
Van Praag, H.M. (1993) 'Make-Believes' in Psychiatry or The Perils of Progress. Brunner-Mazel, New York.

16 Merton Sandler

The place of chemical pathology in psychopharmacology

Why did you go into psychopharmacology?

I didn't even realize I was a psychopharmacologist until many years after I had become one. It's strange but true. I started among the monoamines long, long ago and by chance. The chance was that David Hay, now Sir David, Alan Goble and I were on the house together at the Brompton in 1954. I was doing a short-term research job after a house job there, mostly involving paper chromatography. David and Alan moved to the National Heart Hospital and there saw one of the first cases of carcinoid to be diagnosed in the British Isles; they phoned me at the Brompton and said they needed a bit of biochemical assistance.

So we set about investigating this poor lady, almost draining her of blood. We tried all sorts of bizarre things like doing platelet stickiness tests, borrowing a special machine from Helen Payling-Wright (who died only recently). Principally, we measured 5-HT in body fluids, compartments and blood cells and surprisingly interesting data emerged from this one patient. The main finding was that there was a higher concentration of 5-HT in the right side of the heart, as you would expect from the massive liver secondaries, than on the left. Putting two and two together, we speculated that maybe that was the reason why such patients developed right-sided heart disease. It seems so obvious now but it wasn't then.

So, there I was with an interest in monoamines, when suddenly Michael Pare who was my chum from the Army got a job at the Maudsley; it just seemed that everything at that time, in depression and schizophrenia in particular, had a monoamine dimension – you remember the pink spot . . .

This was when?

Our Army service was 1951–53. Michael Pare was the medical specialist at Shorncliffe and I, having done one year in pathology before I went into the Army went in as a specialist in pathology knowing virtually no

Based on an interview previously published in Sandler, M and Healy, D. (1994) The place of chemical pathology in the development of psychopharmacology. *Journal of Psychopharmacology*, **8**, 124–33. Reproduced with permission from the *Journal of Psychopharmacology*.

pathology – can you imagine it? I was given a path lab and 15 technicians and almost nothing to do; well there were about 15 investigations a day including haemoglobins – I really was bored out of my mind. Anyway Mike and I became friends. We had very many wild ideas – we were both terribly untrained in research methodology and made many mistakes. We started off and wrote four papers, doing heroic things like starving for three days and trying to work out a new liver function test. We kept our urine and found odd chromatographic spots in it – nothing at all to do with liver function but somehow connected to starvation. That was our very first paper, called 'Starvation Aminoaciduria'. And then there was a lot of marching backwards and forwards for the poor bloody infantry over 50-mile routes so cases of 'March Haemoglobinuria' came our way. Soon we wrote a second *Lancet* paper 'Aminoaciduria in March Haemoglobinuria'. We started off in style I suppose.

As I said, when I came out of the Army and got a job in the Brompton, Mike went to the Maudsley and found that schizophrenia and pink spot were all the rage. Gaddum had pronounced in 1953 that maybe it is the 5-HT in our brain that keeps us sane and that became our signpost in the sky. So, I had the chromatographic techniques for measuring 5-HT and its metabolites. I didn't develop an interest in catecholamines until about 1957. I used to be and still am, I suppose, a voracious reader of the literature. I would work through, for instance, the Spring Edition of Federation Proceedings, with its several thousand abstracts. It was like telling beads, soothing and a bit mindless. And it was there that I spotted that very first abstract of Marvin Armstrong describing how adrenaline is broken down to VMA – its fate had been a complete mystery up till that time.

Very quickly Colin Ruthven and I jumped in and developed the first quantitative colorimetric test to measure VMA in urine. There was a postal strike at the time and I delivered our paper by hand to the *Lancet*. The *Lancet* was really quaint in those days. Very Dickensian. High desks and men standing up and writing at them. You expected to see a quill pen. But that's by the way. They published it within a few weeks, so that was a coup really.

Phenylketonuria had also come along by then – wherever 5-HT popped up Michael Pare and I chased it. I'm trying to remember the sequence of events. I wrote my very first paper on monoamine oxidase in 1956 with Alan Davison – that was monoamine oxidase in carcinoid tumour tissue. I had become a sort of one-man carcinoid reference laboratory at that time. With Alan Davison I'd been looking at inhibitors of aromatic aminoacid decarboxylase and found that phenolic acids of various kinds to a greater or lesser extent decreased 5-HT production by inhibiting 5-HTP decarboxylase; and of course, a clinical condition which produced vast amounts of a range of phenolic acids in the body was PKU. So we approached Sam Stacey, Professor of Pharmacology at St Thomas', who had a good *in vivo* assay system for platelet 5-HT. The speculation came off. Because of the overproduction of whatever it was, there was a deficit of 5-HT in platelets and, of course, we suggested that there might be a similar deficit in the brain, which might be the cause of the mental deficit. But, anybody can speculate. That's what I've done mostly over the years – it's been my favourite occupation.

In order, then, to test Gaddum's 5-HT hypothesis that I mentioned before, we got a series of volunteers – Maudsley registrars – and gave them LSD because of its effects on 5-HT. On another occasion, we gave them 5-HTP, the -5HT precursor, together with LSD. We worked with a German psychologist called Brengelmann, who actually had fought against Britain in the War – this was only a few years after the War. I always felt very uneasy in my relationships with Brengelmann but he had a set of measuring instruments and questionnaires for quantifying the changes with LSD which were the best available at the time. And indeed, there was a significant attenuation of the LSD effect after pretreatment with 5-HTP. But the fifth or sixth Maudsley registrar we dealt with had a bad trip on LSD. He had to be sat on by six male nurses and he didn't recover fully for a few months. This put the fear of God into us. We wrote off to our Medical Defence people but we were very lucky that nothing permanent happened. Those were the days before Ethical Committees. If you thought up an experiment, you just did it and nobody asked any questions. You used your own common sense.

So that was my first toe in the psychopharmacological water. Because of our PKU experiments, we got a bit of drug company assistance, I can't quite remember how, but I think it was probably through Mike being a clinician. It's always been more difficult for those of us in the lab to get money from drug companies than for chaps who actually give drugs to patients. I think Mike had contacts with John Marks, from Roche Products. A splendid fellow and a good doctor. Don't know how he got into drug companies. They were pretty down market in those days. He ended up as Senior Tutor at Girton, having been Managing Director of Roche Products. Anyway, John Marks sent Mike and me to Rome, to the very first CINP meeting in 1957. I'd never heard of the CINP. I didn't even know what the initials stood for when I went to the meeting. Neuropsychopharmacology or whatever they called it hadn't reached my consciousness as a possible discipline – it made no impression at all.

Was that in 1958 – when the Pope gave a talk?

Yes the Pope gave a talk and if you say so it was 1958. We all heard the Pope and he died 12 days after. I thought this was what always happens at international conferences. The Pope gives a talk, he dies – not that that counts. Yes, we were all bussed out to Castelgandolfo and Pope Pius XII made some significant pronouncement in Latin, it may have been broken English – can't remember.

Who was there from the labs, how many clinically, how many from the industry?

I can only think of outstanding personalities that I met there for the first time. Hannah Steinberg was there, perpetually drinking coffee with Philip Bradley and Arthur Summerfield. I remember very distinctly, they seemed so senior and grown up with strong opinions about everything. You always admire these grown up people. I still do.

Michael Shepherd was there.

Michael Shepherd was there, very much so. Aubrey Lewis was too but I didn't get to know him. He was developing Parkinson's disease and had a bit of a fixed stare. He looked a bit like Rasputin. I subsequently used to see him walking on the river bank at Richmond, with his wife, and tried to acknowledge him but he never knew who I was. Different from Sir Hans Krebs, whom I always used to see at the Biochemical Society and he'd call me Sandler in his precise Teutonic manner. The last time I saw him was at a meeting on aggression in Windsor Great Park. I knew I had arrived because, for the first time Krebs called me Merton! Then he died twelve days later. I seem to have this effect on people.

Really, I rode in to Rome as it were on the back of Michael Pare. We had our first drug company dinner. God, was it an eye opener. In the villa of Mussolini's mistress, Clara-somebody-or-other – was it Petacci? It was splendid. Roche had really pushed the boat out. This taste of the *dolce vita* and the faint whiff of corruption was the thing I remember most about that Rome meeting. There were some nice buildings around too.

Why do you say an eye opener?

I'm a little provincial Jewish boy from Manchester, of immigrant stock. I was the first one in our family to go to University. There was no question of Oxford or Cambridge or anything like that because there wouldn't be kosher food and there would be non-Jewish girls. So I went to Manchester medical school and lived at home. I led a narrow and cloistered existence. It was the Army really that opened my eyes to life outside provincial Jewish Manchester. Does this explain this eye opener stuff?

Yes. On what areas did the first CINP meetings focus?

I can't remember the topics of the symposia at all. Probably over my head. I remember giving my own paper. It went all right, not too many questions.

Who do you recall as being the key people? Who made psychopharmacology . . .?

Joel Elkes was very much there. Very smooth, very much an operator. Thought of himself as a philosopher and he gave this appearance of being an elder statesman even though he was quite young. He was a figure that I remember. I never got to know him properly until, I suppose, 10 years after that. He never replies to my letters. It's a great character defect. Or perhaps I keep forgetting to put on a stamp . . .

I think I met Seymour Kety first in 1961 when I first went to the United States of America. Seymour, at that time chief of the lab of clinical science at NIH, gave me lunch and had all his disciples around him — what a galaxy they were. Julie Axelrod, Irv Kopin, Joe Schildkraut, Sol Snyder, Dick Wurtman, Joe Fisher, all now famous names in their own right or even Nobel laureates or Nobel candidates. It was funny because sitting round the table, there were 11 or 12 of us and we were all Jewish. I don't know what attraction psychopharmacology or neuroscience has for this group of chaps. Even out of the 10 Presidents to date of the BAP, I calculate that 5 have been Jewish which is a much higher proportion than their representation in the country. I've no idea why. Have you any speculation?

No. Of all of them who has had the most impact?

Well, I think there are two kinds of bright chap around. There are the mathematical or analytical chaps who go deep into one thing but almost invariably lack creativity and the other is the sort of not so mathematically bright individual who sees connections between things. I suppose I think of myself as a hanger-on in the second group.

Now Sol Snyder, even though he's been wrong many times, I'd put almost at the top. He probably combines the best of both groups. He's the exception. Then there's Julie Axelrod, slower thinking I would say but he just gets there, strips down concepts and sees through to the heart of them, sees what is real and what is mythology. I think this is a Jewish trick, as a matter of fact, this ability to see through to the reality, but I may be wrong.

What about Brodie?

Brodie, who was born in Liverpool incidentally and who many consider to have been the father of biochemical pharmacology, was a distant relation of mine as a matter of fact. He was a crazy man. He used to take uppers and downers all the time. He used to take amphetamines in the day time and barbiturates at night to make him sleep. He worked frenetically with the amphetamines — he would carry on until 2 am, 3 am in the morning and get his co-workers along to the lab at that time — it was nothing for Brodie to ring people up at 12 o'clock at night but he never got in until late morning or early afternoon. One way and another, I saw a lot of him but I never got on the same wavelength. Axelrod, in fact, was for many years Brodie's technician and he treated him like it. Axelrod is a sweet man.

I met Axelrod at that same seminal CINP meeting in 1958. How could I have forgotten this, when you asked me who struck me most. Well, I got on this bus back from Castelgandolfo or one of the outings and I sat next to a rather shabby and self-effacing man, wearing a sort of flasher's mac even though the sun was beating down. One of his eyes was covered over. We started to chat about our work. I was cocky. The PKU work and 5-HTP work was going rather well. And he said 'Oh, I'm working on adrenaline metabolism and it's not going well at all'. I thought to myself that if ever anyone was cut out for failure, then this little guy was. He seemed to have nothing going for him. Twelve years later of course he won the Nobel prize.

I thought the same the first time I heard Hans Kosterlitz at the Physiology Society, probably some time late in the 1950s. Kosterlitz used to give what seemed to me terribly boring papers on the action of morphine on the gut. But this was the springboard for his discovery of endogenous opiates. I'm always wrong about these things – mixing up personality with talent. Axelrod was still Brodie's technician when I met him. He eventually got his PhD at the age of 45 and after that he gradually untied the shackles. Some say that Axelrod was responsible for many of Brodie's key experiments. It's difficult to say. I'm sure Axelrod himself would make no such claims because he's so decent and modest.

Some people say all the good work in Brodie's lab got done when he was on holiday.

Well, that may be. Brodie did have many flashes of insight and was a flawed genius I would say. You can't knock him completely. There was a lot that was good about him, but he did tend to exploit people and pick the young one's brains. Perhaps we all do.

Seymour Kety now is a very different kettle of fish. Very charming and diplomatic and formidably influential. He was also very brilliant. Perhaps the Kety-Schmidt approach to bloodflow measurement in the brain, which is where he made his scientific name, wasn't a big enough problem, as far as Nobel prizes were concerned. Given the right problem I'm sure he would have won one. He's still working at NIH, even though he's over 80.

Do you think in the end Kety's role was more an organizational one . . .?

His main achievement possibly was as the brilliant head of the Laboratory of Clinical Science in its heyday although you must remember he was deeply involved in the Danish Schizophrenia project and that was very important stuff too and he was the founding editor of the prestigious and influential *Journal of Psychiatric Research*. I always swore I would never edit a journal because it was a mug's game but after an hour of Seymour's blandishments across the trans-Atlantic telephone, I was talked into being his successor. Thank God I've just managed to pass it along after 10 years. Joe Schildkraut was my co-Editor-in-Chief. Joe had published his monoamine hypothesis of depression to a fanfare of trumpets, in 1965, but this theory had been foreshadowed by work Mike Pare and I had done in 1958.

Yes. Now tell me about that. I've always wondered about it. You seemed to have the amine theory all worked out at that point – at least implicitly?

Well, Mike Pare and I were the first to give 5-HTP and DOPA intravenously anywhere to anybody. We used them to try to cut down the lag period of response to MAO inhibitors in depressive illness. We did a trial of iproniazid because it was bright and spanking new, you see, and we reasoned that if it was just blocking monoamine oxidase, the action must be because of the excess amines that were produced. The only ones we knew of, of course, were noradrenaline and 5-HT. So, we got hold of some of the precursors because we knew that the neurotransmitters wouldn't cross the blood – brain barrier and we treated depressed patients with them. During the lag period, the 2–3 weeks until the MAO inhibitors started to work, we gave them 5-HTP or DOPA intravenously to see if we could shorten the time before response occurred. It didn't work. In retrospect we didn't use enough. Thank goodness because we would have probably sent their blood pressure over the top.

We published our clinical trial of iproniazid in depression. Our amine ideas, disguised under the title of 'A trial of iproniazid in the treatment of depression' languished but Joe's got the full PR treatment and prospered

I've always thought it all comes down to good PR, what do you think?

Yes, yes. Joe's paper is one of the most quoted papers in the world now. Ah well, you win some, you lose some.

Do you want to comment more on the role of PR in the whole thing. because it does seem to me that people who coined the snappy phrases Type I, Type II . . . who market their ideas, get places where others don't – even if they're wrong.

You are absolutely right. I agree with you all the way. The Americans have lived in a marketing climate for longer but we seem to be getting used to it now. We no longer have to talk ourselves down to the same extent and British understatement still needs to be banished. Nate Kline, perhaps the most prominent American psychiatrist of his day, called a press conference even before he gave that first paper to the American Psychiatric Association on iproniazid in the treatment of depressive illness.

Nate Kline, who died in 1982, was a great romantic. He liked reciting poetry and had an inexhaustible supply that he would quote at the drop of a hat. Everybody seemed to like him but I felt uneasy with his flamboyance. Perhaps because of it, he had his face on the cover of *Time* magazine as one of the 10 best known men in America – not one of the 10 best known psychiatrists. When he wanted to reduce his private practice because it was getting out of hand, he doubled his prices overnight to $1000 a throw. His private practice increased substantially when he did that. It was quite incredible. I owe a lot to Nate Kline. I owe about 10 Caribbean holidays to him!

Tell me about that. That was the Denghausen Group . . .

Yes, Mrs Denghausen was a depressed upstate New York millionairess and Nate Kline was her psychiatrist. I think, from memory, he had her on tryptophan and it seemed to work for her. One day, when she was slightly less depressed, Mrs Denghausen said to Nate 'What can I do for medical science' and Nate told her that doctors need to meet with other doctors without being worried about leaving their wives. So for fifteen years, she funded this meeting and 12 or 15 international chaps, of Nate's choice, plus their wives, met on the beach, on a different Caribbean island every year. It wasn't a joke. It was a proper meeting. We started at 8.30 am and carried on until 1, when drinks were brought out on a tray.

There was just a blackboard on the beach under the palm trees. We all took turns to make our presentations, interrupted all the way. We couldn't get away with a loose sentence or phrase – a pretty high calibre bunch. I set up a lot of research collaborations through this Denghausen meeting and got lots of ideas. I came in five years after it all began. Arvid Carlsson joined the year after me. I remember Bernie Wagner, a pathologist, and Biff Bunney there. Sol Synder was asked but he never turned up. Jules Angst was there – a bit like Eugene Onegin. Linford Rees and Alec Coppen had been there from the start.

Tell me how did the BAP come about?

The BAP came about almost casually. We were all lying by the side of a swimming pool in Palm Springs, where that year's ACNP meeting was being held, when I remember David Wheatley saying to Alec Coppen and me what a wonderful thing it would be to have a British College of Psychopharmacology. David Wheatley was the guiding spirit. He liked to go abroad; he loved the sun and foreign beaches and was captivated by the ACNP, which always met in exotic places. So was I. That was in 1971 or 72. We thought about tactics and how to organize things and the name of Max Hamilton cropped up. I don't know who spoke to him. Max certainly wasn't there at the meeting. I don't even know whether Max was allowed into America at that time.

Why?

Max had been a communist party member, though he resigned after Hungary. All his organizational strength derived from his party training so for many years he could not go to America. With Max it was policy rather than personality. He learnt this directly from his party days. Although Max could be an abrasive fellow, it was probably because of his political colouring that he was unpopular with the British psychiatric establishment and never made it on the London scene. In the opinion of many, Max should have been the successor of Aubrey Lewis at the Maudsley.

Who else was involved in the start?

Anthony Horden, Ronnie Maggs, Philip Connell who did such a model investigation of amphetamine toxicity. Everyone thought before that time that amphetamine didn't really do you any harm until Connell published his monograph. Really a fine piece of work.

You said Max was the person that pulled it all together.

I say that David Wheatley was the driving force. He had the intelligence to know he had to have a front man. David was only a general practitioner – and you know how hierarchical we tend to be in Britain. A very successful general practitioner. He was well in with the drug companies because he used to mount very successful clinical trials for them. He was slightly flamboyant but very capable. To my mind he was the driving force. He got his people into place and must either directly or indirectly have spoken to Max. He later did a magnificent job as BAP secretary.

I wanted to talk to you about the great schism in the BAP.

I was on the very first council. A lot of bitterness emerged and the situation became polarized between the non-medics and the medics. The non-medics – as now – thought of themselves as pure, good scientists who don't get besmirched by drug company handouts or anything like that. To some extent the tension is still there in the background and is always liable to re-emerge.

Max brought us all together with his cunning ploy as I said before, of policies before personalities and he was right, I suppose. He'd had a vast experience at manipulating chaps in the party. He talked it through with us at great length and somehow he did weld us all together. But it was a pretty close thing. We had extraordinary general meeting after extraordinary general meeting, well two or three, and they were dismal. The West Hall of the RSM, long before the RSM had been upgraded to its present splendour, was a shabby place, especially on a Saturday morning. I seem to remember the lights weren't on, for some reason.

I seem to remember, too, that Philip Bradley led the revolt, ably assisted by Ian Stolerman and to some extent Malcolm Lader. After the armistice, the second president, by agreement, was Alec Coppen. And then for the only time in the Association's history, there was a fight for the third Presidency between Philip Bradley and me and I lost. After that bitter lesson, we agreed the Presidency should be decided by tacit collusion between past presidents.

One of the other things that happened was that 'Academy' or 'College' were thought to be bad names and so we became an Association for Psychopharmacology.

Was the election bitter?

Well, perhaps I remember it being bitter because I lost, I don't know. Anyway Philip Bradley and I are good friends and I duly became the President after him.

David Wheatley never featured prominently in office, was that because he would have been seen by the non-clinical people as the kind of person who was too associated with the industry?

Well, people are very status conscious and would rather see a professor as president than a GP. But David was secretary at a crucial period and did a magnificent job. In my opinion our symbiotic relationship with the pharmaceutical industry has enriched us and has never got out of hand.

There are virtually no general practitioners in the BAP now.

David was special. He was a member of the Royal Medico-Psychological Association before it turned into the College. So he automatically became a member of the College.

He says you were the person who brought the BAP together. It actually began poorly, as you've said, and it took some putting together, a taking by the scruff of its neck and he points to you as the person responsible.

Well, that's extremely kind. I did work hard at it. It was a bit of a ragged nest after the fighting and there were still a lot of ruffled feathers and sourness. I myself started off in the opposite camp to Philip Bradley and it took time to feel as we do today about each other. I still pull his leg, about Birmingham mostly, which isn't my favourite place in the world.

What did you actually do to sort things out?

I don't know what I did. I suppose that a touch of enthusiasm and talking to people on a one-to-one basis helped. A sense of humour. I think I tried to stop people being so bloody pompous and intense.

There was a period during the 1980s when the BAP was a fun group between yourself and Sid Levine.

Yes. Sid is marvellous, isn't he. I think that's important. I think it's been good for the membership. I hope we don't become too serious ever.

One of the other ways things could have gone, of course, would have been if Philip had organized a branch of the CINP here in the UK. If he had, would we have ever had a BAP?

No, there wouldn't have been a BAP. Many people say we made the wrong decision anyway, to start off with the BAP. We should have started a Biological Psychiatry Society. The conceptual focus on drugs to the exclusion of biological psychiatry in general was really a bit of a misnomer for a society that in some respects has really been a Biological Psychiatry Society. There are still people now who would prefer a Biological Psychiatry Society.

What about the 1984 meeting and the fuss over the St Pierre Park Hotel? There has been this issue with all psychopharmacological organizations that if they go down the large conference centre route, they become just a club for clinicians.

Oh, that's something that really worries me quite a lot as a matter of fact, the hold of the drug companies on academic psychiatry. We all know about free lunches.

Do you want to talk about that?

No, not very much, because I too have many mouths to feed, alas. Without the drug companies we would not be able to conduct our research. Until the last phase of the Thatcher period, I was usually successful in taking money from drug companies without strings, but you can't always do that. You've got to produce the stuff they want sometimes, especially if you want larger sums. It's a great bind. I'm perfectly aware of the ethical arguments but what alternative is there? The universities are bankrupt. The MRC is broke and the Wellcome people are peremptory and idiosyncratic, or at least they were with the old regime.

If you think of a group like the BAP, there are at least six different groups in it – a clinical group, a psychology group picking up the kind of work that someone like Hannah Steinberg was doing back in the 1950s with healthy volunteer work, the industry and the basic scientists, particularly the animal people. Then there's been your area, chemical pathology, and the chemists, the people who have the time and imagination to be able to see receptors and what drugs will bind to them. Any thoughts on which groups have been most influential?

No, no because they've all blended very well. It's remarkable really that it has worked. Our industry representatives have been self-effacing and discrete to a man. The Americans, the ACNP, were also well aware of the problem but they had the good idea of making the industry pay through the nose for corporate membership. It's good. The CINP, of course, has been heavily infiltrated by trade and commerce which is sad. Of course you can't have a meeting for 5000 souls without someone actually paying for it.

What about blind alleys? The field has tended to be dominated by people who sell ideas well – Schildkraut and the amine hypothesis for instance. To some extent the way it came out and the impact it had, stultified things, I think. Take your work for instance. My impression is that what you were doing during the 1970s increasingly became orthogonal to the mainstream and it seems to me that was because the mainstream suddenly didn't seem to be going anywhere any more. It seemed to me anyway that if there was going to be any development it would have to come from without.

In my long research career the only lesson I've learnt is not to get too fixated on ideas. It's very easy to start thinking about ideas as something of your own and you try to cling to them then and not see the bad spots. Come to think of it, I've learned one other lesson: a rat is not a man! If you really want to know about man, you can get some pointers from the animal world but only pointers. Yes, I think we have had many blind alleys because strong personalities hold ideas too long. The famous Spanish histopathologist, Ramon y Cajal, once said, 'I wish to warn young men against the invincible attraction of theories which simplify and unify seductively'.

In terms of this field, can you pick out people and ideas which you think have been counter-productive?

Yes. Starting with Henry Dale and his one-cell-one-transmitter hypothesis, that held everything back for ages. And then there's Freud and the whole psychoanalytic movement, which is still hanging around.

What about the amine theory. Do you think I'm being a bit harsh on the amine theory?

No. Obviously the monoamines have a role but . . . the thing is you've got to be humble and you've got to realize just how little information there is. There is a jigsaw puzzle but with only two or three pieces of the whole picture in place. You can turn them around one way and you get one picture and if you turn them another way you get another. It's easy to link this to that if you have a vivid imagination. But it may not be true.

The industry has a role in imposing orthodoxy, hasn't it? It prefers to produce drugs for example where it knows what exactly they are going to do rather than produce something dramatically innovative.

Yes, industry is conservative. Of course, me-too drugs are the safest financially. I think most people within the industry understand this and that the way forward lies via getting a new drug quickly into man, then watching like a hawk for unexpected side-effects as pointers for new types of drug action. Because one man's side-effect is another man's new drug action.

Who else has been of importance?

Another important chap who never got into this clinical area at all, who is still alive and well, a neurochemist to whom we all owe a great debt to was Derek Richter. A shy retiring man but very talented. One of the very early neurochemists.

Why do you say you owe a lot to him?

I was talking both on a personal level, because I have been a friend of his for some years, and on a biochemical level because he was one of the original workers on monoamine oxidase in the 1930s with Blaschko who died only very recently. And then there was Judah Hirsch Quastel who had a major impact in the early days of neurochemistry. Quastel worked on many fundamental aspects of neurochemistry and biochemistry, on the conjugation of benzoic acid, for example. Things that are now taken for granted. And the same with Richter.

You've been a very public figure in psychopharmacology. Any particular reason?

The reason I suppose I've been involved in so many meetings, national and international, probably stems from the scientific isolation that I've lived in all the years at Queen Charlotte's and this isolation, in a way, has been beneficial because it means that I have had to look elsewhere for intellectual stimulation in a way that I wouldn't have had to do had I worked in Cambridge or Oxford or wherever.

My great regret is that the fax wasn't invented earlier but even so, I have been a pretty inveterate traveller and have made a lot of telephone calls. All this activity has resulted in many international friendships, particularly in the United States, I suppose. So I think of myself not necessarily as a scientific citizen of Hammersmith but just as a scientific citizen. I still talk science into the middle of the night with the same excitement wherever I am wafted by the scientific winds.

Of course, I'm terribly grateful to Queen Charlotte's. I've been a neurochemical cuckoo in their nest but they've been extremely kind to me over the years.

Why did you end up there?

Oh, expediency and opportunism, my dear boy, purely that. I was a lecturer in chemical pathology at the Royal Free Hospital. I had already started on my monoamine way in those days, of course, but my chief said 'well, there's a consultant job going at the Queen Charlotte's, you won't get it, you're too young, but show them that you think yourself up there with the toffs' and so I got my application together. Ridiculously, I got the job, although at the interview, I did everything to wriggle out of getting it. They asked 'are you interested in obstetrics', and I said 'not really'. When they asked 'What are you interested in?' I said 'I'm interested in monoamines', but I also said 'I just follow them wherever they go and if they go down into the uterus, then I will follow them into the uterus'. They took me at my word.

In fact, I came up with a monoamine hypothesis of toxaemia almost immediately and I don't completely disbelieve that even today. It's just that more exciting things cropped up soon after I got to Charlotte's.

Although we found a deficit of monoamine oxidase in human placenta in toxaemia even in those days, it may well just be secondary to fibrotic changes in a toxaemic placenta – I don't know. We never really pursued it further, I'm sorry to say. Anyway the papers came tumbling forth – our department produced twice as many as the whole hospital put together – perhaps more.

At the Cambridge meeting on the History of Psychopharmacology you threw out some very provocative comments about the MAOIs, that some of them are MAOIs but aren't actually antidepressants and there are related compounds that may be antidepressants and aren't MAOIs – do you think MAO inhibition is necessary to their antidepressant action?

You are right, of course. I suppose I have never accepted revealed truth in anything and just because a compound has been dubbed a monoamine oxidase inhibitor and because it does have monoamine oxidase-inhibiting properties, it doesn't necessarily mean that it works because of that monoamine oxidase-inhibiting ability. Take deprenyl, for instance, the monoamine oxidase B inhibitor now used extensively in the treatment of Parkinson's disease because of its possible neuroprotective properties. Well I'm quite convinced that its neuroprotective ability doesn't derive from MAO B inhibition. Other selective MAO B inhibitors don't seem to possess this particular action. The point is that every individual drug has multiple properties and abilities, despite its official classification. We have shown with deprenyl, for instance, that there's a significant increase in superoxide dismutase activity in patients or rats treated with it. I can put up a good case for superoxide dismutase being neuroprotective.

But that's another story. I have argued over the years that the beneficial effects of the monoamine oxidase-inhibiting drugs in depressive illness may not depend completely on their ability to inhibit MAO A. Their effect on this enzyme is maximal within hours but lightening of affect may not be observed before several weeks have elapsed, so there's something else there.

What about the tyramine conjugation deficits that can be found in people who are depressed?

That's very interesting and the finding has held up well, although we still don't know the mechanism. It's not for the want of trying, I have to tell you. I can give you a long list of things that it isn't. It isn't a deficit of phenolsulphotransferase. As a matter of fact its very interesting that we stumbled on that because it led us to some really hard science. We were able to show for the first time that the human phenolsulphotransferase enzyme had multiple forms – PSTM, M standing for monoamines and PSTP, for which dilute phenol was the first substrate we identified. We found that the two forms had different substrate specificities, different inhibitor specificities, different pH optima; just like monoamine oxidase A and B.

Do you think it was the lack of a Bethesda-type PR campaign that prevented the tyramine test being more widely known? It has always hit me that it was a very clear piece of work – one of the few biological findings we have and nothing has been made of it.

Well, it's quite difficult to do. Even the most intelligent patients – even doctors – have difficulty collecting accurately timed 3-hour urine samples. You have to be supervised and there's no way round this – otherwise mistakes are made. That's probably the main problem. Other people have confirmed it of course – Donald Klein and his group, for instance, and others, but people still sort of sniff a little bit, don't they?

Why? Is it just a matter of timing? The idea of a DST test in a sense was there before Barney Carroll but somehow it clicked into place at that time and bingo there's this industry that grew up out of it.

And it doesn't mean a thing that test, yet it still persists; ah well, never mind.

Do you think it comes back partly to the idea that there was a US sales component?

Yes, I think so. Really the new generation of psychopharmacologists have to learn to be their own mouthpiece, their own trumpeter, their own PR man. I think this is important. We tend to be diffident and hide our light under a bushel over here.

Another area you've been involved in, indeed led the field in, but which hasn't received as much outside attention as it perhaps deserves, has been in trace amines. Can you tell me something about trace amines?

Alan Boulton, in Canada, and I myself, on this side of the Atlantic, have both been a bit obsessed, over the years, with all the monoamine substrates of monoamine oxidase that weren't catecholamines or 5-hydroxytryptamine – I mean the tyramines and octopamines, phenylethylamine, phenylethanolamine, tryptamine, etc. They are all present in the brain in low concentrations but that's only because they haven't got specific storage mechanisms. The turnover of octopamine, for example, seems to be just as large as that of noradrenaline. Both our teams have identified a number of changes in these systems in different types of mental disorder but we've only scratched the surface. There's plenty of room for further study. Alan wanted to call them 'microamines' but Earl Usdin and I thought that inappropriate and put forward the name 'trace amines' which stuck.

One of the other areas you've been involved in the last 10 years that I've always thought looked awfully interesting and I've been surprised it hasn't had the impact that I thought it would have, is the whole story from tribulin to isatin.

Well, tribulin is a bit of a tangled skein. You see although we have identified the main MAO B-inhibiting component in tribulin, there now seems to be at least one major MAO A-inhibiting component too. We've recently found, in addition, that isatin, the MAO B-inhibiting component, has a strong action on a quite unrelated receptor system in the body and we're trying to get to grips with the implications of this too.

Another complication with isatin is that it's generated endogenously in the brain but it is also produced in large amounts by the gut flora. Our crucial experiment was in germ-free rats, which excreted relatively small amounts in their urine compared with conventional controls. I've been interested in gut flora all my life. They're terribly under-rated things, gut flora. If you ever have any bizarre or anomalous effects or unlikely compounds in the urine you should immediately think of drugs or gut flora. My colleagues in the lab smiled when I said we've just got to do these experiments with isatin in germ-free animals but then these beautifully clean data emerged. It's a very expensive business – breeding germ-free animals – but it's difficult to approach certain problems in any other way.

So, we've been involved with that but one thing that I would have liked to have spent much more time on, because I think it could have been so desperately important in our over-crowded society is aggression. You probably don't remember that we did a study which got a lot of media coverage on prisoners from Wormwood Scrubs in 1977 where we found an increased production of phenylethylamine or, rather, of its major metabolites, in aggressive psychopaths. Now, most of the phenylacetylglutamine and phenylacetic acid in the urine, in fact, comes from gut flora so we don't know, even now, that these patients had an overproduction of phenylethylamine as such. If you block phenylethylamine degradation with a monoamine oxidase B inhibitor like deprenyl, you get a very substantial increase in urine output of phenylethylamine, from 2, 3, 4, 5 μg per 24 h – it's as low as that you see – to something like 80 or 100 μg per 24 h. A very respectable increase but not when you consider the amounts of the major metabolites, phenylacetic acid and phenylacetylglutamine, in the urine – something of the order of 100 mg per 24 h. So, this is another aspect of the gut floraness of things and it just makes life that much more difficult.

So whether our Wormwood Scrubs multiple murderers with large amounts of these metabolites in their circulation really did produce larger amounts of nature's amphetamine, phenylethylamine, is still an open question . . .

They weren't on MAO B inhibitors?

No, we didn't get a chance to put them on MAO B inhibitors. We speculated and proved that it was true, that the aggressive alpha male in a monkey pack, the pack leader, had a high circulating phenylethylamine metabolite level. We still don't know what it means, but we had a nice trip to St Kitts in the Caribbean to perform the experiment. I'd be terribly interested to pursue it. It may just be that they get more constipated – the aggressive ones for all I know.

Anyway, there is a phenomenon here that needs further investigation. We would have needed the full collaboration of the prison services at the time but they were very difficult. Did I ever tell you about this? The very first paper on the aggressive psychopaths from Wormwood Scrubs came about by accident. I had to go to a very boring dinner at the Royal College of Physicians and I got stuck at the end of a table. The chap opposite me hadn't turned up so I only had the chap sitting next to me to talk to. I asked him what he did and he said he was a psychiatrist at Wormwood Scrubs. So I plucked from the air a fact I'd read that 80% of the murderers in North Carolina had been taking amphetamine at the time they committed their murder.

Really.

Yes, well in fact it was very obvious in retrospect but I had never heard of amphetamine psychosis at that time. They must have been amphetamine junkies who flipped and became paranoid amphetamine schizophrenics. Anyway the Wormwood Scrubs psychiatrist started to get interested and I remembered that we had a test for phenylacetic acid and that phenethylamine is closely related to amphetamine. If you block phenylethylamine degradation in a rat – if you give them a monoamine oxidase inhibitor and administer phenylethylamine – you will get a typical amphetamine-like response.

So I started to generate a hypothesis, you know, as one does after the second drink and he said 'well, perhaps we should test this' and I said 'I'd love to, and can you get some blood'. So he got a dozen of these bloods from a selection of homicidal maniacs and a dozen samples from meek and mild controls and, lo and behold, we had a paper. We sent it off to the *Lancet*. My collaborator promptly got into trouble from the prison service because he hadn't had proper permission to do it. They were scared stiff because experiments on convicts are tricky things.

When I tried to go back to Wormwood Scrubs, the doors were closed. I couldn't get any more samples. Anyway, three or four months passed. I happened to find myself at a dinner party and there was a very brash but personable young man sitting opposite. I was reciting the story and the frustrations of science and all that and this young man, whom I vaguely recognized, said 'well, I might be able to help'. I said 'do you have any useful contacts' and he said he was in the Cabinet and the Home Secretary was his friend – it was Norman Fowler, looking terribly young, like a school boy, in 1977. And he said 'send me the documents of the case, send me everything you've got, and I'll promise to have a word with Willie Whitelaw'. He was quite fired by all this, really.

Anyway, nothing happened for another three or four months and I despaired. Then all of a sudden, a phone call came and he said, 'It's Norman Fowler – you're all right, just apply'. So we got another set of samples with the same result but then our psychiatrist retired and it all got difficult so we went to the monkeys in the Caribbean instead, hoping some time to get back to Scrubs but we never did. But aggression, it's such an important thing isn't it and with these so-called anti-aggressive drugs being developed, I don't know if I believe in them or not. The serenics and all that. Terribly interesting.

Eltoprazine?

Yes, I've been interested since it started and I know quite a bit about it. Eltoprazine may be serenic; at least in a peculiar rat model, the rat maternal aggression model, it's very good. It also has one other unfortunate action, however. It not only blocks aggression but it blocks the sex drive too. And I think Barry Everitt will tell you that these two drives seem to be very closely related. I always remember Barry giving a brilliant paper at a Sardinian meeting when he was trying to disentangle them by producing suitable brain lesions. He never could do so though. I can't remember the details of his experiment except I think this was my first very positive impression of Barry Everitt. A beautiful experimentalist.

Oh yes, aggression is so important. I'm sure if I'd have been able to take the blood of Adolf Hitler or James Jones in Guyana or what was this nutter in Texas called, David Koresh, they would all have had high circulating levels of phenylacetic acid. In terms of aggression, Robert Maxwell, for example, might well have been an example of this. Robert Maxwell was such a charismatic man. As I told you I edited the *Journal of Psychiatric Research*, a Pergamon journal, for 10 years. This meant meeting Robert Maxwell. Well I had first met him in 1973 . . .
I liked him tremendously.

This was the problem, wasn't it?

Tremendously likeable man. I first met him in 1973, at night time, in Strasbourg Castle. I think it was the third or fourth Catecholamine Symposium. It was a very Shakespearean scene in the courtyard, with torches blazing, a crowd of extras milling around. Somebody took me and half a dozen others along to introduce me to this great big chap. Of course, I remembered our meeting clearly because he was famous or notorious but it never crossed my mind that he could possibly remember me.

Well, in 1982, having taken over the editorship of one of his journals, I found myself invited to one of his annual jamborees in June at Heading-ton Hill Hall. They were great affairs with brass bands and drum majorettes and he used to arrive in his helicopter. Well, there he was sitting outside his tent literally, with nobody whispering in his ear and I went up to make his acquaintance and said 'You won't remember me' and he said 'I do – you're Merton Sandler, you've just taken over the *Journal of Psychiatric Research* and I remember meeting you in Strasbourg in 1973'. I was impressed by that.

Hearing you go through the range of things you've done, I'm aware how little chemical pathology I know or was trained in and how much risk, I think, the rest of us non-pathologists run, as a result, of re-inventing the wheel. I'm sure that in five years time people will trumpet things they wouldn't be trumpeting if they knew about gut flora. But it's not a fashionable area at the moment is it?

No, it's not a fashionable area. I think one has to have a lot of luck in science and suddenly some big finding will come. A lot of luck. You're right, who has heard of what I do except for a few specialists in the area really. I suppose we were the first with the multiple forms of monoamine oxidase and that sort of thing. But I'm not a popular folk hero like Marie Curie or Brian Leonard. I don't think cults of personality have much to do with science, though.

What about your interest in migraine?

Ah, yes . . . migraine has played an important part in my professional research life, purely by accident as most of these things are. It happened by chance – I got a phone call one day from a lady called Edda Hanington who was Assistant Scientific Director of the Wellcome Trust and she was passionately interested in migraine. Now it had been known for centuries that certain foods can initiate migraine attacks in certain susceptible people. She pointed out, in a seminal paper, that cheese was one of these triggering substances and suggested it did so by virtue of the tyramine it contains.

She was wrong, of course, about tyramine. It doesn't seem to initiate a headache attack, according to work that was subsequently done over the years. However, my mind is not completely closed. When my colleague Richard Peatfield gave tyramine intravenously to certain migraineurs, some of them did get a headache.

But it was an important question in 1967 and even though Hanington is likely to have been wrong, a lot of people took up the baton and became enthusiastic about the whole chemical background of migraine. As Popper has said, 'Fertility is the result not of exactness but of seeing new problems where none have been seen before, and of finding new ways of solving them'. One of the most important things about Hanington was that she worked for the Wellcome Trust, so when she got on the phone to me and said biochemically speaking 'Help help', it was important because there was money to prime the pumps. So that's how I got into the biochemistry of migraine.

And, in fact, following this lead, we were the first to find that there's a platelet monoamine oxidase deficit in migraine. Two kinds of platelet deficit, as a matter of fact. During the acute attack there's a transitory deficit but about 25% of males have a permanent decrease in platelet enzyme activity. There's been intense activity once more in the past year or two in this area, spearheaded by us but also by Kathleen Merikangas in Yale and Naomi Breslau in Detroit because it turns out that there is a substantial increase in psychiatric morbidity in migraine and up to about 20% of patients have a major depressive illness at some time in their lives. This has now been put on a quantitative basis and studies of the genetics of this phenomenon are proceeding with full molecular biological cooperation – maybe some answers will now emerge.

Do you not think the whole fuss these days about the 5-HT is something of a 5-HT bubble?

Of course, my dear boy. 5-HT is important, I've never said that it isn't. I've earned my bread and butter from 5-HT over the years and I wouldn't really knock it. Even so, 5-HT is all right in its place but there are many other things that the seven groups – so far – of 5-HT receptors connect to. What has amused me over the years is the sheep phenomenon in science. Everybody follows my leader in science. Some American publishes a new paper and it gets the full Bethesda PR treatment and all round the world, the little chaps in their journeyman laboratories follow and write their safe papers and of course the safe papers are accepted. It's the papers that change science that we all have difficulty in placing. Most science, unfortunately, is safe science.

You have to have safe science to get a grant, alas. I really mean that. If you want to get a grant, then you must not stray too far from what the last man has produced. I don't blame the referees when they've had no experience with a new concept – or rather, I don't know if I do or not! If you haven't got enough knowledge of an area and if you're spending public money then to be safe, you turn the project down. Where Leonardo would get his money from if he were alive today rather worries me. That's a big problem David.

Select bibliography
Sandler, M. and Healy, D. (1994) The place of chemical pathology in psychopharmacology. *Journal of Psychopharmacology*, **8**, 124–33.

17 Floyd Bloom

The place of neurophysiology in psychopharmacology

When I first went to do psychopharmacology research with Brian Leonard in Galway in 1980, pretty well the first thing he did was to give me a copy of your book The Biochemical Basis of Neuropharmacology *(Cooper, et al., 1970) and said 'read this – this is all you need to know'. More recently, looking through bookshelves, I've noticed your* Brain, Mind and Behaviour *(Bloom, et al., 1985) and been impressed by it. But the next encounter with you as it were was when you were invited to give the BAP guest lecture in 1987 (Bloom, 1987). The lecture included large amounts of neurophysiology, which I know nothing about, and dealt with alcoholism, which is not my area, but it still remains for me one of the best Guest Lectures I've ever heard in any forum – hence the interest for me to include you in this group of interviews; more than most people you seem aware of the need to reach out – to communicate to people outside your own area where things are at.*

I could certainly understand how it must seem that way. There must be some of that in that book. Both of those books, however, were really not planned to do that when they began. *The Biochemical Basis of Neuropharmacology* was going to be project with a man who led the neuropharmacology course for graduate students at Yale University – one of my many Italian mentors in neuropharmacology, Dr Nicholas Giarman. Unfortunately Dr Giarman died as the book contract was being signed so Jack Cooper, Bob Roth and I agreed that we would do the book strictly to honour our departed friend's memory. We had no idea whether it would be a successful book or not but it encapsulated the lectures that we would have given in that course in that year and we wrote it strictly in the way we would have given it. Students seem to have liked the conversational tone of it all, so it's caught on and we have had a great deal of fun doing it together. It really started out not to become an icon of the field but really just to honour our dear friend's memory and that is the only dedication that the book has ever carried – to our friend, Nicholas Giarman.

The Brain, Mind and Behaviour book came up because of the television series 'The Brain' for which I was one of the science advisors. They had contracted for a book that would be used by junior colleges and community colleges to teach a course on the brain as viewed in modern scientific terms and the person who had agreed to write the book defaulted. With a relatively short amount of time they paid me a generous sum to try and take on this project. The first edition was not completely successful because it is like one of our US postage stamp things; we never got to see the galley proofs for the figure captions so many of them were just totally wrong. None of the reviewers picked up on that; the person who reviewed it for the *New Scientist* gave it such a thrilling review that I was so pleased to have had that review.

But it is the kind of book that will appeal across a wide range or interests and even to people not in the field at all . . .?

That is exactly who it is written for, for people who were interested in the brain but had not had anything more than, say, a good high school course in biology. We had to speak in very plain terms and bootstrap our definitions as we got into it. But I have enjoyed it and I must say it has salved some of my feeling of responsibility for not being in an academic institution, for being in a research-only institution.

Yes, that was one of the points I was going to make; it seems odd in a sense that one of the people I think of as being one of the best communicators in the field, who has the capacity to communicate to people on the street, is you and you aren't in a university. Silvio Garattini is another such person.

Yes, right. Well, you know it is a matter of how you parse your time. I find being at a research institution gives me more concentrated effort to focus on the research and I do these other things in my private time. I enjoy that but I don't necessarily have a lingering interaction with students the way you would if you were giving a course. You know, tastes are a matter of personal judgement and I find this quite acceptable. I am sure you have had the same thing; you go to some place that has read your book and people will comment as you did or bring their copy of it to have you sign it

It isn't only those books though. A flyer for Psychopharmacology: The Fourth Generation of Progress *(Bloom and Kupfer, 1994) came in through the post about a week before I came over. This is at the opposite end of the spectrum. Far from for the man on the street this is the bible for most of us within the field.*

This again is a matter of love more than it is a matter of desire because this College means a lot to me. It was a major maturation point when I was elected for membership in that College and then I became its president. The previous three versions of the text had very good reviews but they weren't organized so when David Kupfer and I took this on we tried to do it in a way that would provide a logical skeleton. No matter where you were in your life's education you could find an entry point and then navigate through the rest of the book – we are hoping for it to work out that way.

You've introduced the issue of your involvement with ACNP; do you want to tell me more about all that?

Well, it was the same gentleman that I mentioned to you before, Nicholas Giarman, who was the person for whom we were doing the course and his close companion and collaborator in many years of research on serotonin, Daniel X. Freedman, who became one of my closest mentors in my scientific career. Both of them invited me to go; the first year I was a post–doctoral fellow at Yale and that would have been 1965. I was elected to membership in 1968 and I had a chapter in that very first book, 'The First Generation of Progress' so it goes back quite a way.

ACNP actually began if you look at the historical volume In the Beginning *(see Glossary) with a bunch of clinical investigators really concerned to get to grips with the issues raised by all these new drugs but it's changed character a lot; do you want to pick that one up?*

It was a very exciting time, probably a unique time in the history of brain research because we had drugs that seemed to cure mental illnesses and they produced very similar behavioural effects on animals and so that gave us an entry point. It was really the foundation of modern neuroscience because it gave us a way to connect the chemistry of the brain with the physiology of the brain in a way that you could now sort of think you had insight into the nature of mental illness. That was impossible before until the drugs provided the tools to do that. So studying the mechanisms of action of those tools became a very exciting opportunity and you could sense that in the field.

But it's funny, at that inaugural meeting my mentor, Daniel X. Freedman, was a member of that audience and yet I cannot find a single word attributed to him. Another of my Italian mentors, Erminio Costa, said a few things, he was associated with Dr Brodie. But I mean in this text he is associated with Dr Brodie quite a lot too. You really should interview Erminio too. He really is another pioneer. Erminio left Italy because the opportunities were here. He worked at the Himwich laboratory in Galesburg, Illinois which was one of the pioneering brain chemistry labs in that era. He then moved from there to Dr Brodie's Lab, all of which really put him in a place to see much of this in the happening.

Anyway, to your question, ACNP from the time that I knew it was a relatively small organization, 400 or 500 people. Non-participating guests were relatively rare. What has happened through the years is that the guest proportions have risen and because there are just so many good people in the field, we have relented on our membership size. It used to be that it was sort of a fixed size, set at around 400, so somebody had to die before somebody else could get in. Now I think we have closer to 700 members and we elect on average about 20 a year depending upon the whims and choices of the council. So it has grown and now the meetings maybe have a 1000 people at them and you can't really feel that you know everything that is going on in all the nooks and crannies of the meeting the way you once did. But science has matured. I mean there was so little to talk about in the early days – the facts were so few that we could spread them out, now there are so many facts and so many specialized interest groups.

One of the things I have heard about ACNP, which is what you hear about BAP also, is yes we have far more detail far more specialization but that there is a problem, almost a crisis, in that a greater and greater number of people are coming along to meetings and finding less and less on the programmes that seems accessible to them – you sometimes hear people say they don't understand even titles of many of the lectures or posters when looking through the programme.

Exactly. So what we have done for the last four years is have a teaching day specifically to provide – I don't like to use the word remedial education – but that is basically what it is. It still has not caught on to any great degree and we still hear that complaint because in part we don't school our presenters enough. I think if we worked with the presenter so that they actually understood that they had to simplify their language because they are talking to people who are not active in the sport although in the audience there will be people who are very active in that sport so that's the kind of problem that arises. I think scientific societies in general have not paid enough attention to that. The teaching day is good but then there are going to be people who are either too busy or too proud to go to a teaching day but who still would really welcome the thing and that's part of the motivation for Cooper, Bloom and Roth and for *Brain, Mind and Behaviour* – to say those things not in a demeaning way but I think really they are not that complicated if you really understand what you are talking about. It's just too easy to slip into codewords and buzz words that you forget what the origin is.

This is still a very clinically orientated college and if it doesn't connect back to mental illness in some way it seems to me that it could be any place. The years that I was there I tried to remind people that this was not the Society for Neuroscience. The Society for Neuroscience meets separately. This is the American College of Neuropsychopharmacology so good science is welcomed but it needs to be good science within the goals of this college.

There is a fear in recent years, in BAP, that it could break apart; the clinical people might feel that well there isn't anything left for us here, let's go back into the Royal College of Psychiatrists. Now you've recently had the American Society for Clinical Psychopharmacology formed by Don Kline for something like the same reason.

Exactly. Two of the previous presidents. Don Klein from Colombia, and George Simpson from Philadelphia, both were founding members of that because they felt that there was not enough clinical. They still come to ACNP and I guess that there are enough people that it really won't destroy the College. The college under the Presidency of Roger Meyer did a very self-critical examination of where it was going and it was decided that things really weren't so bad even if these people pulled out. Really, what the feature of this is, is not clinical only but the clinical/preclinical interface. And so in *Psychopharmacology: The Fourth Generation of Progress*, that's exactly what we tried to do. We tried to make it so that the preclinical scientists understood the nature of the diseases that they thought they were working on and the value of the drugs that they were using as tools and the Clinical Pharmacologists would understand the background at whatever level they chose to grapple with it. So we have introductory chapters and then we have more specialized chapters and very special-ized chapters but they all are self-referential. So if you want to know more about something or if you want to find out where something was introduced you can find the chapter where it began and hopefully that will keep that momentum going because I feel that's the real strong feature as it has been from the beginning of the discovery of these drugs.

I would just like to ask you about one or two more people that you've mentioned – Daniel Freedman. Why was his role in the field so important?

Well, you can get a flavour of the man by reading some of the obituaries and by reading the wonderful article that was written about him when he was the president of the American Psychiatric Association. That would have been in about 1982 or 83. He was among the very first well-trained psychiatrists to go to NIH, to learn modern methods of neurochemical analysis and apply them to the field of interest. His particular drug of interest was LSD. And the work that he and Nicholas Giarman collabor-ated on was the way in which LSD and other hallucinogens changed the brain's metabolism of serotonin and norepinephrine.

If you look around at who the major figures are in biological psychiatry on this side, they will often have one direct link to Daniel X. Freedman or maybe two but everybody felt as though they were linked to him because in addition to his kind of wisdom and experience he was a delightful person. He was always nurturing. I learned more about organiz-ing people and being critical but gentle at the same time, when I was on the study section of which he was the chairman. Although we weren't so close when I was first at Yale he offered me my very first job, when he moved to the University of Chicago to be Chairman and it was a very difficult moment to say 'no I didn't want to live in Chicago even though it would mean working with you'. But he made Chicago a very respectable place in psychiatry.

Later we served together again and became even closer. He went to UCLA and I felt like he was sort of in my backyard. When I got married again he was my best man. But on top of this he was everybody's best man. If you'd been to his memorial service, well, in fact we had an even more delightful occasion we had had for his 70th birthday, when the American Psychiatric was here in Washington, a rather large *festschrift* and the people were organized to make presentations according to the eight lives of Daniel X. Freedman as a scientist, as a teacher, as a mentor, as a philosopher, as a prophet, as a Government advisor, as an analyst because he was also trained in psychoanalysis as well as in biological psychiatry. His editorials for the *Archives* and his management of *The Archives of Psychiatry* had made it in our view the premier journal. And the person who took over the editorship, Jack Barchass, was a medical student who worked for him.

When I first came to Yale I worked with George Aghajanian and George was a direct lineage to Danny. And my co-editor of *Psychopharmacology: The Fourth Generation of Progress*, David Kupfer, was a resident at Yale when I was a research member of the faculty and that's where our friendship began and he remembers those days as shaping his career. The rich texture of biology that was intermingled as a matter of logic and course with the presentation of psychiatric concepts was what made that area a unique area. And I would say that today Yale is still one of the strongest centres for biological psychiatry.

You're touching on a point which is of interest to me which is that in the UK, psychopharmacology generally happened outside Oxford, Cambridge and the Maudsley. The innovative centres were in Aberdeen, Birmingham, Bristol, Cardiff, Merton Sandler's unit, Alec Coppen's unit, but not Oxford and Cambridge. Whereas, here, Yale and Harvard seem to have had much more say in the whole thing?

Although there is *The Handbook of Psychopharmacology* that Les and Sue Iversen edited, that was when they were still at Cambridge and before they went to Merck. And Marthe Vogt who was at Babraham in 1954 – she was really an originator.

That was in 1954 before the field actually took off.

The psychiatry part was outside and I think that's what maybe flavours ours a little bit more conceptually was that the psychiatrists here wanted to learn neurochemistry and so they built around themselves these basic science units. And I don't know what the structure was at Oxford and Cambridge then. The man who has been the head of psychiatry at Cambridge, Sir Martin Roth, has certainly done for Alzheimer's disease what these other people did for psychopharmacology in the United States so it certainly can happen but I think it just takes the right leadership. It is a very interesting observation.

I have this theory though which may be at odds with some of what has actually happened in the US, which is that the drugs and techniques that we introduce in an area like psychopharmacology subvert an approach towards science which is theory driven – you have a drug like LSD and it blows most theories out of the water immediately. So if you take the approach that being scientific is all about having good theories and maybe you chuck your theories out if the observations don't support them that won't work in psychopharmacology. When you introduce PET scans, for instance, people say well look we've got a new way to look at things, let's forget about the old theories and look and based on what we see we'll try and come up with some view that might fit the data.

I have no evidence that would say that that is an incorrect hypothesis. The people who I know, in my generation, in the UK, are very much of the same kind of approach that I have but that's perhaps because they came to the NIH for postdoctoral training and so we all were sort of milled through the same process that said that tradition was okay but the unexpected was the thing to expect. And so even if you didn't have a hypothesis, since you knew you had a very incomplete description of the phenomena and there were multiple ways to look at it, the first thing was to sort of flush up what you really thought you were seeing when you saw this.

Before there was dopamine to look at, all of the actions of reserpine were explained in terms of norepinephrine and then serotonin and then dopamine. So then it became very complicated. Which neurotransmitter is really responsible, which depletion really counts for making them depressed? So it's been a time of constant surprises and constant regrouping of hypotheses and most hypotheses are taken with tongue in cheek or many grains of salt because . . .

Except by the industry who get hooked on the amine hypothesis for instance and build their drugs according to one hypothesis. We have ended up with an awful lot of D2 blockers we don't get . . .

Clozapine is perhaps an example of a drug that breaks a little bit of ground and there are second generations of that one. But yes I mean it has been trial and error. In the day of that *In the Beginning* discussion, when the FDA requirements for testing drugs on humans were much less, then drugs moved pretty rapidly from a drug that did this in animals, without toxicity data, to let's see what it does to people. And if you read the original descriptions of the antipsychotics they thought they were going to see something entirely different and it was the clever clinicians who detected that there might be some place for this particular medication in that disease rather than this disease. Rather than treating battlefield shock it was really good for sedating disturbed people and that really led to a lot of rapid developments and modification of the drug molecule.

Let me just chase this further because again your work, in some respects, stands in contrast to how the field has developed. If you look back to the early meetings, for instance the one that was organized by Silvio Garattini in 1957, and you look through the programme, there was a lot of electrophysiology happening. Now that's very much classical science and it's functionally orientated and behaviourally orientated. Electrophysiology has at least in the UK, except for one or two people, really been lost. By the end of the 1960s there was very little work of that kind really happening. But you're one of the people here who has maintained that line of work, a more classical kind of approach – there's continuity in your work from Olds and Milner, Killam and Bradley through.

An interesting line. I started as a physiologist and my entry into the NIH system was as a physiologist and I think my training in internal medicine makes me sort of sensitized to functional questions. So it is not just knowing what the content of a particular biochemical is or the way in which its chemistry is changed; I want to understand how cell communication has changed and how systems of interaction are changed and really I would like to be able to understand how it's working in human brains. So, yes, I purposely have indeed tried to maintain a focus on functional questions.

That came through extremely strongly in your BAP Guest Lecture. The interest in it was that you actually talked about the effect of alcohol on the functioning of groups of neurones and through perhaps taking a more molar rather than a molecular view you seemed to be able to connect things in a way that was very exciting.

I have to. Maybe I don't call them hypotheses but I definitely have to construct scenarios in order to understand which experiments are really the most important ones to do next. There are so many things that can be done. So being able to bring yourself back to some scenario . . . If I knew that then I could perhaps reframe the orientation. I like to do an experiment that will really change things or at least tell me that I'm on the right track. If I do little experiments that don't really test the boundaries of the concept then I haven't really learned a great deal. It's busy work and it's probably publishable and interesting to somebody but it's not interesting to me if it doesn't help us advance where it is that we are going.

What about alcohol and alcoholism, where do you think its at?

I think it is at a very interesting time of departure because we have stopped focusing on what makes people intoxicated and started to focus on why do some people have difficulty controlling the termination of an alcohol consuming episode. What is it about individual differences that perhaps snookers people into becoming dependent on alcohol when others can walk away from it. And that same question I think pervades most of addictive drug research and maybe other behaviours that go under different titles like risk taking behaviours more generally.

For instance, take the work that is being done in France by Michel Le

Moal who works at Bordeaux. He has just reported that animals will self administer corticosterone; that they like the feeling of having high plasma steroids. We don't understand how they sense those but they will self-administer steroids to the level that their steroids would go when they are stressed – as though there is something about what we call 'stress' Well, you know the soccer game that we were talking about is a great example of that. If you watch human performance under times of war or times of sport and conflict, people perform at a level of physical and mental ability that they can't reach at other times. It seems that there is something about that. That to me is more interesting than why people are alcoholic. It seems to me that if I understood what it is about risk-taking, what it is about apparently self-destructive behaviour that has some mental reward-ing, even though perverse, capacity to it that to me would be an interesting insight. I think that's where alcohol research is now turning the corner to asking. Our animal models are being shaped in such a way that we can understand the importance of environmental cues in shaping repetitive drug consuming behaviour and that layered onto the genetic basis, which for alcohol research is perhaps the strongest of all of the addictive phenom-ena – you can breed animals to readily become dependent on alcohol so in theory you can understand the biochemical nature of what's different about them from the starting line that they came from. Which genes had been enhanced, which new combinations and how did they emerge. All that's going to be a Nobel prize in the next decade. And I think that is going to be a really splendid piece of mental construct on which to build.

The whole alcohol, drug abuse area is almost the murkiest of all in terms of the mad, bad kind of views of human nature.

I love to talk about substance abuse when I go to psychiatry depart-ments. I think it is the current best set of biological data and animal models of direct relevance to human mental illness. And whether you call it a mental illness on the order of schizophrenia or depression, there is certainly a strong component of substance abuse layered onto schizo-phrenia. If you look at any group of addicts, you find a very high proportion of people who are schizophrenic. There is a very clear overlap with depression, particularly with alcohol; alcohol, depression and anxiety track together in serious ways. And maybe a route of insight into the real nature of those biological problems will come from studying the addiction part since we don't have any good clues to get into the other part.

Any ideas what the answers will be? What are your current ideas of what it is that is actually happening in the brain?

In addiction, I think it's . . . at one level it's kind of simple. The brain is constructed with natural reinforcing mechanisms so that actions that are necessary to sustain the individual and the species of that individual will happen – the probabilities become very high. So we have these rewarding circuits. And the drugs that we call the drugs of abuse – I mean broccoli is not a drug of abuse.

No but it's got an awful lot of natural benzodiazepines in it. Maybe you've picked the one vegetable you shouldn't have!

Broccoli? I don't know. I was using it in a totally different way, David. You remember President Bush made popular headlines by saying that now that he was President he didn't have to eat his broccoli. Because to many Americans, broccoli, cooked the way mothers like to cook broccoli, is sort of like green library paste – it has no interesting features at all. I didn't know about the benzodiazepines, that's interesting, but for the most part you don't catch a lot of people abusing broccoli because it doesn't have any immediate reinforcing value and it doesn't have any value that you can remember afterwards – 'I felt really good after I ate that green stuff'. Whereas with really potent drugs that are abused there is both an immediate change which plays upon these chemicals which the natural reward circuits use and builds in an apparent feeling that that was really good, let's do that some more. I think it's through trial and error that human history has evolved these ways of intoxicating ourselves. Crack Cocaine is new but the principle isn't and Opium goes back thousands of years. Every society on the planet that can distil something has made an alcoholic beverage. So that goes back a long way.

But a lot of other things don't catch on; I mean you don't catch people abusing broccoli no matter what the time was. So I think that people have naturally selected by experimenting a lot and again it's this interesting apparent correlation with the experimenters, the pioneers, the ones who are out looking for things – let's try this! Maybe it is because they got a special rush out of this in the same way that Michel Le Moal's mice now are getting a rush out of the natural hormone of stress. Putting yourself into a kind of predicament and bailing out is a unique learning experience.

It's the survivors that get to share their wisdom with the rest and that carries with it a kind of philosophic mastery of the situation, so they became the medicine men and the more powerful people. They prepared the concoctions. The early forms of these medications had religious connotations – they put you in a mood to communicate with God and so a belief in the consumption of something that had magical qualities right from the beginning. So it has carried a place in our culture.

Some people would say that it's been the pharmacodynamic aspects of the improvement of these natural social medications that led to the addictive state – that it wasn't until you could really distil a more powerful beer that people had enough alcohol in the beer to make intoxication a problem. When it was low as in mead beer you didn't get enough out of it. So you got the very low threshold kind of stuff. A similar argument is that it was the discovery of the syringe that led morphine to be injected in a way that gave a rush that put the other rushes in the shade. In the same way when tobacco was used for cigars and for pipes you could only absorb it through your oral mucosa and so the amount of nicotine you got per puff was relatively low and it was long lasting. But the refinement of a different kind of tobacco leaf, with the process that makes it acid instead, led to the inhalation with cigarettes, which then gives a very powerful direct intra-arterial kind of injection to the head. So the pharmacodynamics have changed completely the use of what once was a more subtle form of pleasure. When you chew coca leaves, it's not a whole lot different than chewing gum with a lot of sugar on the outside. You got a little boost but it was slow and long lasting. But smoking it or injecting it gives something that is quite different and that's what leads to these powerful addictions.

So society as a group were of a mind to say that these plant roots have a pleasure value but tampering and tinkering has refined the critical elements; in a way that is not much different to what we would do if we went to Indian or South American Folklore to look for drugs to treat cancer. We would find the roots and the poultices that they would make and then our chemists would try to extract the critical features out of it and make a pill that you could take. Except, here we have done it in a way that is not treating any obvious illness and so we call it self medication.

And that causes all sorts of problems.

So I think anybody could be an addict. Some people might be addictable more than others because of their environmental situation. Yesterday we had a symposium that would strongly suggest that there has been a latent strong genetic theme in other forms of addiction that hasn't been recognized because we haven't followed people long enough to see it. But there is a strong concordance in monozygotic twins and in blood relatives of people who are addicted. So there maybe something there that hasn't been well recognized. And I think that, plus environment, gives us a large part of the apparent variability as to why people become addicted and how do you decide which ones they are.

Let me move back to things I probably should have asked you to begin with. You went to Yale and then you went to NIH and then to Scripps, can we go through what took you to each of these?

I started really at Washington University in St Louis. As a medical student, I did neurophysiology research. I stayed there for my internship and first year of residency. As part of our residency programme, one of the criteria for advancement to the upper levels was to be the winner of a research associateship at the NIH and so I applied for that and got that kind of a job and that's what led me into CNS research. It was such a powerful and exciting time that I choose not to complete my residency.

NIH at the time had Julie Axelrod and Seymour Kety there.

Yes, I was in the National Institute of Mental Health at the part that was at St Elizabeth's Hospital. Julie Axelrod was there and Seymour Kety. Costa was in the Heart and Lung Institute. In our part of mental health, we had a laboratory of neurophysiology that had in it Wade Marshall, who was a more classic macro-electrode neurophysiologist, and a lot of very hard core biophysics type people who were working mostly on spinal cord and didn't care very much about any neurone above the spinal cord.

Dr Brodie was in the Heart Lung Institute. Being at St Elizabeth's Hospital I was somewhat outside of that circle. I would come over for lectures three or four times a week. I guess, of all those people, I worked the most closely with Ed Evarts who was the head of another laboratory in mental health. He was trained as a psychiatrist but was a very good neurophysiologist and interested in mechanisms of sleep and how the brain activity shifts during sleep. He devised some of the earliest methods for recording from animals that were awake, certainly with unanaesthetized animals that were free to perform and do things. And he taught the research associates basic modern neurophysiology. I had only taken physiology as a medical student five years before but even then things were taking off rather rapidly.

So you said that things were so interesting that you actually gave up clinical practice . . .

Yes, I chose not to go back to finish my residency. I had been very interested in hypertension as a career and reserpine was a very interesting drug to me. So what I agreed with Dr Salmoirraghi, he comes back into my life many times, he was the person to whom I was assigned as a research associate. And he had taken into our labs a technique that started with David Curtis in Australia and John Eccles used a bit in his final days on the spinal cord, a technique called microiontophoresis, where the drugs were contained in one of the compartments of a multi-barrel micro-electrode and then you would use the electric current to essentially spritz small volumes out onto the surface of cells. It was a way to test the potential actions of drugs you thought might interfere with neuro-transmission.

There's a few people who claim they began microiontophoresis – Philip Bradley, for instance, was in there at the start.

He was one of the first as well. I don't really know who was the first. Certainly Phil Bradley has a deserved pioneering role in the field. He started with Joel Elkes to look at actions of LSD and other drugs and Elkes was the organizer of the group at St Elizabeth's Hospital. He was recruited from Birmingham to do that by Seymour Kety. The group that I joined when I was a research associate was called the Clinical Neuropsychopharmacology Research Centre and Salmoiraghi was the neurophysiologist of that group. The kinds of electrodes and the kinds of drivers that Dr Bradley's lab used were of a different quality and the kinds of answers they were able to derive were more limited because they were very coarse instruments. I mean they were maybe five times bigger – and the drivers that they were using couldn't generate the kinds of current you needed to get through high resistance small electrodes. So their results were somewhat confusing. David Curtis I think did it a bit more meticulously and by the time Salmoiraghi did it, he was certainly not the originator, but he was in the same way the Japanese didn't invent the autocar but they sure made it a lot better, I think that's where he would see himself as. Trying to refine the controls and trying to refine the kinds of questions that you would ask.

Before then people would publish data that a third of the cells went faster, a third of the cells went slower and a third of the cells didn't do anything. In the first volume of the review of progress for the ACNP, I wrote the chapter on spritzing; you will see a lot of that kind of data . . . but that was a transition point. From that point on we tried to get people to point their electrodes at places where it would make sense rather than just pointing at cells that were easy to record from. And it was that that drove me to do histochemistry because it was a way to put the chemistry at the level of the cells. So it wasn't just what did norepinephrine do on any old cell but what did norepinephrine do on the places where norepinephrine-containing nerves provided the synaptic input.

So you moved from there to Yale in the 1960s.

Well, after I finished the first two years at NIH, it was to devise a method of bringing to the physiology chemical information that drove me to Yale to work with a man named Russell Barnett who was recommended to me by my Dean at Washington University as somebody who really understood how to do histochemistry and understood the chemistry part of histochemistry. So I went there to work with him to work out chemical reactions that would allow us to see where neurotransmitters were located in reference to these things. And I stayed there for four years, from 1964, ultimately joining the faculty.

So in essence to some extent trying to do some of the same things that Fuxe and Dahlstrom and people like that were doing over in Sweden.

Exactly, 1963 was when their papers started coming out–1962 was their very first one on the use of reserpine to deplete the catecholamine and serotonin content of the brain and this formaldehyde fluorescence idea was terrific. It was like light microscopy and it was not very good light microscopy and the freeze-thawing procedure caused the tissues to be severely disrupted. So a lot of us looked at those pictures thinking that there must be an awful lot of structural artefact up there. My question was a slightly different question. I wanted to see it with the electron microscope because synapses are really not identifiable at the light microscopic level. At least in those days they weren't. Now with antibodies against proteins that mark synapses specifically you can get pretty close to electron microscopic information at the light microscope level. My desire was electron microscopy.

I had spent three or four months in the final days of the NIH period working with Keith Richardson, who had been the Chief Technician for the EM Lab at University College London but couldn't get tenure because he didn't have a PhD, so he was essentially driven from England and found work at the NIH where he became the Chief of the Laboratory of Neurocytology. A wonderful, wonderful man, who had such massive strong hands that he could do things that a very few people could do. Making his own glass knives. He taught me all these splendid primitive arts of electron microscopy and so I was very much convinced that electron microscopy held the answer to how to identify synaptic contacts with particular neurochemicals. And that was the approach I was taking with Barnett.

George Aghajanian and I worked together. He was a postdoc coming back from the army. His interest was in serotonin; mine was in norepinephrine and so together we worked out some of early methods to employ reuptake as a way of labelling nerve terminals with radioactive molecules. And that followed right on the heels of a paper that Axelrod and Potter did at NIH, when they gave it intravenously. They could see it taken up by the nerves of the pineal. That was the first demonstration of norepinephrine nerve terminals at the electron microscope level. So we said, well, if they can do that, we should be able to put it directly into the spinal fluid and see it in the brain, and Les Iversen and Jacques Glowinski were doing that biochemically with Axelrod at exactly that same period of time. So it made perfect sense for us to try to exploit it for electron microscopy and it worked.

George Aghajanian has been another very influential figure.

That's right. George was sort of Danny's extension studying the physiology and the biochemistry of LSD. And they came up with some very interesting hypotheses. George also trained at Edgewood Arsenal during a time when many of the cholinesterase inhibitors were secret classified weapons and as part of that he worked out blood assay methods for LSD and was able to correlate the duration of the hallucinations with it. He has spent much of his career trying to work out the neurophysiology of LSD actions in the brain as well as morphine. He was the first to observe that the locus coeruleus neurones were hyperactive when addicts withdrew. And the whole line of treatment of drug addiction has been based upon that. A very quiet, soft spoken man who has turned down many opportunities to leave Yale. He loves Yale. He loves the New Haven environment and he loves to play golf on Wednesday afternoons on the New Haven Golf Course and that's a comfortable life for him.

So I stayed there for four years. While I was away the NIMH broke away from the NIH and became a separate and hierarchically equivalent thing. The first Director of the NIMH was Stan Yolles, who emphasized service and health care delivery as well as the research arm. And so everything moved up a ratchet and the old section of neurophysiology was now the laboratory of neuropharmacology in the National Institute of Mental Health. Salmoiraghi recruited me back to have a section on histochemistry because he understood the importance of that and then he immediately became the Director of the division and so I moved into his job as Chief of that laboratory and I was able to work there very effectively for the next eight years.

So that took you through to . . .

The end of 1975 is when I got tired of government life. Salmoiraghi had left to become commissioner of mental health research for the State of New York and unfortunately my performance as lab Chief gave me his job as division Director and the person with whom I worked in the hierarchy was the head of the whole programme wanted me to become the permanent Director and I didn't want to be an administrator. I wanted to do research.

People had been offering me jobs for many years. The Salk Institute had sort of ambivalent connections to brain research. They were working on nervous system research, trying to do molecular neurobiology at a time when molecular cloning techniques hadn't been invented yet. And so they were spending a lot of valuable time deriving cell lines and doing very meticulous things in cell culture but they weren't interested in the brain. They were interested in cellular and molecular phenomena. They didn't understand the importance of the brain.

Jacob Bronowski had come there and had done the 'Ascent of Man' series and there was a reawakening of interest on the board's part to grapple with some of these more complex areas of neuroscience. So the President of the Salk Institute, Frederic de Hoffman, came to me saying that the Institute were interested in having a laboratory and did I have any interest and what would it take if I did. My standard answer to people at that time was we needed a million dollars to buy the equipment and set up the labs. Everybody else would say well I understand what you need but we can't afford that. He said let me get back to you on that. Three days later he called me back and he said I don't have the whole thing but I've got commitments for nearly a third of that and if you would be willing to come with me on some visits to foundations and various places I think we could put this package together.

My wife had died and I had two kids and I wanted to change the environment. So this seemed like the right way to go. Within a year we had the package put together and I was accepted by the faculty as someone who could be appointed as a Professor and we brought the group.

It was an exciting introduction for me to science architecture because before then I had only ever lived in labs that had been built by other people for other purposes. Now the Salk Institute is itself a piece of architectural splendour. Dr Salk himself, who had great interest in the brain and behavioural phenomenon, took great pride in the layout of this building and Louis Kahn had designed it for the maximum scientific flexibility. They wanted my labs to really meet the needs of what was going to go on. We didn't really have enough money to fill out the first 8000 sq ft, so we only built up to about 6000 of the 8000 sq ft at the beginning. So they sent an architect, who had designed other labs at the Salk Institute, to the labs in Washington and he spent two weeks photographing every step members of our group took, every hand movement that they did, to try and get things together. He would draw up these plans and come back and I would say no this is not right because this needs to be closer to that and that needs to be closer to this and he did that three or four times and finally he threw up his hands in frustration and said what you need is a laboratory that's shaped like a Kodak Carousel. I said what do you mean by that and he drew it – he said you need these things in the middle and everything else should fan out from there. I said fantastic, let's build that.

So we had a lab that had virtually no square walls in it at all. We had the computers which were very expensive in those days but the computers were the central tool to making neurophysiology expandable – so we could do it on a grander scale. At St Elizabeth's we had two rooms to do electrophysiology; in the new lab we were going to have six. And they were all going to run off of a central computer that would run the program and batch it out to each of the rooms. It was a very efficient way of doing it. The rooms were all colour coded – it was fantastic. But first I had to get Dr Salk to agree because all the other labs at the Salk Institute were square labs and here was a lab that was essentially a big cigar box with a Kodax Carousel at one end and everything else was a big wide open laboratory and it was magnificent. He looked at it for a while. He was a little resistant. In the end, he said well this just proves how great a design Louis Kahn did because it will accept even this so we were able to build it. It was exciting it really was.

How did it go trying to build up your own laboratory?

I went out six months ahead of time not really knowing how we were going to finance the continuing operations. I had dowry money that would keep us going for three years but I knew I had a ticking clock. In three years I had to make the thing self-sufficient. And so I hit on lithium as the thing to work on. This was because we knew how to evaluate sensitivity. We could look at changes in thresholds for neurotransmitters. We knew how to localize the best neurotransmitters and with lithium you didn't have to worry about drug metabolism, you could just simply administer the lithium in the food pellets. So we got the first two grants going in that way and it looked like such a nice formula that we then said well lets just substitute the word alcohol for the word lithium – we can measure blood alcohol in exactly the same way and we can look at these other things and that one worked.

During the time I was coming across the country was when John Hughes and Hans Kosterlitz identified met-enkephalin. The first six months that I got to the Salk Institute, Roger Guillemin who was in the lab next door, was also busy using his technology of peptide purification to look for other opioid-like compounds and he had identified alpha-endorphin and later gamma-endorphin.

I didn't have a lab yet so I took his peptides and went to David Segal's lab at UCSD and we were looking at the behavioural effects of these on animals and that directly led to a strong interest in these opioid peptides. So the third grant that we did was on the opioid peptides. The grants all met with success and they were all funded and so we were able to get fully funded within a year after getting to the Salk Institute. And from then on other grants just sort of naturally spun off.

I had made an arrangement with George Koob, who I had met while he was still in Washington. He went to the Iversen's lab to do a postdoc, combining biochemistry and behavioural pharmacology, and we recruited him back and he filled up the behavioural part. And we purposely picked a name for that group that was the Arthur Vining Davies Centre for Behavioural Neuroscience and the behaviour emphasis was there. The idea was that the cellular and molecular events should lead to understanding behaviour.

You've also had a range of strong people go through?

Well, I have been very pleased, one of our very first people who was at St Elizabeth's, when I first came, Roger Nicoll, was just elected to the National Academy of Sciences. Barry Hoffer is honorary Doctor of Science from the Karolinska for his work in brain transplants and explants. George Siggins is the editor of *Neuroscience Letters* and a very well recognized person. Bob Robinson is Chairman of Psychiatry at the University of Iowa. Efram Azmitia is Chairman of Neurosciences for the State University of New York in New York City. Gary Aston Jones is the Head of the Division at Hahneman University. So people of mine are all over the place.

One of the other key people in the field has been Erminio Costa.

Yes, because he started at a time when all we could measure was norephinephrine and serotonin and a little bit of this or that. He has always maintained a desire to improve the skills for measuring things and the ways under which they are measured and he has continuously led the field into what the most important technologies are that we could bring to bear to make it more sensitive, more accurate and more rigorous. So mass-fragmentography is one example. High performance liquid chromatography, he was one of the very first to devise assay systems using that technique. He was one of the very first to use molecular biology in neuropharmacology and among the very first to use patch-clamp analyses in molecular biology. And his concepts of the allosteric interactions of excitatory amino-acids and his natural benzodiazepine displacing peptide, those were novel concepts.

Have we gone too far down the cloning route? Up until recently there seemed to be some hanging together of the functional aspects of things and the biochemical aspects of things. But now with cloning, it seems to me we are producing all sorts of different receptors and the industry has gone down the route of saying well look let's just produce a drug that binds to this cloned receptor and to hell with any other way to produce drugs. Then move them as quickly as possible into man even without going through an animal model procedure. Are we entering a new reductionist era?

Well, you raise a lot of important and interesting questions. I mean the idea that you could build a drug properly to select for a receptor that has been cloned I think is a concept that hasn't been demonstrated. I don't know of any drugs that have been synthesized because we don't really have three-dimensional understanding of the cloned receptors. We can make these nice models of seven transmembrane domains and you can do a lot mutational studies that tell which parts recognize the transmitter and you can try to design drugs for them. But that's not really chiro-chemistry based on computerized reconstructions of enzymes that you can crystallize, where you can design for example in the case of the angiotensin converting enzyme inhibitors, a drug that really fits into the pocket and sees the metal that's critical and blocks the activity.

There are a lot of companies who are trying to do that but really it is a very long and drawn out process. How do you decide which receptor you really want to invest your coins in. And that's where the lack of understanding of the pathology seems to me to come to the foreground. We have some feeling that we know which receptors are important because of the me-too drugs we already have. So unless we want to have more of those drugs acting in the same kind of indirect ways, I mean they make mental health better but do they do it by fighting the disease or by assisting the natural reparative processes that the mind has? And I don't know that we know the answer to those kind of questions. Are they failures of the system or are they representatives of different kinds of diseases?

It would be interesting to ask that question to Herb Meltzer because he took clozapine on when other people weren't willing to invest in it. It was a very peculiar drug and he has now shown that medication-resistant schizophrenics actually can benefit from this drug despite its problems with bonemarrow abnormalities. So there are now three or four new clozapine-like drugs that are trying to reassemble the same mysterious combination of receptor features.

To an extent there seems to be some failure of nerve there at the moment in that we were going down the route having pure and purer drugs but the compounds that were being introduced weren't any superior. And what's happened with clozapine is that we've gone back to a dirtier drug which proves better.

A dirtier compound which through its dirtiness may actually achieve what it is that we are looking for. Now maybe there is a clozapine receptor for either norepinephrine, dopamine or serotonin, but probably not. And probably this is some kind of combination and so you know the older style way of starting with the behaviour and trying to get drugs that would have . . . I mean buspirone came that way. It was a drug that didn't look like a good anti-anxiety compound but somebody had the clever insight to follow it through and that's where the combination is. I am all for cloning but I think people need to be able to do behavioural pharmacology and we need to have a better understanding of the disease.

I'd rather invest my nickels in understanding the disease than in cloning more receptors and, interestingly, Les Iversen has taken that approach in his labs at Merck. I was on the committee that assessed the approach his unit took and I would say that he will get a splendid rating by our committee. It's true he hasn't come up with drugs but coming up with drugs is not easy.

I don't know if you read the stories in *Nature* or *Science* about the relationships that Scripps has had over its arrangement with the Sandoz Drug Company. It is an interesting feature of the field. A Congressman named Wyden, who is a Congressman from the State of Oregon, is in charge of a committee that was looking into drug pricing and at just about that time we announced that in 1997 we were going to have a 10-year relationship with the Sandoz Corporation – that we would give them options to patent discoveries and in return they would give us on the order of a $30 million base per year and in addition would fund research that might help refine some of the discoveries that they would be patenting. The Congressman took exception to this as giving away our discoveries so that this company could make millions off the drugs that they would develop. Well, the point is that none of the discoveries that we would make at Scripps are going to be pills. What we are going to identify are principles of how cells interact and where diseased cells may interact differently. Starting from that and making a medication that people could take safely requires maybe 10 to 20 times the amount of money and thousands if not hundreds of thousands of man hours of investment and time and a lot of luck.

In the same way Leslie Iversen has done some splendid research and although they may not have anything that is on the market today they've got things that are going to be on the market and they've built a system which is likely to generate things that will be on the market. Merck didn't have that kind of a presence in CNS research, before. They had some lucky hits but mainly they had L-dopa and some other things that they had licensed in. The process of going from discovery to getting a drug that works is a very arduous one and only companies with enormous resources can afford to stay in there long enough to wait for a new one to come up. Hoffman La Roche hasn't had a new drug in the benzodiazepine series and it's not from lack of trying.

The Private Research Institute is something that is very, very different that you find in the US that we don't find anywhere in Europe. Certainly not in the UK. The only person who has got anything comparable in Europe is probably Silvio Garattini. What is it about the US that produces these kind of Institutes?

I guess the Mayo Clinic was the first to have its own Research Institute because of the feeling of those physicians that having research done on site would give them an edge over people who had to read about it some place else. And because medical research has always grown up with the feeling that good clinicians can be good researchers – you know from Banting and Best who recognized diabetes and went into the laboratory to try to understand what principle of the body was at risk here. There has been a strong relationship between medical researchers and medical practitioners and so it was very natural for the Mayo Clinic and the Cleveland Clinic to have such an arrangement.

The Scripps Clinic was born in an era after the discovery of insulin when it seemed appropriate to have a scientific institute backing it up. The Salk Institute is slightly different in that the Salk Institute has no clinical facility. It was just a private research facility that sprang from Jonas' participation in the field trials for polio vaccine. The 'March of Dimes' said well if he can do that let's give him a place where he could do that for other diseases. That was the origins of it. I think private generosity charitable giving in our country is perhaps more organized to do this kind of thing than it is in other places.

Certainly you do produce very strong Institutes that can produce independent science. One of the arguments that Silvio Garattini would have is that if you work in the University, you can't really be independent. You have to fit in with government priorities and other such constraints.

Well, see we don't do that particular kind of research as much. In fact in this country a lot of clinical pharmacological trial research is done by people at Universities because it is easier for them to get those grants or contracts to do the research than to get the Federal ones at the moment. What I like about the private place is simply its independence. We can work on whatever we choose to work on provided we can raise the money for doing it. I mean that's the other risk is we don't have an endowment so being able to succour us through times of crisis requires a kind of relationship such as the one that we've had with the Johnson and Johnson Company and now that we have worked out the details the one we'll have starting in 1997 with the Sandoz Corporation.

When did you move to Scripps?

I moved to Scripps in 1983 so a little over 10 years ago. I moved because I had some growing pains. I had some feeling that the kind of work that I wanted to do was becoming too behavioural and perhaps too much involved with kinds of questions we have discussed – addictions and alcoholism – and if any of our work was really going to be valuable I thought it needed to be in a clinical environment. So being dissatisfied and looking at other jobs at the time, the people at the Scripps whom I had known for quite a while, and actually I was doing a collaboration with Richard Lerner, who has now become the Director; we were doing some the the first molecular biology asking how many genes are used in the business of the brain. So when he heard I was looking at other jobs, he said 'well why don't you come over here, I can get Johnson and Johnson money to help start you off' and I did. And it was terrific; its been terrific ever since. We have now grown from 8000 sq ft to more than 60 000 sq feet. We have a department of close to 250 people with a faculty of about 30.

There can't be too many larger shows anywhere outside of industry.

I think in terms of kinds of skills we bring together, which run the gamut in classic neuropharmacology – plus, purposefully, a very strong emphasis on neurovirology and neuroimmunology.

What role does the industry play here? There's a range of views across Europe from Germany where it's a very respectable career to have been a scientist within the industry to the UK well you're not a real scientist if you work within the industry – you really have to be in the University system to be a proper scientist. The attitude in the States here seems to be more open than in the UK.

I think it's just based on realism. On the one part industry is a pretty creative place to work particularly in start-up industry, where you can be dedicated to a very small frame of activity and you have the promise of good money and the opportunity perhaps for even an enormous amount of personal wealth should you succeed. And so that makes it quite honourable, especially when jobs are not available any place else and you want to work and you want to have state of the art equipment to work with and you want to have contacts with good consultants who can keep you on the straight and narrow.

It's not a bad life. Between Scripps and UCSD there must be 100 start-up companies that are based on ideas that have come from our research laboratories and where lots of postdocs are working very effectively in an environment that is very nurturing for them and they move up the ranks. As other companies spin off there are opportunities for them to take what they have learned and move on. So it's becoming a quite reputable area. And there are people in this college both in CINP and the ACNP, Paul Greengard is one, who spent a long time in industry and came out. Larry Stein, who is Chairman of Pharmacology at UC Irvine, spent a long time at Wyeth and came out. And I think people are moving back and forth; Sam Enna who is now Chairman of Pharmacology at Kansas went to Nova when it was growing and came back out of Nova to the academic area. I would think the transition is becoming more flexible, more dynamic. It used to be that people would stay in industry for long periods of time. But that's not everybody's cup of tea so it is quite natural for people to move on from time to time. Leslie Iversen will be another chapter in that history when he takes whatever his next job will be.

In the UK, when people look at the US, they say 'you guys get ahead because you're able to throw vast amounts of money'. Are there vast amounts of money here — has the for 'Decade of the Brain' made any difference?

Well, there really hasn't been any more money for brain research as a result of the 'Decade of the Brain'. It's a nice banner to carry at the head of our crusade but I don't know where it is going. I don't want to hop out of the army but personally I don't think it's the right way to do it. The people who are leading it don't want to come up with a plan. I think we can't convince Congress that we know where we are going unless we have a plan to get there. And just saying we need more money for brain research because its going to answer questions in the abstract is not convincing anybody. It certainly doesn't convince me. I couldn't get a grant to do it that way.

So we have to do more than just appeal in this way we have to get involved with the lay organizations, the NAMIs and the NARSADs — they're the ones who have the relatives with mental illnesses that need solving. If addiction were less of a dishonourable disease, there are a lot of people out there who could spring to the defence of why this kind of research needs to be advanced rapidly. Take AIDS, which is propagated mainly by dirty needles among addicts at the moment, I mean clearly if we're going to spend all that money on AIDS and we don't deal with the real problem that's . . .

Why people use needles.

Exactly: this is a behavioural disease. So, anyway, I think the 'Decade of the Brain' has not culminated anything and even though it does sound really nice practically it hasn't changed the situation. There is a lot of demoralization in the young troops at the moment because the criteria for getting a grant funded are so high that you may as well play the California lottery to get a grant. The funding levels are less than 10%. So your chances of getting funded are poor. It just has to be of such infinitely superb quality and what that does it channels you and it eliminates a lot of risk taking, a lot of creativity, at least on paper. You might do that work once you got the money but you can't express yourself in the way that you once could do so and in which creativity even by itself was a redeeming virtue on a grant application.

So in that sense the Europeans may over-rate what we can do. And there is a lot of splintering among our groups. There's a strong resistance to the kind of research that I enjoy which is sort of team research. Tinkering in the back room by yourself is unlikely to discover the kinds of answers needed for a problem like AIDS. What is it that causes the neuropsychological impairment of AIDS. That's why we have put together the neurovirology, the neuroimmunology and the classic pharmacology. Because nobody is looking at the degenerative disorders of the brain in a way that would model on the classic techniques that we have used in the past. We know nerve cells are dying. We don't know why. What's in there that is making toxins that are killing nerve cells? The answer to that may be reflective of why people lose nerve cells in schizophrenia which we don't really understand.

The European school of thought is strongly integrative – you produced the worlds' best tissue pharmacologists – all these receptors being cloned need tissue pharmacologists and system physiologists to put them back into living organisms. Physicians are about the last link we have as integrative biologists. Most programmes in pharmacology and physiology are totally molecular at the moment. Opioid peptides wouldn't have been discovered if Hans Kosterlitz didn't know how to do the Guinea Pig Ileum and the Mouse Vas Deferens. The classic skills of screening compounds – they are going to be more important and the premium will be high because there is nobody left teaching anybody how to do that except you guys. So forming an alliance with the classic schools of British pharmacology I think is a very critical thing to do.

To more or less finish up with where in some respects we should have started can I ask you why you went into medicine?

It went like this. I went to a rather small high school and when I was approaching the end, we didn't have career counsellors. Everybody in the city of Dallas went through this generic system of aptitude testing after which you were mailed the results and that was to indicate your career path. So my results came back that I should be in public relations, advertising and journalism and that I should stay away from hard science.

That fits what has happened perfectly to some extent in terms of communication doesn't it – maybe not the journalism?

Unquestionably. So I went home and I told that to my father and I said they gave me this list of schools and the one that looked really neat to me is the University of Missouri School of Journalism. He said Floyd you're going to go to medical school. After you get through medical school you can do anything you want to. But the only way that a Jewish boy growing up in Texas is going to be able to secure a life for himself is to be a physician. My father was a pharmacist, worked with doctors all his life, wanted to go to medical school but because of an illness he had to drop out of school. Then he needed to earn a living because it was depression time, so pharmacy was an easier route. And all of his life working with doctors he thought that the only thing his son could be and many Jewish families wanted their sons to be doctors. My son the doctor is a long-running Jewish joke in the United States.

Maybe aptitude tests aren't so useless after all.

It was definitely right. While my father was still alive and I would be interviewed and point that out, he'd always say what are you talking about, I never said that. But I can remember the afternoon very clearly.

Select bibliography
Bloom, F.E. (1987) The emerging pharmacology of ethanol. *Journal of Psychopharmacology* **1**, 227–36.

Bloom, F.E., Lazerson, A. and Hofstadter, L. (1985) *Brain, Mind and Behaviour,* W H Freeman & Co., New York.

Bloom, F.E. and Kupfer, D. (1994) *Psychopharmacology: The Fourth Generation of Progress.* Raven Press, New York.

Cooper, J.R., Bloom, F.E. and Roth, R.H. (1991) *The Biochemical Basis of Neuropharmacology,* 6th edn. Oxford University Press, Oxford.

The changing face of psychotropic drug development

I was born in Belgrade and I have spent my childhood and adolescence there. Pharmacy and medicine were the tradition in my family. As a matter of fact one of the first pharmacies in Serbia was founded by my great-grandfather Antoine Delini, a French physician who apparently came to visit the country and then never left it. To study medicine was for me therefore obvious and natural since very early. I went to medical school in Belgrade.

Why did you leave Belgrade?

My decision was primarily influenced by a stay in Dusseldorf, where I had lived and spent some time studying and working. I would have probably stayed there, but life plays some tricks – the man I was in love with lived in Belgrade. Since he didn't want to leave the country, I came back to marry him. But thereafter and for many reasons, my decision to leave was firm. Among these reasons the beginning of my involvement in reseach was certainly an important one. I came to Switzerland in 1966 and this has been my home since then.

Did your early research have anything to do with the CNS?

Primarily not. When I finished medical school, due to the fact that there were no immediate positions in the Institute for Child Psychiatry, in which I wanted to specialize, I started a training in pharmacology at the Institute of Pharmacodynamics in Belgrade. The project I was working on was related to the investigation of some plant extracts and their allergenic properties. How we got a sample of metoclopramide, a benzamide derivate with a request to have a look at the compound, I don't exactly know. But my debut in psychopharmacology is related to this drug, a predecessor of sulpiride. Since metoclopramide was used for treatment of gastrointestinal disturbances, I was interested to see if it has some protective effects on reserpine-induced ulcers. I found that indeed it had. But I also noted some slight central activating effects. In order to understand this interaction with reserpine I went to study the literature about the mechanism of interaction with reserpine. And that was my debut in psychopharmacology.

You can imagine that there was not much to find in the literature at that time, since the very first papers about psychotropics started to appear only in the early 1960s. But my interest in these drugs and their mechanisms of action was awakened and to me it was suddenly evident that psychopharmacology was what to do next. But where? Who was strong in the field at that time? There was practically no university research in Europe. Most of the research was concentrated in the pharmaceutical industry. Geigy Laboratories in Basel was therefore the obvious choice because they were among the leaders in psychopharmacology and famous because of the discovery of imipramine.

Who was there?

The head of CNS Research was Dr Walter Theobald, who died in March 1995. He was the pharmacologist and essentially the 'biological' father of imipramine and the series of its analogues (desipramine, clomipramine, insidon, carbamazepine). He was the one who initiated the clinical studies with these drugs.

When I came to Geigy I intended to stay there only for a limited period of time, to learn about the backgrounds of psychotropics and then to go back to clinical practice. This period, however, never ended.

My first task was in the general screening laboratory. It was a very good start. Everything I did and had to do made sense to me. General screening combined all the techniques available at that time by means of which psychotropic properties could be identified. Among them, however, the one I credit with major importance was the general observation technique. I learned how to observe from the late Clara Morpurgo. I owe her most of my interest in psychopharmacology and my education in basic scientific principles. She was an exceptional personality, creative and pragmatic at the same time and a born scientist. Unfortunately she left Geigy about a year after I came, otherwise I would have probably progressed much more rapidly under her guidance. But so I had to learn everything by myself, by trials and errors and own experiences. There were no teaching facilities, no handbooks, not even monographs about psychotropics.

With Clara Morpurgo I worked first on the elaboration of a standardized, so-called drug-interaction test battery and operationalized observation technique in mice, which could be suitable for rapid and reliable recognition of various classes of centrally active compounds. The method was published in one of the issues of *Drug Research* in 1968. For a long time we have successfully used it as a routine procedure. Clara Morpurgo also encouraged me to start the development of animal models for testing psychotropics. Brain lesion-induced catalepsy in rats as a model of Parkinson's disease, conditioned hyperthermia as a somatic counterpart of anxiety, and several others that I have elaborated later on, were based on some principles that I have learned from her. These models were extremely useful, because they were not necessarily dependent on a preconceived hypothesis of the mechanism of action of a drug.

That's not the way drugs are found anymore.

No, all these screening techniques are more or less abandoned today and replaced by *in vitro* receptor binding assays or other molecular biology techniques. But at that time there was nothing else. We knew almost nothing about the functioning of the brain. Not even DA receptors in the brain were known at that time. All these discoveries came later. So the only instruments you had at your disposal were your eyes, your observation, your imagination, a search for analogies and extrapolations of what you saw in animals to clinical situations. It was a fantastic time. The observation and the search for analogy with clinical phenomenology were essential. There was an extraordinarily tight bond with the clinics. Nobody needs today to be medically trained to do research in psychopharmacology, but then – without that medical knowledge it was almost impossible to translate experimental findings to the clinical situation and vice versa.

How did clinical training count?

Well, we operated with simple and maybe very naive analogies from today's perspective. We thought, if you can produce convulsions in men, well by the same means you can produce convulsions in an animal. If you have a treatment against convulsions in men – and we went to the laboratory from the clinical observation – then any drug that you discover to have anticonvulsant effect in animals will have to exert the same effect in man. Cardiazol or electroshock convulsion were for instance models for petit-mal and grand-mal seizures as reserpine-induced depression was a model for testing antidepressant properties. There were also simple behavioural tests, like for instance the fighting mouse or the isolation-induced aggression as tests for anxiolytics. By testing and analysing a large number of drugs, by comparison to those already known to be active in the clinic, we elaborated a spectrum of activity that we supposed a new drug had to have. There was not much biochemistry. The interest in a compound was decided upon the spectrum of action in animals, upon quantitative or qualitative differences to a standard and assumptions about analogies. The fact that this was an efficient approach is illustrated by the number of major antidepressants that were developed during this period.

It was the only way to begin?

It was the only rational way to begin. It was an extraordinary way also because it was combined with so much learning about behaviour, about the mechanisms which control it and about CNS physiology. The investigating drugs were also a means to investigate the pathophysiology of brain functions. Geigy did not have a specialized CNS biochemistry unit, as was the case with Ciba. The importance of biochemistry increased only after the merger of the two.

Maprotiline was a Geigy drug or a Ciba drug?

This was almost a parallel discovery. I first worked on maprotiline in Geigy. The compound was synthesized by Dr H. Schröter and I have tested it (Delini-Stula, 1972). By intuition almost, because its particular biochemical profiles was unknown to us in Geigy, Dr Theobald proposed it for development. But I think Ciba had a priority in the patent application by about three months and Geigy had to abandon it. Anyway, after they merged it didn't matter who was the first.

An awful lot of people at that time operated by hunch. Brodie seems to have been a man who went on a hunch.

Absolutely. Why for instance did Dr Theobald selected Insidon for development − a drug which was unimpressive in the screening and did not even do much biochemically? I remember the discussions about that. An extraordinary simple philosophy was behind that − we have imipramine and we know what imipramine does. *Ergo*, we will look now for variations around the spectrum, a little more of this, a little less of that! Amazing, isn't it! So, Insidon impressed by its 'softness' as an antidepressant but it had more marked anti-aggressive properties.

Why did Ciba and Geigy merge? And what was the atmosphere at the time?

The atmosphere was very dramatic. Probably because it was the very first big merger of that kind. There were even suicides. The shocks produced today by mergers, economic crises, loss of jobs and functions are also dramatic, but I haven't heard about casualities of that kind. But, at that time the fact that you lose your job or position due to such an event was perceived as catastrophe by many people in Switzerland. Geigy staff probably suffered more than Ciba since the dominance of Ciba was obvious and their more authoritative management style was felt immediately. This was also the case in the CNS department headed by Professor Hugo Bein.

His is a very famous name.

Yes, he was a very famous name. He was also a very authoritative and sharp-minded person.

Tell me something more about the different management philosophies of the two companies?

Geigy was rather a family enterprise, where I felt there was a lot of respect for people's individualities. I am talking about what I have experienced; some may have seen it differently. Geigy was perhaps conservative and rigid, but rather human, at least I experienced it that way. Ciba was larger, with a stricter hierarchical order, and it was more impersonal. Anyway, the time in Ciba was quite different from the one I have spent in Geigy. Professor Bein left perhaps a year after the merger. After him none of the heads of the Biology Research Department were really CNS men having any psychiatric experience or background in the field. We in our CNS department managed somehow by ourselves.

The department was large and encompassed the CNS psychopharmacology group, which I was in charge of, and the CNS biochemistry group. Luckily, the collegues I had were all talented, dedicated and creative personalities. Retrospectively, it was the most productive period of my life, if you judge by the number of CNS compounds that were in the development between 1975–85. Ciba was among the first to have highly selective noradrenaline and 5-HT reuptake inhibitors as well as selective MAO-A inhibitors, even though the company never succeeded to introduce any of these into the market.

How were the 5-HT reuptake inhibitors discovered?

Their discovery is the best example of concept-guided development. It was based on Carlsson's findings of differences in the potency of various tricyclics in inhibiting noradrenaline and 5-HT uptake and his hypothesis of the role of noradrenaline and 5-HT in the control of mood and drive – for example, that 5-HT might be more important for mood regulation than noradrenaline. The idea to look for a preferential or selective 5-HT uptake inhibitor as a better antidepressant was therefore almost obvious. So we put a lot of efforts into screening 5-HT-reuptake properties of drugs. Ciba had an excellent biochemistry group and, as I said, I consider myself lucky to have had the chance of having such good colleagues as for instance Laurent Maître (who was also the head of the CNS department), Peter Waldmeier and Peter Baumann to name just a few. We collaborated intensely with each other and I still believe that this is important, because biochemistry alone, without integration of functional testing, cannot provide the necessary bridge to the clinic.

But it was a period where people were thinking about serotonergic and noradrenergic depressive subtypes.

Yes, therefore drugs with selective 5-HT- or NA-uptake inhibiting properties were also considered as a means to identify possible subtypes of depression. We already had a highly selective NA-uptake inhibitor (oxaprotiline) in development (Delini-Stula *et al.*, 1982) and we thought it will be important to have its counterpart – for example, a selective 5-HT- one. Also other companies had started the same programmes in the early 1970s. But I believe that we were among the first to really have one, CGP 6085 (Waldmeier *et al.*, 1977). The drug went into human pharmacology testing, but was cancelled, last but not least because the decision-makers in the company did not share our confidence in this type of drug. Curiously enough, the company always insisted and asked for drugs which will not be me-too, but through all these years they never really had the courage to persist in developing a really novel drug.

Why, what went wrong?

Laurent Maître and Peter Waldmeier may remember even better the tedious discussions and our fights for the novel projects and for each of the drugs we proposed for development. But, I believe the essential problem was that the research was mostly managed conservatively, by those who were unfamiliar with medicine in general and the CNS field in particular. There was nobody there who understood the complexity of psychiatric research, experimental as well as clinical. The eternal question was: 'What is the proof that you are right? Where are the facts?'. But, if you have a new concept how can you have the evidence without clinical experience? How can you have hard facts after early clinical trials ? How do you explain the pitfalls of bad study designs and a lack of statistical significance in a clinical trial or the importance of reproducible findings by experienced clinicians to those who believe that the only truth is $p < 0.05$? We were helplessly trapped in a circle of the most ridiculous types of reasonings. That's how, for instance, oxaprotiline, the most selective NA-uptake inhibitor, was killed, a drug which was certainly clinically efficient and very well tolerated, as it was recently demonstrated by a retrospective analysis of data. But, what I regret most was the fact that levoprotiline, the inactive enantiomer of oxaprotiline, was not pursued and properly clinically tested.

Now levoprotiline is an interesting story.

Levoprotiline was a unique means to test how correct the hypothesis of noradrenergic involvement in depression was or, more precisely, how important are presynaptic mechanisms for antidepressant properties. Biochemically, with respect to the effects on monoamine metabolism, the drug was inert (Waldmeier et al., 1982). But it showed antidepressant properties and similar efficacy to oxaprotiline as well as tricyclics in several comparative clinical trials. We desperately argued for a rigorous placebo-controlled trial to prove its antidepressant effects, but never had it approved. You realize the importance of such confirmation – it might have been the breakthrough in our concepts about the depression and mechanisms of action of antidepressants. The frustration related to the levoprotiline story, with all the other frustrations due to the loss of so many promising compounds, was a final impetus for me to leave the company. Somehow I couldn't deal anymore with what in my opinion was a mismanagement of clinical development also.

I had started to increasingly involve myself in clinical research during the last five years in Ciba because, perhaps arrogantly, I thought I could influence it for the better. Nevertheless, of the almost 20 interesting and active CNS compounds in the portfolio, Ciba succeeded in bringing none of them out. The last development failure, as far as I know, is brofaromine, a selective MAO-A inhibitor, discovered in our screening in the early 1980s. This is a rather tragic and upsetting balance of accounts if you consider the excellence of CNS research in this company. Every new concept or finding of importance emerging from the basic CNS or clinical research was immediately implemented and further elaborated. We had a certain freedom in exploratory research which is practically non-existent now. Apart from benzodiazepine research, there was no other area where we were not actively engaged and at the front. From this point of view it was really a fantastic period.

You began to go back and train in the psychiatry?

Yes, because I wanted to follow and clinically test myself the drugs, which I thought are so precious for the further progress in the field. Essentially, I have never lost the contact with the clinic. In between I had sabbaticals at Psychiatric University Clinics in Basel and Zurich where I had the chance to work with late Paul Kielholz and Jules Angst, respectively.

What was Paul Kielholz like? He was a seminal figure in developments.

Yes, he was. Somehow his name and his personality fit very well together. You have never met him? He was impressive with his tall, fatherly figure and extraordinary charisma. The patients adored him; many feared him. It is difficult to say why it was so. When you talked to him you always had the feeling that he was able to see through you. He had this kind of slightly amusing smile as if saying – you know, everything is fine, don't take the things so seriously. That was also his attitude towards science and biological psychiatry. It's nice to have a bit of neurobiology, but don't take it too seriously. I don't think that he cared about beta- or alpha-receptor regulation concepts, or even really understood much of the biochemistry. He was down to earth and concerned with clinical practice all the time. But he was an authority and somehow he managed to put his mark on biological psychiatry, without – I ought to say – a truly scientific achievement.

Concepts like masked depression?

For instance. He put it forward because it thought it of practical import-ance for everyday clinical practice. He didn't like things which did not appear to have immediate clinical relevance. His classification systems were meant as a help and guidance to the practitioners. He didn't care about their scientific validation. His classification was very influential in Europe but he was also interested in concepts like target symptoms and he picked up on the idea of the MAOIs possibly causing suicide because they affected catecholamines.

Many of the things that he has postulated were designed to guide psychiatrists in their daily work. This was a didactic approach, based on his observations and his clinical intuition. But, there is no evidence that they are really correct.

No, there isn't, they were speculative concepts almost, but the idea of target symptoms and suicidality caught on despite the lack of evidence, which maybe says something about his powers of persuasion.

Yes, but also it reflected his cautious attitude. In clinical practice, the primary thing in his mind was not to harm and not to compromise anyone and not to compromise himself. So he didn't want therapeutic failures or problems or anything which might throw a shadow on the reputation of his clinic. For instance, his assumption that MAO inhibitors, or any kind of antidepressant, which lacks sedative properties would promote suicide was based more on intuition, but was accepted as a fact by almost everybody without ever any scientific evidence that this is true. This was the power of his personality and authority.

You also trained with Jules Angst?

Yes, I have spent some time in his clinics too. You can say that if there are two fundamentally different personalities then they are Paul Kielholz and Jules Angst. Kielholz didn't care about scientific precision or even maybe scientific truths, while Jules Angst was careful about every single scientific detail and believed only in facts. Paul Kielholz was a very social person and politically engaged. Jules Angst was rather withdrawn and exerting his influence at a different level. His contribution to psychiatry is remarkable, it will remain and will be referred to and quoted after a hundred years, which I doubt will be the case with many Paul Kielholz contributions. So you see the difference.

You came be in charge of research medically?

When in 1987, due to one of the reorganizations at Ciba, our Clinical Neuropsychopharmacology, that is, our Phase I/II, group was integrated in the Clinical Research and Development Department, I moved entirely to Clinical Research. Geographically it meant from Biology Research on the one side of the road to the Clinical Department on the other side of the road. But it was like being transferred to the other side of the ocean. There were profound differences in the hierarchical structures, management attitudes and styles between two departments. In Clinical Research, there was more rigidity, bureaucracy and, I am sorry to say, a lack of professionalism in the management of clinical studies. When during one of many restructurings of the Department the responsibility and authority of the heads of the groups was transferred to business-orientated managers without a medical background, I perceived that as a programmed disaster.

But did this affect CNS specially?

Perhaps CNS only, but I don't know exactly. Anyhow, CNS is the most difficult and complex research area. You don't have objective and well defined measures of mental states and their changes. Today the credibility is given to numbers, to 'hard' facts. But, can you explain a schizophrenic mind with numbers only? Medicine trains you more than any other science to operate with an interpretation of integrated observations, with 'soft' signs and a quick synthesis of personal experiences with given reality. I firmly believe that you will never be able to make a proper diagnosis of a mental disease only based on 'numbers'. This applies also to the understanding of the meaning of, let's say, Hamilton Scale scores. Can you justify the efficacy of a drug simply on the basis of a HAMD score? Well, you cannot develop a drug if you blindly consider the HAMD score difference as the only 'evidence' and, above all, without ever having experienced a depressed patient. You cannot do a good clinical trial if you don't have an understanding of clinical reality.

The introduction of Good Clinical Practice principles in Ciba at that time was certainly a must and none of us in clinical research has negated the importance of it. But somehow I think there must have been a big misunderstanding of what GCP means and of how it should have been implemented. Many of the control systems, which were imposed on us because of the lack of trust in our performance, ended up in increasingly rigid bureaucratic procedures and delays of decisions. They turned out to be rather counter-productive, inhibiting and demotivating. Well, I couldn't cope with that. I couldn't work for the lack of success. Luckily, when my decision to leave was almost ripe, I got the offer from Roche.

That's a bit like moving from AC Milan to Inter Milan, isn't it?

Not entirely. I was moving out of Basel. Roche opened a new International Clinical Research Centre on January 1 1990 in Strasbourg. On January 2, I was there in a position of responsibility for the CNS research unit.

Why outside of Switzerland? Was the industry slowly leaving Switzerland?

I don't think this was the primary idea. I think the idea was to have a clinical research centre within the European community in order to be more flexible and to have easier access to experienced people from different countries. My task was supposed to be a building up of a research programme in schizophrenia – it was quite a challenging task for me. There is a lot of research and development in depression, justified, of course, but much less so in schizophrenia. I had felt that this is a field where a lot more research should be done. My project was related to one of the partial benzodiazepine agonists (bretazenil), which accidentally was shown to have some antipsychotic properties. The whole story about benzodiazepines and their antipsychotic potential has been a matter of debate over decades. So I felt there was something challenging to do and to learn about the benzodiazepines. All the methodological problems of clinical trials in schizophrenia also interested me.

Was Willy Haefely involved? He was one of the key people, who for some reason isn't known about so much?

Willy was a very good friend of mine and of course he was involved. He was the Head of CNS Research in the Biology Department in Roche. He was also another exceptional personality. I think there wouldn't have been any deep understanding of benzodiazepines without Willy Haefely. He was their father. An extraordinary mind. Very creative. If you have an image of a scientist as he should be then in my eyes it was very much Willy Haefely.

It's curious, if you read the books, people talk about Leo Sternbach but while he was involved in discovering chlordiazepoxide, Willy Haefely was the benzodiazepines.

I think I already said this. Essentially it's a very strange thing that there is a reference to the chemists who have synthesized a drug but hardly any to the biologist who discovered its potential. That there is reference to the chemist is perfectly all right. But the work done by the biologists, the astuteness of observations, the creative mind which sorts something meaningful out of the observations so that you can go further – nobody ever mentions that. The merit of the biologist who is sitting, observing and investigating the effects of the compounds and providing the conceptual framework for their development, as was the case with Willy Haefely, is rarely adequately praised. Now, whether he was right or wrong in some of his hypotheses that's a matter of debate, but I think this is irrelevant. Even the wrong concepts are stimulating. You go and find what is wrong and so it means further research and progress.

Anyway you entered the area with the issue of the partial agonists . . .

Yes, and the project went very well. But, unfortunately, two years afterwards Roche's interest in developing bretazenil for schizophrenia just faded and the project was abandoned generally. I have the impression that classical psychiatric indications are slowly losing their importance for big companies because I believe, they are not considered as very profitable. The development starts to be cumbersome and costly. The management sees only the difficulties and maybe perceives that at the moment in this area there is a kind of a steady-state. There is nothing conceptually really truly new. And maybe this is discouraging them from investing in this kind of research. Nowadays you have a very tedious and long road ahead of you if you want to develop another antidepressant, neuroleptic or tranquillizer. So there is a loss of interest in the classical CNS indications.

In a sense, then, we're at the end of an era, aren't we?

Well, yes, I would guess it is so. I don't know whether the extent of changes in the CNS field is as dramatic in other companies as the extent of change that I have perceived within the three big Swiss companies. Ciba–Geigy, a leader in antidepressants, abandoned research on antidepressants by 1986/87 or maybe even earlier. There was no further active research in antidepressants. In Roche the same thing is happening in the benzodiazepine field and in Sandoz, I guess, in neuroleptic research.

Why did Roche run with moclobemide when Ciba for instance didn't develop brofaromine?

The climate in Roche and the climate in Ciba were not identical. In Ciba the changes to 'business-orientated' research and development started very early, already in the mid-1980s. When I came to Roche in 1990, the structure and organization were different. But it doesn't mean that there were no difficulties in developing moclobemide. Nevertheless, personal authorities still counted. First of all, there was Mosé da Prada who discovered moclobemide's properties, then there was Willy Haefely and Roman Amrein, head of CNS Clinical Research. They were very strong and dedicated personalities who believed in the concept. In Roche, at that time, the opinion of such personalities was still respected.

But they had to cope with the legacy of the MAOIs?

Certainly. This had a big impact on the development and acceptance of the drug. The disbelief that a MAOI-type of drug, even if novel, will be accepted in USA, was probably decisive for the attitude of Ciba. I believe that unless there is the trust that you will have the USA market and have a sizeable profit, the big companies do not want to engage in the development of any drug. The costs of the development are just extraordinary and without that market the return-upon-investment is probably uninteresting. Roche certainly has the same attitude today, but to have the USA market was apparently not so decisive some years ago. The research succeeded with moclobemide really at the very last moment.

Has there been a problem in marketing moclobemide in that its the only RIMA?

This is of course unfortunate for the drug, because it is hard to argue about a drug class if you have a single compound only. From the scientific and research point of view every drug measures itself against another one. This helps to acquire a better knowledge, to improve and validate the concept, and to gain the confidence of the users. It is a pity that Roche has no follow-up development. What they intend to do I don't know.

Let's turn to the European College of Neuropsychopharmacology. Were you involved from the start?

Yes. The idea of founding the ECNP came from Per Bech and Carl Gottfries, who proposed this at the 25th Meeting of the Scandinavian Psychiatric Society. In 1985 they invited a group of representatives of other societies to Copenhagen where the proposal and the first outlines of the College were discussed. At that meeting the late Ole Rafaelsen proposed me as a member of the constitutional board, that is, the Executive Committee. That's how I came in. The idea about ECNP was enthusiastically accepted at that meeting. Also I have identified myself with it completely.

What did people hope to get from ECNP?

First of all I think there was a need to have a platform within Europe, a kind of forum of those people who have contributed here in Europe, in one way or the other, to the research in the field. There was CINP, of course, but CINP was not representative of Europe and not any longer what it was in the beginning. A kind of exclusive club where everybody knew everybody. The meetings are now huge – 5000 persons or more and the activities not transparent any more. The second reason was the existence of ACNP, which is a very influential society and not only of scientific importance in giving direction to the research in the field. ACNP is representative of American opinion and politically important. In Europe there was no counterpart of the ACNP, and the CINP circle was not a proper platform to profile European biological psychiatry. So many of us felt that we needed a society where we can unify our experience and promote European standards and concepts. A society which will be a partner for discussion with our American colleagues.

There was also more and more an impression that European biological psychiatry was overwhelmed by American psychiatry. Of course, that's a development, but we should not forget that many of the 'American' ideas had been generated essentially in Europe. We are facing a very curious situation. You generate the fundamental things and they are taken overseas and all of a sudden you have to digest what they portray as their own creation. Isn't this a frustrating situation? I think all these motives were behind the idea of ECNP. There was also no association at European level, which would have been the one to give direction to young scientists, to give them the opportunity to profile themselves within Europe and compete with the Americans.

How did it happen that I was the first President-elect? After the meeting in Copenhagen we decided to organize the first ECNP constitutional meeting in Brussels which took place in 1987. At that meeting the general assembly elected C. Gottfries as a President, Per Bech as a Secretary and me as President-Elect, based on number of votes that the proposed candidates received. So that's how it happened. But at the following congress in Göthenburg somehow things went in a different direction and many decisions of the Brussels assembly were not respected. All of a sudden some other forces entered into play and nobody was prepared for that.

Other forces being . . .

It is a very delicate thing to talk about and people may think that what I say is because I was disappointed. This is really not the case. The procedure at the Göthenburg meeting was just irregular. There was a lot of manipulation behind the elections at that general assembly. Anyway a new Executive Committee was formed and another President elected. I understood that maybe what was wanted was a bigger and more influential name. I am not such a name for sure. A few of us who were initially in the Executive Committee couldn't however accept how the original idea of ECNP changed under the new presidency. We found that it turned out to be just another kind of society but not with the profile it was meant to have at the beginning. Maybe now the things will change again because there are new people in the Executive Committee.

It certainly hasn't become an ACNP-equivalent yet.

Definitely not. It doesn't have anything so distinctive as the ACNP has. It's just another society. Sometimes they have good meetings, sometimes bad meetings. But there is no specific attraction or motivation for any young person to think that it's a particular achievement to be elected a member of ECNP.

Where did the idea for a European Committee for standardization of clinical trials in Europe come from?

The idea came again from Per Bech. Initially we (Per, Jenny Wakelin and myself) were a sub-committee group of ECNP. But since we received no support for our activities from ECNP, in 1990 we decided to work independently. We wanted to find a way to promote standards of CNS clinical research in Europe in harmony with Good Clinical Practice requirements, European and FDA guidelines, but also considering the application of the newest scientific achievements. There wasn't any support for this kind of initiative in the ECNP. ECST is aimed to deal with clinical methodological problems generally. We felt that's what is really missing. The meetings that we have since 1991 in Strasbourg confirm this. I have proposed Strasbourg as the meeting place because I was there and I could really help to organize it. Those who participate in our meetings are quite enthusiastic about it, because our approach isn't academic but orientated towards practical solutions taking into account the newest findings.

It's one area that needs to go forward – the area of clinical trial designs and methods . . .

Definitely. I believe that there is a big gap between what the research can do and what can be proved in the clinic. A gap that is very difficult to bridge. The industry had a restrictive policy with respect to truly research-orientated trials but without industry you just can't do much.

One problem for ECNP is that at almost the same time the Association for European Psychiatry was formed and surely it would have always been hard to get two European organizations to start up at the same time. Another thing, as you said, is that the companies are beginning to leave mental health for the neurodegenerative areas.

I feel that we are facing almost evolution-like dynamics in the field. You had the time of big developments in psychiatry. Now we have a phase where we are as in a steady-state with our biological concepts. I don't think, with these kind of concepts that we have now, we can do much more than what we have done. Obviously you enter then in a phase of apparent decline. Perhaps the research will have to go again in the 'wrong' direction and then there's hope that there will be a turning point for something very new to emerge. But at the moment the pharmaceutical industry restricts developments and experiments. Even those who are big in CNS have limited their involvement. They support only those projects which appear to be the most profitable from the marketing point of view. There is more and more stringent selection as to who and what will be supported. The flourishing phase is certainly over. The new introductions nowdays are essentially drugs which are 10 or 12 years old or more.

Nobody works on animal models anymore. What are the implications?

Or very few and they are farther than ever from clinical reality. There are very few medically trained people in this kind of research today. Many learn about mental disorders from the DSM classifications and then believe they know what the diseases are like. They believe that if you have a drug which attacks receptor X, this will solve the problem of treatment, but that is naive. You can't progress without animal models from my point of view. But they need to have some construct validity and predictive value. You cannot really know what will happen in a living organism if you are only testing *in vitro* or in some isolated biological systems. This is so obvious. But creation and validation of conceptually novel models needs new drugs, clinical testing and decades of work.

You could argue that the only way now that we could actually find new antipsychotic agents or antidepressant agents would be by going down the neurodegenerative route because people will be trying to produce something completely different, which may co-incidentally . . .

Indeed, but you have to have the chance to test them and to go back to the models. On the other hand, because there are such restrictions now on the use of animals in research, you also have a problem. You have to justify every animal that you use so you just don't want to get into this trouble. But I really strongly believe that we will not be able to make any really new discoveries without a certain liberty of exploration, without preconceived hypothesis as to what you should find. With all the limitations imposed today by public opinion, authorities, rigid clinical development schemes and lack of resources, I am rather pessimistic about serendipity.

You were involved with AGNP, the German Society, before ECNP; what was it like?

I liked very much the AGNP because it was a small society. There were about 200 members, a number which was kept constant for years and years and among them were all the grand names of German-speaking psychiatrists. AGNP was influential because actively involved in political life, in taking the positions about actual issues and research activities via its working groups. It's a very active society but very transparent in the organization. What I liked about the society was that you could come and talk informally about your findings at the meetings. Everybody knew everybody. AGNP is a tradition, which maybe you also see in the BAP but hardly in any other societies, which are starting to be so huge and anonymous. AGNP as a platform for communication was very productive. From this point of view I like the kind of societies which really keep a certain standard in the membership and remain somehow modest.

The influence of industry on these things is mixed, isn't it. You've got to have the industry to produce the drugs and you've got to have the industry to support the various different societies

This is always a kind of partnership. The problem is that everything becomes so commercial, everything is business-orientated – there is no more real partnership just for the sake of the science. It's partnership just because there is buying and selling. Why was this different in the past? Because I believe that there was a period when the industry, science and the clinic lived in a system of mutual exchange and support without so much money directly involved. The clinic needs good drugs, but clinicians seem to be obliged to buy and promote every sort of rubbish because there is money involved. That's where there starts to be a problem.

Is what you're saying the industry needs clinical people to be independent and they're not?

I'm certainly for an independence of mind and objectivity. I am working for the industry but I want the freedom to be independent in my scientific opinions. If a drug does something which I think should be said that it does, I want it to be said. I never wanted to change my opinion just for the sake of the market sales. But it starts to be a problem that a lot of things are presented in a way which suits the marketing, but not scientific objectivity. That's where I think some people may be selling themselves.

Select bibliography

Delini-Stula, A. (1972) *The Pharmacology of Ludiomil in Depressive Illness* (P. Kielholz, ed.) Int. Symp. St. Moritz. Hans Huber Verlag, Bern, pp. 113–23.

Delini-Stula, A., Hauser, K., Baumann, P., *et al.* (1982) Stereospecificity of behavioural and biochemical responses to oxaprotiline, a new antidepressant, in *Typical and Atypical Antidepressants, Molecular Mechanism* (E. Costa and C. Racagni, eds) Raven Press, New York, pp. 265–70.

Delini-Stula, A., Vassout, A., Hauser, K., *et al.* (1983) Oxaprotiline and its enantiomers: Do they open new avenues in the research of the mode of action of antidepressant?, in *Frontiers in Neuropsychiatric Research* (E. Usdin, M. Goldstein, A. Friedhoff and A. Georgotas, eds) McMillan Press, London, pp. 121–34.

Waldmeier, P.C., Baumann, P.A., Wilhelm M., *et al.* (1977) Selective inhibition of noradrenaline and serotonin uptake by C 49802-B-Ba and CGP 6085 A. *Eur. J. Pharmacol.*, **46**, 387–91.

Waldmeier, P.C., Baumann, P.A., Hauser, K., *et al.* (1982) Oxaprotiline, a noradrenaline uptake inhibitor with an active and inactive enantiomer. *Biochem. Pharmacol.*, **31**, 2169–76.

19 Gordon Claridge

The psychopharmacology of individual differences

In your 1970 book Drugs and Human Behaviour, *you said that psychopharmacology is a meeting ground. One of the people who came to meet there in the early days was Hans Eysenck. Can I ask you about your view of Eysenck's work and theory?*

I came across Eysenck first when I was an undergraduate because I did psychology at University College London and he taught personality theory there. That was from 1950 to 1953. I was impressed by him. He was one of the few people, who you could say gave a really systematic set of lectures on this subject. I was really impressed by what he was saying — that there were ways of approaching personality scientifically. To be honest I can't remember whether the drug part of it was in the theory at that stage but the point was that a drug postulate was intrinsic to the theory in a sense . . .

That was the McDougal idea, the idea that there was a factor X corresponding to introversion and extraversion . . .

Well, it was really the idea that there were biological bases to personality and the fact that you can examine that in two ways. You could simply select people who were introverted and extraverted and see whether they differed on some major biological measure, factor X or whatever it was. Or you could use drugs which shifted people along the introversion – extraversion dimension and see whether you could make people, as it were, more or less introverted or extraverted on these biological measures. That wasn't exactly part of Eysenck's published theory in 1950. The drug postulate actually came out rather later, so he probably wasn't talking, at least in print, about it at that time. But from the very beginning, at any rate as far as I'm concerned, there was a natural connection between what you could do with shifting people's behaviour temporarily with drugs and the sort of permanent differences in their behaviour that related to

Based on an interview previously published in Claridge, G. and Healy, D.(1994) The psychopharmacology of individual differences. *Human Pharmacology*, **9**, 285–98. Reproduced with permission from *Human Pharmacology*.

personality. So that was really how I got into Eysenck's theory as an undergraduate and then, after a while, I went to work for him.

The idea that a psychologist should work with drugs has recently been an almost alien one; were things very different then or was this just Eysenck?

I don't remember there being any problem about that. One had very relaxed relationships with medical people who necessarily had to oversee the work. I never had any problem with that. I suppose Eysenck was a fairly influential figure research-wise and was able to recruit medics to facilitate the research – so it was a slightly protected environment in that respect and I'm not sure what it was like outside to be honest. One was all rather caught up within this 'Eysenckian industry', as it were and didn't pay too much attention to what was going on outside! I suppose this kind of research was a slightly unusual thing for a psychologist to do, but it just flowed naturally from the kind of approach Eysenck had to individual differences (Eysenck, 1963).

Looking from here, one of the key things that happened during the 1950s which appeared to give the drug postulate a kick-start was the work by Charles Shagass on the sedation threshold. What impact did that seem to have then?

It had a great effect on me and I took some credit I suppose for doing quite a lot of work on it for Eysenck and developing that particular theme within his department. The other thing that came out of the sedation threshold of course was the link to an experimental psychopathology of abnormal behaviour. It brought home the point that a lot of individual differences in drug response, as they relate to normal personality, were just part of a bigger theory about relating individual differences to abnormal states. This was the connection to psychiatric disorder, which is fundamental to Eysenck's theory. Any work which went on that was connected, say, to drug response of psychiatric patients was automatically relevant to work on individual differences in normal personality – and vice versa. So the sedation threshold work, which was very much an attempt to find a diagnostic test for psychiatric illness also had a relevance to what Eysenck was trying to say about normal individual differences.

I got involved in that because my role in Eysenck's department was to look at the psychiatric end of things. I was attached to the Army hospital in Southampton most of the time that I worked for Eysenck and so I got interested in the psychiatric side. That led me to look at Shagass' work, which Eysenck drew my attention to, and I developed an alternative way of measuring the sedation threshold with Reg Herrington. Working in isolation in this army hospital without very much knowledge of the literature, we decided that there ought to be another way to do it instead of using the EEG. So we developed this very simple technique of getting people to double numbers while they had injections of sodium amytal. We often said afterwards that if we had read the literature on the sedation threshold we would never have done it because when we looked at it later the methodological problems were immense. Nevertheless we just steamed on and decided to do it and in actual fact it worked quite well (Claridge and Herrington, 1960 and 1963; Herrington and Claridge, 1965).

You were working with Eysenck from when?

Well, I did my PhD in what in those days was called mental deficiency, then called mental handicap and is now called learning disability. I did that with Neil O'Connor on a quite different topic although I did actually apply some of Eysenck's ideas to temperamental differences among the learning disabled. I then, after a short time working as a clinical psychologist, went to the army hospital at Netley, associated with Eysenck's department. This was between 1957 and 1961.

When you say 'within the Eysenck group', as it were, who were the key people in the group?

Well, almost all the people who were working on the individual differences side of things, at some point dabbled with drugs. There were people like Irene Martin, for example, who has just retired, and Harry Holland who sadly died. There were also studies by Treadwell and Rodnight on another sedation threshold procedure, using nitrous oxide. Most of the people who actually worked for Eysenck at some point were pushed towards having a look at the effect of drugs. You must remember that I was actually in an outpost in Southampton, so a lot of people who went through briefly I didn't know.

Individual differences as construed by Eysenck – what are they for a jobbing psychopharmacologist.

Basically what Eysenck believed, and still does, was that you have a number of personality dimensions, the central one of which is introversion – extraversion, and people range along these dimensions, which are mostly genetically controlled and hence reflect different sorts of nervous systems. In the case of introversion – extraversion, he used the concept of arousal to articulate that – that introverted people have rather arousable nervous systems and extraverts have rather less arousable nervous systems. So it's a kind of temperamental theory of personality. The other dimension, neuroticism, which is seen as a sort of amplification factor – if you're neurotic *and* introverted you're very aroused. And then the P-dimension – psychoticism is a very recent addition, which in my view Eysenck hasn't really said anything very useful about in terms of biology. But that's the basic theory.

He tied the introvert/extrovert dimension to the reticular activating system and the neurotic one to ANS reactivity, didn't he?

Well, to limbic system arousal – or 'activation' as he called it. He distinguished between these two ideas: arousal connected to introversion and activation to neuroticism.

What about the P axis? Nobody seems very happy with it; on the other hand it does seem to have a certain empirical validity.

Well, in so far as it refers to another domain of psychiatric disorder and the one that's sort of left over from the others, I suppose, one would expect some correlation with psychosis. In fact other approaches to the question have been more successful, particularly the schizotypy concept. This also has to do with differences among normal individuals but it was derived from direct observations on schizophrenia rather than as a more abstract factor developed from a personality theory, as in Eysenck's case. There are several things that are weak about Eysenck's P—dimension. For one thing psychiatric patients don't score very highly on questionnaire measures of it. Secondly, it's very unformed at a biological level. And finally insofar as a biological basis is proposed – that it has to do with aggressiveness – it seems quite inappropriate as a major theory of psychosis: I don't think anybody who knows anything about it would say that the crucial feature of, say, schizophrenia, is extreme aggression. Quite to the contrary in fact.

What came out of the work for you? Can you give me a flavour of what it was like working on the sedation threshold?

Well, I did two sorts of experiment with drugs and personality which fitted in with Eysenck's drug postulate. The first used the 'fixed dose' method. Here you take a laboratory test which has been shown to differentiate, say, between introverts and extraverts or anxious and non-anxious patients and .then, with a small dose of sedative or stimulant, try to shift the subject's performance on the test. In this way, according to the theory, you should be able to make the person temporarily introverted or extraverted, or anxious or non-anxious, by mimicking the underlying biological status of these personality factors. I did a number of experiments like this. But I didn't find that approach very interesting or very informative. I'm talking here especially about introversion – extraversion. I always felt it was a somewhat naive approach to understanding a complex personality dimension like that.

It was much more exciting with the sedation threshold, where you give a varying dose and where the amount of drug is itself the measure of the individual difference you are looking for. I think Reg Herrington and I – and incidentally he should be given a lot of credit for the work –

found a very simple, usable and reliable method of measuring these drug differences. We showed some quite dramatic differences between subjects within psychiatric populations; we were able differentiate major groups of neurotic patients and apply the sedation threshold usefully in schizophrenia research. At that time it seemed to be a rather exciting development.

Why did it not catch on?

Well, of course it's a fairly drastic technique for a start. It's not an easy matter I suppose to give people sub-anaesthetic doses of barbiturates. It involves putting people to sleep at sometimes quite high doses, which raises an ethical question. From a diagnostic point of view I suppose you could argue that it doesn't add that much information. Perhaps it is interesting from a research point of view but one might ask whether psychiatrists really need to inject their patients with massive doses of barbiturates to find the kind of information about their mental state that the sedation threshold can give.

I wonder about that. It makes sense to say that we have extraverts and introverts and that they handle conflicts in different ways but one of the interesting things – for me anyway – is that for some reason for the last 20/30 years we've been reluctant to diagnose hysteria – as if we don't want to know about the extraverts and their reaction style. If we had a test that would detect our hysterics better, it might be useful.

I suppose from that point of view, yes. What is interesting to me, having now moved more towards teaching undergraduates about psychological disorders, is how much of the literature, in respect of the neuroses, just focuses on anxiety and reactive depression: in Eysenck's terms, the more introverted, neurotic type of individuals. I raise the issues of hysteria and psychopathy in tutorials and lectures but it doesn't really ever catch on. There isn't a *Zeitgeist*, as it were, about it – if you talk about hysteria, people think of it as some kind of historical anachronism. But there are people of that sort of personality still around and, yes, it would have been interesting to have kept some sort of objective test procedure for differentiating hysterical forms of neurosis. The thing is, again, people find it difficult to believe when I tell them this, but when I worked in the army hospital we actually had very, very dramatic cases of hysteria.

We have it still . . .

What I can remember about these people is that the sedation threshold procedure did put them out like a light. There was no kind of deception about it. Their sensitivity to barbiturates was amazing. In fact what was so interesting was the very large variation that you could find among psychiatric patients: some, the highly anxious neurotics and obsessive –

compulsive patients, had massive resistance to barbiturates, and others, the hysterics and psychopaths, were supersensitive. But the sedation threshold did seem to die out. Possibly because of the ethical difficulty in the end. But then a whole lot of test procedures like that died out. A lot of psychophysiological research actually didn't lead to any practical test measures in psychiatry really.

What else died out . . . ?

Well, I'm thinking of things that correlated with the sedation threshold, like galvanic skin response and some EEG measures – and a lot of other laboratory procedures, like perceptual tests, that Eysenck pioneered as measures of personality and psychiatric disorder. I think that in normal personality research it all faded out because it turned out to be much more complicated than Eysenck suggested. But I'm not sure that it's the only reason in psychiatry. One of the strong points about Eysenck's theory that I found, especially using the sedation threshold, is that it does work well in extreme psychiatric populations; like differentiating between disorders that partly represent exaggerations of underlying normal personality traits.

One or two other possibilities for why things fizzled out are that the drugs that formed the basis of the theory – the barbiturates and amphetamines – became much harder to use and secondly the fact that the antidepressants, when they came along, turned out to be sedatives rather than stimulants, at least the tricyclics did; was that a problem?

I think what happened with the emergence of the antidepressants and so on, was that there wasn't really a simple theory that could be locked on a theory like Eysenck's. It was after all a very straightforward theory dealing with classical stimulants and classical sedatives and I think antidepressants didn't quite fit it. And Eysenck's theory you must remember has never been very physiological. It was pseudophysiological. He could handle these rather gross classes of difference but I think once other drugs came in then the theory wasn't able to accommodate them. And there weren't other people around with that kind of sweeping vision so that he had to do it instead. Others worked along similar lines with drugs but it's been on a much more limited basis you see. So I think Eysenck was telling, and has continued to tell, a fairly simple story about fairly simple differences in the temperament aspects of personality. And drugs were just one part of that programme.

If you look back at the programme for the first two or three CINP meetings, Eysenck was a guest speaker, which probably seems extraordinary to biological psychiatrists now. But when he came out with his drugs and personality article in the Journal of Mental Science *in 1957 he was really in a sense one of the few people at the start of the psychopharmacological era who had a cogent theory that was there to be tested. Were you aware that, quite apart from the work he was doing in the UK, that he was such a big name in psychopharmacology, was there a feeling that psychopharmacology was the emerging branch of psychology in a sense, or is that going too far?*

I don't think actually Eysenck went down very well in America but he was very influential in Europe and I know that a number of German psychologists and psychiatrists and others were very taken with his work. My own interest at that time which I suppose was coloured very much by Eysenck was in those parts of psychology that were interdisciplinary. I was interested in psychosomatics, psychopharmacology, anything which connected psychology to other disciplines. My own view was that that's how science should be and I think Eysenck thought that too. Psychopharmacology would not be taken over by psychology but simply that there were shared concepts and methods. It didn't seem particularly odd to me that there should be that kind of interchange between naturally adjacent subjects and I think the fact that Eysenck was talking in these conferences was some recognition of that.

Who from the psychiatric side was working in this area? What about Malcolm Lader?

That's right. He's one of the outstanding figures when you think about it. He was very accepting of psychology and he was looking at the same sorts of things really, for example, the galvanic skin response and things like that in anxiety and in response to drugs. This was very close to Eysenck but had more influence in psychiatry than Eysenck did. I suppose the reason Eysenck may have become less popular, was a general thing about him, which is that he has tended to try to put forward fairly sweeping and over-simplified statements that lost credibility. This has also contributed to his reputation as too much of an academic psychologist, such that gradually what he says seems less credible and valid to psychiatry. It would be interesting to know Malcolm Lader's views on that period. He was certainly the one who stands out as doing parallel research.

When did that particular period end?

For me it ended probably some time in my early Glasgow days – I continued to follow the literature but there wasn't very much after that. Around the time of my book *Personality and Arousal* in 1967, there was a sense that a lot of people had lost interest. I carried on with the sedation threshold for a while because the other offshoot of that was an application to anaesthetics. The idea that you could titrate people's dose levels as it were, how much anaesthesia they would require for an operation.

Has anyone tried to do that on a mass screening basis?

Not that I know of although I did it on an experimental basis. I worked with an anaesthetist and we measured sedation thresholds using premedication. We found some correlation with personality but they were all rather complicated relationships and it never caught on. Interestingly, not all that long ago (two or three years ago), somebody in the Glasgow Behavioural Science Department came to see me and they were working on that. There seemed to be a sort of residual interest in trying to index differences in anaesthetic levels, but it was more ongoing anaesthesia during the operation than trying to work out tolerance levels beforehand.

There were one or two other people playing around with methods of monitoring. But I think it was then beginning to get detached from the personality aspect as far as I could see.

Where did your interest in LSD come from?

Actually that goes back to when I worked for Eysenck at Netley. He sent me to Netley to specifically look at neurosis to try to develop experimental measures for differentiating dysthymics and hysterics. But I was rather naughty and got interested in schizophrenics in the end. I started to use some of the tests I'd been using in the neurotic group with the schizophrenics; this included the sedation threshold. And so my interests shifted more and more to the idea that you could apply the same kind of ideas to psychosis. Eysenck had already done that – so that was nothing very novel. But he hadn't published much on it and certainly nothing on the P-scale at this point. Nevertheless, it was in his early theories that you could map dimensional models on to the psychoses.

So I got interested in psychosis and when I went to Glasgow I had a sort of half—formed idea that you could apply to schizophrenia the drug postulate idea of shifting behaviour with an appropriate drug. And that's how I got interested in LSD. If you could show differences between schizophrenics, say, and normal people in a particular measure, like galvanic skin response, then it ought to be possible to produce a drug model of that physiological effect with, say, LSD or mescaline or whatever. That's what I did. When the drug was legal I gave LSD to normal volunteer subjects to see whether one could produce a temporary nervous system state that was like that which I believed might be true of schizophrenics.

I had originally done a lot of work on schizophrenics looking at what I considered, and still consider, to be the crucial thing about their nervous system. Which is that they seem to be in a chaotic, 'dissociated' sort of state – some parts of brain function seem to be disconnected from other parts. At the time, I formulated this in terms of an arousal model: that schizophrenia was a dissociative brain state due to a failure of some kind of homeostatic mechanism, leading to peculiar patterns or profiles on psychophysiological measures of function.

One thing I did some work on to test this was the galvanic skin response and a perceptual test called the two—flash threshold. I found that the association between these measures in schizophrenics was very peculiar – and unique to them. So I then gave LSD to normal subjects and produced the same effect in them. I believe that that was a good model for schizophrenia, although admittedly the underlying physiology was obscure. But the thinking behind the method was identical to Eysenck's drug postulate: manipulating the nervous system with an appropriate drug to produce a state – in this case 'psychosis'—— which replicated the state to be found naturally in some people.

Was there any correlation with psychoticism or anything like that?

I didn't know because the P-scale wasn't around at that time and schizotypy research hadn't properly emerged either. But, in retrospect and reading the literature since then – although there isn't a lot of it because of the problems with LSD – I think there is a good reason to believe, yes, that the reaction to LSD is coloured by the personality and had the P-scale or some equivalent been given, that would have come out; that is, the LSD effects would have been greater in people high on a psychoticism scale or schizotypal traits. That was certainly my strong clinical impression in just looking at subjects and looking at the literature since then.

In a sense if you ask me when the period ended, I would have said somewhere around 1972 and your article on the schizophrenias as nervous types (see References). What reaction did you have at that time? It was a very clear statement of a particular point of view . . .

Well, it's interesting you should ask me that because I have more recently published a sequel to it.

Yes, I was going to pick up on that a bit later.

Well, the reaction to the 1972 article was actually rather favourable. It was accepted in a psychiatric journal (Claridge, 1972). It was reprinted in the *Annual Review of Schizophrenia*. Yes, I think the psychiatric response to it was quite favourable. That was a period when people were perhaps less settled in their views about these questions. There was a sort of transition period between the Laingian period and a more biological era. I think people found it quite an interesting contribution which contrasts rather with its sequel (Claridge, 1987).

Contrasts in what way?

Well, one of the 1987 referees, I might say, was quite rude. Indeed I had a great deal of difficulty getting it published. It was rather insulting. I had to answer all these insulting comments.

What was the problem. If you were to publish your 1987 article now, when the whole field of psychiatric genetics has swung toward a more dimensional approach, I think there would be a very favourable response.

So feelings have changed rapidly, haven't they? I think that's probably true but I have to say that at the time the paper was published, the dimensional view was rather sneered at actually. It was seen very much as a psychology view. Schizophrenia had been pulled into a discrete medical model and there wasn't very much room for dimensional ideas. They looked too much like reversions to Laingian concepts, which was quite wrong in that what I was putting forward was a very biological concept actually. But nevertheless they were interpreted I think as rather antimedical. But there does seem to be a shift back now and schizotypy is the flavour of the month and it's beginning to take off a bit.

It's curious the way things go. There are Zeitgeists and fashions . . .

Yes, and they seem to move rather rapidly in a cyclical manner . . .

Who else is working in this area? There are clearly the schizotypy people and psychobiologists like Cloninger and Van Praag who have recently been putting forward dimensional theories of personality.

In schizophrenia research I would think of the American schizotypy people but in the area of more general personality research I would think of people like Marvin Zuckerman who produced the concept of sensation seeking. He's an obvious person. The other person in this country is Jeffrey Gray. His work has obviously been very much part of the dimensional tradition. In the case of Eysenck's original two-dimensional theory, he was important not only because he shifted the axes around but also because of his work to establish the proper biological basis for these axes. And of course he used drugs to do that (Gray, 1982).

Do you want to comment on that. Are you one of the people who thinks that rotating the axes was a good idea?

Well, I think it actually says something about the whole style of Eysenck's theory. You see I think Eysenck's theory is more limited as a theory of personality than he would claim. I think it is really a theory of temperament rather than personality. In other words I believe there are, for example, some fairly fundamental differences in reactivity, which you can see even in small babies and in animals. It is very biological therefore and undoubtedly in my view there are substantial genetic determinants to what I would call our temperaments and that Eysenck has rather elaborated too much into a theory of personality which I think is a broader term. Jeffrey Gray's theory seems to me to fit that temperament idea rather better. The concepts he rotated the axes to − anxiety and impulsiveness − seem to me to fit onto the brain rather better. Differences in fearfulness and anxiety make sense as basic temperamental differences which are going to be related to some brain system, whereas differences in introversion and extraversion and so on don't seem to have quite the right sound about them as temperamental concepts or so I think . . .

Too much top down rather than bottom up . . .?

Yes, that's right. I think that Jeffrey's way of dealing with it is more plausible really because it not only fits the notion of these basic biological influences but it also fits the notion that these theories are more to do with temperament. They are much more limited actually than Eysenck claimed. They are not so predictive I suspect of a wide range of social behaviours but they are predictive of some rather extreme psychiatric states. It is very significant that if you take, say, people who have had chronic neurotic anxiety the theory works very well. This shows up in the sedation threshold results. It reflects some basic difference in nervous system responsivity relating to anxiety as a temperamental trait. Similarly with the psychopathic state or hysterical personality, where you're picking up on some deficiency in that respect, with theories like Eysenck's and Gray's − and hence with tests like the sedation threshold − you are not saying anything about, and shouldn't pretend you're saying anything about, the more subtle aspects and traits of personality that stem from this disposition.

There is some independence of personality from temperament?

Yes. They − i.e. personality traits − belong more with other sorts of personality description I would say.

You mention Jeffrey Gray's work with drugs.

Well, I think in a way that Gray's theory was the salvation of Eysenck's theory in a biological sense in that Eysenck's own theory was sort of stuck with a rather old fashioned pseudophysiological view of personality. His concepts were initially Pavlovian and then based on rather gross psychophysiological concepts. Whereas Jeffrey Gray attempted to get at the real brain even though it was in a rat. In so doing he rescued the theory, which was in danger of becoming a kind of phrenology I think. If you look at Eysenck's last statements about the biology of personality he split the brain into two bits which relate to the two dimensions, a very simplied view of it all.

I think in rotating the axes, Gray also made the theory more usable in terms of the sort of behaviours that flowed from dimensions of personality like anxiety. It always struck me as an awkward, and, probably for psychiatrists, not very helpful statement, to be told 'Here we have a patient who is high in neuroticism and low in extraversion' as a description of an anxious neurotic. And that may be one reason why Eysenck's theory is not employed very much in the psychiatric setting. It doesn't seem to say very much whereas at least Gray's attempt to relate it more to the underlying anxiety mechanisms might I suppose say something about potential drug effects, for example.

Are you aware of people like Cloninger in the US and Van Praag in Holland who have tried to construct a 3-axis system, each of which is tied down to a particular neurotransmitter?

It seems all a bit over simplified to me somehow. That's one thing that has led me away from these ideas. I'm not so convinced anymore that you can dimensionalize people's behaviour in these ways and say, well, that's that transmitter and that's another transmitter.

People seem to be going a step too far?

Yes, too reductionist and too simplistic. It seems to me that if you select your evidence you can construct these schemas but there is a lot of cleaning up of the evidence in order to do this – I think that's even true of possibly Eysenck's theory itself – an attempt to arrive at just a few descriptors which map neatly onto some biological descriptors might be altogether too low-level really. It partly comes down to factor analysis and what interpretations you draw from that.

Maybe the factors in factor analyses of personality questionnaires are just artefacts and people and the brain just doesn't work this way. You can't take a factor in isolation and say that it is 'due to something'. Factors are statistical concepts pulled out, as it were, for the moment in order to look at what's making up the variation. I've thought about this quite a lot in the past about Eysenck's dimensions and other dimensions because they are not very dynamic. They are a kind of static, cross-sectional view of individual differences in a population but it's not clear how these would begin to interact, as they necessarily have to, in order to describe the ongoing behaviour of the person. You've got to construct other principles to do that. So that seems to me a possible serious flaw in these dimensional type theories.

I can think of similar examples closer to my own research on schizophrenia. If you consider, say, positive and negative symptoms, you can take schizophrenics and you can certainly factor out behaviours and say, well, there are positive symptoms and negative symptoms in schizophrenia. In fact in my view that isn't likely to be true. It's more likely to be a dynamic thing with positive and negative symptoms alternating or forming part of a dynamic process of psychotic behaviour. You arrive at these clusters or dimensions simply because you are analysing a number of measures taken at one point in time. But that doesn't actually represent the real dynamics of the state.

I'd like to ask you about the LSD research going on during the late 1950s, early, middle to late 1960s. Was that a good idea. Did we learn anything from it?

My own view is that it's a bit of tragedy that it stopped. There were mostly two reasons I guess. One is that it became an illegal drug and I suspect that scientists were rather relieved that they didn't have to bother with it any longer; and anyway, at that time the 5-HT-LSD-psychosis connection didn't seem all that convincing to make them think otherwise. And the second reason was the arrival of the amphetamine/dopamine model, which seemed to add up to a neat uncontroversial story: schizophrenia, antipsychotic drugs, and so on. Incidentally, I don't think these two reasons are unconnected and that the amphetamine/dopamine model has been sustained long past its 'sell-by date' by the lingering unease about drugs like LSD and their connotation as street drugs.

Which is clearly wrong.

Which is clearly wrong, but it seemed to catch on and it sort of eclipsed the LSD story. But the latter anyway was getting messy because of the street drug use and it being made illegal. Though I understand people were using it therapeutically until quite recently.

Very peripherally. It dropped out of the mainstream very, very quickly.

Yes, in research. I think it was a tragedy in a way and I think it will subsequently be realized that if we had continued with LSD or at least drugs of that general type, drugs which were psychotomimetic, then we would have found out more about schizophrenia than we have with amphetamines. My own view is that there was a failure even to address the question of what I would call face validity. If you went out to look for a drug which mimics a natural state it seems to me that you would look for a drug which patently did that. If you give anybody a small dose of LSD, well most people anyway, you're going to produce something which is pretty weird and psychotic in general and that's always seemed to me the mimimum requirement for choosing a drug model of psychosis. There may be other requirements obviously but the first requirement is that you have to have some kind of face validity. This has never struck me as being the case with amphetamine. You can make people paranoid and so on with large doses of amphetamines, or even with small doses of amphetamines in highly sensitive people, but it's not actually a natural psychotomimetic.

Yes, that's interesting. For 30 or 40 years housewives were using amphetamines and there really wasn't a problem. They certainly weren't becoming psychotic and then all of a sudden it became a big issue and amphetamine psychosis was described and everybody became so concerned about this drug that very few people would be happy to have it nowadays. It's rather strange that this can happen, isn't it?

Well, I think it's an interesting example of the way thinking proceeds in science. People seize upon things to fit in with existing preconceptions. They selectively attend to certain kinds of evidence. It's almost a kind of delusional process, theory-building in science, and that's a good example of it – selectively fitting things together because they make a good story. In the amphetamine case, if you looked at it calmly it would never strike you that it was an obvious thing to do. It would have been more obvious to stick with a set of drugs like mescaline, LSD and the other psychotomimetics. And there's no point in saying, well, it's not a very good model because schizophrenics have auditory hallucinations and with LSD there are visual hallucinations, because that is not quite as true as lots of people made out. Anyway, even if it were true you're still nearer to the psychotic states than you are with amphetamines. But it disappeared.

What role do you think people like Hoffer had and the research they were doing? They were doing some studies with LSD, which between one thing and the other contributed to the idea that research was happening in this area which was unethical, that's a bit strong but . . .

Well I think that just added to it and I think science does very much follow social attitudes. There was a sort of serious, I suppose, biological side to the research, then there was the street use and then there was a sort of semi—scientific research in the middle. There was quite a lot of research like that on LSD, which had a sort of legitimacy I suppose, but which in the end it helped to kill LSD off. Some of it was actually quite interesting. There's a lot of stuff written about LSD and things like creativity but people who had more biological ideas didn't see the need to look at this stuff in order to understand psychosis.

It wasn't just the fact that LSD was made illegal. It was the fact that it actually did have an interesting experiential component to it, don't you think? There was a whole literature of that kind which was sort of on the borderline. Some of the therapeutic stuff, where it had been given to patients like alcoholics, didn't have much basis to it. This was all tied up to psychodynamic interpretations, uncovering layers of personality and all that kind of stuff which, as you know, has always been dubious in certain areas of psychiatry.

I think it just drifted away on a sort of sea of psychedelic ecstacy in the end and . . . I collected together some references recently because my undergraduates were asking about it. The research did seem to stop quite suddenly and, even when it was there, there was this funny mixture of research. It was either serious research or it was vaguely suspect in some people's eyes. It didn't fit into the neat kind of pattern of the amphetamine/dopamine theory which psychiatry needed at that time. They needed to establish a firm, very biological view of schizophrenia.

Can I pick up on the point you make that LSD was associated with research on creativity – it was also associated with research on religious experience, wasn't it, and because of that I think it was inevitable that it would be seen as fringe work.

Oh, yes, absolutely. It seems to me that the history of psychiatry has been very much a fluctuation between an attempt at a hard scientific, genetic biological theory and this experiential thing. This is a tension that has always been there and the 1960s, with Laing and so on, was very much a time when the latter really took over. And although LSD obviously did have potential for people working on it to talk about it as a biological model, it fitted too much the Laingian thing to ever survive unless somebody had come up with a real breakthrough. So, yes, I don't think psychiatrists were generally able to accept that within the climate that was emerging at that time. They needed to reject Laing and all that stuff. It's interesting what's happening now is that it seems as though we're growing up a bit and people aren't quite so polarized in that respect.

I think you're right. As you were saying earlier people like you and Malcolm Lader were quite happy working at a common interface during the early 1960s. Then we have Laing and all of a sudden, as you say, a tremendous polarization.

Well, it was really a three—cornered thing, wasn't it, if you include Eysenck? On the one hand, you had Eysenck and Laing, both opposed to the medical view of mental illness. But in other ways, of course, Eysenck and Laing were in entirely different camps. Parts of Eysenck's theory can fit in well with the medical model, the heavily biological part. It's the other parts – the dimensional view of illness – that set Eysenck in opposition to the medical establishment and which in a peculiar sort of way and that particular respect put him closer to people like Laing.

There doesn't seem to have been much of an LSD research network in the 1960s, which is interesting in its own right.

I did my research completely in isolation in Glasgow. I had a series of psychiatric colleagues in the Glasgow department and they were into that kind of stuff. They took all of the psychotomimetic drugs and we decided to do this experiment on LSD. It was partly an attempt within, well put it this way, the Glasgow department had had Laing there and there were a number of people in it who, although overtly saying that they didn't really go along with his views, nevertheless had a sneaking interest I suspect in the kind of experiential bits of what he was talking about. So they would experiment with these drugs. It was all perfectly legitimate of course and anyway there was a feeling at that time that you needed to know how schizophrenics felt. You therefore needed to take something like LSD to find out, which I actually believe is true.

So some of my colleagues were taking these drugs because they felt they would give them insight into schizophrenia. I slotted into that quite well you see because I was interested not only in taking it to find out that too but also doing an experiment on it to see whether one could replicate the 'dissociation of arousal' effect that I had got with schizophrenic patients. I don't actually remember to be honest reading a great deal about . . . well, I read the usual stuff, but what I mean is I don't remember meeting anybody who had written for example at that time. I knew about Peter McKellar although I didn't actually know him well but I knew he was interested in LSD.

What about the Bradley and Elkes group during the 1950s?

Oh yes, indeed. I was very aware of that. In fact I was very much persuaded by Bradley and Key and all those people in Birmingham that LSD was a good model. Indeed, I still use their papers and results in lectures here. They are classic papers. Certainly they convinced me that there were similarities between the experimental effects of LSD and what happened in schizophrenia. And there was Mednick who was writing about this – he had a learning theory of schizophrenia.

What's striking about Bradley and Key's description of LSD effects in animals in their 1950s papers – if you read them out of context, what you would think you were actually reading would be an account that schizophrenics had given of their perceptions and cognition. So that's what struck me about it.

The disappearance of LSD is a story that needs to be told.

Oh yes, why it disappeared so abruptly hasn't been told. It's not just a case of a better hypothesis taking over from a worse one.

Do you think it fits in with the shift from the democrats to the republicans in the US and the general closing down . . .

I didn't want to say that.

No, but time-wise it does fit. You wonder about these things.

A more rigid kind of attitude you mean . . . you're probably right. There is a kind of openness of experience about LSD and that's lacking in certain periods. It may be reflected politically.

There are echoes in the story about mesmerism. It was associated with the French Revolution. An awful lot of people around the time who were actually signatories of the revolutionary papers and so on were mesmerists and of course once the revolution began to eat its own children then mesmerism was one thing that went. It ended up proscribed for the better part of 100 years.

Yes, that's interesting.

Reading through your book on Drugs and Human Behaviour, *one of the things that I'm struck by is that most of the principles of what you could call cognitive neuropharmacology were there then. It's become a bit of a growth industry again in the last five years with a range of groups trying to explore the impact of drugs on cognitive function and rediscovering principles like asymmetrical transfer, but they're all there in your book – it's either marvellous that you had all of this then or disappointing that we seem to be reinventing the wheel – depending on your point of view. But that's another research programme that went into decline in a sense – the idea of looking at neuropsychology with drugs in human volunteers quite apart from using LSD.*

Yes, I think that's probably right. From the individual differences point of view of course that might have been because the individual differences effects within normal subjects can be quite complicated and didn't stand up – you got tired coping with all sorts of interactive effects, so I think that may have been why people stopped doing it.

But looking at some of the things you talked about in the book. You talk about the effects of chlorpromazine on continuous attention tasks. This hasn't much to do with the individual differences framework as such, has it? In this area, the funny thing is that there was work happening in the 1950s and 60s and all of a sudden it stops and it's now being picked up again – so there's an interesting hiatus where you've got references from the late 1980s and the 90s and from the 1950s and early 60s and nothing in the 1970s or early 80s.

Yes, well. I'm just trying to think what happened. Part of what happened might have had to do with what happened in psychology generally. Of course neuropsychologists have always been very concerned with looking at brain abnormality and all of that stuff has certainly been a strong theme. Then there's always been a strong theme in strict cognitive psychology, the work of Broadbent and Baddeley and others at the Applied Psychology Unit in Cambridge. But for some reason, they weren't particularly interested in drugs or physiological manipulations other than sleep.

Combining these two in cognitive neuropsychology, I agree, is relatively new. This is attempting to bring brain functions more specifically into cognitive psychology. Well maybe it simply is that up till now cognitive psychology has always been a bit of a black box kind of discipline. People didn't really want to talk about the brain. They'd rather draw flow diagrams between black boxes and maybe the lack of interest in drugs was because, if you don't bring them in, you don't have to address brain questions and maybe it's only since the brain has been brought into cognitive psychology that it's been possible or interesting to take up this kind of work again.

That's the only reason I can think of – that it reflects to some extent the rate of development in different areas of psychology and over a period there was no place for a pharmacological dimension because the pharmacological dimensions had been largely accommodated within the individual differences framework, which faded out for other reasons.

Schizotypy is the other area – when did you begin to move from individual differences framework into schizotypy?

Well, I see schizotypy as individual differences. As I said earlier, my interest in the basic ideas about schizotypy, although it wasn't actually formulated in that way, goes right back to when I worked for Eysenck in the 1960s. When I talked to schizophrenics for the first time as a young researcher it seemed to me, although people had warned me that they were on another planet, actually sometimes they seemed to be like any other people I had met.

It struck me that maybe this dimensional idea that Eysenck had could actually be applied to schizophrenics in their better phases. Of course they could be totally mad but quite a lot of the time they were perhaps like Laing had said, perhaps more interesting to talk to than the people in the officers' mess, which I think is what he said about his own stay in Netley – because he was also there. So, that's really where it started.

I got quite interested in the notion of some continuity between schizophrenia and the normal personality at that time. And then when I went to Glasgow, the LSD experiment in a sense attempted to shift some people into a temporary state with drugs. So the logic was just the same as with Eysenck's original drug postulate applied to introversion – extraversion. But then there was a sort of gap because I couldn't find any measures of the dimension itself. Of course if I'd been a little less insular I might have looked to the States because Meehl was writing quite early on about just this idea of schizotypy but I wasn't actually aware of it.

Eysenck then came along with the P-scale and so I started to use that and got quite interested in measuring psychotic traits in normal people. He then spoilt everything by changing the P-scale in a way that seemed to weaken it. By this time, I had come to Oxford and I had a young undergraduate, somebody called Reichenstein, who I will never forget because she said she wanted to do a project measuring schizophrenic traits in normal people. I hadn't told her about this – she just came along to me and said she thought schizophrenic traits could be found in normal people and that she wanted to try and work up a questionnaire to measure these. I sort of sat back in my chair – it was amazing really that she should have arrived at this on her own. So she then constructed this questionnaire, which was the basis of the schizotypy measures that we then developed here. Then of course the whole thing took off. I discovered lots of other questionnaires and other questionnaires since then have been constructed. And now there's an explosion of questionnaires.

When did you become aware of Meehl?

Well, not more than about seven or eight years ago. Quite recently. The schizotypy scene was a very scattered kind of thing. Last year I went to a conference in Italy which Adrian Raine and Mednick organized and it was the first time any group of people had come together to talk about schizotypy. That was really quite interesting because the work had been done in scattered little bits and nobody had really brought it together.

Having discovered the schizotypy literature and developed our own questionnaire which we thought was better than the P-scale, we nevertheless adopted the Eysenckian strategy towards research. This was to describe the individual difference at a personality level and to find some sort of underlying biological measure of it.

Do you want to comment on the measures?

What we really did and are still doing was to examine a number of different paradigms. For example, I got very interested at one point in the augmenting – reducing effect on EEG, described by Buchsbaum and others in the States and I used that for a while. Then I had a DPhil student – Paul Broks – who was interested in work on interhemispheric differences. He wasn't interested in schizotypy actually but I persuaded him to use our schizotypy scale. He was pessimistic but he did an experiment with this and found differences in lateralization in relation to schizotypy. And then I had another DPhil student who I tried to push in the same direction but he wouldn't be pushed. But Steve Tipper was in the Department at that time, the negative priming man who you know well. It seemed to us that the cognitive effects you get in negative priming experiments were a natural kind of description of some of the things that go wrong in schizophrenics – a failure of cognitive inhibition. So we looked at it in schizotypy.

That kind of model then goes all the way back to your interest in selective attention from the 1950s.

Oh yes, absolutely. The only new thing about it really was the hemisphere perspective, which was not very represented, if at all in the 1960s scene. Anyway, we looked at various aspects of schizotypy, including a study of relatives of schizophrenics and drug manipulations. For example, Tony Beech and I looked at the effects of chlorpromazine on negative priming, which shows that chlorpromazine strengthens negative priming. In other words it had an effect consistent with the findings in schizophrenia and schizotypy of a weakening of negative priming. So as a strategy, that in a sense goes right back to the Eysenckian drug postulate applied to an individual differences problem. I think that there is something to be learned from using this kind of two—pronged approach – too much research is isolated. I always remember a colleague of mine, Peter Broadhurst at the Maudsley hospital in London who was a Professor of Psychology in Birmingham for many years. He was a behaviour geneticist and his view was that whenever you did an experiment on individual differences, say measuring negative priming, you ought always to do it on twins because you can then answer two questions at once. You can answer the question does negative priming in this case relate to schizotypy and you can also answer a question about the genetic component in the individual difference you are studying. I have always remembered that because it seems to me that that's another example of where you can efficiently join together research approaches on the same topic.

Can I raise the question of behavioural genetics – your mentioning it prompted in me the reaction that psychologists are supposed to be liberals who are all for nurture and geneticists are all conservatives who are all for nature, etc., etc. but it is a case of trying to bridge that divide, isn't it – the most productive opportunities lie there.

I think that's right. I did once do a twin study on the sedation threshold with that sort of thing in mind, trying to see whether there was a genetic component to the sedation threshold. So I was very much into that sort of stuff in those days, trying to link all the psychos: psychogenetics, psychopharmacology, psychosomatic, anything with psyche in it I was quite interested in because it seemed to me that there's where the contribution of, or a strong contribution of, psychology might lie. Not isolating itself from other areas but trying to see where it could connect up to those areas. And I was very impressed when Brian Leonard came here recently to talk about psychoimmunology, which is another example of the same thing.

Your work with LSD and the sedation threshold reminds that one of the interesting things about psychopharmacology for me is that it's one of those sciences which is not theory driven. There's always been new compounds coming out which don't fit into the theoretical framework and you've got to reconstruct things because of them. But Eysenck's work was different in that it was one of the few things that was theory driven.

It was highly systematic, yes, and thought out but it became slightly restricted. But there were some quite extraordinary phenomena investigated. I spent my first few months working for Eysenck, I remember, sitting looking through a handbook of experimental psychology looking for any phenomena which could possibly show individual differences between introverts and extraverts. Because according to Eysenck's theories if you take any piece of behaviour it's bound to be influenced by inhibition or excitation, which were the individual differences concepts he was playing around with at that time. So I spent a whole term just reading, picking out things like time judgement and all sorts of curious phenomena like that which were bound to show individual differences. And if you thought about it you could always find a reason which fitted into Eysenck's theories. A lot of it was like that and there were some extraordinary phenomena studied. There was a thing called Bidwell's ghost, for example.

What was that?

It's a phenomenon where if you present, say, a green stimulus, as a flash of light and then you mask it with a white stimulus you see the complementary colour; you never see the primary visual image at all. So it's really the suppression of the primary visual image and it's called Bidwell's ghost. According to Eysenck, the extent to which this occurs should be correlated with extraversion and be affected by stimulants and sedatives according to the drug postulate. So he had this Japanese student doing that and somewhere in the literature in one of his books I think on drugs that came out of Eysenck's laboratory is an experiment on Bidwell's ghost. So almost any experimental laboratory phenomena was up for grabs, as long as you could make some story about it being affected by inhibition or arousal.

One of the things about working in a department of experimental psychology, a general department, that I've come across in the last 20 years here, is the lack of interest in that fact from the point of view of experimental psychology. Because the point about Eysenck's theory is that it's both a theory of personality and a theory simply about individual differences. So if you look at it and say, okay, we tried to explain introvert and extravert and we were using things like Bidwell's ghost to get into the biology of that. That's one view of it. The other view is if you are an experimental psychologist and you're doing experiments on Bidwell's ghost, there are big individual differences and Eysenck would claim that this theory or that kind of theory could explain these. It's interesting how very few experimental psychologists are interested in that fact. Mostly the effort is directed only towards the phenomenon itself. Nobody really pays attention to the individual variation.

One of the interesting exceptions to that is Steve Tipper because when he was working here on negative priming, he did get interested in the individual differences side and this ties up very nicely with an area like schizophrenia research. But that isn't recognized very often. Some years ago I gave a seminar in the department here and tried to make that point but mostly people are wanting to get rid of the individual differences – they regard it as part of the error variance and a bit of a nuisance.

What about the future?

I think that clearly you can't turn the clock back and for ethical reasons it is quite difficult perhaps to visualize, for example, giving people LSD and measuring negative priming. But I think if there were some ways round that it would be important to take them as I'm sure that looking for animal models in schizophrenia is only one approach. Inevitably I think one has to try and look for human models. I mean we know a lot about anxiety and I think that is because we have models of anxiety in humans as much as in animals. With all due respect to Jeffrey Gray (and I think he would probably agree) you have to supplement animal work with work on humans – I think that that needs to be done with schizophrenia somehow. The obvious way is the use of some kind of psychotomimetic substances other than LSD. There may be other methods. Non—pharmacological. For example, I have had somebody working on out of body experiences in my laboratory and that may be a non-pharmacological method; and I suppose sensory deprivation is another but the thing about drugs is that you can control the situation.

To some extent anyway

Select bibliography

Claridge, G. S. and Herrington, R.N. (1960) Sedation threshold, personality and the theory of neurosis. *J. Ment. Sci.*, **24 106,** 1568–83.

Claridge, G.S. and Herrington, R.N. (1963) An EEG correlate of the Archimedes spiral after-effect and its relationship with personality. *Behaviour Research and Therapy*, **24 1,** 217–29.

Eysenck, H.J. (1963) *Experiments with Drugs*. Pergamon Press, London.

Herrington, R.N. and Claridge, G.S. (1965) Sedation threshold and Archimedes' spiral after-effect in early psychosis. *J. Psychiatric Research*, **24 3,** 159–70.

Claridge, G.S. (1967) *Personality and Arousal. A Psychophysiological Study of Psychiatric Disorder*. Pergamon Press, Oxford.

Claridge, G.S. (1970) *Drugs and Human Behaviour*. Allen Lane, London.

Claridge, G.S. (1972) The schizophrenias as nervous types. *British Journal of Psychiatry*, **24 121,** 1–17.

Claridge, G.S. (1987) 'The schizophrenias as nervous types' revisited. *British Journal of Psychiatry*, **24 151,** 735–43.

20 Malcolm Lader

Psychopharmacology: clinical and social

Looking at the interviews you've done so far, I think there are some things you have missed.

Such as?

Let me start with how science is organized here and I think probably it's the same in other countries. There is a small echelon of very influential people, who usually have the letters 'SIR' in front of their names and often 'FRS' after it. They take a strategic view of British science and they'll be invited both formally and informally to give advice to politicians. Now there is no psychopharmacologist in this country at that level.

Below that is a second echelon of people who are involved in the tactics of research. They sit on grant-giving bodies and are influential because research needs money. And the money is controlled by relatively few people. To see who has been influential you look at CVs as to whether the person has been on the MRC Neurosciences Board, the Wellcome Mental Health Board, the Mental Health Foundation or one or two others. These people have a view on the tactics of research, so that if somebody comes up with a particular project it will be referred to one of them. But they won't be able to influence whether there will be a shift of psychiatric research from social to biological, etc. Then there's the third group of people below that who are used occasionally as referees and so on. Now many of the people that are highly regarded within psychopharmacology are not so regarded outside because they have not been on these grant-giving bodies. Appointments to grant-giving bodies are essentially by consensus of a whole group of people, mostly from outside the field.

People outside the field often determine the status of those within it?

Yes, psychiatry and psychopharmacology have not been regarded as cutting edge subjects until quite recently. I think there's a change now with neuroscience coming in but that's only been in the last 10 years. Before that it was regarded as very much an 'also' ran. I have been asked by my pharmacology friends, why did you go into psychopharmacology, why didn't you come into cardiology or gastrointestinal pharmacology like the rest of us? But in my case I did a PhD with a classical pharmacologist and that made all the difference. There was no way I was ever going to look at pharmacology or psychiatry again in the same way.

Who did you do your PhD with?

Well, I did the usual intercalated BSc in Physiology with a gastrointestinal physiologist, Professor Gregory in Liverpool, who was probably one of the leading people in that area and a first-rate scientist. There were only two of us doing this BSc so we had a lot of individual tuition. I developed an interest in doing research in that year. The other thing which happened, which also cast a fairly long shadow forwards, was that I came across a book edited by S.S. Stevens, called *The Handbook of Experimental Psychology*. When I read that, I realized that psychology could be a scientific subject and that psychologists were often better scientists than doctors were. It showed me that you could quantify psychological phenomena and I suppose I spent my career taking that forward.

Anyway, I finished my medical degree. In Liverpool, then, there was no psychiatry and I didn't like the medical setup. I got a good qualification and I decided to go to London. Looking around for a job, I was taken on by Professor Schild who was a classical pharmacologist, famous for all he had done on the quantification of antagonism techniques. He had a grant with Michael Shepherd and Hannah Steinberg from the NIH and they took on three of us – myself, Lorna Wing and J.D. Montagu.

After a golden period with healthy human volunteer work, Hannah Steinberg must have been moving over to animal work at this point.

Yes. Her early nitrous oxide work was superb but she had moved over to animal work and she wasn't all that interested in the work that I was doing. Michael Shepherd oversaw the clinical side of it. Heinz Schild said to me just go off, you know, and measure things in man and look at the effects of different drugs. I said 'well, measure what?' and he said 'measure conditioning effects'. So I read the literature and I found that although there was a vast literature on conditioning effects, there was very little on what happened to unconditioned effects. They had gone straight into conditioning as a sort of paradigm of 'neurotic illness', which I suppose in a way it is for some neurotic states like post-traumatic stress disorder.

Anyway, I thought I'd better try and work out something about unconditioned responses and I did habituation work using some physiological measures, such as skin conductance. Now if I'd have taken advice on this I would have been told you don't have enough precision. I just assumed that we knew what we were doing. Professor Schild was a gut-bath man in his own research. But it worked. It wasn't clear until our first study that skin conductance was measuring sweat gland activity. Using this we did formal bioassays which were the first bioassays ever done in psychopharmacology.

This involved doing what?

Measuring skin conductance responses to a series of unconditioned stimuli and measuring habituation. It followed a logarithmic course, so I just used a logarithmic transformation and got a regression line on it and then you could use this as a measure of alertness, arousal or whatever you wanted to call it.

But all along we wanted to use these techniques in patients and in about 1961, I started to take these techniques to the Maudsley. Lorna Wing was already there doing some other research. I brought these techniques down and we worked together I think for the next two years. We produced a lot of material and got a Maudsley monograph out of it. She was delightful to work with, very patient and a very astute clinician. The third member of the team, was actually probably the most senior and that was J.D. Montagu, who was very good on technical work and I learnt a lot from him. I also learnt when to stop developing techniques because you can go on and on. He had the most magnificent technical knowledge but sometimes he lost sight of the fact he was actually going to apply this technique. The three of us together I think were a good team.

Then I had to decide what I was going to do in the longer term. I'd been speaking to Michael Shepherd about this and he said 'I think you need to do proper psychiatric training' and I agreed. So I applied for and obtained one of the training registrarships at the Maudsley. There wasn't any question of going anywhere else. I had seen the place and it seemed such a critical mass of research, mostly social research – which was Aubrey Lewis' interest. Between John Wing, George Brown, Michael Rutter and Jim Birley, a whole group were working on the social side. I was taken on for the clinical course and I thoroughly enjoyed it. It was an experience in those days with people like Gene Paykel and Bob Kendall and lots of others. I went on the rotation in the usual way.

Was there much pharmacology research?

There was very little pharmacology. Some was being done by Ted Marley but it was very basic psychopharmacology. Dick Rodnight was a biochemist and he was interested in psychopharmacology but the Biochemistry Department had tended to move onto metabolism and phosphorylation.

One of the things you did which is fairly unusual from a training point of view was to get involved in writing the first book on clinical psychopharmacology.

What happened was Michael Shepherd had been asked to write the textbook and he invited myself and eventually Dick Rodnight to collaborate with him. I think it's fair to say I wrote much of it but it was an excellent training because it meant that I laid a foundation for a width of knowledge in psychopharmacology. Up till then I had been very focused and narrow which is what you have to do if you want to establish a reputation in research. I was looking back recently at what I said about benzodiazepines and I was suspicious of them even then. I regarded them as safer barbiturates but not without dependence potential.

There was also the influence of Aubrey Lewis who is terribly maligned by his inferiors. If you were a junior to him he was very considerate in almost all ways except that he worked on a different level. I'll give you an example – when I coming up to the DPM he was asking what was I revising. I said I was reading Jaspers and I didn't think much of it, 'it's all very philosophical' and he said 'what edition are you reading' and I said 'well, it's the translation, the English'. 'Oh no' he said 'you must go back to the first edition because that was when he was just out of the mental hospitals and in fact it's much more psychiatric'. The problem is that there was no translation of the first edition and my German isn't good enough to sustain a heavy textbook of that sort. But it didn't occur to him that anybody wasn't fluent in German, French, Spanish and so on.

But he was a very kindly man. What he did was to make psychiatry respectable. Up till then, there were only a couple of Chairs in the country. Most medical schools shied off setting up departments because they didn't think it was respectable and there was no academic basis to it. What Aubrey Lewis had to do was to cut through all the undergrowth, take away all the speculation, all of the poor science and start to put it on to a proper basis. He's been criticized because he didn't do a great deal of original research, and there's some basis in that, but nobody could have done much in the way of original research until the ground was cleared and he did that. He clarified our concepts of what is mental health, what is mental illness and what we mean by diagnosis. What he would have thought of DSM-IIIR, I can only shudder because he was a great iconoclast.

So I did the three years, got the DPM, actually with distinction and then I knew I wanted to do research. Schild and Shepherd had gone to the MRC and suggested a Psychopharmacology Unit. The MRC had turned that down, on the grounds that neither of them was a recognized psychopharmacologist. Schild was certainly a distinguished pharmacologist but not a psychopharmacologist. Michael Shepherd was a most able and distinguished psychiatrist, but again I can see how he would not be regarded as having the right background for a Unit of that sort.

Anyway, I was in this package that went into the MRC. Harold Himsworth, the secretary of the MRC, was a great one for picking people out and pushing them forward. He phoned Aubrey Lewis, who had been my PhD examiner, and said is there anything worth salvaging from this and I presume Aubrey Lewis said 'yes, salvage Lader'. The next thing I was being interviewed by Harold Himsworth – this was in 1966, just as I was finishing the DPM course. I sat in a very low easy chair with

Harold, who was about 6'6', towering up above me, asking me questions about this and that and what I wanted to do.

They took me onto the external staff which was a very odd thing to do. The external staff of the MRC is really a place where you put people who had left other Units that had closed down – it was a temporary parking place while they sorted something out, but they put me onto it. They would never upgrade it to a Unit and I've stayed on the external staff ever since, with a core support, a couple of technicians, a secretary, statistician, a couple of senior lecturers and clinical people and it's been a sort of a mini-Unit, but not actually called a Unit. It's very unusual. I only have an honorary status with the University and honorary status with the Institute of Psychiatry. And I have to put in the usual programme of research every five years and they ask me for a report on the previous five years and so on.

One of the curious things is that Aubrey Lewis, Michael Shepherd and Linford Rees who was at the Maudsley still in the late 1950s were founder members of the CINP.

Yes, that was right. You have to remember that there were relatively few real psychopharmacologists. What we had were clinicians with an understanding and a very great interest in psychopharmacology because it was the topic of the time. You have to remember all of the psychotropic drugs practically were discovered in the 1950s – lithium, chlorpromazine, both groups of antidepressants, LSD, and so on. It was very vigorous from that point of view. The problem was there was no basic science to support it. It was an empirical subject. We knew nothing then about 5-HT – it had only been found in the brain a few years before. So there was a great distance between what was happening empirically and clinically on the one hand and what was underpinned by basic sciences on the other. That's why psychopharmacology tended to be either clinical or empirical animal psychopharmacology, the sort of stuff that Hannah Steinberg was doing but again without the link to the neurosciences. The CINP was essentially set up by clinicians who wanted an international forum in which to develop the subject and who also wanted a way of promulgating the use of drugs in psychiatry. They had their own agenda.

You also have to remember that the United States was not interested in drugs. I was lucky, we had almost a 30-year clear run in the 1960s and 1970s, when the Americans were not doing much psychopharmacology. It was only then that they finally gave up their flirtation with psycho-analysis and moved into psychopharmacology, and of course with their resources they've swamped the subject. I'll give you an good example from addiction, which is an area I'm interested in. The MRC spend about £32 million a year; I suppose Wellcome spend the same again but NIDA and NIAAA together have a budget of $800 million a year. Even allowing for population differences and for the fact that some of their research programmes have a service element, which we don't have, we can't compete with funding on that basis. We have to be very selective as to what we do.

About 10 years after the foundation of the CINP, Aubrey Lewis said that if you asked him what had been more important for psychiatry, the advances from social research or from psychopharmacological developments, he would have to say the social developments – a point that has been echoed by Michael Shepherd even quite recently. It seems curious that a lot of the early clinical trial work was done at the Maudsley by people like Linford Rees, Brian Davies and Michael Shepherd but then somewhere in the early 1960s, the Maudsley seems to have turned away from psychopharmacology to the extent that Michael Shepherd and Edward Hare became notable sceptics about drug treatment.

Yes, but you can argue that in fact they were being rather realistic about a lot of things. Look at the problems we have with people with schizophrenia in the community, how difficult it is. We are having to reinvent the wheel – how do we give community care, do we have compulsory treatment orders? The long-term outcome of schizophrenia may be somewhat less severe because you space out the relapses but the deterioration is still there. The patients don't function as well as they might. With antidepressants you get a 30% placebo response and a 70% drug response. There's only a narrow value between them and then we see the problems with the benzo's and so on. And of course with lithium – I mean have we really stopped people coming into hospital with their hypomanic attacks?

So we have to be careful that we don't overvalue the psychotropic drugs that we've got. After all, for the first 30 years we were just producing more haloperidols, more chlorpromazines, more amitriptylines, more diazepams. It's only recently, with the development of receptorology and molecular biology, that you can tailor drugs much more. It's only now that we are in a position where we can develop say 5-HT-1 full antagonists and predict what sort of things they would do. That is where other branches of pharmacology were in the 1950s and 1960s.

You say there were no proper psychopharmacologists. What about proper clinical psychopharmacologists – I see you as being one of these.

There weren't any. There are quite a few now who take a training in psychopharmacology but there were very few in my time. There are a lot of people who you think of as psychopharmacologists who have no formal training in pharmacology. You see this when it comes to matters to do with pharmacokinetics and other strictly pharmacological aspects of the subject.

You also said that during its golden period in the 1960s and 1970s, clinical pharmacology looked down on psychopharmacology.

Yes, clinical pharmacology developed rapidly. A lot of very able people went into it partly because general medicine has always been crowded and this was a way of getting publications quickly and also taking part in the development of whole groups of new compounds. The pharmaceutical industry exploded in the 1950s, 60s and 70s, starting with the antibiotics but there were lots of other areas – beta-blockers and later the alpha-blockers. Because of this there were able people who decided positively to go into clinical pharmacology and do a PhD. They were then able to leap-frog up and their abilities were such that they ended up sometimes as clinical pharmacologists or sometimes back in the mainstream of general medicine in important and influential positions.

That didn't happen with psychiatry. Although we had the drugs, we didn't have the rationale in the same way. We had no idea how anti-depressants worked. Now there were of course surprises in the other parts of pharmacology, no-one predicted that propranolol would be an antihypertensive but they did predict it would have anti-angina effects and that was a powerful prediction. There was a feeling that psychopharma-cology reflected psychiatry and psychiatry has always had a low reputation with general physicians and neurologists. It hadn't developed that much and that of course I think really was inevitable owing to the complexity of the science at the moment.

Have these problems anything to do with our difficulties in making up our minds whether we should take a categorical or dimensional approach to mental illness? The dimensional point of view was much more common back in the 1960s. Your work on skin responses, naturally led into dimensional viewpoint. What happened? Gordon Claridge suggested that the fuss around R.D. Laing made people very wary of that kind of approach.

I think Laing had no real influence on UK psychiatry. His influence was in parapsychiatry, or metapsychiatry. People who were not in the pro-fession but wanted to have some influence on it – the antipsychiatry brigade.

No, the reason that the categorical view of psychiatry took off was nothing to do with the subject itself. It was entirely to do with the American health care reimbursement system. If you want to get paid for seeing a patient you had to attach a categorical label. You can't attach a dimension. You can't say I've treated someone who has the following dimensional problems – although that's actually what you do. I think if you are dealing with a patient, the best shorthand way of doing it is to have a dimensional formulation. But of course I accept that in this day and age that people get paid by insurance companies and that accordingly treatment is going to be dictated by what label you hand that particular patient. That's what happened in the United States and that's why DSM-III has taken over. Having produced that, the next stage was that the pharmaceutical companies, in order to get licenses, had to have a definable indication and that was obviously going to be DSM-III or DSM-IIIR. This has reinforced the categorization of psychiatric syndromes – I think prematurely. But there are things where science is over-ridden by business interests.

One of the things that was big in the 1960s was psychophysiology and the general area of psychosomatics.

I was working in psychophysiology, essentially because I wanted measures that I could use to increase the precision of the clinical ratings. In fact, in that Maudsley monograph I increased the assessment of sedative actions by an order of magnitude over even very careful clinical ratings. This was a way of getting additional precision to do the sort of things which a classical pharmacologist wants to do, which is dose-effect curves, inter-actions, isobols and things of that sort.

I used psychophysiology because you couldn't use the EEG, which was potentially much better but it's more complicated and you couldn't quantify it in the 1960s. It was difficult enough to quantify heart rate and skin conductance. You would spend hours with a ruler analysing paper traces but by simplifying the experimental paradigm, and just using uncon-ditional stimuli, I could quantify responses. Now these happened to be autonomic measures and that inevitably meant that psychosomatic conditions were going to be relevant, although I was never myself overly interested in psychosomatic aspects of it. I was certainly interested in the idea that some of these psychophysiological measures could give you an insight into psychosomatic conditions. For instance, there was the idea that if you get a hypertensive reaction as part of a sudden response to a stress then maybe eventually that hypertension will fix. That's probably what does happen. But the problem was that psychosomatic medicine was one of these rather fringe topics. There were a lot of respectable people in it but the meetings that you went to were quite odd. There wasn't a lot of science and I used to try and keep my distance. I was never a member of the Psychosomatic Society although I spoke at a few of their meetings.

On that score, one of the things that hits me is the power of business and politics to redefine psychosomatic syndromes. I'm thinking at the moment of hyperventilation which has become panic disorder.

Well, not totally. We always used to say if you go back far enough and look at German literature at the turn of the century, you're sure to find that someone described panic disorder and everything else. After all we are not the first people to observe phenomena. That's why, for example, it's very interesting why schizophrenia isn't well described before the 19th century but apart from that we are very often reinventing the wheel. What we are also doing is moving the wheels round and putting them on different corners of the old tramcar.

But there's a large group of people who have fluctuating types of symptoms and what you label them is neither here nor there. They respond to stress with physical symptoms and they are inconvenienced by them. Some of those physical symptoms will set up a vicious circle like hyperventilation or the perceptions of palpitations and you get the catastrophic interpretations and so on.

Can I switch to the foundation of the BAP? Whatever the reason, whether the Maudsley was pro- or anti-drug, when it came to the founding of the BAP, it was very much founded by non-Maudsley, non-Oxford/Cambridge people, why do you suppose that was?

I started off by saying how British science is organized, where the influence is and how the money goes. Societies like the BAP and the other one that I was involved with, the Society for Studying Addiction, which is much much older, don't have much direct influence on that. What they can provide is a forum where people realize there may be a hiatus and they start to do something about it. But it has to be the senior people who realize that. So I've been a member of the BAP from the start and I've been President and so on but I've no illusions about it being a very influential body.

One thing which I don't think anybody's mentioned to you about the original founding of the BAP is that amongst all the other issues such as calling it an Academy, advertising it in the *Lancet*, the meeting at the RSM, keeping it very much clinical, there was a suggestion that it would have a closed membership. That was anathema to me because when you work in an academic setting you have youngsters doing PhDs who want to go to these meetings and want to become a member. The one thing I was not going to join was a closed membership society. A quite small number of members were being talked about originally. To me that would have been a great disincentive to the youngsters. What happens with a closed society is that you pack it in with clinicians who've got an interest in psychopharmacology for 10 years and then they move on to something other and block the places. So that was why I was against it.

Has this happened to the American College?

Well, yes. I know some very good younger psychopharmacologists who can't get into ACNP because it has a closed membership. It doesn't allow the subject to develop. Coming back to the lack of Maudsley involvement, it just happened that way. Firstly there wasn't a lot of psychopharmacology there. There were Ted Marley on the basic side and John Stephenson at that time. Barry Blackwell had moved on to the United States and then there was myself. So it wasn't that the Maudsley was against it; there weren't many people in the Maudsley interested.

The most senior person in the 'opposition' was Philip Bradley. We had meetings up in Birmingham with Ian Stolerman who was working with him, Channi Kumar, who was much more involved in psychopharmacology in those days, and we actually got more people outside the academy to oppose it than were inside the academy to support it. It was almost a 2:1 ratio. A lot of people in industry thought they were going to be taken for a ride – that the Academy was going to say that all clinical studies had to be done by members of the Academy on an accreditation basis and the industry of course didn't want that. They could see a rip-off coming.

I think Max Hamilton hadn't originally realized what was going on. But he then realized he had perhaps been given too optimistic a picture and he back-pedalled on it. At one stage he was almost ready to resign as President unless there was a resolution of the conflicts. And then we did have some compromise. If you look back at the Constitution there was an associate membership, which I insisted on. There was no limit to the number of members. We changed it to an Association which was much more UK term, than Academy.

We thought it had all settled down until of course everything cracked open again at the Guernsey meeting, which I boycotted. It seemed to me again that this was the old guard coming in, the clinicians, and saying we should have a nice prestigious, expensive meeting in Guernsey. That's why the meetings ever since have been in slightly seedy university settings but they've been very successful meetings. I don't think you'd get that kind of attendance at hotels in Guernsey or whatever.

The division between the higher paid clinicians with an interest in psychopharmacology and people who regard themselves as professional psychopharmacologists still lies below the surface. You also have to remember that half of pharmacologists work in industry. That was something else that was forgotten by clinicians who were interested in psychopharmacology. Psychopharmacology is unusual in that half of card-carrying pharmacologists work in industry so you have to have good representation of that constituency.

Another strain emerged almost from the start in that quite a few people saw the BAP as the biological psychiatry section of the Royal College, in exile as it were and there has been something of a tendency ever since if things aren't going right for some people to say well let's up sticks and move back into the College.

The major influences on the Royal College, of course, were social and more recently psychodynamic; drugs were never very influential. I think it would have been a mistake to have set up a psychopharmacology society as a biological psychiatry section manqué. There is obviously a close relationship between them but there are large areas of biological psychiatry that have nothing to do with drugs.

But the BAP has been a biological psychiatry society almost rather than a psychopharmacology association. At BAP meetings we get sessions, for instance on neuroimaging, that are not directly to do with drugs.

That's true but also we have a lot of straightforward psychopharmacology as well. You have to have a balance because the drugs are going to be used in a biological psychiatry context. Beyond that they are used at two other levels, one is by general jobbing psychiatrists who obviously have to know about therapeutics although they don't have to know that much about psychopharmacology. You can give an antidepressant perfectly adequately and competently without knowing what it's doing to the amines in the brain. And of course increasingly a lot of psychopharmacology is done in primary care but there are relatively few general practitioners who have any interest in how the drugs actually work. GPs have never been members of the BAP.

You mentioned the benzodiazepines and you also said that way back in the 1968 textbook, you hedged your bets then as to what the role of these drugs would be; do you want to give me an overview of how the benzodiazepine saga evolved and why has it been such an issue in Britain — perhaps more than anywhere else?

There are several reasons. First, if you look at the literature in the 1960s, I wasn't out of line in saying that they weren't the major step that the drug companies were trying to make them out to be. It was in the 1970s that I parted company with the mainstream people who were then saying these were safe and effective drugs. In the UK, the usage was amongst the highest and my original worry about the benzo's was that this amount of usage cannot be justified and therefore maybe this was coming about because the drugs were producing dependence even in normal doses.

Peter Tyrer and I started questioning what was happening about 1975 to 1978. The issue caught on the United Kingdom because a group of us were quite vociferous about it, and because GPs were beginning to notice themselves that there were problems. The UK had a strong antipsychiatry movement and probably an even wider antiscience movement, and the media were looking for a whipping boy. People were saying that 'my life's been destroyed since I went onto Valium or whatever'. Professionals were prepared to give quotes and saying these were dangerous drugs. No professionals of the same status were prepared to say that this was all nonsense. John Marks had a try but he was regarded as tainted because he had just retired as managing director of Roche.

After television picked up the story, the press took it up and then of course eventually the lawyers took it up and although we think of the United States as the country where the lawyers chase the ambulances and so on, in this country, we've had two or three big firms of lawyers who specialized in negligence and they took up the issues. They saw that there was possibly some mileage in it. Whether or not they had compassion on their client or not was immaterial. It was part of their job to push their clients' claims as much as possible.

The net effect is still patchy because although we've made an impression on the precribing of anxiolytics, prescribing hypnotics has hardly altered and yet the problem is a very similar one. A lot of elderly people are particularly affected.

But why a particular thing suddenly takes off in one country and not another is fairly difficult to predict. France should have had much more problems because they've got twice the usage that we have. The United States are much more consumer conscious but there's a big lobby there which says they're not actually using enough benzo's. What they gloss over is the fact that because you get anxious doesn't automatically mean you have to have a benzo. But there's a different perception of the issues over there as well and I think the pharmaceutical industry have become much more subtle in the way that they get people to espouse their cause.

Do you want to comment on that further? There's been a recent book, Toxic Psychiatry *(see Glossary) which has made fairly sweeping claims in that regard.*

I haven't read the book but I know the sort of things that were said. The pharmaceutical industry, of course, is a very big and very successful industry. It works on wide profit margins. But it's high risk. It takes $200 million to develop a new drug. A company is often developing a drug at the same time as its other competitors are and often a company is not first in the field. So in the past they worked hard to get the support of the opinion formers in order to get some penetration of their compounds – people like you and I and all the senior members of the BAP.

Now what's happening of course is that things are changing. The days when consultants would write a prescription and the GP would say well that's interesting and start using it himself have gone. The GP wants to know what the cost of it is. The drug companies have the problem of how to penetrate the GP market without being able to use the specialist as their spearhead. Obviously drug companies are not charitable organizations; they have a legitimate right to promote their products within ethical limits. But companies vary. We talk about the pharmaceutical industry but that's an over-simplification. You've got big companies, which are very energetic and they will hold meetings and they will try and dictate who they have on a particular meeting agenda. You have others who are 'no-touch' companies. *They will give the money without strings; all they want is an educational spin-off. Then there are others in between. In the development of drugs, they may or may not take advice.*

When it comes to marketing, there are rules and regulations about this but there are subtle ways to influence you. If you're giving a lecture and you've been flown half-way round the world by a company, not many people will stand up and say that the company's products are inferior to another company's product. They are, at least, going to say that amongst the products worth prescribing are A, B and C even if they are perhaps a little less likely to use the compound of the company who is supporting them. It's human nature. So the thing to do is if you don't believe in the company's product, not to accept the invitation . . .

Chasing the benzodiazepine issue somewhat further, what appears to have happened is the media seem to have got their teeth into this story and perhaps through it into the idea of the medical story generally. What impact do you think the media are having on the practice of medicine more generally now.

I think the influence of the law is even greater. Patients are much more ready to sue. I do some medico-legal work and one is asked to comment as to whether it is worth going to legal aid. I find increasingly that some of these claims are totally unsustainable. Even if some damage was sustained as a result of the drug treatment, the drug treatment was perfectly routine.

What happens, then, is that the hazard of legal action makes you become more defensive in what you are doing. I will give a lecture this evening on benzodiazepine withdrawal and someone will ask 'well what do I have to do to stop my patient suing me'. I think what you have to remember is the sheer nuisance of being sued – it's so time consuming. People who have had this problem say they'd do almost anything to avoid going through that again. There's no substance in many of the complaints but you have to get the notes out and prepare a defence, speak to the solicitor for the Medical Defence Union and so I think that people do try and avoid that as much as possible.

The latest concerns in this regard have centred around temazapem, with apocryphal stories about little old ladies sending their husbands down to the pub to sell their supply. Is there any truth to this – and just how dangerous is temazepam?

The evidence we have seen on the Technical Committee on the Advisory Council on the Misuse of Drugs at the Home Office would suggest that benzodiazepines in general, but in the UK temazepam in particular, pose major problems in the addiction field. Temazepam was originally formulated as liquid-filled capsules, the contents of which could be easily injected. Addicts used it as an adjunct to opioids such as heroin, to smooth out the effects of cocaine and amphetamines, to give them courage to commit the offences needed to sustain their other habits, but increasingly as a primary drug of addiction. A substantial proportion of temazepam addicts inject, with all the subsequent dangers of transmission of HIV and hepatitis. These arguments led us to recommend stricter scheduling of temazepam but this recommendation is still under consideration by the appropriate government departments. Needless to say, cost consideration has raised its ugly head. Meanwhile, temazepam is freely available and indeed there are stories in the literature of little old ladies selling on their temmies in the pub. However, world-wide the problem is flunitrazepam, Rohypnol, which is taken either by mouth or quite often by snorting.

Some countries have already banned this compound. I find the whole addiction field quite fascinating but my research forays into it have been focused on a few aspects.

One could argue that neuroleptics cause more severe and more substantial problems than the benzodiazepines.

Yes, but schizophrenic patients are not likely to have a voice or to have access to MPs in the same way and the benzo's are very widely used. A lot of people know about them. Something like one in three women and maybe one in five men have taken a benzo. People know someone who's taking them and they can identify with somebody who's having problems. So you're dealing with something that is very widely used and that gives the newspapers and the media a head start.

Then there are, of course, the 'villains of the piece', the drug companies, who are busy promoting these drugs. There's also the idea that they are promoting these drugs for the worries of everyday life, whereas the neuroleptics are used mainly for serious mental illness. So there's the idea of the medicalization and the trivialization of psychological responses. Then there's the political dimension – that it's all due to social and political problems! There are other reasons which I can reel off. Women, for example, take them twice as frequently as men, so there's the idea maybe that we are dealing here with something that male doctors give women to keep them quiet! The media interest has all died down in this country now but it's coming up in other countries I'm told.

You've been prepared to be quoted in the media; do you not think that in handling things through the media you cannot expect to get what you want across?

That depends. The media varies. I always make myself available. If I give a lecture, and somebody from the newspaper phones up and my secretary takes the number, when I phone back I can often sense the surprise in the reply 'oh, you phoned back'. They don't expect that. Once you do that and you're prepared to talk sensibly about it at a fair length and let them go through all their questions they will often, and this happens to me quite frequently, they will say, can I fax you what I am going to write. Now you can't ask for any right of veto or any influence on what they say but you can correct matters of fact and they want that. They don't want to be get a reputation of someone who is loose with the facts. Like barristers, journalists are instant experts for 10 minutes or 10 days or whatever. But you have to take the risk that they may misquote you.

If you get quoted right three times for every time you are misquoted that's fair. But you've got to know how a journalist works and the constraints they're under. You can't go away and say 'oh, I'll think about that for three days'. It's dead in three days. When a piece of news comes up, you've got to either comment on it or you say I'm not the person that you want for this and try and give them somebody who is. They've got a job to do. When you get them on your side, they are very helpful.

Are you saying that the stock response that journalists are only in a story to sensationalize it is too paranoid?

No, it depends on the media or the newspaper. You don't expect *The Sun* with its readership to use the same sort of headlines as *The Times*. If you get a medical or science correspondent, it doesn't mean they'll have a technical background. I often ask how much technical background they've got and if they say 'I've got a PhD in pharmacology', obviously I can put it into such and such terms and leave it to them to de-jargonize it. If they say 'well I don't know anything at all', I say 'well bear with me and I'll try and explain it as simply as possible' and you talk about chemicals in the brain. But that's part of my job. I've never lost sight of the fact that I'm paid by the public to do research. The least I can do is to commit myself to telling them what I am doing, or what is going on in my particular area of expertise.

One of your more recent interests has been in sudden death in psychiatric hospitals, which seems to have something to do with the dose of neuroleptics being pushed up. This seems to have an awful lot to do with clinical practitioners acting empirically and not on the basis of any training in psychopharmacology, which leaves them open to the idea that if a small dose of the drug is useful, a larger dose will be more useful — it's very much ad-hocery.

But it's for us to do the research and educate them. This is what has happened with the benzo's. Doctors don't give indefinite prescriptions anymore. We need to educate our junior staff and those of our colleagues who are using high doses of neuroleptics; and we need to point out that there some dangers. Chlorpromazine should not be used. In cases that I have seen, its pharmacokinetics tend to become unpredicable at high dose – especially when other drugs are mixed in.

This is part of a wider problem of polypharmacy involved in treating disturbed patients. You've a responsibility to the nursing staff and carers not to have a severely psychotic patient who becomes aggressive. Our practice is to use benzo's for sedation which is more logical.

It's for us to identify a problem, to do the research into it and then to give appropriate advice. That's why I wrote a paper in the *British Journal of Psychiatry*, although it was all anecdotal. If somebody does die unexpectedly on a neuroleptic, the first thing you do after trying to resuscitate is to take a blood sample and see what the blood levels were. It is a legitimate role for a clinical psychopharmacologist to look into these problems. Our colleagues who have got the day-to-day problems of dealing with these patients may only see one case in their professional lives, they're not going to be able to work it out.

Between benzodiazepine guidelines and neuroleptic dose guidelines, what about the issue of guidelines? These are obviously needed but are we at risk of choking off progress with all these rules?

I've been 'guilty' of introducing guidelines. Guidelines are only as good as the people you can persuade to give up a day or two to sit and develop them. And even then they are only guidelines, they are not rules and regulations. We know that diazepam is only licensed for four weeks' use but if you go on for five weeks you justify that. It's only when you're doing something for which there's no body of opinion to support you that you're on your own. Guidelines are just a consensus – what most people would do but there can be quite a substantial minority that does it differently.

Has the development of biological psychiatry and its codification in DSM-IIIR led to something of an Anglo-American cultural imperialism in psychiatry?

With the amount of money that the Americans have to do research they are always going to dominate – once they get interested. As I've said before, we had a good run for our money in the 1960s and 1970s, until they woke up to psychopharmacology. The decade of the brain came along, then, and they could just throw money at projects. They have budgets which outrank ours severalfold so we've got to be very specific. Not quite niche research because we are still doing better than that – but I think we ought to be coordinating things a lot more in this country if we are to continue to compete with the Americans.

They waste a lot of money but some of it sticks and some of the things they do are extremely competent. Some of it's very imaginative and some of it isn't. But even the unimaginative work is done with such controls and so on that it's very important. The clinical trials they do influence the field because they do them so well.

You've also been very heavily involved in the Society for Addiction. Can you tell me about your involvement in that?

Yes. I've always been interested in addiction. You can't work in psycho-pharmacology and not realize that a whole group of compounds of various types are addictive. You can't compartmentalize these things. The problem is that, clinically, working with addictions is a very difficult thing to do. I greatly admire the people who manage to do it.

When I got more involved with benzodiazepines, it became quite clear that there was a whole area of addiction that I had to work into. Hannes Petursson and I did some systematic research into addiction – tolerance to compounds, withdrawal, challenge tests. That was all in the second Maudsley monograph that I wrote, which is widely quoted. Then my friends in addiction said why don't you come and help us out. There aren't many pharmacologists in the addiction field. I was put up for the

Presidency of the Society for the Study of Addiction and I was gratified by that and I had 10 years which I really enjoyed.

In a way, my strength was that as I wasn't really fully in the field, I could stand back from all the tensions of this group and that. I could balance alcohol against drugs of dependence and nicotine and so on and still pursue my own interest in benzo's. The Society, I think, quadrupled its membership under my Presidency. Its financial situation is now 10 times better. But it was an example of a Society that was ripe for development. Now you've got psychologists and sociologists and all sorts of people who go along and it's no longer dominated by the medics. That's to its advantage.

The problems you deal with are sort of an unwritten chapter in psychopharmacology in this country. All the focus is on the antidepressants, neuroleptics and minor tranquillizers but the down side is not covered.

A lot of people who are first-rate pharmacologists, working in the addiction field, are in the United States. They do not regard themselves as psychopharmacologists, which is unfortunate but it reflects the organization of the topic. For example, in the United States, the NIMH is separate from NIDA which is separate from NIAAA, although I think these two will be pushed back into the melting pot soon.

Over here the addictions have been separated out and of course the Royal College of Psychiatrists has had an addiction section for a long time now. There is a lot of addiction work which throws light on the aspects of psychopharmacology. For example, dopamine is a common thread. Nevertheless, psychotropics like the antidepressants, which are not addictive, lead us to believe that they can be studied separately, so that many in psychopharmacology have nothing to do with the addictions and this is unfortunate.

What about the LSD story? There was a certain apocalyptic quality to that. It came, it created psychopharmacology, and then it vanished.

I'm not so sure about that. LSD was an interesting area. There were groups of people who were particularly interested in it. There was some speculation, some hypotheses which developed from LSD, but you also have to remember that we didn't have much idea what LSD did and a substantial body of opinion developed among academic psychiatrists that the LSD phenomena did not resemble schizophrenia. Some elements are the same but so what, there are other drugs which produce hallucinations – you can give anticholinergics and get hallucinations. There was a feeling that this was not an appropriate model for schizophrenia. So it was side-tracked and the people who went on pursuing it were regarded as not being justified.

The second thing was the therapeutic aspect of it for which there was enthusiasm. Patients given LSD were always the poor prognosis, difficult to define patients; patients with personality disorders, patients with alcohol problems of various kinds. When it was given to anxious patients and schizophrenic patients it was a disaster and it became marginalized as a result. And then we started to get reports of abuse on LSD. A few people jumped out of windows and the whole thing had very worrying implications. A few people continued with it in a desultory sort of way.

I was in a meeting last year 'Fifty Years of LSD' to honour Hoffman. There was a small group of people there of his age, in their 70s and 80s, who had used LSD extensively and spoke of it with a certain nostalgia – how they'd found it useful. When you asked them what did it actually do, there were no controlled studies and they had no great specificity of what it was doing. It was quite obvious that whatever the scientific aspects of LSD, which were very important – the 5-HT story and so on – the therapeutic aspects had really been exaggerated, the side effects had been ignored and so on. And interestingly at this meeting, there was nobody who had dealt with the topic of LSD misuse. So there was a very curious sort of flavour to this. I wasn't involved with LSD because it had reached its peak in this country in the 1950s and by the 1960s it was already discredited. But it was interesting. I could get an insight into what had been very important. My only regret was that the man who could probably have thrown more light on it than anybody had died earlier that year. That of course was one of the greatest of the real psychopharmacologists, Danny Freedman. He had worked with LSD, as well as most other things. A first-class mind.

Finally, following on Valium and LSD, fluoxetine has become the latest media drug. How do you read that?

The fluoxetine story is a very interesting exercise illustrating all the influences which impinge on the pharmaceutical industry, the prescribers of drugs and their patients. The United States is the biggest drug market and if a drug is successful there, views about it tend to be very US-orientated. Fluoxetine has been very successful despite increasing numbers of competitors and despite a temporary setback with the exaggerated concerns about suicidality and aggression. More recently, the claims that fluoxetine can change personality remind one of the old controversies about amphetamines and LSD in the 1950s. My view is that there is a significant prevalence of minor and moderate chronic depression in the community and these are people who are being helped by what is an effective antidepressant. The media hype reflects the wide use of fluoxetine and also the search by Americans for perfection in mental health.

Select bibliography

Lader, M.H. and Wing, L. (1966) *Physiological Measures, Sedative Drugs and Morbid Anxiety.* Maudsley Monograph, no.14, Oxford University Press, London.

Lader, M. (1972) The nature of anxiety. *British Journal of Psychiatry,* **121,** 481–91.

Lader, M. (1978) Benzodiazepines – The opium of the masses. *Neuroscience*, **3**, 159–65.

Petursson, H. and Lader, M. (1984) *Dependence on Tranquillisers*, Maudsley Monograph, no. 28, Oxford University Press, Oxford.

Shepherd, M., Lader, M. and Rodnight, R. (1968) *Clinical Psychopharmacology.* English University Press, London.

21 Herbert Meltzer

A career in biological psychiatry

Why did you go into medicine?

Why did I go into medicine? I came from a family of very bright people but who didn't have the opportunity for higher education. The first really educated person who came into my life was the general practitioner who treated my family. He was someone I esteemed greatly. I had a couple of serious illnesses when I was a kid. Once I got rather extensive second degree burns, which he helped me survive. I was thought to have a heart murmur, which probably was not the case. Nevertheless, it led to a certain amount of contact with doctors and a genuine respect for the profession. As I grew older and took science courses in high school, I started to think of myself as potentially going into medicine. I registered as a pre-medical student when I began college at Cornell University in 1954.

I was also very interested in philosophy at the time and as one could go into medicine in the States without a science degree, I continued to take the more introductory level science courses offered for pre-medical students, along with philosophy. I took the pre-med organic chemistry course at the same time as I was taking a course in logical positivist philosophy, which was the dominant approach to philosophy in the United States at that time. I found this type of philosophy very arid and stultifying, while the organic chemistry was brilliantly taught and very exciting. I perceived the opportunities it provided for creativity and for synthesizing general principles; the mastery that seemed possible completely engaged me. A kind of game got started between myself and the professor – could he come up with reasonable questions that I wouldn't get right and somehow I did get them right. At the end of the course, I easily decided to become a chemistry major, although I still thought I'd go into medicine.

However, I got completely caught up with chemistry and by my senior year in College, I had great difficulty in deciding between a career in medicine or chemistry. I applied to both medical school and graduate school. I was awarded a prestigious fellowship to study chemistry at Harvard and I decided to do that. However, I had also been accepted to Yale Medical School which I had applied to because it was the only medical school in the US which required physicians to write a thesis. I started at Harvard Chemistry shortly after Watson and Crick had won the Nobel prize for the double helix. I took a course with Watson and one with Crick. I loved the work and did exceedingly well but I became almost clinically depressed about losing the opportunity to become a doctor. I decided in the middle of the year that I really should go to medical school and do medical research rather than pure chemistry. There was something about the relationship between physicians and patients that was really very important to me. My chemistry adviser was a man named Robert Woodward who had also won a Nobel prize – many people thought of him as the most brilliant organic chemist of the 20th century, maybe of all time – but his laboratory was like a factory, very hierarchical, with no chance to interact with him. That certainly diminished my interest.

So I decided to go back to medical school. It was a difficult year of transition. My father died at that point and I needed to earn some money to continue in medical school but I had also exempted out of most of the first two years because of my graduate and undergraduate work and I began to work in psychopharmacology instead.

Who with?

I worked with Daniel X. Freedman and Nicholas Giarman. Actually this wasn't my first experience in psychopharmacology. In between graduating from Cornell and beginning graduate work in chemistry at Harvard, I worked for a summer at Lederle Laboratories in New Jersey, searching for new classes of MAO inhibitors.

This was 1958?

This was the summer of 1958. I was free to explore their entire library of compounds. Nobody really knew enough about monoamine oxidase or about principles of rational drug design to do anything other than approach this task empirically, but I made some educated guesses which worked out rather well. Through this experience I got caught up with the potential of drugs to treat mental illnesses. I read McIlwain's textbook on neurochemistry (*Biochemistry and the Central Nervous System*) at that point. I developed the probably false notion that all that was worth knowing about neurochemistry at the time could be summarized in 120 pages. This was rather seductive in that it seemed it could be easy enough to learn enough to contribute to this field which was just in its infancy – contrast that with the current situation!

When I began medical school at Yale, after the Harvard experience, I had time to work in a lab for a stipend to earn part of my tuition. I was hired by Jack Peter Green who was studying biogenic amines in mast cells. In my second year, I went on to work with Daniel X. Freedman and his collaborator Nicholas Giarman, who was one of the leading pharmacologists of that era but who was killed in an car crash a few years later.

Dan Freedman and Tom Detre were both assistant professors in Yale at the time and while I had this excellent lab experience with Dan and was thinking more about going into basic science, my first clinical clerkship as a medical student was on Tom Detre's very famous unit at Grace New Haven Hospital, called T1. Tom was a most talented and charismatic clinician, with a strong interest in psychopharmacology. I was greatly impressed by his way of interacting with severely ill patients. At the end of that three-week clerkship, I decided that I wanted to be a psychiatrist. I knew that I wanted to continue doing basic research into brain and behaviour but that I also wanted clinical training. This was the final resolution of the dilemma that I became depressed about in college, when trying to decide whether I should become a laboratory scientist or a clinician. What I had found at Yale Medical School at that time seemed to be the perfect synthesis.

What was Freedman like at that time?

Freedman was then a young assistant professor of psychiatry, who was very eager to move psychiatry from an exclusive descriptive and psychodynamic approach to the biological domain as well. However, his basic neuroscience knowledge was limited. I remember that shortly after we met he took me out to dinner to 'pick my brain' about the relationship of LSD to serotonin. I remember coming home from that dinner feeling elated, like some important rite of passage had taken place. It was the first time that someone at a faculty level had identified within me an intellectual contribution that I could make. Dan, even then, had the habit of identifying young people who he thought had some promise and then really nurturing them. That would have included people like Jack Barchas, Malcolm Bowers, Floyd Bloom, George Aghajanian, Donald Cohen and many others.

I worked with Dan throughout medical school. He was certainly one of my idols and became and remained very important to me. After my internship, I went to the National Institute of Mental Health in Bethesda, as a Clinical Research Associate in the laboratory of Jack Durrell, something I may return to. After two years at NIMH, I decided that I did not want to stay there permanently. I felt that I would do better at a University, with more independence, than as a junior person in a big lab. I wrote to Dan for a letter of recommendation. I'm sure it contributed to offers I received from Harvard, Albert Einstein, Cornell and other places. Dan had moved from Yale to the University of Chicago to become the first Chairman of Psychiatry there. Prior to his coming it was a department with no national identity. He had already recruited a number of outstanding people when I asked him for a recommendation for one of the schools on the East Coast. He said that he would be happy to do so but he asked me to also take a look at Chicago. I accepted out of a sense of politeness. I had no interest whatever in going to the Midwest, which I barely knew. In that era Chicago had a terrible reputation as a city.

I flew into Chicago on a lovely crisp Autumn Sunday afternoon, checked into a University guest center on the Midway, a rather beautiful boulevard lined with campus buildings. I had a few free hours before I was supposed to meet Dan for dinner. I walked across the campus to look through a Gothic cathedral, which seemed out of place. I opened the doors of what is Rockefeller Chapel and the Chicago symphony and Chorus was performing the Bach B Minor Mass. I was absolutely enthralled with Bach at that time and I stayed and listened to it until it was over. By that point I had decided whatever might happen during my visit, I would be agreeable to an offer.

Dan and his wife Mary took me out to dinner to their private club. There was an assistant dean, who he had managed to dragoon into spending an evening with this raw recruit. I forget who else was there. They got me slightly intoxicated and the next thing I knew I was calling my wife and saying . . . we should come to Chicago. I spent 17 generally very satisfying years there until I could no longer continue clinical research but that is another story.

In the UK, I don't think Dan Freedman has had the impact of someone like Seymour Kety, for instance, but between the editorship of the Archives of General Psychiatry *and his work on LSD he really was one of the seminal figures.*

From a scientific contribution point of view, he was significant but not the overwhelming influence that Seymour Kety has been. What was seminal about Dan were the numbers of young people who he brought into research. Any number of leading researchers were considered to be one of 'Danny's boys'. Its these people, who he mentored and nurtured and, secondly, the standards that he set at the *Archives of General Psychiatry,* which were his great legacies, more so than his LSD research. He was able to create an aura around the Archives, that Europeans may not have appreciated. People put up with some of the most outrageous things just in order to get their papers published in that journal. He constantly escalated the requirements. He would sometimes get seven or eight reviews of a paper.

Instead of the usual two or three.

Yes. People would then begin to write little novellas for these reviews. I recall receiving reviews, which might be five or six pages each. Of course, there were often significant differences of opinion among the reviewers. Dan would give you some guidance about which points he thought were the ones you should attend to if he decided to accept the paper. There is no question that that became the new standard for the field of psychiatric research. No other journal in psychiatry prior to that time had that level of expectation.

About the time I went to NIMH, Kety produced two reviews in the *New England Journal of Medicine* and in *Science* on the sorry state of schizophrenia research, debunking pretty much all that had been done and setting new standards for what should be reliable research designs. In that sense, the achievement of both was complementary – one as an editor, one as an investigator and critic, establishing new standards of excellence.

He worked incredibly hard. He generally didn't come in until 10 or 11 in the morning but then would work till midnight and beyond. He hardly ever ate. He smoked constantly. I probably have increased vulnerability to lung cancer just from the time I spent in his office. Once he started talking to you, it could go on for hours. He would do his editorial work on the journal in bursts – for two or three days steady, once a month. I think he probably had some mark on the wall behind his desk where he piled the incoming articles. When the stack got to a certain height, he would begin to work it down. He usually dictated his letters and then scribbled corrections on the draft. He had the most incredible, unintelligible scrawl but was blessed with a wonderful typist who could decipher his remarks. I don't know if you've ever had any letters from him or heard any of his talks. Some of it is unintelligible; it almost seemed like he had a thought disorder at times and then sometimes his writings and talks had the most incredible elegance and wit. The editorials he would publish in the Archives could be extremely polished, almost Jamesian, with incredibly complex syntax, puns and multiple levels of meaning. At other times, he could be off-the-wall. and even embarrassing. But he really was a great man.

Do you not think it's possible that his reputation for his work on LSD has only been temporarily eclipsed because the LSD story went underground and there was no longer any referencing of the work that had been done?

The LSD model of schizophrenia, of course, fell from grace and was replaced by the dopamine hypothesis and in many ways that LSD research pointed towards the 5-HT-2 receptors that has certainly been important for my research on atypical antipsychotics.

The other way that Dan was terribly important to the whole field of psychiatry is that he had an immense influence in Washington and among foundations. There is no doubt that he really helped to give shape to the NIMH, as it existed until 1994. He was the *éminence grise* for so many of the NIMH directors. Herb Pardess would have acknowledged this with great gratitude. Dan and he would be on the phone constantly. I'm reasonably sure he discussed all the major decisions that affected NIMH with Dan. Dan was also constantly testifying before Congress and had great influence among the Foundations. He was the number one consultant to search committees for Chairs of psychiatry and for evaluating existing programs. So, his influence was pervasive and is sorely missed now that there is a real crisis in American psychiatry.

Let me ask you about an earlier crisis first. It seems extraordinary to me that US psychiatry in the 1950s and 1960s was so controlled by the analysts and yet a few key people like Nathan Kline, Kety and Freedman were able to go to Congress and get them to part with huge amounts of money to set up psychopharmacology research programmes.

Yes. Although American academic psychiatry in that era was dominated by psychoanalysts, many of whom were Europeans who were escaping the war, these people were not narrow minded. Dan Freedman owed his career to Fritz Redlich and while Redlich probably knew little about the biological basis of behaviour, he respected it and really thought that it was important to the future. They did not simply wish to turn their departments into psychoanalytic institutes. I received job offers from a number of these Chairmen, in 1958, who were keen to bring a biological orientation to their departments. There was so much benefit developing from the new antidepressants and neuroleptics that one could easily make a case for increased research in mental health.

Can I take you back to the period at NIMH and ask how that looked to you at the time?

Well, it was fascinating. I had trained in psychiatry at Mass Mental Health Centre, which many people thought had the leading psychiatric residency programme in the States. It was an amazing place from 1964–66, when I was there. It was dominated by psychoanalysts, who were totally committed to psychodynamic psychiatry. Even their approach to schizophrenia was psychoanalytical.

Who were the key figures?

The key figure was Elvin Semrad. He was thought of as the leading spiritual and intellectual light by hundreds and hundreds of the brightest young American psychiatrists who trained there. He had an astonishing ability to establish a relationship with severely ill psychotic patients – to get them to talk about themselves to whatever extent they were capable. He genuinely believed, or so he taught us, that psychotherapy could have a major impact on schizophrenia and that neuroleptic drugs could be a barrier to real recovery.

This was even after chlorpromazine?

Chlorpromazine had been introduced to Mass Mental in the early 1960s. In fact when I was a second-year resident, I was appointed chief resident on an ongoing NIMH-sponsored study to compare psychoanalytic psychotherapy and thioridazine in the treatment of schizophrenia. The grant was for a seven-year project, in which three cohorts of very chronic schizophrenic patients were transferred to a research unit at Mass Mental, for two years for on the couch psychoanalysis, four times per week – with periods of thioridazine or placebo on a double-blind basis to see if thioridazine had an effect. As I said, I was the chief resident on the fourth year of the project. To cut a long story short, the results showed that psychoanalysis and thioridazine was so superior to psychoanalysis and placebo that the project was terminated at the end of that year. The study proved the drugs worked. However, one could argue that it was never really a clear test of psychoanalysis because the people who were administering this treatment, despite being experienced senior analysts, were really participating in this study to meet the expectations of the hospital director rather than out of genuine interest. So they really just went through the motions, often missing appointments and letting patients sleep on the couch.

Who actually conceived of this study?

The project was initiated by the Head of the Hospital, Jack Ewalt and the Director of Research, Lester Grinspoon. It had a great impact on any further research in the psychotherapy of schizophrenia.

Philip May did some work in this area as well.

Yes. Phil May did the famous Camarillo State Hospital study, which produced similar finding on the benefits of drugs versus psychotherapy in schizophrenia. What was important to me at Mass Mental Health Center was the opportunity to spend hours listening to and trying to relate to psychotic patients to identify the contribution to their psychosis of their experience in their families and elsewhere. To some extent we were expected to concentrate on 'here and now' issues but the main focus was expected to be on childhood. I will never forget presenting a patient I had worked on to one of my supervisors, Dr Susan Van Amerangum, one of the leading figures of Boston psychiatry. I had carefully collected whatever information I could about what had been happening in this patients life at the time of the onset of the psychosis and what was happening in our relationship but the main thing she wanted to know about was the history of his toilet training.

It seems remarkable that an institution as psychodynamically orientated as the Mass Mental Health Center was at that time should have produced so many eminent psychopharmacologists, or at least psychobiologists. Eric Kandel and Ed Sachar are striking examples.

On the schizophrenia unit that I described, I participated in research with Ed Sachar who was in the midst of his brilliant work on increased activity of the HPA axis, during psychotic turmoil. Eric Kandel was just beginning his life-long research on *aplysia*. I was assigned to Eric for supervision of one of my outpatient treatment cases. I remember distinctly finding him the most helpful of my supervisers. He was less analytic, as you might expect, than the average person there, but very intuitive and clever. That's the wonderful thing about psychiatry; I don't know how long Eric continued doing clinical work, but he might have done so for some time because it was such an essential part of the identity of a Boston psychiatrist. Clinical skills in psychotherapy were the most highly esteemed. The pressure to become a psychonanalyst was immense. I count myself very lucky that I was able to break away from that culture and go to the NIMH. Many of my fellow residents, who remained in Boston, joined the Psychoanalytic Institute and became training analysts. The potential many had to be scientists was never developed, although there were exceptions, including Richard Shader, Robert Liberman, Roger Meyer, Richard Wyatt, Dan Weinberger, Joel Kleinman, David Reiss and Carl Salzman.

Norman Weiner, who became Chairman of Pharmacology at Colorado, was at Mass Mental Health as was Joe Schildkraut and Gerry Klerman. Gerry was Semrad's assistant. We didn't have any real didactic training in psychiatric except for a course Gerry was permitted to give on the history of psychiatry. Gerry was the role model for the clinical investigator who was beginning psychopharmacology. He was developing the field at the time and publishing in highly respected journals. Although I didn't work with Gerry directly, I knew much about what was going on in his depression research in terms of standardized diagnostic assessments and the collection of biological measures by Joe Schildkraut and others. This certainly influenced me in my later career.

We were supposed to learn it all from our direct clinical work and supervision. I look back on it as both the worst and the best of training. What I most value was the experience of being with patients who were very disturbed and becoming comfortable relating to them.

So, I don't regret having trained there. It's an enormous challenge to do clinical research of the kind that I've done. I've always felt that in order to keep clinical staff motivated over the long run, they have to believe not only in the worth of the science you're engaged in but in you as a clinician. Unless you are a first-rate clinician, you will quickly lose their support, which is essential if patients are to participate in research projects. I have heard about examples in research institutes, where staff actually sabotaged the clinical research simply because of their hostility to the clinical chief of the unit, which stemmed from his insensitivity and indifference to patient well-being.

When I went to NIMH, Jack Durrell was there. He was considered to be the most outstanding biological psychiatrist working in schizophrenia at the NIMH. He was Seymour Kety's chief clinical investigator. He introduced me to a completely different approach to treating schizophrenia. It violated every single principle that I had been taught at Mass

Mental Health Center. There was no individual psychotherapy, intensive involvement with the families, different types of group therapies, nurses as co-equals in the treatment enterprise, education about the illness and drug treatment. At first I was horrified by it. I thought that it was almost malpractice. Then, to my astonishment, the first cohort of patients I worked with in this manner improved amazingly. Perhaps, I didn't say it clearly enough when I was talking about Elvin Semrad was that in teaching us to do psychotherapy with schizophrenics, he also discouraged the use of antipsychotic medicines. When we did use them, it was almost out of a sense of failure, that there must be something wrong with our ability to establish a relationship and to understand what patients were feeling and thinking. What I found at NIMH was the integration of drug treatment with family and social therapy – what we called milieu therapy – with biological research and excellent results. It was really exciting.

Who was responsible for introducing this?

Durrell was. He was a fine scientist and an outstanding clinician. There is no question that that experience shaped my ultimate ability to do clinical psychopharmacology. The psychosocial programme I developed for patients on clozapine was all foreshadowed by his example. Ironically, Dr Durrell got into a conflict with the directors of the Clinical Centre at NIMH. He was told to stop his clinical work and to continue his laboratory work; he refused to do this and left the NIMH. He established the prototype in Washington of what became the Psychiatric Institutes of America, an enormously successful chain of clinics and hospitals. Unfortunately, he never continued his biological research.

After he left, his unit was reassigned to Fred Snyder, a sleep researcher, and I was put in charge of the clinical programme. I worked on that Unit for another year and a half. I trained Richard Wyatt and David Kupfer to be my successors. I often said that I came down to NIMH for research training, and I certainly got that, but even more so I learned clinical psychiatry that became the basis for what I went on to do in Chicago and Cleveland.

Beyond what I previously said about the Chicago Symphony and the ambiance of the University of Chicago, the key factor that made me accept Dan's offer to join a brand new department rather than go to a more established place was that I was offered a 12-bed inpatient unit at the Illinois State Psychiatric Institute, with which the University of Chicago had an affiliation. That offered me an opportunity to institute the clinical method that I had learned at NIMH and provided a base for my research in the biology and treatment of schizophrenia and major depression.

Tell me more about the research there.

Well, it goes back to my first research project at NIMH. I was seeking a neurochemical deficit in schizophrenia. I came across a paper by Hanns Hippius, the Professor of Psychiatry in Munich, in which he and a colleague, Bengzon, reported that schizophrenic patients had increased creatine kinase (CK) activity in their bloodstream. They proposed that this enzyme was leaking out of the brain and that its loss might be the cause of schizophrenia because of the role of CK in energy metabolism. I studied some newly admitted psychotic patients at the NIMH and replicated the finding (Meltzer, 1968). It would take a long time to describe all the studies I did subsequently because I got intensively interested in the mechanism. I was able to show that the form of CK in the blood was coming from skeletal muscle and not brain. I set up various animal models to study the process. The best model that I found for this enzyme leakage from skeletal muscle was the combination of restraint stress plus phencyclidine (PCP) (Kund and Meltzer, 1974).

When I went out to Chicago, I was still very much involved in this study. I was able to get an NIMH grant immediately to pursue it. The Research Unit I set up was to study this phenomenon in the acute stages of psychosis. I had an animal lab also in which I continued to investigate the cause of skeletal muscle damage. This is how I did my first serotonin research because the best model of Duchenne-type muscular dystrophy at that time was the combination of intraperitoneal serotonin plus aortic ligation. I pursued this finding in a great many directions.

I've been a scientist who has followed my intuition fairly freely rather than stay with a narrow research agenda, although I would argue that I have been able to keep my focus but with the freedom to follow the best approach. I think Sol Synder does the same thing. He has told me that he will do 10 experiments for every 1 that really works. I'm not sure what my ratio is but I am willing to take risks.

An interesting result of the neuromuscular work was my discovery that plasma CK activity varies as a function of race. Black people normally have higher plasma CK levels than Caucasians. This was important because relatively small elevations were used to detect the carrier state of muscular dystrophy. Black women were being falsely identified as carriers on the basis of CK levels that were normal for them. I still see this work, which is 25 years old, quoted from time to time.

Gradually though, I got more into the direct study of neurotransmitter hypotheses of mental illness, especially serotonin and dopamine. The critical thing that intervened was that Edward Sachar, who was Chairman of Psychiatry at Columbia at the time, called me to collaborate with him on some neuroendocrine research that might provide a test of the dopamine hypothesis of schizophrenia, by studying basal serum prolactin levels in unmedicated schizophrenic patients and controls (Meltzer, Sachar and Frantz, 1974). We set up a wonderful collaboration that lasted until he had a stroke about five years later. The prolactin work that I did with

Sachar led to the first experience I had with clozapine. I was the first to report that clozapine did not stimulate prolactin secretion in man.

I began to pursue a number of independent leads, particularly around the serotonergic system. I developed a whole lot of animal models, based on neuroendocrine effects. That's really what got me into the intensive study of serotonin receptor subtypes from a functional point of view. Another thing that happened was that I was among the first three investigators in the US to use fluoxetine to treat depression. The very first patient I gave it to developed a severe dystonic reaction (Meltzer *et al.*, 1979). I thought he had received haloperidol instead of fluoxetine, that there had been a nursing error in what he had been given but it turned out that it was fluoxetine. That led me to the study of the interactions between serotonin and dopamine neurotransmission. What I am focused on now in relation to schizophrenia and depression is still the interaction between the serotonergic and dopaminergic pathways.

So how did clozapine come into your research?

A pivotal event was my treatment of a near-fatal case of tardive dyskinesia from one of the Illinois state hospitals. This woman was down to perhaps 60% of her normal weight due to her inability to eat on her own, or to be fed by nursing staff due to the severity of her truncal movements and problems in swallowing. I treated her with clozapine which I had permission from Sandoz to use. She really had an astonishing, life-saving improvement in her tardive dyskinesia.

This was when?

I think that would be in the early 1980s. This case was the last of many studies with clozapine which led me to work with Sandoz to help plan the strategy to get clozapine approved by the FDA – even on a restricted basis because of its ability to cause agranulocytosis. There was clearly a need for other people who were similarly disabled or who could not respond adequately to the standard antipsychotic drugs to be treated with clozapine.

The prolactin research with clozapine was my first human study with the drug. Before that, I did several studies in animals, which showed that it elevated serum prolactin levels. Clozapine produced an unusual type of prolactin elevation in the rat. Whereas haloperidol produced large increases that were prolonged – up to 4 hours – clozapine produced brief increases for 30 minutes of equal magnitude despite the persistence of adequate plasma levels. Gary Gudelsky and I showed that this was due to clozapine's ability to activate hypothalamic dopamine neurones. Clozapine stimulates, for example, large increases in extracellular dopamine in the frontal cortex and to a lesser extent the nucleus accumbens in awake, freely moving rats.

A major characteristic of my research style has been to try to integrate pre-clinical and clinical studies. Thus, the patient I described with the dystonia led to my basic research on serotonin and dopamine interactions. Equally there are a number of preclinical observations that have generated clinical ideas also. As I indicated, I have done so to satisfy my need to have both in life. It's something I still enjoy. I find it hard to imagine doing clinical psychopharmacology without being really up on the literature of what's happening at the cutting edge of basic research.

There is an argument though that the basic research is beginning to take off explosively and it's hard to know just what relevance an awful lot of it has to do with clinical practice. Groups like ACNP and BAP seem to be having problems because the clinical members are going to the meetings and finding that the programme has become almost completely incomprehensible.

That's true. But the clinical person who is really doing something creative has to understand what's happening in basic science. It's less and less easy to do but more and more necessary. That's why I particularly believe in the research centre concept. I was among the first group of awardees of an NIMH-supported clinical research centre when the belief finally surfaced that efforts of that nature shouldn't all be concentrated in Bethesda. The Center I direct started out as a small enterprise and it's still only relatively small but my group has more PhD bench scientists than clinical investigators. I still direct some aspects of the very basic research, usually working with fellows or a fellow, who I can support in the lab to work with one of the PhDs. I would think that without being part of that kind of an enterprise I couldn't keep up with the field.

How many research centres are there in the country?

In the field of mental health, there are now approximately 20–25 centers. It started with seven in 1977. Of the original seven there are five of us left. Each center has its own mission. There is a suicide centre, an adolescent centre, child centres, mood disorder, brain imaging and so on. Mine is devoted to studying the biological and psychopharmacological bases of schizophrenia and mood disorders. The dual focus stems from my earlier work with the neuromuscular system because those kinds of abnormalities were characteristic of both mood disorders and schizophrenia. I'm an anti-Kraepelinian in that sense.

A Unitary psychosis person?

Yes. While I believe there are clear differences in these disorders, I also find there are many abnormalities that they share in common. My colleagues Helio Elkis of Brazil and Lee Freedman and I have completed a meta-analysis of the literature on CT and MRI scans in schizophrenia, major depression and normal controls. We found essentially no difference between the two patient groups on brain scans. One has to be able to explain these commonalities. However, there are unique features. We've been recently looking at the striatal D-4 receptor abnormality that Phil Seeman reported in schizophrenia. We have partially replicated his findings but we found no such difference in patients with mood disorders.

Let me take you back then to the Chicago. You say that you were there for 17 years, why did you leave?

I left because the governor of Illinois, James Thompson, decided that research in the Department of Mental Health was of extremely low priority. He converted the Illinois State Psychiatric Institute, which had been a well-funded and protected research base, into a community mental health centre. My colleagues and I couldn't continue to do research because of the lack of funds and the clinical burden. When the opportunity was offered to me to occupy an endowed research professorship at Case Western Reserve University School of Medicine, I was ready to accept. I decided Case would provide an excellent environment for the research centre. The move went exceedingly well. However, recently, continued access to inpatient facilities has become a problem. Inpatient research is very costly and requires subsidies from the government or the hospital system. No one wants to pay for it any longer. I believe the research enterprise will suffer greatly because of this.

That brings us back to a point you made earlier about the current crisis in American psychiatry, how do you see that?

We are losing ground in psychiatric research in general, and psychopharmacology in particular. The most serious problem is the amount of money that is available from the National Institutes of Health to fund research grants. When NIMH was incorporated into in 1992 or 1993, it lost a great deal of money for complicated reasons. Now priority scores have to be in the 10th percentile or better to get funded whereas the 20th percentile or lower was funded at one time. The actual number of grants that are being funded is much less.

The second way in which research is being undermined is the move towards managed care, as part of health reform. Huge insurance companies are gaining control of the medical delivery system. This has cut down the availability of hospital-generated monies for research purposes. Once great hospitals are becoming little different than community hospitals. Only a very select group of academic centers are able to fund a centre that needs an inpatient base to continue. The third way in which research is being cut back is that the pharmaceutical industry is also retrenching.

The one good development, which is something I am very much involved in and proud of, is a non-profit fund raising group called NARSAD – the National Association for Research in Schizophrenia and Depression. I helped to found NARSAD, eight or nine years ago, along with Herb Pardes, Sam Keith, Will Carpenter and several other people.

It's the first successful means of letting the general public and particularly people of means know that they can, through contributions, really advance the treatment of the seriously mentally ill and our understanding of mental illness.

We started, I remember, hoping we could raise $100,000 to fund three or four small grants of about $25,000 each. This year we able to provide about $6,500,000, for two fairly large programmes. The largest is called 'The Young Investigators' Program' and is for people who are just finishing their PhD or residency training and assistant professors who haven't gotten a grant yet. We also have a programme for Established Investigators with grants, who are seeking money for some novel ideas that they couldn't get funded at the federal level. I think we now have a national identity. The prospects of getting into the $10 million/year range are really quite good. There isn't any question in my mind that the success of NARSAD has enabled many talented young people to enter and then remain in research.

I take a great deal of pleasure in the fact that clozapine is one of the major reasons that wealthy people in the US with children who have serious mental illness have been motivated to contribute to NARSAD. The story I hear over and over again is that after years of unsuccessful treatment with standard drugs that a physician finally put their child or relative on clozapine with excellent results and that out of gratitude and recognition that research does make a difference, they are willing to give substantial amounts to money to NARSAD.

Well, that's a good note on which to revisit the clozapine story. At the stage you were doing your prolactin work had it been killed by agranulocytosis?

In 1976, I wrote what people told me was a very influential review with Stephen Stahl, of the dopamine hypothesis of schizophrenia, which was published in *Schizophrenia Bulletin* (Meltzer and Stahl, 1976). After that, I began to pursue novel drug therapies for schizophrenia, for example, dopamine autoreceptor agonists as potential treatments. I studied the effect of alphamethylparatyrosine, an inhibitor of dopamine synthesis. I also began a search for clozapine—like drugs without agranulocytosis. I identified a very interesting drug called melperone (Meltzer, Fang and Young, 1980). Clozapine was going nowhere until 1985 when John Kane and myself and Gil Honigfeld and Jack Singer from Sandoz thought about how an approach could be made to the FDA to gain approval for its use in tardive dyskinesia, based on cases like the one I described previously.

You were able to get hold of clozapine from Sandoz for this lady; how were you able to do that?

The agranulocytosis was discovered first in 1975 after a group of elderly patients from a small area of Finland died. It was immediately withdrawn from use world-wide. But as is now very apparent, if you withdraw people from clozapine, they may relapse rapidly and severely. We don't really understand why that is but it is a difference from other drugs. It's like taking insulin away from a diabetic. They often won't respond as well to a typical neuroleptic drug as they did. As a result many people were put back on it. Sandoz would probably have preferred to completely end its availability but did continue to provide it on a 'compassionate need' basis. I would say that myself, George Simpson, John Kane and Nathan Kline were among the few still using it in the US but to a very limited extent. My experience with it was sufficiently positive that I felt obligated to participate in the effort to seek FDA approval. Therefore, Sandoz, with the help of John Kane and myself, put together a New Drug Application, which was submitted to the FDA and which was rejected.

By whom?

Paul Leber and probably others at the FDA rejected the positive recommendation of the Advisory Board to approve clozapine because there was no controlled trial to establish its freedom from tardive dyskinesia. The next step was to provide a controlled trial, which was 'Study 30', designed to show its superiority to chlorpromazine for neuroleptic-resistant patients (Kane et al., 1988). Sandoz was willing to take the considerable risk that clozapine could be shown to be more effective than standard antipsychotic drugs.

They must have put a lot of money into it?

I would estimate that that study must have cost between $5–7 million. Even if it was successful, there was no certainty that the drug would be approved by the FDA or that it would be widely utilized. Other limitations for developing it were that it only could have five years of patent life and that Sandoz might be sued if somebody developed agranulocytosis and died. Sandoz also anticipated that it would be used in only a small number of patients. Fortunately they went ahead with the study and fortunately it was approved.

Why did they go ahead?

Well, I've been told that Sandoz agreed to support the study because the FDA was interested in clozapine, despite or maybe because of their rejection of it for use in tardive dyskinesia. I was also informed that the FDA used its leverage with Sandoz based on non-clozapine-related issues to urge them to do this study. So in a very positive way there was a collaboration between the FDA and Sandoz to see that a controlled study with clozapine was done. Not only did that study lead to the approval of clozapine but it showed the potential for other drugs to do as well or even better and it became a great tool for understanding the brain just as did chlorpromazine in its day.

What do you remember most about the trial?

The moment I remember most was the interim analysis which was done when the first 150 patients were completed. The four principal investigators had a meeting in New York City together with the project statistician, John Patin. The results were presented by John and Gil Honigfeld. They showed an astonishing effect of clozapine compared to chlorpromazine. The effect was so strong that even if the two drugs were only equal in effectiveness in the second half, there would still have been a significant advantage for clozapine.

After I returned to Cleveland from that meeting, I called the lab together and said we must drop virtually everything else we were doing and focus on clozapine studies to understand its mechanism. I concluded it was going to revolutionise the field and I believe I was correct in this regard.

When you said that it was going to revolutionize the field, there was a paradox in that, in a sense, it was back to chlorpromazine. For 20 years people had moved down the road of more selective D-2 blocking agents and all of a sudden you've got this dirty drug, which proves superior.

At least for the present, that is how it would appear. Conceptualizing what clozapine does clinically, it takes treatment-resistant patients and brings them to the level of non-treatment-resistant patients. Some people become astonishingly better just as some people with schizophrenia get astonishingly better after haloperidol treatment. However, there are other things that clozapine uniquely does that differentiate it from chlorpromazine such as no extrapyramidal symptoms, no tardive dyskinesia, no prolactin elevations, and I think, most importantly, it improves some aspects of cognitive function (Hagger *et al.*, 1993).

You've stated we need to draw a distinction between the antipsychotics and the neuroleptics. Do we?

I think so. The capacity to produce parkinsonism and akathisia are major and immense drawbacks for an antipsychotic agent. Probably as many as 50% of schizophrenic patients under routine treatment conditions become non-compliant within months of starting medication. Most people believe that's due to extrapyramidal side effects. So an antipsychotic drug which doesn't produce them is going to be so much better tolerated. There's all sorts of evidence to suggest that continuous rather than intermittent treatment with neuroleptic drugs is going to lead to the best long-term outcome. Therefore, you have to have a drug that doesn't produce intolerable acute side effects or delayed onset side effects like tardive dyskinesia. Some day we're going to have antipsychotic drugs that do this.

The other neuroleptics are effective across a range of disorders, the major affective disorders, OCD, is clozapine any good for conditions other than schizophrenia?

Clozapine is quite effective in a range of disorders. We have published several reports showing that clozapine is effective in treatment-resistant manic – depressive disorder and treatment-resistant psychotic depression. We've also confirmed that it's very effective in L-dopa and bromocriptine-induced psychosis in Parkinson's disease. It probably doesn't help OCD; in our hands, it makes OCD worse. There are actually some older studies using clozapine in classical major depression as an antidepressant and it was effective.

So, we are back to the unitary psychosis concept.

To some extent, yes. I've recently written a paper about the implications of psychopharmacology research for the unitary psychosis hypothesis. The fact that drugs like clozapine are effective across the spectrum of mood and schizophreniform illnesses, is supportive of this view.

How does it work, if it isn't working by blocking D-2 receptors on their own?

Well, I've provided a lot of valid evidence, in my view, that blockade of the 5-HT-2 receptor is an important element but I no longer believe that all of its advantages are due to that property. I think there could be a significant contribution from 5-HT-6 and 5-HT-7 receptor antagonism, possibly D-2 and D-4 receptor blockade and possibly its ability to modulate the cholinergic system. Other investigators highlight its strong alpha-1 and -2 adrenergic blocking activity. Clozapine is the ultimate 'dirty' drug of psychopharmacology, at least for the present, and that may be its genius.

If that is the genius where does that leave us? The industry at the moment is predicated on purer and purer drugs. Molecular biology and receptor cloning is all about getting a drug that will target just one receptor system.

That strategy has much to recommend it. We do need drugs that are incredibly selective for obvious reasons. They are indispensable but clearly, in the case of schizophrenia at least, they may be less effective as drugs. There is much evidence that strong 5-HT-2 and weak D-2 receptor blockade, as is present in risperidone, sertindole and olanzapine is useful to decrease extrapyramidal symptoms. However, I believe that these drugs will show significant differences from each other and clozapine. They will have very different clinical profiles because of the differences in their relative affinities for receptors other than the 5-HT-2A and D-2 receptors.

The catecholamine theory of depression and the dopamine hypothesis of schizophrenia really made the field respectable but did they also hold things back.

They provided a structure and the hope that we were on the right track. It has turned out that the original versions of these hypotheses were seriously in error. They sought to explain too much. That is particularly true for the catecholamine hypothesis. Its amazing how long the dopamine hypothesis was not seriously challenged given all that we know to be incompatible with it.

One of the hunches that I have on that was the industry is highly conservative and once they start on a line of drug development – to inhibit catecholamine or 5-HT reuptake or to block D-2 receptors – they keep doing that and that keeps a theory in place even though the field should have actually moved on.

I remember attempts in the 1980s to move beyond the catecholamine hypothesis into the endorphines and the opiates as well as an attempt to develop drugs related to GABA as antipsychotics. But the failure to find anything of therapeutic value brought the field back to dopamine. An early version of the serotonin hypothesis of schizophrenia, as explored in the 1950s and early 1960s, died because of the failure to validate any evidence for psychotomimetic indoleamines in urine and blood or post-mortem specimens from schizophrenics and the absence of gross effects on the behaviour of schizophrenics of enhancing and diminishing sero-tonergic activity.

Would you have needed to have that validation? You could argue that the LSD model had much more face validity than the amphetamine model – after all, housewives were having amphetamines during the 1950s and they weren't going psychotic.

I may be less than objective here but my feeling is that psychopharma-cology really drives the field. There's a great scepticism about the biological abnormalities reported in schizophrenic patients, particularly in this era of neuroleptic treatment. And besides that, there is the enormous problem provided by the probable heterogeneity of etiology and pathophysiology. We all give lip service to this issue but then many people proceed to forget it and keep expecting to find group differences between schizo-phrenic patients and controls. I wrote a paper once on sub-typing of schizophrenia and how to use this concept to study the biology of schizo-phrenia. The heterogeneity view suggests you must follow single cases or small groups of cases, which may be biologically similar. Once you start to examine a whole consecutive series of schizophrenic patients for common biological deficits, you're bound to find great variability.

The biological marker strategy has proven exceedingly difficult to work with for this reason. I'm sure it's one of the things that makes the search for a genetic marker so appealing. In order to find a principle, if you will, from psychopharmacology that is as sustainable as was the dopamine hypothesis has been, is very desirable. For example, as we speak, there's a lot of interest in the possibility of a specific novel dopamine abnormality in schizophrenia, in the D-4 system. This stems from Seemans' research which was stimulated by the demonstration of the greater effectiveness of clozapine versus typical neuroleptics in schizophrenic patients rather than from animal research. I'm convinced that animal models of 'schizophrenia' are of secondary value. Schizophrenia is the quintessential human brain disease. It is going to be exceedingly difficult to obtain a useful animal model. We can model certain components of the disorder, i.e. stereotyped behaviour or catatonia, but the essence of the disorder, the cognitive dysfunction and loss of volition, is very hard to model in animals. One can use animal work to generate hypothesis but these ultimately have to be proven in man.

Before clozapine, you were systematically working your way through the options in terms of treatments active on dopamine receptors but with clozapine a real passion seems to have entered into the picture for you.

That's true. I had treated individual cases through the years, maybe half a dozen, that had responded exceptionally well to clozapine after doing poorly with a variety of treatments. But it is a tribute to the power of the randomized control trial, as I said, that only when I saw the outcome of the first half of Study 30, showing the superiority of clozapine over chlorpromazine, was I truly convinced that it was exceptional enough clinically to push forward with it and, secondly, that it was urgent to study the biological basis for this. This redirected my energies and eventually led to the serotonin hypothesis of its mechanism of action.

Serotonin has been an enduring interest, along with dopamine – serotonin interactions. The first major breakthrough that I had in this regard was understanding the basis for the time course of clozapine—induced prolactin increases in rodents. The prevailing idea about the mechanism of action of clozapine was that D-1 receptor blockade was the important feature. I tried to check that hypothesis by studying other atypical antipsychotic drugs. At that point in time I had used a variety of antipsychotic drugs, which had atypical properties in man – I'm not sure if many other people had as much experience. So I could approach it on the basis of both clinical experience as well as the basic research I had been doing. I also had the advantage of having the extensive statistical support provided by the clinical research centre. A research fellow from Japan and I, Shigehiro Matsuhara of Hokkaido University, were able to study about 20 putative antipsychotic compounds with D-1, D-2 and 5-HT-2 activity. Ultimately we were able to show that we could an identify an atypical antipsychotic drug on the basis of the D- 2/5-HT-2 model.

For a long time, I believed that all the clinical advantages of clozapine had to be due to one biological mechanism. I rejected the possibility that its spectrum of advantage for treating both positive and negative symptoms in the absence of tardive dyskinesia, EPS and prolactin increases, could be due to many different receptor affinities in the right balance. Now I have reluctantly come to think that this possibility may be correct. I now believe that there are multiple mechanisms that clozapine directly or indirectly calls into play, which account for its advantages.

Clozapine has clearly transformed the way you see things and it has given hope to a great number of people but you still seem very open on the issues. You encouraged me at one point to seek publication for an article asking whether we can we afford it. A lot of people, in your position, approached by someone like me who really hadn't had the opportunity to see the benefits you had seen, might have tried to kill the piece.

Well, I must say that I didn't try to kill it or encourage you not to seek publication because I felt that there was a need for debate about the issue. Under some clinical circumstances, the greater effectiveness of clozapine could cost so much that one could rationally say that it's not worth it (Meltzer *et al.*, 1993). I'm not so fanatic about seeing patients do better that I think there's no limit to the amount of money that should be made available for what might be a small advantage. There are health systems that might provide excellent care for schizophrenia in which clozapine might not be a cost-effective treatment. I think one of the great deficiencies in psychiatry right now is that there are too few people studying cost effectiveness issues.

Can we do it? We're being forced to but can it validly be done?

Oh I think we can. My son, David, has an MD and a PhD in economics. He did his PhD with Gary Becker of the University of Chicago, who won the Nobel prize in Economics in 1992. I've just seen a paper that David co-authored on the cost effectiveness of prostate cancer testing. He's a real professional at it; I am strictly an amateur. But I see the way that it could be done if people had the proper training. I realize that the approach has an enormous amount to recommend it but the methodology, as it applies to psychiatry, is still rather limited.

One approach would be a cost utility study which I think is the best approach to apply to schizophrenia. In a cost utility model, different people who have a stake in the issue, whether it's the patient, the family or society, indicate measures of value. This might be the number of years of one's life you'd be willing to sacrifice in order to be free of the symptoms and social dysfunction of schizophrenia. This approach to pharmacoeconomics works best in a very complicated situation like schizophrenia, where there are many offsets to a particular advantage. That approach, if it were applied to antipsychotic drugs would allow schizophrenics, who I think often provide reliable judgements, or their families, to say how much it is worth, for example, to have freedom from the risk of tardive dyskinesia versus the possibility of getting agranulocytosis, seizures or increased weight gain, on the negative side.

With that approach, given the greater cost of clozapine, we could come up with how much we would be willing to pay for each unit of utility, each meaningful increment in benefit. In a world where the rationing of health care is becoming more prevalent, there are crucial decisions that should be made on the basis of that kind of information or similar considerations.

Now to get back to my personal style: why would I encourage someone with a different idea to publish? Actually, I've always had the feeling that if I was wrong about something, I'd rather discover it myself. In that sense, encouraging somebody else to produce something that's different to what I believe would be somewhat inconsistent. The only reason I might have been tempted to discourage you would be my passion for clozapine. I really think it's grossly under-utilized and I would not like to have it under-utilized for the wrong reasons, one of which is the idea that it isn't cost effective.

The cost-structure of the English health care system, however, is entirely different to the American one. The costs that are attached to the treatment of mental illness in England are almost an order of magnitude lower than in the US. If that's really how little it costs to treat schizophrenia in England, then you have to respect that it may not be a cost-effective treatment. But that is not the case here in America. I have completed another study in which I have looked at the cost of treating the non-treatment-resistant schizophrenic patient versus the ones who are treatment-resistant. I can still show a cost-effective benefit of clozapine in non-treatment-resistant schizophrenia, although it's very slight compared to what is possible in treatment-resistant cases, which are extremely expensive to treat in the United States.

In the case of England, one of the things that I think is relevant is that in a public sector model, there is this great tendency to underestimate the cost. The full costs are hidden from the public. I almost think it's deliberate. It's the exact opposite in a private sector model where for financial reasons, both for maximum reimbursement and to lower taxes, the public and private sector are motivated to overestimate their costs. In the study that I did, I had to use what I considered to be unrealistically low figures of what it cost to treat a patient in the public sector because they wouldn't really charge any of the administrative costs for running the system. I think that is the case in England, where many aspects of running the health services are hidden, so that it looks like an amazingly efficient system.

One of the curious consequences about the issue of the cost of clozapine is that in the UK, at least, one of the things you hear people say is that it was only with clozapine that psychiatry began to be taken seriously – because of its costs.

Because of the costs! That's appalling. Nevertheless, if that is what it takes to be taken seriously, I'll accept it. There are amazing stories in the States about the impact of using clozapine. One of the low or high points, depending on your viewpoint, was that I was chairing a symposium, just as clozapine was being introduced, at the annual American Psychiatric

Association meeting in New York City. There was a ballroom full of people at the Marriott Marquis Hotel, 2–3000 people. John Strauss, of Yale, had just started to speak. All of a sudden, the doors of the auditorium opened. In streamed about 150 people from the New York Chapter of the National Alliance for the Mentally Ill screaming, 'clozapine is obscene', carrying banners and completely disrupting the meeting because they were so upset about the price of clozapine. They wouldn't let Strauss continue. I somehow got the leader of this group, a man named David Jaffe, to quiet down by making an agreement with him that if he would wait until the talk was finished, I would give him time to address the audience. There were police gathering at that point and it could have become an ugly scene at any time. Jaffe got his group under control and Dr Strauss finished. Then Jaffe got up and gave a really passionate speech about how because of the price at that time, many people who wanted it weren't going to be able to get it. He got more than a polite round of applause from the audience and then left.

I don't expect that I will ever do anything else in my life that would be nearly as gratifying as the work I did with clozapine. I have had many experiences along the way with people whose lives have been transformed by it. A patient of mine, whose picture was on the cover of *Time* magazine several years ago, was a street person who had been in jail and who is now the produce manager of a supermarket in my neighbourhood. He's engaged and living a very satisfactory life. There are a lot of people in the first group of patients we started on clozapine who have not been hospitalized in nine years. To be a part of that is what I dreamed about as a College student.

However, I am very mindful that we are far from doing what we need to do with regard to serious mental illness. My goal right now is to study the phase of schizophrenia prior to the appearance of psychosis. I believe that there is a neurodegenerative process that is taking place at that crucial time.

That might be picked up by screening?

That's what we're working on. We think we can do it. We are intensively working with patients and families to recapture the events of that time. I believe there may be some process that may involve stress—induced glucocorticoids, and probably glutamate in some way, to cause a condition called apoptosis – progammed cell death. This is the only thing that we know of at this point that would explain how you could have a degeneration of neurones without there being signs of gliosis. The brain is remodelled during adolescence. Ironically this was prefigured in my neuromuscular work. I saw evidence that there had to be a dying back of neurones to explain what we had found plus a sprouting of other neurones to recover the function of the muscle fibres that were left. Even then, I wrote that it might be possible that some process like this could be happening in the central nervous system. This now seems a possibility. It turns out that all the 5-HT-2/D-2 compounds are causing effects on CK activity in psychotic patients, not all of them but a surprisingly substantial number of them. So maybe I'm going to have a chance to go back and hopefully finish up the story where my career started.

Are we talking about something like a nerve growth factor as being important in the treatment?

Well, let's say if there is this process of neurorestructuring that has gone awry in schizophrenia, then a variety of factors that guide neuronal connections could turn out to be very important. In the case of the cognitive dysfunction that may be central to the disorder, the majority of the damage may be present at the time of the first episode. This suggests a need to identify and treat patients before they present in the emergency room in a delusional, hallucinatory state. I believe that the positive and negative symptoms emerge from the cognitive dysfunction. Because of this, we have been doing a lot of work on pre-morbid function in people at risk for schizophrenia. Some aspects of that process could be modelled in animals. We know that neuronal loss takes place during very early adolescence, before most people become schizophrenic; most of the remodelling in the brain is supposed to be over by ages 12 or 13. But it's probable that a small but significant part continues later. This is based really on a theory which was developed by Peter Huttonlocher at the University of Chicago. It has never been adequately studied in primates or rodents. If that's when pathology is beginning in schizophrenia, our animal research should focus on it like 'a laser beam'.

From the outside it seemed that with DSM-III, the psychiatric profession changed and went biological but with clozapine on the front cover of Time *as well as* Listening to Prozac, *this change of culture has reached down to street level. Would this be a fair statement?*

Biological psychiatry never took over the field as much as one would think. We may have been very visible in terms of the media but if you ever attended an Americian Psychiatric Association meeting, you would realize that the majority of American psychiatrists are more interested in psychotherapy and the like. Someone I know, with a history of recurrent depressions, recently suicided; prior to her suicide, she was treated by one doctor with psychotherapy and another doctor with drugs. That reflects the old bias against drug treatment. The psychiatrist who did the psycho-therapy wouldn't use drugs because he didn't know enough about them or thought it would interfere with their relationship.

How can that attitude remain despite the work of someone like Klerman to show that the psychotherapy and drug therapy can be additive?

Yes, but you have to understand where the prestige is. Tom Detre used to say that society sees us as druggists. And at Mass Mental Health Center, the goal was not to become an academic, or do research in a laboratory, or do clinical trials, it was to be a psychoanalyst. What's really transforming this situation is the way mental health care is being structured by huge insurance companies and managed care – who will pay physicians only to do pharmacotherapy. They fund 10/15 mins with a patient once a month for a review of drug treatment. They will not pay adequately for psychotherapy. That will be funded only by someone being willing to pay for it out of his or her pocket. That aspect of the psychiatrist's professional life will diminish greatly. The American medical student is turning away from psychiatry because of poor reimbursement and because they don't want to do just pharmacotherapy.

I am concerned that the rate of progress in the next several decades is not going to be the same as what we have had in the past. The next generation of psychiatrists is going to be much smaller. It's a rather pessimistic view but I do think you are on the right track in chronicling what has been a really golden age of psychopharmacology. I hope it's going to continue in some way in the future because there is still so much to do. Clozapine and the other new drugs are a real advance but they are only palliatives. My goal is to stop this disease before it ever expresses itself. If I can achieve something toward that in the next decade, I will really feel very fulfilled.

Select bibliography

Hagger, C., Buckley, P., Kenny, J.T., et al. (1993) Improvement in cognitive functions and psychiatric symptoms in treatment-refractory schizophrenic patients receiving clozapine. *Biological Psychiatry*, 24 34, 702–12.

Kane, J., Honigfeld, G., Singer, J. and Meltzer, H.Y. and the Clozaril Collaborative Study Group (1988) Clozapine for the treatment-resistant schozphrenic: A double-blind comparison with chlorpromazine. *Archives of General Psychiatry*, 24 45, 789–96.

Kuncl, R.W. and Meltzer, H.Y. (1974) Pathologic effect of phencyclidine and restraint on rat skeletal muscle structure: Prevention of prior denervation. *Experimental Neurology*, 24 45, 387–402.

Meltzer, H.Y. (1968) Creatine kinase and aldolase in serum: abnormality common to acute psychoses. *Science*. 24 159, 1368–70.

Meltzer, H.Y., Sachar, E.J. and Frantz, A.G. (1974) Serum prolactin levels in unmedicated schizophrenic patients. *Archives of General Psychiatry*, 24 31, 564–69.

Meltzer, H.Y., Young, M., Metz, J., et al. (1979) Extrapyramidal side effects and increased serum prolactin following fluoxetine, a new antidepressant. *Journal of Neural Transmission*, 24 45, 165–75.

Meltzer, H.Y. and Stahl, S.M. (1976) The dopamine hypothesis of schizophrenia: A review. *Schizophrenia Bulletin*, 24 2, 19-76.

Metzer, H.Y., Fang, V.S. and Young, M.A. (1980) Clozapine-like drugs. *Psychopharmacology Bulletin*, 24 16, 32–34.

Meltzer, H.Y., Matsubara, S. and Lee, J-C. (1989) Classification of typical and atypical antipsychotic drugs on the basis of dopamine D-1, D-2 and serotonin2 pKi values. *Journal of Pharmacology and Experimental Therapeutics*, **24 251,** 238–46.

Meltzer, H.Y., Cola, P., Way, L. *et al.* (1993) Cost effectiveness of clozapine in neuroleptic-resistant schizophrenia. *American Journal of Psychiatry*, **24 150,** 1630–38.

The role of behavioural pharmacology in psychopharmacology

Did you do pharmacology in University?

No. I did a medical biochemistry degree at the University of Birmingham from 1956 to 1959. It was a unique course in that those selected for it, of which there were only a maximum of six for any one year, were interviewed and the interview was primarily to find out those people who at a very early stage had an interest and a flair for research. Birmingham was essentially a research department, where there were something like three to four times as many postgraduate and staff members as undergraduates for the three-year course. The other unique thing about it was that all of us had to get an ordinary degree in chemistry as part of our three-year honours degree course and at the same time had to attend several of the basic science courses and some of the clinical courses that the medical students attended. The whole idea was to equip us as bench scientists but with quite a strong orientation towards clinical applications. It was the only course of its type in the country.

And what led you from that to pharmacology?

Well, it was a joint department of medical biochemistry and pharmacology. In the final year of the BSc course, we had a course in neurochemistry with Brian Ansell, who was the senior lecturer in Philip Bradley's department. Philip Bradley was unique, as you know, he was the only Professor of Neuropharmacology in the country. So we had a two-month course, including some practical work, where I came into contact with both Brian and Philip. There was just something about the CNS and the brain that I found exciting – it was nothing more than that; it was just a feeling that this was interesting.

An opportunity came then, once I got my degree, to do a pharmacology project. A grant came from the Tropical Products Research Institute, which was part of the colonial office in London. Alistair Fraser, the head of department, was a World Health Organisation adviser on tropical diseases and he had very good contacts with things like the colonial office and so consquently this grant came into the department.

It was a grant for a postdoctoral fellow together with one PhD student. The post/doctoral fellow was a biochemist called Stan Sherrit, who's now working in the pharmacology department in Newcastle and he took me on as a research student. Basically he was not a pharmacologist and right from the very beginning, his approach was a biochemical approach. We had to look at a number of tropical products from Jamaica which were being used as medicinal plants. One of my first jobs was to screen about 100 plant extracts, which were sent over from Jamaica to us for testing.Now that was extremely important because it meant that I had to learn – there was no-one there to teach me – how to screen plant extracts for pharmacological activity. It was a case of self-teaching. I had only had a small amount of specialist training in pharmacology. I had done quite a bit of neurochemistry because between times I had also gone down to the Institute of Psychiatry, to McIlwain's Unit, and done a short postgraduate course with Henry McIlwain and Richard Rodnight. And that taught me how to approach the neurochemical aspect but not the pharmacolological aspect. So really, for the first year, there I was in a laboratory which was not primarily orientated to the broad areas of pharmacology but having to produce results and therefore you learn with your fingers and that's precisely what I did.

One of the plant extracts came from the Jamaican shade tree called *Pithecolibium samanth benth*. This contained a number of alkaloids which were being extracted very crudely and used for treating unspecified mental illness but also for lowering blood pressure. We managed to work with a chemist in the University of Jamaica who isolated and partially purified some of these and he sent us the semi-purified alkaloids which I started working on. I then had to do a general pharmacological screen for activity on the gut, on blood pressure, on the cardiovascular system and so forth but then I could also now start looking at the brain because some of these alkaloids were convulsants and this really led me right into neuro- and psychopharmacology. So, I could then use all my experience in the area of neurochemistry to look at how the alkaloids were possibly affecting intermediary metabolism and so forth which was very important when understanding how the convulsants work. And at the same time from the pharmacological point of view I could start actually looking at antagonists and so on and get some idea as how these things work. You have to remember that we had no idea how convulsants were working.

In fact my first paper on the pharmacological properties of these alkaloids was published in *Nature*. In those days it was very easy to publish in *Nature*. Now you can't publish unless it's in the area of molecular biology, which nobody understands and it's probably irrelevant anyway. In those days it was a much more genuinely broad journal for science, representing a range of different areas and scientific interests. That's where I published my first article and including the first self-experiment.

One of the tests I did was a local anaesthetic test. You could do this on the response of the guinea pig to pain following a subcutaneous infusion of the putative local anaesthetic and we found that this compound did apparently reduce the response to pain. We then looked at a standard frog preparation and again the same thing happened. So we thought that it may be a local anaesthetic and what my supervisor and myself did was to send a sample over to the hospital to get it sterilized and then we each injected one another on the forearm to see what would happen and indeed we did find that it was a local anaesthetic. The problem was that we noticed that the numbness continued for a long time. In fact the numbness led to a necrosis. What we had done was to kill off the nerve cells and skin.

Because these alkaloids were going to form the centrepiece of my PhD, I also got training in toxicology because there was a section of the department specializing in toxicology. So it meant by the time I had finished in Birmingham I got a bench training – hands-on training in biochemistry, specializing in neurochemistry, general pharmacology, general toxicology and some neuropharmacology. No psychopharmacology as such. But the other important thing was also working during that time with Michael Chance.

He had a subdepartment of animal ethology as part of this department of pharmacology and toxicology, biochemistry and mental biochemistry – Euan Grant, John MacIntosh and Michael Chance. Now in the area of ethology these people have really been very important and they are still going. Basically what they did was have colonies of wild mice and wild rats and they were actually for the first time really looking at the behaviour of these animals from a social point of view. So, social ethology.

Where did they get this kind of idea?

It was very revolutionary at the time. Michael was trained originally as a pharmacologist but he was interested in ethology. Euan and John were trained as zoologists. So they came to the department of zoology to work with Michael to look at social interactions in wild rats compared to white rats which are highly inbred and probably don't show a lot of the complexity of behaviour that you see in the wild. They had runways and so forth with glass fronted one-way mirrors in front, so they could observe the animals in as natural as possible environment, looking at their interactions and different types of behaviour. They worked out, I think it was dozens, if not a hundred or more, different behavioural interactions which had meaning for the animal. This was long before computers. They had a system of coding to code different behaviours – when a strange male, for example, was put in a runway with the normal host male and that sort of thing. Now they took this one stage further because they then introduced drugs like barbiturates – you've got to remember this was all before the benzodiazepines and so forth, so there weren't that many. Or leptizol, for example, a stimulant, and then looked at the effects on drug-treated animals with normal animals, in terms of social behaviour.

They showed me all these methods and what I tried to do was to simplify the methods to try and make it practical so that we could possibly bring a new dimension into drug testing in terms of the effects of drugs on social behaviour in mice. It wasn't terribly scientific on my part but it probably was, in retrospect, extremely important in bringing out the whole idea of studying the sort of behaviours which are relevant to the animal and then looking at drug effects on those complex social interactions – both acute and chronic drug effects.

What Chance and his colleagues were trying to do was to simulate what was happening in the real world of the patient. Because they also had, at the Uffculme Clinic in Birmingham, which was a psychiatric clinic, an opportunity to spend some time there looking with one-way mirrors at the behavioural patterns of patients. So there was a psychological dimension to this as well, which they then tried to see if it would simulate in any way in animals. This whole concept, retrospectively, I think was very very important because it did bring into this whole business of animal studies the idea that they are invaluable but only invaluable if it has meaning for the real world of the patient.

Who else was in Birmingham at the time. Obviously Philip Bradley . . .

Philip Bradley, Brian Ansell . . . Joel Elkes had left many years before . . . Brian Key was there. If you look back at the original work on chlorpromazine on the reticular activating system, for example, it was Bradley and Key, who did it all. I knew these guys personally. We would have coffee together. Even as undergraduates, we were treated as though we were postgraduates. There was no such thing as staff, technicians and students. It was a small department. We all had coffee together and therefore you were expected to have opinions. And in our training, for example, right from the second year onwards, there would be weekly seminars and we were expected to perform at least twice a year, in front of the whole class and staff, including the professor.

Among the others there was Robert Schneider, who really taught me what pharmacology I know. He was a colleague of Edith Bullbring, a German Jew who came over here in 1936. Interesting Quaker background, so not a religious Jew, but who was the only trained pharmacologist in the department. His interest was primarily in gut pharmacology but he taught me the discipline of setting these things up reproducibly and in fact we did several practical demonstrations together for the British Pharmacological Society.

Alistair Fraser I think was extremely important to me for two reasons. One his dedication to science. An extremely powerful figure. Very old fashioned in many ways. Quite authoritarian. What he said went; this was an empire and he was in charge of the empire. No one ever doubted what he said. He insisted on high standards of research. None of us were ever allowed to present, for example, at a British Pharmacological meeting or anywhere like that unless we had been before the Professor. And it was always sound criticism. We were all taught right from the very first seminar as undergraduates, there are ways to present – you don't read and this sort of thing. So these standards of scientific and written communication were all part of the training.

How about clinical people like Alec Jenner?

When I started my PhD, that Unit was already breaking up. It had contained Alec Jenner, Alan Bolton, Peter Ramwell, again a biochemist. There were several technicians who were quite important on some of the early papers but again not known internationally. But Alec was really the centrepiece there – the circadian rhythm hypotheses all started there – he then went on to Sheffield. Now I didn't know Alec at all until much later on when in fact the Brain Research Association started with John Dobbing and people like this. The Brain Research Association was one of these anarchic organizations which was set up during the late 1960s, which aimed to cross-fertilize all the neurosciences from clinical right the way through.

An early BAP?

Well, it was much wider than the BAP. It brought in neuroanatomists, neurosurgeons, neurologists, some psychiatrists, a lot of behavioural people, in the area of what would be brain and behavioural research now. Memory men, Steven Rose, for example, was very much involved in the early days. It's kept going but it's not as active now, not as well known but at that time it was quite important and Alec had a sort of peripheral interest in that, so that's really where I met Alec.

The guiding spirit behind the BRA I suppose would be John Dobbing who was the Professor of Child Development or something like that. He was a clinician but he also had a lot of interest in neuroscience. There was John Smart and Jen Sands at Manchester and they were very much involved in developmental psychology but looking at the behavioural aspects of development in animals and this sort of thing. Patrick Wall, in London, you know the famous pain man, was involved, and Derek Richter.

Even as late as the early 1960s you had a bunch of the physiologists really not being prepared to concede that chemical neurotransmission was for real despite the work of Marthe Vogt, John Gaddum, Derek Richter and others.

That's right, but they had no impact on me at all. The impact came from the biochemists. For example, Crawford who was working in Gaddum's old laboratory in Edinburgh, was for a time working in the Queen Elizabeth Hospital in Birmingham which was allied in a way to our medical school. Robert Schneider knew Crawford and Robert's chief technician learnt how to set up the fundus-strip preparation to measure 5-HT and I then learnt the fundus strip and how to measure 5-HT. At that stage I didn't know what the hell 5-HT was. It was something to do with the gut. Edith Bulbring's work on peristalsis had implicated it. That to me was the importance of 5-HT. It was the gut.

At that stage we all knew about D-receptors and M-receptors from Gaddum's work. But the neurotransmission angle only came in, when we actually tried to understand what these alkaloids were doing and with talking to people like Brian Ansell and from going down to McIlwain and Rodnight's department.

Henry McIlwain's name is one that comes up every so often; was he important?

McIlwain was a wonderful eccentric. A very shy man but with an intense love of science, very dedicated as a teacher. If you look at neurochemistry in Britain at that stage there was only one unit and that was Henry's unit in London. In terms of the really fundamental work on brain slices, for example – there's the McIlwain chopper which we still use for producing extremely small 1 mm squares of brain tissue – then there was basic work studying respiration, studying intermediate metabolism and studying the effects of drugs on intermediate metabolism. That was all Henry. If you look at the *Biochemical Journal* in the 1930s, 40s 50s, it was all Quastel or McIlwain. It was all *in vitro* work but nevertheless very important in laying the basis for looking at drug effects on metabolism – that not all drugs are working just on receptors, this is also is a consequence of that.

The only other group was the Richter group, which by the nature of the MRC was very much concerned with clinical aspects. To my mind that was an enormous weakness that there wasn't more cross-fertilization between these groups. And I think personalities could have come in there because McIlwain was an extremely retiring sort of person. He wasn't the sort of guy you could have a joke with. He was quite reserved. Quite removed from his students but a very dedicated teacher.

He would run these courses that would last for a month to six weeks and I was lucky enough to be sent on one of them. It was 80% bench training. Now this is the difference between what is happening now in universities and what was happening then. Neuroscience is a practical science and a lot of it gets worked out on the bench and if you can't bloody well do it, go and do something else. So all of us were trained as bench workers. You thought with your hands.

What about the frustration a great many of these people, I'm thinking of Derek Richter in particular, had in terms of getting the clinical people to cooperate?

I think that's true but one thing to my knowledge never happened, even at biochemical society meetings, because I used to attend Biochemical Society meetings, particularly the neurochemistry group, which was another very important way for us youngsters to move forward – you had the Brain Research Organization and you had the Neurochemical Group of the Biochemical Society which was very active then – these were the sort of, if you like, professional groupings that we were allied to but you very, very rarely saw the Richters and McIlwains coming together in terms of symposia and saying well now we're going from the brain slices through to man.

Richter did try and put together a few meetings through the 1950s doing just that, trying to bring Elkes and the physiologists and the biochemists together in one place.

This is true but these were international type meetings. They didn't have an impact on us. We couldn't go. There was no money. Nothing whatsoever for us to go. So unless we were very lucky to have a head of department who says 'well, look there's a course now would you like to go on that course, or I'll send you on that course'. By and large even going to Pharmacological Society meetings we paid out of our own pockets. You just lived cheaply and hoped for the best. So in terms of the impact on people at the bench level, you read it in the literature and so forth but these meetings didn't have much impact.

So, that was basically the Birmingham period. As I say, having to teach yourself, I have always felt was extremely important. You make terrible mistakes but you learn to think. You learn to challenge yourself at the bench and this was what we were all encouraged to do. You do the experiment and then argue a case against your peers within the group and they spared nobody. And that I think led to scientific independence and a critical faculty. If you weren't critical someone else was going to shoot you to bits and sometimes it was extremely tough. The Birmingham experience was probably the most important thing I had ever done. Being in that sort of atmosphere, which I have never been in since. I've always been the loner since that time. Never had that sort of intellectual stimulus and cut and thrust which you can get with dedicated scientists who are really turned on by what they are doing and excited about science. It was a unique experience which I think is largely dead now for all sorts of reasons and I think it's a great pity for young people.

Was there the same atmosphere throughout the UK at the time or was there anything particular about Birmingham? It did feature as one of the centres for emerging neuroscience . . .

I think there was a lot of optimism in Universities then. I can't judge – I was only at Birmingham and Nottingham in the UK for any length of period but I think there was a totally different attitude. There was a lot of optimism. Money was going into the Universities. The Robbins report had come in the 1960s and the whole idea was that you've got to open up Universities by putting money in and by looking at the whole educational system – why is it that the percentage of working class children going to university has not changed since the middle 1930s and yet we have free education and all the rest of it. What the hell's going on and this was the first time that a Labour government attempted to try and redress this. I think that was reflected in the whole ambience of the University.

Admittedly, we had a big advantage because all of us knew once we had got that degree, we were getting jobs and that made it worthwhile. Although I don't honestly think it would have made a difference because that's the way we were. That was the ambience of the University. You weren't doing the degree to get a job. You were doing the degree because you bloody well wanted to do it. And you were selected for those courses right at the very beginning because that's what you wanted to do and you didn't want to do anything else. For example, the year I was in, there were five of us: everyone is a Head of Department or a Head of a big Clinical Biochemistry lab. And that's the way it went until Fraser died – he had a heart attack and they amalgamated the department – and the whole thing changed.

From Birmingham you went to Nottingham.

Nottingham was a pretty clapped out University, at least as far as science was concerned. There was a School of Pharmacy obviously set up by Jesse Boot, and the major Chair in the School of Pharmacy was endowed by Boots. The School of Pharmacy was in temporary buildings. I applied for the lectureship and in fact I think I had just done my oral in Birmingham, when I was called for interview and offered a full lectureship in pharmacology in the School of Pharmacy. Jimmy Crossland was the Reader of Pharmacology. He had worked with Derek Richter way back in the old days in the Whitchurch Hospital in Cardiff. He was renowned for his work on acetylcholine in the brain and I suppose because of my interest in the CNS and I knew of Crossland's work, never having met him, I went there and I was very pleased to have a job so quickly. Basically I was responsible for some of the CNS teaching on the biochemical aspects of pharmacology which is what I did for six years.

I suppose to some extent out of my PhD work on the chronic effects of psychotropic drugs, and at that time Crossland had a vague interest in sedatives and barbiturates, we developed, I think for the first time, an animal model of barbiturate dependance by using sodium barbitol which is a long-acting barbiturate. We used it in drinking water whereas before people had been injecting the stuff, which gives you problems with central depressions and so forth. So really what I did was to start low doses in drinking water and then increasing the dose over a period of 2–3 months until you got totally dependent animals.

Then the trick was to actually look at what happens to the behaviour and again this was totally a novel area. So I started doing work on multiple t-mazes. Now these experiments would take two or three months, every bloody day, including Saturdays and Sundays. You would have to go in and work and by that time we were living in Nottingham and I had two kids and the kids would be on the back of the bicycle and one on the handle bars, going in to feed the rats on Sunday. But it was again broadening the behavioural studies and including also what I had learnt of the biochemistry. So, for example, I did quite a lot of work and published it in biochemical pharmacology on intermediate metabolism, ATP, phosphocreatine and so forth, during dependence and withdrawal and seeing how the biochemical changes in high energy phosphates correlated with susceptibility to seizures and that sort of thing. Now at that stage we had just got the fluorimeter, a very old fashioned . . .

That had come in just then?

No, they had come in earlier but they were only becoming available for more general use during the 1960s. The spectrophotometer was still being used for doing all our enzyme assays but the spectrophotofluorimeter was where you would produce a specific fluorophore which would fluorescence when specific wavelengths would activate it and that enabled us for the first time to accurately measure serotonin, dopamine and noradrenaline in brain. Before you could only measure those by a bioassay. We were using the frog rectus abdominus muscle, for example, for measuring acetylcholine. And in fact it is still the most widely used method for measuring nanogram quantities of acetylcholine in the brain. There is still not a good, replicable HPLC or fluorimetric method for measuring acetylcholine in brain tissue.

So, the spectrophotofluorimeter was a real advance. They were still considered to be fairly sophisticated instruments in the middle to late 1960s. We were lucky in Nottingham to have one first and one of the pharmaceutical chemists was particularly interested in fluorimetry for doing spectroscopic analyses and we used it then to measure noradrenaline, dopamine, serotonin by using column chromatographic techniques but also using solvent extraction techniques. So you're talking about methods that were very laborious and retrospectively not terribly accurate but that was the best we had at the time. Our work involved looking at chronic drug testing, looking for behavioural correlates of the chronic treatment and always looking for neurochemical correlates of the behavioural changes produced by drugs. I had three PhD students when I was at Nottingham, all of which have done well subsequently.

Another important thing during the Nottingham period was that I had my first sabbatical in the German Democratic Republic which was again a very interesting period. Politically I was still very active; this was an intense Cold War period and so on and as academics it impacted on us. I had been investigated by the Special Branch when I was an undergraduate at Birmingham – totally illegally. They actually raided my room. In fact some of the staff at the University actually protested about this on my behalf. So we were in a very vulnerable position. In Universities we were still safe. But outside the University it was a totally different matter. So I was more or less told there were certain jobs that you will not get so don't apply.

But anyway during the latter part of the 1960s, I was in contact with the Physiology Department in Birmingham, with Peter Ramwell and Ian Bush, who was the Professor. They had gone and taken their whole team to the States, to the Worcester Foundation and they were doing very very interesting work on the neurophysiology of steroids. During my period on staff in Nottingham I had looked at the chronic effects of ACTH on behaviour and showed for the first time that not only does one lower the seizure threshold but that you get a facilitation of learning and memory with steroid hormones. With the contacts with Bush and Ramwell and so forth I thought it would be very nice to follow up this whole business of the action of steroid hormones on brain.

They arranged everything for me – a six-month research programme, money, everything. A letter came through and so forth. So I went to the American Embassy and showed them all, yes, fine, Dr Leonard, now I want you to fill in this form – and like a fool I was honest and on the form was 'have you been or have you ever been or are you a member of these organizations?' 1. communist party; 2. the British–Soviet Friendship Society; 3. Campaign for Nuclear Disarmament, etc., etc. to which I put tick, tick, tick, and three minutes later the man came back and said 'well, Dr Leonard, we've got too many goddamm commies in the United States as it is, this is going to take a long time'. So to cut a long story short I couldn't get to the States. And I was pissed off because as I say I was due this sabbatical period and I thought what the hell do you do. So through my other political contacts I was told well look there's a very interesting man in Leipzig who has spent two years working with Derek Richter.

Who was that?

Dietmar Biesold. He was probably the best-trained neurochemist in the whole of the East block and he was trying to maintain international links. So I thought about it and thought why the hell not. So I went there and spent six months actually working with the Brain Research Institute in Karl Marx University in Leipzig. I was the only pharmacologist but I had training in biochemistry and this was grand. What we were working on was a very interesting area of neuro-ontogenesis, in other words, looking at the whole neurochemical development of the brain in the rat. Looking from one day old rats right the way through to adolescent rats, at the actual developments in hexokinase, for example, and shifts in glucose metabolites as those enzymes mature.

Now being a pharmacologist with an interest in behaviour I was of course interested in not only learning all the enzyme techniques but also then I introduced some basic behavioural methods into their group for assessing development and also looking at drug effects. This was a contact which I maintained and I still maintain with that group, which is still going despite all the appalling things that have happened since the wall came down.

Biesold himself was very much an anglophile but he was very patriotic. He was one of the few people who had left the party in 1953 following the Workers' Revolt but because he was so good professionally and he had all the contacts and so forth they couldn't do much with him and so he was more or less allowed to carry on as Head of this Neurochemistry Department in the Brain Research Institute. Eventually he became Head of the Brain Research Institute and maintained international contacts right through the worst of the Cold War. He had Westerners from France, from Finland, from Holland, from Britain and from Ireland, actually going in and working in his lab and some of his youngsters coming out and working in their labs. He also maintained what I would call the best aspects of socialist thinking at that time in terms of open and critical discussion of what was going on around him; indeed, as well as highly critical discussion of what was happening in science in the West, which he knew.

When you came back you moved into ICI. My impression is that working within the industry in Germany and Switzerland from the late 19th century was very respectable. However, it was not so respectable to work in the industry in the US or the UK. In the US that began changing, only during the 1940s or 1950s. My impression is it changed even slower in the UK. Did you think when you were moving over to the industry in 1968 that this was the end of the academic career in a sense of being able to move up the University ladder or in terms of being able to be appointed to offices within academic societies, etc.?

At the time I must say I didn't plan things like that at all. The thing that motivated me then and now is research and where can you do research. By 1968, certainly, the Department in Nottingham was very sterile; nothing much was happening, there were no grants coming in. It was quite an authoritarian structure as well. I personally felt that I ran the risk of becoming like so many British academics before and since – frustrated so you give up – after all there's nothing to make you work. You do your bit of teaching and that's it. You've got a good job, a pension at the end of it, long holidays if you want to take them, which many of them did within that Department.

And so you either then accepted that that was going to be the future and you just specialize in growing roses and flitting around at home or alternatively say enough is enough, I've had my experience with teaching and okay I want to do something else – full-time research. This was the only way open at that time to do it. I had been to talk with Alec Jenner about the possiblility of going to an MRC Unit and there was nothing.

Everything was very insecure – grants, postdocs, senior postdoc fellowships; okay, you get them for two years, three years, maximum five years but by that time I was married with two kids, I wasn't willing to take that risk without security. Therefore when the job came up with ICI, I took it.

They didn't know what they were taking on but they gave me a lot of freedom. I can't remember ever in the three years that I spent there doing any screening work or any work of any possible use to them. Basically they wanted somebody to come in and set up what we called neurochemical pharmacology. David Greenwood was the other youngster with me at the time. David had come from the University of Dundee. He was trained more as a pharmacologist. I had unlimited facilities for doing work, a couple of technicians to work for me and I could travel. This was a situation that I had never had before.

I think I published over the period I was in industry, both in Britain and in Holland, something in the order of nearly 80 papers. I intended that deliberately. If a compound had been patented and I couldn't publish something, I wasn't going to touch it. So everything was done with a purpose and it was great fun. On the scientific side it was very productive but in terms of the politics it was appalling.

What came out scientifically?

Well there were two areas. I had long been interested in hallucinogens and this was work that I started in Nottingham. Along with one of the PhD students, we found one or two interesting things. One was an endogenous substance that modulates behaviour. This was a compound found in all mammalian brain, including human brain, that had two effects on mice – in a low dose it produced a sort of coma and in a high dose it produced convulsions. I published a number of papers in *Neuropharmacology* on this material. The best we could do in terms of identification was to establish that it was as a glycopeptide. We still don't know what it was but a fairly low molecular weight glycopeptide.

At that time I had linked up with David Shaw, in Derek Richter's Unit, to get human brains from schizophrenics who had committed suicide and from control examples. And we found that there were differences in concentrations in this material. But the trouble was we never managed to identify it chemically. I never managed even in ICI to get the chemists to come along with us and tell us what the hell this stuff was. And I wasn't competent to do this. So that's where it stayed.

The other area that I was interested in while at Nottingham was drugs of abuse. Now that started with the early barbiturate stuff and then we started looking at LSD and hallucinogens. And that's where I started really getting into the whole business of neurotransmitters and changes in brain dopamine, etc. So I continued that in ICI, where we had facilities to do all these sort of things – anything you wanted to do in terms of machinery, rats and things.

The work on hallucinogens there had an interesting connection with Porton Down, which I didn't know anything about. I was just told when I got there 'oh, you're interested in hallucinogens; that's interesting, well would you like to look at these different types of substituted tryptamines?'. It was wonderful. I had a whole pile of about 20 different substituted tryptamines and they said 'we know nothing about these things at all; why don't you look at them'. So I did and published a lot of biochemistry on them in *Biochemical Pharmacology.*

Then I had a telephone call from a guy from Porton Down, one day. And he said 'oh, I hear you've been doing some work', so I said 'yes, it's quite interesting, I've sent the results in for publication'. 'How would you like to come down and talk to us about it?'. This was really very interesting because I thought with my politics and everything 'Jesus have they not twigged'. So I said 'yes, I'll come, no problem at all'. And I did. And I got into Porton Down and I was shown all around Porton Down. Everything was very hush hush as it is in places like Israel. And being political I naturally played stupid and asked questions about it. This was the Cold War period and the whole thing was being shared with the Israelis and so forth, so I found that very exciting. Obviously there was a direct link between ICI and Porton Down for this type of research and I had come in on the periphery of it.

But anyway, to cut a long story short, what I did then was to start some work on viloxazine, which was just coming in. Viloxazine was purely a spin-off from the beta–adrenoreceptor antagonist programme which Jimmy Black had started way back in the year dot with propranolol and so forth. In fact there was bugger all drugs in ICI at that time. They were still making their money on halothane, propranolol and one of the lipid lowering agents. They had virtually nothing else and their patents were going to expire so they picked up viloxazine fortunately. Dave Greenwood did a lot of the basic work on viloxazine and because of that I started getting interested in antidepressants and I thought this was an area that we should now be going into.

It was at that stage that I had a run in with the senior management at ICI over my politics. I was asked by a left-wing newspaper to comment on the annual report for the Association of the British Pharmaceutical Industry, as a pharmacologist. So I did and it was published in London and within less than 24 hours I was in front of the Research Director. Very red faced, very angry, he threw down a photocopy and said 'what's this?'. My name, Brian Leonard, was on it – not Dr Brian Leonard, and no address. Brian Leonard, Research Pharmacologist. They traced the whole thing through from Millbank, the Headquarters in London, to me. 'What's all this?'. So I said 'it's what I consider to be an objective commentary on the Association of the Pharmaceutical Industry report, which I was asked to do' and I said 'I don't think it's got anything to do with ICI, ICI's not mentioned. My title's not mentioned. Just a pharmacologist. I'm a private individual'. 'You work 24 hours a day in the industry, your only loyalty is to ICI, don't forget that. You are not going to get on very well in this company are you?' and that was it. I said 'well, I think what you've just said is totally illegal and that I have a right to my own opinions".

So, within three months I was in Holland. Mike Barratt who was Head of Pharmacology when I first went to ICI had left less than a year later and gone to set up a Pharmacology Department in Organon in Oss. Mike, shrewd politician that he is, realized when we met at a Pharmacological Society meeting in the summer, that I wasn't getting on too well with the management, and he said 'have you ever thought about going abroad?'. I said 'not really' and he said 'Holland's quite nice and they've got an interesting set up, very different from ICI, why don't you come over some time and have a look?'. So I went and looked and what they wanted basically was someone who would set up a Biochemical Pharmacology group to work with the behavioural people on a drug, which they couldn't understand, but it seemed to be an antidepressant, called mianserin.

I like the Dutch. Very tolerant people. Again very good facilities and certainly status wise they seemed as if they were going to treat you seriously. And there was a chance which I never had in ICI of really linking behaviour directly with the biochemistry and setting the whole thing up. The real challenge for me was to establish how the hell mianserin worked. The drug had been found purely by chance in a clinical setting on volunteers.

How?

It was developed originally, based on animal models, as an antimigraine drug. And it was a very good antimigraine drug. Sicuteri tested this in Italy; he was one of the many people involved in the serotonin hypothesis of migraine. He had shown that it was something of a serotonin receptor antagonist. Okay, it was clinically effective but it was shown to have a very sedative profile and a slightly hypotensive effect.

As it had an obvious sedative profile, the question was what's it doing in the brain. It was known to be an antihistamine and the suggestion was that this was just an antihistamine effect. Anyway it was then tested by Turan Itil in New York, who was very very much sought after then because he had a method of analysing the power spectrum of the EEG in volunteers and he could show that standard antidepressants produced a certain change in the power spectrum of the EEG. And he looked and said that the effect on the volunteer EEG is almost identical to imipramine; 'had the company ever thought of looking at mianserin as an antidepressant?' Organon said 'no, because it doesn't do anything to do with the reserpine reversal test'. That was our thinking at the time – totally mechanistic. Anyway, this led to an open study in depressed patients which showed it was antidepressant. It then went further and one of the first double-blind studies was done in Cork in Bob Daly's department.

So this caused a problem – we had an antidepressant that was not working like a MAOI or a tricyclic in any of the animal models or other tests. How could this be explained?

It has always hit me that whatever mianserin's credentials as an antidepressant, its effect in dismantling the orthodox theories and promoting new thinking has always been underestimated.

Mianserin I think is totally underestimated for its importance in the whole area of depression research. Because it was really the first genuine atypical antidepressant. There had been iprindole but that wasn't very potent. Mianserin was well established as an antidepressant. Its anticholinergic profile was negligible; our pharmacology department had shown very early on that it had virtually no cardiotoxicity. It was genuinely the new article.

So, working with the behaviourists and basic pharmacologists and so forth, we thought 'what the hell is going on with this compound'. So I was worked on the neurotransmitter end of things and Henk Rigter and Henk van Riezen worked at different aspects of the behaviour and it was at that time that we realized that we had to look at chronic animal models of depression. We had got it all wrong. The reserpine model was just rubbish – all this acute stuff was not relevant because we had already shown that there were differences between the acute effects and chronic effects of mianserin on the turnover of amines in brain. Something was happening which could only happen chronically.

So this led you to the olfactory bulbectomy model?

Yes. It was just at that time that Keith Cairncross early in 1973 had come on sabbatical from Australia to Manchester and Henk van Riezen had met him at a British Pharmacological Society meeting, invited him over to Organon and we all got together and had a chat. Working as a PhD in 1971, Keith Cairncross had shown that when you removed the olfactory bulbs of the rat, there was a hyperactivity which could be attenuated by chronic but not acute treatment with amitriptyline and also there appeared to be changes in noradrenaline.

Why would you ever do something like that?

Because if you look back, there's a literature that goes back to about 1911, to Watson working in the States. Presumably one of these experiments done purely by mistake. Anyway he had damaged the olfactory lobes of the rat and found that the animal became irritable and pugnacious. We now know that that rat was probably much more damaged than just the olfactory lobes. It had damaged the frontal cortex and therefore as a result cortical damage and so forth you got these changes.

This was followed up by a woman in New York called Pohorecki who looked at what happens to the concentration of noradrenaline in the ipsilateral amygdala area when you remove one olfactory bulb. She found out that it lowered the noradrenaline content, suggesting that whatever was happening, the lobes in the rat were not just involved in olfaction, it was much more important than that. There was a lot of behavioural and physiological literature, showing that the lobes in the rat were part of the limbic circuit, unlike in the human and higher mammals when they are not – they are solely involved in olfaction.

Keith Cairncross who was a psychologist knew that sort of literature. He was also interested in pharmacology and so he started to bring this together. It was a very very important finding. Now he came to see us and Henk van Riezen and Henk Rigter learnt how to take out the lobes. It seems difficult but it is very easy once you know how and I then started working with them on the biochemical consequences. So we formed a team looking at all aspects of the behaviour and biochemistry.

Basically we started to establish it as a model. But we only ever used it very much as a research model. What we did find at that stage was that mianserin was equally active as all of the tricyclics and MAOIs in normalizing the hyperactivity and also some aspects of passive avoidance learning, which is defective, after bulbectomy. These were very laborious experiments. You were talking about two treatments, two to three weeks, every day. Industry hates that sort of experiment because it means weekend working. It means special handling. It means a totally different approach which industry doesn't like. These are research methods.

The whole area of models seems to have gone out of the window recently as we have plunged into molecular biology and all that. Do you want to comment on whether we really need models or not? Is it because, other than screening models such as the Porsolt test, they are not suited to the needs of industry? There doesn't seem to be the same interest to build up complex models of behaviour where you are trying to correlate aspects of behaviour with biochemistry and trying to understand the interaction between the two.

I've got many, many criticisms of industry but one of them as a scientist is the pure scientific reductionism that what we are seeing now – you know, mental illness equals an abnormality of a specific receptor type in a specific brain region. Now this is bullshit. The brain is much more complex than that. But if you take that philosophy to its logical conclusion, all you need to do is to have a laboratory devoted to *in vitro* cloning of receptors and targeting particular receptor types. Whether that has any relevance whatsoever you will only find out maybe four or five years down the line when you put the compound into man.

You see what they are doing now is they are short-cutting. They find a specific ligand for a specific receptor type in a test tube. They short-cut, doing the minimal amount of toxicology, the minimum of acute behavioural testing, the minimal amount of pharmacokinetic analysis and then they get the compound into man as soon as possible. Now sometimes that can work – I mean from a statistical point of view it can. Whether of course it has any relevance to what you've been doing on your binding and grinding of receptors is another matter. But in 9 cases out of 10 it probably won't work because that is not the way the brain works and it doesn't lead to any deeper understanding of the psychopathology of the illness for which you want better drugs.

These are all short-cut reductionist methods which were starting when I was in Organon and where the whole structure changed within Organon to meet good laboratory practice standards – so the bureaucratization came in to the industry then.

Good laboratory practice means what?

What that means is, whereas before, when you submitted your data to the regulatory authorities, they would examine the basic data reports and that sort of thing but as long as the stuff had been written up reasonably well that was basically the end of it. With good laboratory practice which largely came from the FDA in the United States, in order to get a drug even considered by the FDA, good laboratory practice had to be fol-lowed, even in Europe. Now that meant that all notebooks, every piece of data had to be available. It meant that at any time officials could come from the FDA, walk into the laboratories and say I want to see your data on A, B, C and D. So everything now had to be carefully recorded. And not only carefully recorded but in a certain way. So there was a total bureaucratization of the laboratory. This was coming in when I was leaving to go to Galway in 1974. Towards the end of my time I was filling in bits of paper. I was checking that the right forms had been filled in when they were writing data from an experiment and all this then had to be categorized in a certain way to go into the company archives.

So you became nothing more than a bureaucratic pen-pusher and the fun of doing an experiment without a protocol was lost. Very often, you know as a scientist you find observations coming about by accident and then you say 'right, let's quickly do an extra experiment now'. You couldn't do that anymore because everything had to be done by protocol. And so it meant that the research became totally bureaucratized and still is.

So that's I guess why the industry now hives off that kind of research to University labs or other independent groups.

Well, yes, but there's less and less of that. Because if you can get away with this reductionist approach, you just have binders and grinders and you have a standard protocol and you could train a monkey to do it basically. In the end, once you've got the techniques worked out, why do you have to bother about research? And you see there is this argument against all of the animal models – okay, what have they ever told us and not only that they have led us in the wrong directions in the past – as with the reserpine model.

But it goes deeper than that. There isn't even a coordination between the basic science departments and the medical department. So when you get a drug through into clinical trials, for example, you've got all this material coming back for blood testing but the basic scientists have no interest and no look in on that at all. And so there's a distrust. Basically they would never say this, but there's a distrust between the medics and the scientists. Neither understand what the other's doing and couldn't care less. Basically, you can publish your binding and grinding experiments in *Nature* because it's molecular biology. You can clone yet another receptor, great stuff for *Nature* and you've made it from a professional point of view but I think this is an utter disaster in terms of psychopharmacology. If you look at the number of large companies now who are doing what I call really fundamental neuroscience research, there are very few of them. These are the areas that can be cut you see because it's not going to help you ultimately register your drug.

I think all this needs total re-evaluation but there is no way in which this is going to happen in the near future, with the way in which industry is designed and the pressures upon industry by the regulatory authorities. It is not a happy place to be, any more than the Universities are now a happy place to be for research. So that's one of the reasons why I got out even though I had been very happy. It was a very good training for me in terms of research management – running a department. All the managerial skills that you would never have got in the University. It was a very positive seven years in industry which I never regret but I would never want to be back there.

If ICI was odd, the West of Ireland was an extraordinary next move.

Having spent seven years in industry, I knew I was an academic. The only way to make progress in industry is through management in terms of the business aspect. My politics, my whole philosophy, is totally against that. It is the very antithesis to what I believe in. So I went into industry to use it, but it was using me as well if you like.

When I was an undergraduate in 1955 I had hitch-hiked with a friend of mine all around Ireland. Hitching on the occasional lorry and bread cart and asscart and that sort of thing. There is something about Ireland that I've always, maybe from way back, previous generation of the family, that's appealed to me. Maybe it's the sheer anarchy or the community thinking which I liked. Anyway there was an advertisement for a job in Galway and Crossland from my Nottingham days had in fact been doing some of the teaching to fill in over there, because the previous Professor of Pharmacology, who was basically a surgeon teaching therapeutics believe it or not, had died.

I saw the advertisement in *Nature* and I asked Crossland about it and he said it's not only very run down – the Department doesn't exist. And he said whoever is going to take it on is really going to have to put their back into it and get the thing moving. I applied. There were eight of us interviewed. I arrived the night before at 1 am on the last train down. It was a November night, pissing down with rain, as only it can do in the West of Ireland. I had nowhere to stay. I walked out of the train station, up Eyre Square into the Imperial Hotel.

When I woke up the next morning, it was one of those wonderful days, the sun was shining, the sky was blue, it was just unbelievable. And I thought this was my sort of place – you just don't know what the hell's going to happen even down to the weather. So I went to the University and was interviewed by all sorts of people and I didn't know any of them. Four of the interviewees were from the United States, all Irish Americans, most of them senior to me. So I went for the interview and all the rest of it. And there was of course the Irish. I didn't know anything about Irish exams and when I turned up they said when are you going to take the Irish exam?

That night I went back to Helga and the kids who were still living in England and said 'look, I don't think any of this is going to come off but okay lets see what comes of it'. Then I was phoned up by Sean Lavelle, Professor of Experimental Medicine, the other half of the joint department and he said 'by the way you've got through all the faculties, you'll be offered it'. So that was basically it.

I started on 1 September 1974. I had one empty hut. Literally an empty hut. It used to be the morgue for the regional hospital and I think they moved out the altar or something like that before I moved in. Nothing else. One thousand pounds, an empty hut and me on 1 September 1974. I thought this is going to be a real challenge. I must say Organon were very good to me. First of all they bought me a spectrophotofluorimeter. They gave money for other basic apparatus, about £10,000 – a lot of money in those days, to get me started and they have always been very good. But the University was just appalling. I didn't realize just how naive I was at the time.

I had to establish, totally from scratch, a proper scientific course in pharmacology for the medical students and ultimately for science students, with nothing. With not even a staff member. They gave me a technician, who is still with me, Brendan Beatty, since 1974. I managed to get some money from the Medical Research Council of Ireland, who were also very good to me in those days, to take on two PhD students and I got a bit of extra money from Organon to take on a third. So I had three PhD students, one technician and me. It was only in 1978, over four years later than in fact they appointed a lecturer, Jim O'Donnell. Until that time I was virtually carrying the whole teaching load, research load, everything with virtually no money.

So, I knew it was going to be tough and indeed it has been. But most enjoyable. Largely because of the quality of people. They are wonderful people at undergraduate and postgraduate level, and the staff. Now we've got, at the last count, with everybody thrown in with research technicians and so forth, nearly 30 people at the postgraduate level.

Were you at the very first BAP meeting?

I was at the famous meeting in the RSM, chaired by Max Hamilton. There would have been about 70 odd people there. The whole thing arose because a group of psychiatrists, people like David Shaw, David Wheatley, Alec Coppen, Merton Sandler, wanted to set up an Academy of Psychopharmacology. They formed an *ad hoc* committee to do this and they wrote a letter, I seem to remember, I think it was to the yellow journal, more or less saying that this was formed. Now there were obviously the basic science side were rather upset about this.

Why were they upset?

Well, they were upset because they were being excluded. The general feeling was that psychopharmacology is not just the prerogative of the clinicians. Psychopharmacology goes right across the board from basic neurosciences through to clinical science. And here you had a group of clinicians trying to, if you like, take over psychopharmacology in Britain at the time.

People will argue the way things have gone that the basic scientists have gone down the neuroscience route without reference to clinical relevance and in actual fact that psychopharmacology as such really is a clinical enterprise and needs to be very closely linked to what can be demonstrated to happen in clinical populations.

No, I would disagree entirely with that. I think that it's both clinical and basic. The sort of people that were involved, Bradley was obviously leading this, and their work was neuropharmacology – they were looking at the neurophysiology of reticular activating system. My own work in the area of hallucinogens, for example, was looking at both behaviour and biochemistry of hallucinogens to try and really see at the molecular level what was happening and to try and explain this very sophisticated phenomenon that was occurring in human beings as a consequence of taking these drugs. So I wouldn't agree with that at all. I think that all of us thought at that time that psychopharmacology encompassed both the basic sciences and the clinical sciences and here we had a group of well-known clinicians more or less usurping the whole of psychopharmacology and setting up this rather what we considered to be a pretentious Academy of Psychopharmacology to the exclusion of the basic scientists.

Can I push you on this one. The way the BAP has gone, I can agree with you that there needed to be some pharmacologists involved in a British Association for Psychopharmacology because an awful lot of clinical people didn't know anything about pharmacology. But on the other hand if you look at the basic scientists who are now active in the BAP, they don't know anything about pharmacology either – they're neuroscientists and we're getting this tremendous tension within the BAP, between those who want clinical relevance and those who really want a neurosciences society.

Yes, but I think there always has been what you have called a tension, I don't know whether tension would be the right word, I think that's too strong a word, certainly in the past it would have been too strong a word. When the organization was formed, basically we were saying that okay you have to try and explain at molecular level and a systems level what is going on when you give drugs and animal pharmacology and behaviour is relevant to that. In fact what came out of that meeting at the RSM was an agreement that this indeed should be the case and I think everybody recognized the mistake of trying to set up an Academy, largely to the exclusion of the basic scientists.

Anyway, it was a one-day meeting – a very lively affair with Max Hamilton jumping up and down and telling people to 'shut up, I'm in charge'. It was very stormy but at the end of the day everyone agreed that we would move ahead together on this and the basic scientists came in with it and the new constitution was drawn up by Max Hamilton. I don't think I was at the meeting, which subsequently followed, with the adoption of the constitution and so forth. But I was a signed up member from that time. I must say, to begin with, it was a very quiet society. You were talking about summer meetings with 70 people, but of course it has certainly improved since that time and become very influential.

ACNP has recently fractured with Don Klein having set up the American Society for Clinical Psychopharmacology. His line is that ACNP are becoming too much neurosciences orientated and that's fine for the neuroscientists but it's not so good for psychopharmacology proper.

As a basic rat-ologist, I would have sympathy with Don's view. I think that's what all organizations like the BAP have to watch. The strength of the BAP in the past was a balance between clinical and pre-clinical psychopharmacology and it's all too easy now to get into the trap with all this work in molecular genetics and molecular neurobiology to say you can explain the whole of mental illness in terms of some fundamental fault in an enzyme system or transport process or a receptor mechanism. It's a gross oversimplification and it stinks of scientific reductionism, which I think is extremely dangerous in any area but particularly in any area to do with neuroscience. I think it's very seductive as well. It worries me that we would go too much towards basic neurobiology in the BAP and I think it is something which has to be very carefully looked out for. The BAP must be a broad church in other words not a narrow sectarian group of acolytes around a concept in psychopharmacology. That I think has been the strength because I think the BAP as always been a broad church and I'm just hoping it's not going to change.

But increasingly we are getting to the stage of having symposia which aren't constructed so that people make links between areas or else we seem to have much fewer people who have the broad understanding in the field that would enable them to say look you are going to just re-invent the wheel if you keep going down this route.

Well, yes. I think it's complex. Where are the grand old men with the vision — this is basically what it comes down to. You want people with both experience and fantasy and that's bloody hard to find now. I think that that is the way in which scientific research and certainly academic research has gone. That people have been almost forced to overspecialize. One must always specialize in a specific area, obviously to do anything worthwhile, but to overspecialize and thereby exclude things are not directly relevant to the problem which you're looking at at the present time because if you do, it means you can't produce the papers, which means that you can't justify the grants, which means that . . .

You won't get the next grant.

And the University therefore starts looking very carefully at your performance during the year and your support from the University goes down and so on and so forth. And I think it's an extremely dangerous way in which research is going in all academic institutions. I think that is impacting now on what's happening in learned societies like the BAP. So people have not got time to really think in a broad constructive way about what's going on. When this happens at a senior level it has an even bigger impact for the junior level. Because the juniors are not being brought up in an environment of enquiry, of fantasy of chancing a hunch. You've got a project to complete and by God it better work because the grant depends upon it and indeed your next grant may depend upon it, your PhD may ultimately depend upon it. Don't take any chances for God's sake. Just play safe. Now this is bad for science. It's very bad for science and that's what I think is being increasingly reflected in organizations like the BAP, which I think is extremely sad for the future.

You've recently become treasurer of CINP. Had you links there before?

Well, I have been a member of CINP since 1968 and I have been a regular attender at their meetings because I see it as the major international body representing psychopharmacology. It's been a broad church with both clinical and basic psychopharmacology working together for symposia with appeal to both. So to me it was a logical extension. My involvement at a bureacratic level came about six years ago, at the time of the Kyoto meeting when Alec Coppen was President. The CINP is quite unlike the BAP in that it's very much a Presidential organization. It is the

President who appoints the Chairpersons of the different committees and so that whole thing can change from one two-year Presidential period to the next. I think that's a big weakness. It means that continuity need not necessarily occur.

Anyway, when Alec was appointed, he knew that I had been involved for many years in Africa, in Tanzania and Uganda and Zimbabwe, with third-world education. I had raised this at members meetings, on a number of occasions, that CINP was an organization dominated largely by North America, to a lesser extent by Northern Europe, which was not taking cognizance at all of the major problems in third-world countries. It was basically a rich man's club.

There are all sorts of reasons given why nothing was done. One was that it's a relatively poor organization. It was US$ 50 per two years until I became Treasurer which was absolutely ridiculous, considering that you are dealing with only very senior people – you are talking about people with approximately 20 years' research experience with a large number of publications before you can actually become a member. Anyway, to cut a long story short, Alec said, okay, I'm the President, now I want you to form an education committee – we didn't have one before – and you're the Chairperson, you do what you want and I'll back you, which is basically what I did. I had no money – there was nothing in the budget for the committee – so for three years I funded this by talking to friends in the industry and getting a few thousand dollars and the first three workshops we ran were in Harare in Zimbabwe. Ted Dinan and myself did them. We established a basic curriculum across all areas of psychopharmacology, aimed specifically at the needs of third-world countries.

Aimed at whom?

Well, it depends on the country. In the case of Zimbabwe, there were only at that time four qualified psychiatrists in a population of 11.5 million and Zimbabwe was far ahead of most of the black African countries. So when you are actually talking about running courses, you are talking about running courses for mental health ancillary workers – very intelligent, highly motivated nurses, basically, a few general practitioners with an interest, and one or two trained psychiatrists who were basically centred in a capital city. So that's the level of your education. What should you be looking out for when you're using chlorpromazine, when you're using imipramine, when you're using diazepam? What are the real practical problems with these drugs and how should they be used ? What are the side effects and why do the side effects occur? We were trying to establish a rational basis for the drugs which are available on the WHO recommended list. On the basic WHO recommended list you've got something of the order I think it's about 130/140 drugs, that's all. Covering all therapeutic areas. Of those, the drugs in the CNS area are something of the order of 12 or 14 – you've got one or two drugs for the treatment of epilepsy, one or two for the treatment of anxiety disorders, which is basically the benzodiazepines, standard neuroleptics, which would be haloperidol and chlorpromazine, imipramine, basically as an anti-depressant.

So you are really very limited and restricted to what can be done. Even that is a luxury in many places. You would get them in the major centres, but when you are really out on the sticks, although theoretically they should be available, half the drugs are not available. There is a breakdown in supply. Now what the heck do you do when you've got patients going mad and all the rest of it. So Ted and myself found it a real education. I would deal with the basic pharmacology, side effects, drug interactions, and Ted would deal with the clinical applications. It was very labour intensive. We ran these courses over a five-day period and then we would try to get some of the clinicians together to talk about research. Research which is relevant to the country, research which doesn't require big apparatus and so forth. Get people thinking on how to use the material which is available. We did three years of this.

Julian Mendelwicz then took over from Alec Coppen and obviously this was producing some sort of waves within the CINP and so they said, well, perhaps we ought to give you a budget and that's basically what happened. So the committee has been extended and we've increased our coverage to South East Asia, Indonesia, Vietnam, Korea, to the Middle East, Yemen, Egypt, Iran this year, to Namibia and South Africa. We've got very big plans for training trainers in South Africa to help to cover the English-speaking African countries. This has kept going under the new Presidency of Lew Judd. It's been quite anarchic. We've been working all the time with the mental health division of the WHO. Now we are trying to get a proper curriculum going and get printed material and so the whole thing is building up and hopefully we'll eventually have a course structure and all the main continents will be covered in terms of the training programme.

As a result of that I became known to the Committee. The Treasurer's position became vacant in 1992; it lasts seven years. It's the worst position on the executive. For political reasons, geographical reasons, I was nominated as Treasurer and the rest, as they say, is history. The executive consists of seven people – the President, two Vice-Presidents, the Treasurer, the Secretary, the Past-President – that's it. This group meets twice a year and sort of basically to guide the organization.

The educational work you are doing is totally consistent with what I know about you but of course the other way to see it is that you're spreading an Anglo-American cultural imperialism that is pharmaceutical company-friendly and may not be relevant at all.

Oh well I disagree with that totally. The very fact that we're working with the WHO means that we work with drugs that are all generics and we have to be sensitive to the primary needs of third-world countries, in terms of cost of drugs and all these sort of things. And secondly, we don't ask anyone; they ask us through the WHO. So, in other words, a need is identified. We are asked to fill that need and we only go and fulfil that need. That's the way it always has to be with any of these educational programmes and I think we have to be very sensitive about any cultural imperialism of any sort.

Some of the things that we've seen in Africa and in Indonesia in terms of treatment of patients with mental health facilities and so forth are just unbelievable. In Indonesia, we went to one of the State psychiatric hospitals and it was sort of reasonable for a third-world country in terms of the physical structure – very basic but reasonable and clean. But we went into an enormous male ward at 2 pm and all the patients were asleep. We thought this is very strange. These are disturbed, manic patients, acute schizophrenics and of course they had all had whacking great doses of haloperidol in the backside or something like that. They were zonked out and this was the way the whole thing was run and controlled. And then we were shown the ECT machine and we thought, great, have you got an anaesthetist? Oh, no. Raw ECT. Big men hold the patient down – it's 'One Flew Over the Cuckoo's Nest' stuff. This is the way things are done. So that's the level you're dealing with. In many cases, they don't even see a psychiatric nurse; if the patient goes a bit mad you tie him to a tree until he calms down.

So cultural imperialism may be a good thing.

No, I'm not saying that at all that cultural imperialism is a good thing. No, you don't impose; you say well there are other ways of doing things. These are the other ways which can be used and they can be used in a relatively inexpensive way and in terms of the impact it has on the welfare of the patient, it may be much better for what you are doing. So you try and educate by example. What I would like to see, of course, is an extension of the educational programme so that we could have scholarships to take out some of the young trainee psychiatrists from these countries and train them in a really good environment somewhere and then send them back so that in fact you are enriching things. Now, unfortunately, the CINP doesn't have the money and WHO only has limited funds and they contribute nothing in terms of funding. And so this is what I would like to see done. Now whether we would be able to do it by getting funds from charities like the Ford Foundation is something that we are now looking into. I see the programmes and workshops as showing that we are willing to help and that we are cognizant of the problems but it is scratching at the surface and we need to be doing a lot, lot more in terms of really training young psychiatrists, first and foremost.

Can I put it to you that the engine that drives a lot of psychopharmacology, the goose that lays the golden egg, has been the pharmaceutical industry. I'm interested to explore your attitude to the industry given that you're Marxist in orientation.

Well, the world we live in is a capitalist world and the countries that I live in have been capitalist countries, so what do you do. You either look at the reality of the situation or you pretend it doesn't exist. One of the fundamentals of Marxism is you always look at the reality of the situation. That applies to the industry. When we're thinking of psychopharmacology where do we get our money for research from – in an ideal world I don't think a single penny should come from private concerns for the sort of research that we want to do – it should be state funded.

State funded? What about cooperatively funded – the BAP, for instance, should raise its own funds or the psychiatric profession could?

No, I don't even think that. To my mind, the hallmark of a civilized country is its values – its education programmes, its health service and so forth. It sees the need to enrich the intellectual life of the country. This, therefore, means that all basic research, be it medical or non-medical, is funded through the appropriate organization such as the Medical Research Council, the Science Research Councils and so on. In other words projects are peer-reviewed, etc. but this framework does guarantee the total independence of the scientist to carry out work for a reasonable period of time on projects that would otherwise never be funded if you relied purely on funding of the private applied type, where research has to have an immediate pay off in terms of the person funding it. That's what I mean by state funded research. To some extent that was the case in Britain in the good old days before the ghastly Thatcher. Even in Ireland, when I first came 20 years ago, restricted though the funding was proportionately, it was higher than it has been in recent years. That is not the situation now and I don't think in the foreseeable future that will ever be the situation in any industrialized country. What are we left with? We are left with universities which are becoming primarily teaching institutions, conveyer belts for turning out half educated graduates and technicians – not scientists, not intellectuals, whether it be in the arts or in science and I think this is an extremely dangerous situation.

Anyone working in the university is expected to raise funds to support basic research. In pharmacology we are very fortunate in that the industry needs us and the reason they need us that we can do some fundamental research project or long-term research projects cheaply. And the reason we can do it cheaply is of course that we've got highly motivated PhD students, who have within three years to get a PhD and ultimately get a job. So they are highly motivated and reasonably well trained and they only have to be paid a pittance and so you can get work done in a university which you would never get done in industry for that cost. So, therefore, it's not even a symbiotic relationship, it's a parasitic relationship.

Now that doesn't mean we're not grateful. Of course we're grateful and if we don't have that money coming in from private resources we would have no money at all for research and we might as well pack up and go home and just teach. The reality is that without the industry, there would be no basic research of any sort in psychopharmacology because all the other sources of funding by and large have dried up.

Right, now let me be as awkward as I can. On the one hand, you do your work in Africa for the WHO and your orientation as a Marxist all seems to fit into this quite well. However, on the other hand you are very publically seen defending for instance the latest group of antidepressants, the 5-HT reuptake inhibitors, vigorously, even though the evidence that they are really much better than the older generation of antidepressants doesn't appear to convince most clinicians. From knowing you and how you see the issues, I can understand why you see things the way you do but that's not always how things look from outside. For instance, take the question of long-term efficacy of antidepressants. This is important but studies on the long-term efficacy of 5-HT reuptake inhibitors becomes, for the Marketing Department of a drug company, just the way to sell their drug rather than the answer to a scientific question and people like you get used to put forward an industry-friendly point of view. What this leads to among many practising psychiatrists is a perception that people like yourself are doing the marketing of these drugs for companies better than they can do it themselves. It's an ironic and ambiguous position it seems to me.

Well yes I don't see it that way of course. I would never do anything which would prevent me from sleeping comfortably in my bed at night. Knowing the drug industry pretty well, having worked in it and having worked closely with it for well over 20 years, the reputable international companies have no time for the so-called academic psychopharmacologist that can be easily bought and will say exactly what they want him or her to say about a particular drug. Since mianserin we've had lofepramine, we've had selective monoamine oxidase inhibitors, we've got this plethora of SSRIs, so the industry realizes that what is flavour of the month this month is going to be changed next month and if you've got somebody who is constantly changing and saying exactly what the Marketing Departments want, their objectivity is lost. The shelf life of this kind of person is extremely short. And what the reputable drug industry wants, I think, is people who are independent and who will say what they genuinely think about the compound. And it works in their favour, just as much, to protect the integrity and independence of the individual.

But with the debate about 5-HT reuptake inhibitors, you get statements being made by people, even within the BAP, who say that the average clinician shouldn't be using the old compounds and if they don't switch over they will start getting sued. This is not the way for debate to happen. It seems like debate in soundbites. We get you on national radio saying that your average jobbing clinician isn't prescribing the 5-HT reuptake inhibitors, which are a much safer group of drugs, because of the price. But this is not the way they are perceived clinically.

My argument would be, and I put this at more length in fact on some of the other radio programmes this week, is one that I've always said which is that there's no improvement on efficacy in the last 30 years in the area of treating depression – we're all agreed on that – what is new I think is the side-effect profile and toxicity. Now I happen to think that's an extremely important issue to be getting across.

The other big problem is that of suicide. My argument there is an ethical one. I think we should always, as far as possible, consider the needs of the patient first. We can never predict which patient is going to attempt suicide and how they are going to attempt suicide. What we do know is that drug A, a cheap drug, if they do attempt on that there's a higher probability that they're going to harm themselves than if they drug B, which is equally effective as an antidepressant. So leaving everything else aside from a purely moral point of view I feel we should be prescribing drug B.

All of this came out of a long article I wrote in the *Irish Doctor*, where I was specifically asked as a pharmacologist to write about SSRIs for the simple reason there are four of them in Ireland and they're expensive drugs. The media issue has come out of that but in every programme I've said look there are two types of drugs. There's basically the old ones, the tricyclics and basically different groups of new ones of which the SSRIs have received some prominence, but there are others. So, to my mind it's all totally consistent with my philosophy. I want to see drugs used appropriately. I want to see the best drugs being used. I think it comes back to my view in a civilized society we look at cost in the real sense and the cost means taking into account the quality of life of the patient.

But the average clinician doesn't perceive a major advantage to the new drugs. A lot of people will take the Pope maxim, 'Be not the first to take up the untried, nor yet the last to cast the old aside'. Then you have the argument that the studies that lead to drugs being licensed are not independent science. They are constructed to allow the FDA to legitimize certain claims rather than constructed from the point of view of trying to do independent science. So from that point of view, it seems reasonable to try these drugs out on some patients and chat to colleagues rather than go by the so-called evidence. Any powerful lobby otherwise is going to look like it's orchestrated by one of the companies to do the marketing for them.

Yes well of course that's an interpretation. I can't to anything about the way people interpret what my motives are. All I can say is what they are, what the reality is. I'm associated with the National Drugs Advisory Board – all I can say is when you actually look objectively, using the data, most people would independently come to the same conclusion that these drugs are equally effective as the older tricylics and they have the major benefit of being less toxic, safer and therefore better able to fit in with the new concepts of the long-term treatment of depression. You cannot persuade me, as a pharmacologist with a knowledge of toxicology, that a drug which produces a constant tachycardia, for which no tolerance develops is beneficial for the cardiovascular system of that patient. And that is precisely what happens with any tricyclic given at the appropriate therapeutic dose. Leaving aside everything else, from the toxicological point of view, that is bad news. And I stand on that. I'm not advocating any particular new second generation antidepressant. I refuse ever to speak for a particular company or particular drug. I would just talk about a group of drugs. So if you want to ascribe to me motives which I don't have that's fine. I think that the worst thing we could do is to shut ourselves away in a laboratory, talk to rats and write obscure papers which nobody reads. If you're going to appear in the public domain you are going to have people who are going to doubt your motives and say well of course that's the way Leonard goes on and has expensive holidays and big cars, neither of which of course is true.

But on the other hand if the SSRIs went under or if they hadn't impacted at all, an awful lot of companies might have been tempted to pull out of CNS and as a consequence Alzheimer's research programmes wouldn't be as likely to be happening. Do you not think that people like you and me have to be prepared to be compromised slightly to try and make sure that industry don't find the CNS an area that they don't want to be in?

No, I am convinced that the industry looks very carefully at all this and they realize there is so much that still needs to be done to find new drugs for the treatments of different types of mental illness. If they can find anything for Alzheimer's disease, then this would be an enormous break-through, from a medical and a financial point of view, which is why all the money is going into memory research. Every company of any size has got Alzheimer's research programmes going on. The consequence of that to neuroscience, both clinical and basic, is very considerable. That is a positive side, if you like, of the industry. Okay, they're motivated by greed, it makes no difference whether you're selling bombs, soap powder or drugs, the motivation is the same. However, from the scientific point of view, of course, it is extremely beneficial and with the sort of society we are living in, it is the only way that those of us who are basic researchers in the universities can exist. It's a very complex issue, but that's the world we're in. I don't feel compromised by it. I wish it were not that way but changing it means changing society.

23 John Hughes

The discovery of the opioid peptides

Some time back I was interviewing Hannah Steinberg, and she said to me that she felt that one of the key discoveries was the discovery of enkephalin in the brain. This was brought home to her in an unusual way when she went to try and get a copy of Nature *to photocopy a copy of your article and found that the actual pages for that article had worn away – and this was only about two or three years after it had come out. Clearly it was a piece of work that caught the imagination not just for people within the field but of the wider public. Can I ask you how it all came about?*

Well, like many of these things, scientific advances come about because, I guess, the individual scientists get fascinated by a particular problem. Why they get fascinated with that problem is often quite unclear. Okay, some of the truly great may be want to understand the origin of life and so you have Watson and Crick and they went straight for it. The rest of us lesser mortals settle for what interests us, perhaps because of baggage we carry from the university, a particular lecture or a supervisor that really turned us on to a particular subject or particular area. It's difficult to say.

I wanted to work in neuroscience. I knew that when I completed my first degree but I also wanted to do medicine. I tried to combine both. I was at King's College Medical School for a while. But I also registered for a PhD under John Vane and spent three very happy years not doing any medicine at all doing research into adrenergic and non-adrenergic, non-cholinergic transmission in human and animal blood vessels and at the end of that period I realized how ignorant I was – particularly of the new biochemistry of the brain. It was a period when lots of things were happening, particularly in the States.

This was when?

This was 1966/67. It was the time when adrenergic uptake was being discovered and exploited, the biosynthesis of catecholamines, the serotonin story was beginning, the whole of brain neurochemistry. So I went over to the States, to Yale, to learn some of this new neurochemistry. I guess it's your postdoctoral training that sets you in that kind of direction. I therefore became a neurochemist, from having a first degree in biochemistry and pharmacology, a passing acquaintance with medicine and a PhD in pharmacology. I was particularly fascinated at that time by what modulates transmission. Everyone at that time thought there was only a handful of neurotransmitters and therefore the key to how the brain functions must be how these transmitters modulate and how they interact with one another. In fact some of my early studies were concerned with quite an important peptide Angiotensin, which facilitates adrenergic transmission in a number of situations. So that was the state of play when I went to Aberdeen.

Why Aberdeen?

Why Aberdeen? I wrote to John Vane, saying I was coming back from Yale. I had certain irons in the fire; one was to do yet another postdoc in London University, at King's College, perhaps even resume medicine, which was a possibility; another one was to go to Newcastle, where there was a new department of pharmacology being set up. Really I was quite set on the idea of an academic life – it appealed. They were the two I said to John I was thinking about. He wrote back and said well he didn't think there was anything at Newcastle and it would be daft to do another postdoc but Hans Kosterlitz was setting up a new department in Aberdeen and he thought I ought to go there. He put me in contact with Kosterlitz, who actually visited me in Yale. We got on very well right from the start. Kosterlitz was a fascinating man.

Tell me about him.

Well, at that time he was approaching 65 and, very unusually, the university had waived the normal employment requirements because they wanted to set up pharmacology as an independent entity at Aberdeen. The then Professor of Therapeutics and Materia Medica in whose department Hans was at the time wanted this to happen. They all agreed that Hans should be given a five-year extension to his normal tenure. So at the age of 65 he became Professor of Pharmacology in the Department of Materia Medica in the University of Aberdeen.

Remarkable

Absolutely extraordinary. It was a combination of circumstances. This is what the clinical school there wanted. This is what the clinicians wanted. They accepted that eventually it would become a separate department.

Where did he actually come from?

Kosterlitz had been in Aberdeen since 1935 – plus or minus a year or two. He had come over with the rise of Hitler. Although not a Jew himself, he could see what was going on – he had Jewish connections and he was thoroughly disturbed by the whole situation. I don't know if he meant to come over permanently. It may be it was a combination of things. He wanted to work on insulin and intermediary metabolism, he was deeply interested in that, so it just kind of fitted in. I don't know — he's never said that he either intended or didn't intend to go back. As it happened his fiancé came and joined him some years later and they got married. They actually ended up in Aberdeen because one of the co-discoverers of insulin, Macleod, was Professor of Physiology there and he wanted to work with this man. Unfortunately this fellow died within a year of Kosterlitz arriving but by that time, you know I guess the way you drift into things, he had decided to stay on at Aberdeen and make a career there. So from Berlin to Aberdeen and he has been there ever since! He was a clinician of course.

You both met and he talked you into coming to Aberdeen.

I didn't need much convincing it was more a question of could I convince him I was suitable. In those days, although academic jobs were easier to find than they are now, they still weren't that easy to come by. This was obviously a good opportunity. I had never been to Aberdeen in my life. I'd been to Scotland, I'd climbed in Scotland and had a few holidays there but I had never been on the East Coast, apart from Edinburgh. So I really didn't know what it was like. I had no experience of the university. I knew a little bit about Kosterlitz. I had read some of his papers and familiarized myself with his work. But I thought he was a thoroughly nice man and it sounded a good opportunity and who knows if he was going to be retiring in five years time, there might be a job there. One perhaps thinks in that way but little did I know, he still hasn't retired, of course. He's 91 now. He doesn't work in the lab but he still goes into the university to his office each day.

He offered the job and I took it. The first time I saw Aberdeen was when I arrived with our cases, on the train, the following September. And the outcome of that was good. In those days I mean it was much freer, much easier — maybe it was Aberdeen, maybe it was Kosterlitz — he gave me a lab, an office, a technician and quite a chunk of apparatus. I told him what apparatus I wanted and he provided it. Plus I was given a small research allowance. So within a month or two, I was on my feet and doing experiments. Within six months I had written up an MRC grant and got it. So within a year of getting to Aberdeen I was an independent investigator with my own technician.

Obviously there were quite heavy teaching duties. In comparison with now, I suppose you wouldn't call it heavy but there were 30 medical lectures a year, along with the practicals. We set up a first degree programme in pharmacology within a year as the department expanded from three people to four to five people. But I continued with my research on neuromodulation and that's what Hans was interested in. He was interested in the cholinergic system. Particularly using the guinea pig ileum as a model. I was interested in using blood vessels and the vas deferens as a model. And of course the other interest of Kosterlitz's was opiates.

He had had that for some time, hadn't he?

No – he only got interested after Paton and Schuman published their original paper showing that morphine inhibited acetylcholine release from guinea pig ileum – we are talking mid 1960s, early 1960s. He had actually applied that knowledge to the adrenergic system – he'd done some experiments with John Thompson, who was funnily enough the Professor of Pharmacology at Newcastle where I had originally wanted to go. He was my PhD examiner. He was the reason I wanted to go there; Thompson was a very learned man, a very good experimenter and a very nice man as well. A very, very pleasant man – he still is although he's retired now. John Thompson was famous for having developed an isolated preparation of the nictitating membrane of the cat, which is an incredibly tedious preparation which takes anything between an hour and two hours to dissect and put in an organ bath. This is a classic medical student experiment – you can do it *in vivo*; you take the cat and tie the nictitating membrane to a thread and you can show that by stimulating the nerve supply to the membrane you get a contraction that is adrenergic in nature. Well Kosterlitz with Thompson showed that that adrenergic transmission was also morphine-sensitive, which was the first time that that had been demonstrated.

When I joined, with my interest in adrenergic transmission, he was on at me right from the start 'come on, morphine interacts with this you've got to find other models in which this applies' and I'd say 'I'm not interested in morphine, morphine's rather boring. It's okay for a medical class demonstration but . . .'. Anyway, he kept on and I actually had an interest in drug abuse, drug addiction but I was working from the other side 5-HT and LSD and so on.

But it just so happened that there was a young student who wanted to do a PhD with us, from Glasgow, a fellow named Graeme Henderson who is now a Professor of Pharmacology at Bristol. He came to do a PhD with Kosterlitz and myself and we thought about the problem and we said well why don't you look at adrenergic transmission – Kosterlitz hadn't actually measured noradrenaline release, which was my particular forte at the time. So we gave Graeme the task of looking at noradrenaline release from nictitating membrane, which was a very cruel thing to do to a PhD student. It is incredibly difficult preparation – we actually got John Thompson up to Aberdeen to demonstrate it, to show him how to do it but it was still a very complicated, very tricky thing, apart from being expensive as well.

Anyway, Graeme did a first-class job and showed that indeed morphine did inhibit noradrenaline release as you would have predicted from pharmacological experiments but really there was nowhere to go, the nictitating membrane was just too complicated, too expensive. I had been mulling over in my head – you know well let's put him on to see if he can find another adrenergic model that responds so that he can continue his PhD, otherwise we'd have to shift him to something else. He tried a number of preparations without any luck.

It just so happened – I was down at the library one day, I guess this was 1970/71, just flicking through the journals, and I came across an article in *Acta Physiologica Scandinavica* that showed that the mouse vas deferens was quite a good preparation for looking at noradrenaline release but what caught my attention was that they had done a frequency output curve. Now most people didn't do that at that time. This actually measured how much you got out per pulse, at different nerve frequencies, which is one of the things I had been studying, and to my astonishment the mouse vas deferens appeared to show the same output characteristics as Graeme Henderson had shown for the nictitating membrane which was a morphine-sensitive preparation. I wondered if there was a connection there.

So I went back to the lab and said to Graeme you know try this – it's worth trying and just left him alone. A couple of days later I wandered in and said 'did you have any luck with it?' and he said 'oh yes I put up the mouse vas deferens and I put morphine in and there it was inhibiting the mouse vas deferens'. I said 'well that's very good'. In fact it wasn't that brilliant – if you got an inhibition it wouldn't wash out and there were a lot of technical problems which we solved over the next few weeks.

That was really the start of my true interest in morphine because there you had an adrenergic transmission, which was the love of my life at that time, inhibited by morphine. Now this was fascinating and there was also this frequency relationship which we never explored further in fact because we had already got hold of enough things. Graeme was able to make a PhD thesis out it – in fact we got several PhD theses out of that little preparation.

Then – this is the way the scientist thinks – you get an interest; it tickles you, it nags at you and I began asking questions that I guess Kosterlitz had been asking for some time. But it had never occurred to me before – why should there be morphine receptors in the vas deferens; why should they be in the guinea pig ileum for that matter or the nictitating membrane? That was a topic of discussion for a long time between Kosterlitz and myself and others in the group. We knew it was a pharmacological receptor – it had all the characteristics of a classical receptor. And so the idea grew up well that if there is a classical receptor, it's not there to interact with morphine; perhaps it's there to interact with something else.

Now this fitted in with a lot of other stuff that had been going on at that time – work in the States particularly by a fellow called Liebeskind and his PhD student Huda Akic – they had been studying stimulation-induced analgesia in rats. They would insert electrodes into the rat's brain, particularly into the periaqueductal grey matter, and showed that if you apply the right frequency and current you could get a profound analgesia in the rat. They had taken this a step further than other people – they had localized the action. They showed that the analgesia could at least be partially reversed by naloxone and they reported this observation. They didn't draw any conclusions from it – they were very puzzled by it. I'm not even sure now why they did the experiment – except on the basis that morphine is an analgesic so let's try morphine antagonism.

That seemed to me a very strong hint that there must be something in the brain that actually acts like morphine. And you know this combined with the fact that there was this stereosensitive receptor really fired me up. You know this is too good an opportunity to miss – here we've got all the facts and we've got an assay with which we could test this hypothesis. That was really the starting point.

So something in the brain that attaches to this receptor?

I guess it might not have got any further. I did some preliminary experiments which were negative and we were very busy at that time. We had gotten very much into receptor specificity apart from a general interest in neurochemistry. Hans was fast approaching retirement – this was 1972. It is possible that if Hans had retired I might have carried on for a bit and then given up. About that time, funnily enough, a fellow called Avram Goldstein actually had published a paper, in which he specifically raised the question of whether there could be an endogenous morphine substance in the brain. He reasoned with characteristic straightforward logic that if there was, then you should be able to detect it with morphine antibodies so that is exactly what he did. He took brain extracts and did radioimmunoassays for morphine and got nothing and he concluded that there can't possibly be an endogenous morphine-like substance in the brain, which was interesting. I thought this is totally wrong but I might not ever be able to prove the opposite.

However, Kosterlitz being Kosterlitz, approaching the age of 70 decides he wasn't going to retire. He had to give up the headship of the department but he suggested to me that we make a joint application to the National Institute on Drug Abuse – remember this is the time when there was a great push by Nixon to get involved in drug abuse and the problems of drug abuse and NIDA was founded and all these things were going on. So we wrote up a programme grant, proposing a unit for research on addictive drugs, not based at the clinical school as we were then – we would move down to the preclinical site at Marischal College in the centre of Aberdeen. And we got the grant. Quite extraordinary. The university agreed to give me leave of absence – I could keep my tenure so that I could go back to my job if the thing collapsed which was a consideration with a young family.

This did give me the opportunity at last to experiment in a way perhaps I wouldn't have done before. Staying in the university mainstream I might have carried on doing tried and trusted experiments that I knew would yield papers and might actually give me a chair perhaps or at least a promotion. This was an opportunity – it was a clean break. I made it quite clear to Hans I was only doing it because I wanted to search for the endogenous ligand. He wasn't too happy about that.

What was he trying to chase? What was the programme written around?

The programme was mainly written around looking at whether there was opiate receptor subtypes, looking at the development of tolerance and dependence in isolated tissues and animals. Essentially more of the same as what we were already doing in the department but trying to understand the basic mechanisms underlying tolerance and dependence. When you think about it now I mean it was a very kind of amateurish attempt. There was no way with the tools at one's disposal that one could possibly do that at that time.

But often these agencies fund things because they know this is the area that needs to be funded and they hope that during the course of the project you will develop the tools, isn't that it?

Well, that's the hope more or less, yes, but when one looks back and reads the grant application you ask how on earth did we get away with that. There was nothing better at the time. I think ours was as reasonable an approach as anybody's.

I said Hans well look okay I will collaborate with you on the receptor stuff but I really am going to search for the endogenous ligand. No one else need be involved – me and my technician will do the business if you like. 'Fair enough', he said, 'I don't think you'll have much luck'. As it happened we did have luck. It was really incredibly simple in a way once one had decided it was there. You know you have got to be convinced, you really have got to be convinced in science that you're right. This business about the impartial scientist assembling facts in order to disprove a hypothesis is absolute balderdash. Karl Popper could never have been further from the truth. You have got to be convinced.

Deluded almost?

Yes, and I think most scientists are deluded. I'm sure there are those out there that do pose the questions and go about it in a logical way. But I'm not one of that group. I have to believe in something before I do it and I believed in it. Of course it's very dangerous; delusions are dangerous. But I think I was a good enough scientist to recognize that. Now that was the one thing we were very concerned about that even if you did come up with something, how would you prove it really was endogenous. That really worried Hans even before we got any results.

What was the problem?

Well, we were looking for an opiate but we had hundreds of very powerful opiates in the research unit. You know you could be led a really merry dance if they started to infiltrate into the lab, into the food chain and as it happens morphine is in the food chain, in the same way that cocaine is and the benzodiazepines are.

In broccoli – the benzodiazepines are in broccoli.

Well, they seem to be everywhere. So that was a concern. It didn't worry me too much but you know we were obviously going to have to do the proper controls. I started out fairly logically looking for various classes of neurotransmitter. Based on the evidence that time, we were going to be looking for a biogenic amine and really got nowhere. I varied the extraction conditions and tried to make them as general as possible and in fact the extraction conditions I settled on eventually were determined by two things. One was the necessity to extract a large quantity of tissue. It is very easy to take one rat brain, for example, and homogenize it in 5 mls of 0.5 molar HCl, add EDTA and ascorbic acid. That's easy but if you're going to homogenize 5 kg of brain you end up with an awful lot hydrochloric acid, which is very difficult to get rid of – apart from ruining some apparatus as well. So that was a consideration.

We did start off with hydrochloric acid but we got absolutely nowhere. Basically the problem was that we could do extracts of brain and even regional extracts and there were a lot of very depressive substances in there. If you put it on the mouse vas deferens, twitching away nicely there, the mouse vas deferens would just die. You could wash it out but you couldn't show the critical response which was reversal with naloxone. We got one or two indications. You'd put naloxone on and get a couple of twitches but they would die down again. I'd call Kosterlitz and say 'look at that'. 'Ah, you're deluding yourself' he would say and march off and I'd light my pipe and think about it. You know it did happen – every time I put naloxone on. It was true but you would never have got anyone to accept it. It was clearly there.

Anyway, I put all the stuff away over Christmas of 1973, closed the place down, stored some extracts in the fridge and then we all went away for Christmas. We came back and I decided to clear out the fridges. My technician, Helen, said 'shall we throw these out?'. They were negative, they were rat brain, guinea pig brain, rabbit brain and things like that. The research didn't cost much, because when we knew anyone used an animal we would take its brain – they were only interested in testing a blood vessel or something. I said 'well wait a minute, let's just check through them once more'. So we checked through them and to my astonishment, a couple of the extracts gave the same very fast inhibition but when you put naloxone on this time, it didn't just come back for a couple of twitches, it came back and stayed there. And that was astonishing and it was repeatable I mean I must have dozens of experiments with this extract and a couple of others.

What was the difference between this and previous ones then.

Well, I never really followed this up but what I think the problem was is that obviously brain extracts contain a lot of adenosine derivatives and there will be adenosine itself there which is depressant, ADP and ATP, all of which are very depressant. I suspect that plus other substances present in the extract, which had been stored at only 4°, not −20°, I think they had gone off at 4°. We hadn't meant to keep the extracts. They were other experiments and were put back in the fridge, just out of poor housekeeping really – normally you'd put them in the deep freeze. Now if I had put them in the deep freeze, I think you wouldn't have seen it.

Funny the accidents that can happen and shape things, isn't it?

Absolutely amazing. I have still got the slides. I don't think I've still got the tracings because I had a fire a few years back, which destroyed the original data but I've still got one or two of the slides which show that response. Of course, then, it was relatively easy. Okay you could reproduce those conditions but once you had that activity you knew it was there and you could start to do some chromatography which would have been the next stage anyway. We would have got at it probably logically in the end. But at that point we could move on to chromatography and really it was relatively simple then to purify it up to where you had got an extract that certainly wasn't chemically pure but at least it was pharmacologically pure. You could apply it to the mouse vas deferens and depress the response, give naloxone and the response came right back. It was clearly reversed.

That was quite a sense of achievement. And you could show that there was a fairly small molecule by Sephadex chromatography. I quickly showed it was a peptide although I had been convinced it was an amine – you know self-delusion didn't go too far. We did the proper tests, incubating it with some enzymes and they knocked out the activity. To me it was clear that it was a peptide. It was behaving like a peptide on thin layer chromatography. I had had some experience with peptides working with angiotensin which was a help.

So at that point the problem was really how do we keep the lid on this . . .

In terms of keeping it . . .

Not talking about it. I mean I had told people within the Unit. There were various degrees of excitement. Kosterlitz was certainly excited; he was convinced once he saw a full reversal. The problem was keep a lid on it and also what the hell do we do now? We needed large quantities of brain. You know, I made a silly error, one of those absent-minded things but I never thought at that time to look at alternative sources of material. It had to be brain or nothing. Now, in retrospect, if I had known more about the field of peptide pharmacology and biochemistry, I would have known that there are people in Sweden, who were extracting huge quantities of intestines from pigs or cows or whatever, and discovering all kinds of peptides in them. It just never occurred to me to try anything else, not at that stage.

So the problem revolved around finding the species of animal that was large enough, that was accessible and it really came down to either the sheep or the pig. There weren't enough cows slaughtered in Aberdeen to give a decent supply. Sheep were very difficult – they've got very thick skulls, with smallish brains and anyway they weren't really slaughtered on a large enough basis. So it was pigs of which they did quite a few in Aberdeen.

I managed to convince the head foreman in the abattoir, which was an old abattoir dating from about the 1700s. When I say it was old, it was open to the skies. Men worked in the open air at benches. There were some covered areas, the killing areas. The pigs and particularly the cows were hung up in stores, in the open air. There were birds hopping around and so on. In fact the place was in such a poor state it was closed down within a year or so. I guess if it had been one of these prissy places, that was always spick and span, they wouldn't have entertained the idea of someone coming in there and dissecting out brains on a bench.

But they were willing to provide pig brains – pig heads we negotiated first of all. As it was I found it was far too difficult to try and break open a pig brain and so that was going to cost me a bottle of whisky a session to get the guy to help me out. Normally what they do is the animal is killed by a bolt, it then goes through a kind of tumble dryer, which acted as a kind of steam bath where the bristles were rubbed off on a rotating drum on a conveyer belt, then it was hooked up onto a conveyer line and it comes to a man who stands with a huge chainsaw, a bit like the Texas chainsaw massacre, the guy stands there and, as the pig comes through, he starts at the rear end and slices the pig until he just reaches the skull and then he stops. Of course what I wanted was for him to carry on going right through the skull so that I can then get in there and scoop the brain out. That disturbed their rhythm, I can't remember why, well, it was quite difficult to saw through the skull and I think they also liked to sell them intact.

So anyway, a bottle of whisky settled it and I was able to get my hands in there and scoop out the brain and then whip it over to the bench and dissect off the cortex and freeze the rest on dry ice. I'd go there at about 5 o'clock in the morning, cycle through the old town, collect the dry ice from the docks first of all, cycle up to the abattoir and work for about three hours. Come 8 o'clock I'd get on the bike again – I've still got the bike by the way. I had a carrier on the back – I had pinched a discarded supermarket basket, so that contained the dry ice receptacle which the brains went in on the back of the bike. Back to Marischal College, where I spent the rest of the morning pulverising the brains into a fine powder and then extracting them.

So that was the kind of crude mechanics. One was then into 100s of litres of solvent, large amounts of brain – it became a kind of semi-pilot plant operation in laboratories that weren't designed for it of course. That was the real difficulty. That was really quite hard. It took close on a year to get all that sorted out and to get the chromatography going and all that time of course we were also doing experiments with the materials, studying the distribution in brain, using bioassays to get a fix on it. But really it was at that stage – you know there comes a kind of commitment, it's all or nothing. I had stopped all other research, so I wasn't going to be publishing very much, apart from the stuff I did in collaboration with Hans. So you had to be successful or die.

At this point, I almost had a falling out with Kosterlitz. I was certainly very annoyed with him because he had gone across to the States to a meeting of the International Narcotic Research Conference and at the end of this meeting for some reason the discussion had come round to the question of whether there was an endogenous ligand – now we weren't the first to discuss it or even think about it and it was certainly discussed at that conference – but Kosterlitz stood up and said 'well, in our laboratory, Hughes has now shown that there is an endogenous ligand'.

Immediately that caused a furore. It was agreed that they should arrange a further conference, not an INRC conference but a Brain Research Conference, probably to be held in Boston. Kosterlitz came back very pleased with himself and said you are going to be invited to a conference to talk about this and I exploded. I said it was absolutely ridiculous. I think I knew the Americans better than Hans, having worked there.

They're dangerous, aren't they?

Incredibly dangerous. Well, they're competitive. I don't blame them but I knew how competitive they were. An English group of scientists would say 'jolly good, get on with it old fellow'. So I was annoyed to say the least. But the damage was done and I thought I'd better make the best of it. The conference was going to be published in a booklet form; it was called the Neuroscience Research Programme. It was run by a fellow called F.O. Schmitt at an institute in Boston. The meeting was arranged for May 1974. I gave the data – well I went to give the data and before I even got my first slide up – well I put the first slide up showing depression of the twitch – and Goldstein was on his feet saying 'is that naloxone-reversible; is that naloxone-reversible?' I said 'well wait for the next slide'. I had only met him once before at an INRC conference in Aberdeen and he was obviously very het up. He sat through the rest of the session, unconvinced. He was that kind of man. But obviously other people were convinced, very much so.

What happened was there were a number of what were called rapporteurs, at the conference, meant to write up the review articles. You didn't write the paper – they wrote it up for the book. They were busy writing right through the conference and there were several of these scribes from Snyder's lab. Now, I only heard this story afterwards, there was a guy called Pasternak and a woman called Pert, Candace Pert.

The world knows about Candace, yes

They were supposed to collaborate with the writing up and I heard from Candace that Gavril didn't even stay around for the final minutes of the conference. He certainly wasn't going to be writing anything up because he had disappeared back to the lab in Baltimore to repeat my data but also to try and get a headstart on everyone else.

Get their publication out quicker than yours.

Well, I don't know about getting it published but he obviously thought well perhaps we can win here; we'll use the binding assay and we'll show that there's a morphine-like substance by the binding assay which Lars Terenius had at the same time. At the same conference Lars had reported similar data to mine using the binding assay. Except he hadn't taken it as far and he wasn't willing to compete with the Americans. He knew how competitive they can get. He said 'I'm not going to compete John. If you want to compete you can'. I offered to collaborate with him I said 'let's work together, you do the binding, I'll do the bioassay, we'll collaborate'. He didn't want it. He wanted no part in it. Very interesting.

There are different models of science, aren't there? I think it was Phillip Bradley who was saying to me that schooled in the British school of things, science was a collaborative enterprise and he had his eyes opened by some group in Cambridge whom he found were out to compete and this was a big shock to him.

It was different for me. I mean Terenius was a much more established scientist than I. He had made his reputation in the steroid receptor field. He got into opiates via that. He was one of the first, along with Snyder and with Simon, to show receptor binding for which he never got due credit. Pert and Snyder and Terenius and Simon all published in the same year but perhaps unfortunately for Terenius, he was forced by his Head of Department to publish in *Acta Physiol. Scand.*, I think because his Head of Department was the editor or something like that. I can't remember where Simon published. But Pert and Snyder published in *Science* and of course called a press conference at the same time. They knew how to play the game or at least Snyder knew how to play the game.

Whose was the work? Pert or Snyder's?

Pert did the bench work. I mean Snyder has never been anywhere near a bench at all. But there is no doubt in my mind the concept was Snyder's and that Pert would never had got anywhere without Snyder.

This is always tricky. Often quite a few of the breakthroughs are made by the people working on the bench. She would say she was the one who got the idea of using radiolabelled naloxone, without which the breakthrough wouldn't have happened.

Well, that's not true because both Terenius and Simon had already shown how to do it using a different methodology. The advantage that Snyder's lab had was that Snyder had been a long-time consultant for New England Nuclear. He would say to New England 'here's a new biochemical that has just come out; I think you should should tritiate this. I think it will sell well. By the way I want first go at it'. So he was in a particularly privileged position. And that was the case with naloxone. I'm fairly sure that it was he who suggested that naloxone should be tritiated. So they had this unique tool. I don't think there was any particular merit in their methodology. Once Goldstein had shown that you could get binding, however weak, using a particular technology, it was only a question of refining it. Goldstein was the first one.

Ought he not to have been included in the Lasker prize citation, along with yourself and Hans?

Well the problem with the Lasker prize was twofold: one was that they tried to split it between two things, the opiate receptors and endogenous ligands, which of course were quite separate. Now obviously Hans and I had worked a lot on the opiate receptors but if they wanted to give it for the binding and the binding alone, then it should have gone to Goldstein, Snyder, Simon and Tyrhennius.

But I understand they only give these things in three's. Candace Pert makes out that that was the reason she was excluded. Have you read the book Apprentice to Genius *(see Glossary). How accurate is it?*

Reasonably. I think where I do take issue is Pert's situation. We eventually fell out over this. We were reasonably close friends for quite a long time – she had a very extrovert personality, very interesting. But she can get a little too heavy and she really went over the top on this. And I'm afraid what she did was inexcusable. She used politics to try and gain for herself a position on the Lasker prize. She used the women's movement. I mean it was inexcusable. There was not a trace of antifeminist attitude with any of the people involved in this story. Never was, never has been. That was just a clear political manipulation. Not only that she made incorrect statements at the time – she likened herself to be in the same position as

I was. Her relationship to Snyder was the same as my relationship with Kosterlitz.

She was a junior to him, just as you were to Kosterlitz, she said.

It wasn't the case. She was a PhD student, I was an investigator funded in my own right. I wasn't some PhD student, taking orders from Kosterlitz. The work was my design. We were collaborators. Whereas Pert quite clearly was being directed by Snyder. I am afraid PhD students can only have it that way. I'd like to think that PhD students can come up with something novel on their own account that will get recognized, I know of people who have been. Brian Josephson here at Cambridge, for his description of the way transistors work and he got the Nobel prize for that, quite clearly his own work and his own conception and that's a PhD thesis. It wasn't Pert's conception. It was her work at the bench.

A lot of people would feel that the fuss has compromised Snyder, that he may not get the Nobel prize because of it − because Nobel committees don't like a fuss. What about the fact that his lab tried to scoop your work − you said Pasternak raced back home . . .

Yes, Pasternak did and they were obviously in competition and so were many other groups. I can't blame them. I think there was an element of unfair play if you like in the sense of Pasternak rushing back. There certainly was an inordinate delay in the publication of the booklet from that conference and when it did appear there was work by Pasternak showing that they had an endogenous ligand which was never reported at the actual conference. But it was accepted at the conference that you could add material afterwards, which I think probably everybody did. You could argue, though, that he was adding material that wasn't even thought of at the time. It's water under the bridge but it just demonstrates the competitive power of the Americans. They're going to compete and that shouldn't surprise anyone.

And also the public relations aspect of it. They hold press conferences. They even hold them first and then publish in the journal. How important is that because arguably they do end up being the big names partly for that reason rather than because of the quality of their work

Snyder is very controversial. I know him reasonably well. We have never fallen out, I'm glad to say. Sol is an extremely bright man, an extremely good psychiatrist. He probably could have made a name for himself in any area, psychiatry or whatever he chose to go into. As it happened he decided to go into competitive lab work after working with Julie Axelrod. What he brought to that was a kind of flair, in sensing out what was interesting and then putting people on that track. That's what he did with Pasternak, Pert and many other people. I think that's what also, harking back to the Pert controversy, that's what weakens her argument because

Snyder has had a string of successes – a track record. Whereas actually Pert's record on leaving Snyder was very chequered. In fact it eventually ended in disaster.

I mean what she learnt at Snyder's knee was that the way to get on was not actually good experiments, critical experiments, but to publicize them. And I can remember at least two press conferences she called, when she was working in NIMH, one was to announce the discovery of Angeldustin, which was the endogenous ligand for the phencyclidine receptor, which died a horrible death, and there was another one as well, I can't remember what it was, but there was another press conference. And then of course eventually there was peptide T which she was so convinced in herself that she left the NIH to set up her own company, which I gather has since folded.

Going back to Snyder and publicity, he's played the game. He's played the game brilliantly. Some people hate him for it, some people love him for it but the majority of people know him for it, which probably is the most important thing. There is no doubt about it, I mean I don't know how many millions of scientists there are working around the world, you have only got to look at the millions of papers that are published each year, what differentiates one paper from another? Not very much if you really think about it. So if you can get an edge, a competitive edge, why not use it? It just goes against everything we have been taught in this country. It's not the European way either but it is the American way. It's not only Snyder. He's taken it to possibly the ultimate lengths.

Is there an issue here about citation indices skewing the field? People on this side of the water publish in journals that may not be listed over in the US. I mean could you say that the Americans aren't always deliberately not citing people over here but are simply genuinely unaware of work that is being done outside of the US?

We know that's nonsense, don't we? I think there is laziness – that the Americans lay their hands on whatever is close at hand and it tends to be American publications and what they have learned from their colleagues at their own meetings and Europe is a very far away and European representation there is still relatively low.

Plus there is an insular rather lazy attitude and I think plus a degree of xenophobia as well. Of course some nations suffer more than others from this, the French more than anyone else but of course if they will continue to publish in French that really is their problem. It will be interesting to see what happens over the next 10–20 years as neuroscience grows in Europe. I don't think it will ever be quite as big as in the States but it will gain. Will there be a more even balance I don't know. I suspect not.

What was the Lasker prize ceremony like?

Fantastic. I must admit I was and am very naive. When I got a call saying

I had won the Lasker prize, I can't remember how it happened at all now, I think I got a letter from Mary Lasker congratulating me. I thought that's very nice and the money. I must admit I had never heard of it before that. I had had a number of awards anyway and I thought it's nice to get another award. Fine and there is going to be a trip to New York and there is going to be a few thousand dollars in it, that's very pleasant. It was nice to know that Kosterlitz would be going and see Snyder and then I got a call from Candace Pert. I guess I still didn't twig. She was going on and on about you know she had been excluded. This went on for weeks. At one point I just said 'Look, Candace, stop this, this is just a prize. Hans has won some that I haven't won, I've won some that he hasn't won. I can't do anything about it'. I guess I hadn't appreciated then how the Americans viewed the Lasker. I didn't realize that they recognised it as a premier biological award.

So there was a naivety there. I mean I was soon disabused about that and of course by Candace's antics and then by the press interest and then by the ceremony itself. They put us up at, I think, The St Regis Hotel on Fifth Avenue. I had a suite of rooms that I could get lost in. It was actually quite nice because it was the one time that I got to talk to Sol Snyder for three hours solid without interruption. We got together in the hotel, in my sitting room and just chatted. It was very interesting. The ceremony itself was real razzmatazz. I shook hands with Edward Kennedy. Whatever you might think of Edward Kennedy this was to my mind the highest I've got in American political circles anyway. I did say hello to Nixon once but didn't shake hands with him. It really was quite something; it left you with a sense of gosh they do do these things well.

I have never been that interested in prizes to be honest. The other thing that did astonish me was when these awards start to flow in. It had never actually occurred to me that people would want to reward you. Having the Nobel prize in the bag was always a joke rather than a realistic idea – well, I suppose at the back of your mind there is the hope – it's a good enough discovery, they might think about it. But there were all these other awards. It was amazing. Very nice. Some people argue that awards in science are not a good idea I don't know. You can't give an unbiased opinion, once you have won a few. It clearly does lead to some nastiness, there's no doubt about that. And I know there are people in the States that, each time October rolls around, get impossible to live with in the lab. The other thing I hadn't realized is that people actually work towards getting the Nobel prize in terms of politicking. I don't think you can stop people giving prizes so it's a good idea to have as many as we can so at least there's a fair distribution.

The discovery of the enkephalins opened up new perspectives on things. While the antidepressants worked on neurotransmitters that we had previously found in the brain, these were alien drugs, whereas the suggestion with the opiates was that the body produces its own drugs, which made the whole idea of drugs and therapy seem something totally different to what had been before. Before that a drug was a poison, which you hoped to use with art, but after it therapy became a matter of restoring balance rather than introducing poisons. The other thing that changed was the idea that neurotransmission is not all-important – that neuromodulation may be as important. Do you want to comment on this?

I think you are right. It opened people's eyes to a different way of looking at the brain and certainly a different way of looking at drug therapy. There is no doubt about that. Morphine was no longer just an exogenous plant poison, it was something that was tickling the endogenous system and that may well apply to a number of other substances as well. So there was that to it. It opened up a vista as well. We had known about the hypothalamic releasing factors but they were thought of in a very restricted sense and all of a sudden, here is a brain/gut peptide that is not restricted at all. And not only that, it has a whole pharmacology, which we knew about because enkephalins didn't come to us new born, virginal, they came to us with a huge pharmacology, a huge fund of therapeutic knowledge and that was really particularly exciting. It suddenly made people realize that there were mechanisms there that we hadn't even dreamt about. And of course within 10 years we identified another 100 peptides in brain. So it started a lot of hares running.

It seems that in some respects the cream of British scientists of your generation, Leslie Iversen, yourself, Geoff Woodruff and a range of others, have all opted to go into the industry. Now in Switzerland and Germany, even as far back as 100 years ago, it was very respectable to make a career within the industry. But in this country it hasn't been. It became a little more respectable in the US a wee bit earlier than here and interestingly perhaps one of the companies there in particular who pushed the boat as regards trying to do proper research within the industry was Parke-Davis who set up some of the first industrial research labs. Any comments?

I can only speak for myself in terms of why one moved into industry. I was Professor of Biochemistry at Imperial. The job was becoming less attractive as it was for all academics at that time. Because this was the Thatcher revolution. Although I supported many things Thatcher did, one of the things she did was to my mind quite nonsensical was that she took an axe to the university. It was an indiscriminate axe. I recall well at the time the early retirement programme to try and get the dead wood out.

Which of course would have got rid of people like Kosterlitz. He wouldn't have had any chance would he?

What it did was of course it got rid of the good people. The people who wanted to take early retirement were those who knew they could get another job. In fact I applied for early retirement; I was only 35 at the time. I know from my own department that we lost several good people to early retirement. They knew they had got jobs elsewhere or we had to hire them back in various capacities, whereas the people that I really wanted to get rid of, the people who hadn't done it for 20 years, were stuck there. So one was faced with that problem. This idea that there has got to be a linkage between wealth generation and intellectual pursuit, I think is a load of garbage and always has been. No one denies that you have got to generate wealth in this country but the idea that you can take a scientist and somehow harness him in some abstruse way to wealth generation is just barmy.

The only people that can do that are the engineers. If they really wanted to accelerate the wealth-generating process, they should have put money into engineering professions and also a commitment to change the way industry thinks about the scientist and particularly about engineers because for too long we have had an industry which has been dominated by arts graduates, who know their Socrates or whatever, which makes them very good at the boardroom, very good at public relations, very good at listening but bloody hopeless when it comes to technological decisions. Until that changes any fiddling about with the university system is not going to achieve anything.

That was one attitude I had. It was also getting more and more difficult to get grants. I was never unsuccessful in getting grants but I was spending most of my time writing grants to support a very large group of 15 to 20 people. Now on top of teaching, administration and other responsibilities for which one is not paid very much, it didn't seem to make sense. At that juncture in my career, this was 1981, the research was going well but I was open to suggestions.

Parke-Davis came along. The Vice President, who was in charge of research, came and said they were thinking of setting up a research institute in this country, would I be interested in being considered? Had I seen the advertisement in *Nature*? No I hadn't seen the advertisement in *Nature* and I wouldn't have thought of applying if I had have done. They said well perhaps you would like to consider it. I said yes. At that time, they wanted a link with a university and Cambridge was in their mind. It wasn't until 1982 that they actually made a deal with Cambridge and then were able to formally offer a job, which gave me time to think about it.

I thought there was nothing to lose and maybe a lot to gain. I was being offered a chance to build an institute from scratch, in some ways like what we did in Aberdeen but in a slightly grander form this time. There was going to be the academic dimension, so it was attractive that I wasn't going to have to break the ties completely. Quite frankly the idea of developing drugs, discovering drugs, was intellectually challenging and very exciting. I was trained as a pharmacologist and here was the opportunity to do something I couldn't do in academia, to get chemists and biologists together to work on a common problem and they were going to let me choose my own problem as well.

They didn't ask me to come a run a research institute and tell me 'and this is what you will be doing', they asked me well what would you do. I wanted to work on neuropeptides. Neuropeptides were the coming thing. I mean this is 10 years after enkephalins and after Hokfelt's and other people's work. Peptides were there but no one had ever done anything in terms of developing a useful therapeutic agent from them, by and large. So there was an intellectual challenge, a commercial challenge and there was the therapeutic challenge.

It was just really the question of deciding where one was going to fight one's battles, what area were you going to choose. I don't think I had anticipated quite how challenging it was. I knew the industry would want its pound of flesh. I wasn't naive in that sense. I had worked with Parke-Davis many, many years previously, as an undergraduate. I took a year off when I was at London University to work as a technician at their Hounslow Laboratories, which was subsequently closed down when Parke-Davis merged with Warner-Lambert so I was well aware of the pressures in industry and I knew that they weren't going to sink many tens of millions of pounds here without expecting something back. My favourite expression is that the life of a research director is fairly short and can be brutish so enjoy it while you can.

The kind of comment one sometimes hears from others, who may just be jealous, is that scientists can do science but they can't really discover drugs and there is inevitably this tension if a company spends a lot of money on bringing in the best scientists who tackle interesting problems but don't necessarily deliver drugs which clashes with the corporate raison d'êatre. Is there a clash between being a good scientist and being a person who knows how to actually develop a drug. Are the two compatible?

I can't agree that there is a clash. I mean I hope I'm a good scientist and I hope that I'm actually quite good at developing drugs. What I would say is that being a good scientist doesn't guarantee that you are going to be good at developing drugs but the two are certainly not incompatible. You have got to think in a different way. You have got to rise to this particular intellectual challenge, which consists by and large of putting a lot of different strands of technology and people together.

I mean discovering the drug is actually the smallest part. It is actually then what you do with it and how you stay with it. We have a particular drug that we have had in development for eight years now and one we could have given up on many times. There have been disappointments. It has gone into a clinical trial and it has not fulfilled its potential but we have kept at it. We have kept doing basic research with it, we have kept it alive within the company. The idea is to get the compound into man. Just because it doesn't appear to work for the original indication doesn't mean we should drop it. Let's look at the other possibilities. We have done that with this compound and we are now going in a completely new direction.

The classic case, I suppose, are all the compounds active on the 5-HT system which were developed as antihypertensives, because they are antihypertensive in the rat, but not in man. In humans though they actually do do a whole lot of other things.

It is very foolish to think that you can go in a straight line in drug development, very foolish indeed. With the state of preclinical science, particularly in neuropharmacology and psychopharmacology, it is impossible to predict what is going to happen in man. All you can say is given the best of circumstances, we think this drug will have this particular group of properties and that it may be useful in this particular set of conditions. However, until we get it into man and we then begin to evaluate its psychopharmacological profile, we really won't know where we are going. But we can then feed that data back to preclinical investigations once more, so it's a two-way process – it's not a straight arrow. Time might be a straight arrow but the drug development process is not.

Isn't there this problem at the moment that we seem to have hit – Alec Coppen put something of this in terms of psychopharmacology being like trying to hunt for oil – to date, even though we've got very sophisticated geology, the best way to find oil is to dig oil wells and in terms of pharmacology it's to give drugs. In the 1960s we were able to give drugs to people but now we can't with the same abandon. The increasingly sophisticated pre-clinical work gives people the impression that all the science has been done by the time a drug comes to man and we fail to appreciate that so much more needs to be done once it gets to man. But the problems of doing that work in humans seem to be increasing the whole time. It's very difficult to insure work with healthy volunteers for instance outside the industry.

It's a bit easier in this country than in others, particularly in the States. But you only get one bite of the cherry even in industry. You have got to get it right and that's the art of the preclinical sciences – to try and choose your best ligand to go into man with and hopefully keep it there long enough that you get it used so that even if it is not the ideal drug you can have another one waiting in the wings once you have got clinical evidence of some sort. It's a pity you can't go into man in that way anymore.

One of the other problems I think is that no one discovers drugs the old way any longer by putting them into animals either. They go into a binding assay, they go into an enzyme assay, they go into a cell line or whatever but no one does a whole animal screen.

Do you think this is wrong?

Is it wrong? Not from the industry point of view because clearly that was not a very efficient way of doing things but by God did it discover drugs. I am reminded about another drug that we are working on that was discovered precisely that way. Its pharmacology is well described, or at least people think it's well described but we are now looking at it at a molecular level and find it's doing something quite unexpected, which is going to lead us back now, I hope, to a new line of drug discovery entirely. We can now go back and re-invent that drug in a different form for different uses.

So yes there is a place for that kind of pharmacology. I don't know where you do it — I mean it would be more than my job would be worth to suggest to the company that we should go back to taking compounds and randomly putting them into a CNS screen or something like. I don't know how you do it. The way Woodruff and I try to do it is that we look around and see what there is in the literature and try and put two and two together. There are things that turn up that the original dis-coverers don't spot themselves.

On that line one of the other interesting things about a psychopharmacology meeting these days is the secrecy issue — whereby there are things that industry scientists can't discuss because of patent issues, etc.

It's business. I don't believe that there is much that we can't discuss — the one thing is clinical results and that's a shame. It is very difficult to present early clinical data — I mean you are just giving away too much to the opposition. It's an intensely competitive area. On the preclinical side Glaxo, for instance, seemed to be pursuing an open policy a few years ago but now they seemed to have become more secretive again as far as I can see. There is another company I can think of whose Research Director told me that they now deliberately don't publish on anything. They may be right because you know we are all travelling along roughly similar parallel lines — it is luck by and large whether you get to a chemical entity first. Once you get there may be it is a mistake to give it away too soon.

So a sense of balance is needed. There is this terrible balance all the time of commercial advantage against the disadvantage of switching off your scientists. The last thing I want to do is switch these young people off. They are here to discover drugs. They are just as interested in discovering drugs as I am, I know that. Coming back to what I said at the beginning, scientists only do what they do because they are interested. Its like a stamp collector — he collects British Empire because he likes British Empire stamps, not for any logical reason. It's the same with these guys — so you have got to harness their inquisitiveness, direct it to some extent but not too much and that's the fascinating bit of the business. Its not easy to do.

So you are as interested in the art of management as much as anything else.

I try and do both. I still have an active research programme of my own but my main responsibility here is to make sure this place works. And most of all to these people, making sure they keep their jobs and they will only keep their jobs if they discover drugs. That's the hard facts of the world we live in. In the same way as academics only keep their jobs if they keep on publishing. No, it is intellectually challenging. I don't subscribe to any fancy management theories – they come and go the whole time. It comes down to individuals and the way they handle things in the end; there's no particular role model, no pattern that anyone can follow because every situation is different.

Is industry a very conservative force within psychopharmacology? For instance once it was shown that many of the early antidepressants blocked reuptake, industry kept on making reuptake blockers rather than going out and finding out something new about antidepressants?

By and large it is bound to be conservative because of commercial exigencies but also, and I have to say this, because the scientists who work in industry are not the pick of the bunch. There is competent science but they don't do innovative science. The incentive to take risks is not there because if you take risks it means you stick your neck out. Now I'm the kind of guy who takes risks. I can afford to because I'm not bothered if someone sacks me, I know I'll get another job. Now if you're a middling scientist in a middling company are you going to stick your neck out for a drug you can't be certain will work? Time and time again people play it safe. Rather than say bring a line of compounds up for consideration for clinical development, they stall. They say 'well, perhaps we ought to look at this and this'. I know discovery teams that have got 10 or more years working on a particular line of discovery and never bringing anything to the point where it would be put under the microscope or even less into patients.

Now it may not be deliberate. They may not even be conscious that they are doing it. But I can see it happening and to me the mechanism is obvious – they feel uneasy about being challenged. That was the other thing I noticed when I came into the industry. I have adjusted since but I was brought up in the hurly burly of the British Pharmacological Society.

The British Pharmacological Society really is cut and thrust.

Yes, you were brought up to ask questions and give as good as you got and fair enough if you are going to get up and give results you have got to be prepared to defend them. And that's a good British tradition. The Americans do it somewhat differently. They tend not to challenge openly. Within the industry they certainly do it differently. They don't like this cut and thrust; they are not used to academic exchanges; they don't like it and one has to be careful of upsetting sensibilities. That was a difficult one to get hold of and by and large that is why this place was set up or I like to think it was. It wasn't set up to be a mirror image of Ann Arbor, which is our main research headquarters. It was deliberately set up by the Vice President at that time because he thought it would be good to do something different elsewhere and until someone tells me different I consider that's my remit. To be a bit of an iconoclast, to stick my neck out and to do things differently. If you can't take risks here you won't be able to anywhere.

But to come back to what I said earlier, I have to balance the fact that we're a mature organization, after all we've been here 11 years now, against the fact that I have a large number of people here who depend on me to some extent and certainly Parke-Davis for their jobs. So I hope we are not heading down a pathway where oh my gosh we'd better not do that because that's my paypacket at stake but equally we have to be sensible.

Sometimes industry though can all of a sudden create a field – I mean they created psychopharmacology.

Who else could have done it? Clinicians couldn't. They needed the Chemistry. At the end of the day unless you have the Chemistry you're not going to get anywhere.

How have things changed in the last 10–20 years?

There have been tremendous changes. What used to be the old classical approach, which is what I was trained in, has almost completely gone by the board. I'm not sure you can distinguish a psychopharmacologist from any other kind of neuroscientist these days. Everyone uses molecular techniques, everyone is asking roughly the same kind of questions. The role of psychology is an interesting one. I sometimes wonder if the gulf there is much greater than perhaps we suspect. Psychologists seem by and large to be asking different questions from the psychopharmacologists.

Do you think there is a risk of going too much down the neurosciences route?

No. You have got to follow where the science is going.

But how can anyone, at least anyone working clinically these days, keep up with the explosion of knowledge within the neurosciences?

They have to focus on a specific area – obsessive – compulsive disorder or whatever.

But then you don't make the bridge across areas. Are we at a stage where we are going to lose the possibility of having people who can make the connections across diverse areas, who can see the implications of discoveries in one area for development in another? The kind of link that you made between the nictitating membrane and the vas deferens – you'll get people who are just vas deferentologists

Well, I think there will always be individuals who can make these connections. And after all cardiologists don't have a lot in common with urologists these days, do they? There has got to be a linking process, you're right. But one thing I am convinced of is that we are only at the start of the psychopharmacological revolution.

So what comes next? We had that breakthrough in the 1950s and 1960s when all the major groups of drugs were discovered . . .

And nothing since. I think what you are going to see is the true second revolution. Serotonin uptake inhibitors are all very nice but they really are variations on a theme and however useful they may be it is not that significant an advance. No you are going to see the true treatment of psychosis, the treatment of disorders like obsessive – compulsive disorder in a rational way that goes to the heart of what is involved. I think you are going to see a lot of fragmentation of psychiatric disease.

There is going to be a real challenge, I don't know when it's going to come, to medical ethicists, to industry, to regulatory authorities when the first drug that can truly improve memory arrives. I'm not talking about anti-Alzheimer drugs, I'm talking about true cognitive enhancers – noötropics or whatever you like to call them. It will happen as sure as eggs are eggs – someone is going to discover a way of either improving the learning process or improving the retention process. How are you going to control that? Would you even want to control it? You are then into a brand new era, aren't you? You could then actually say that a psychopharmacologist, not only is going to be able to cure some of the worst ills of mankind, but he could actually advance the cause of mankind. I don't think anyone could rationally argue that it would not be a good thing to improve learning or memory?

In the 1960s the public were all for these new drugs that were coming out but more recently there has been this great concern about drugs and even though the drugs we are producing are safer and safer there seems to be more and more concern about what can be trivial side effects or a feeling which people seem to have now got that they are born with a warranty – that nothing should go wrong for them.

The no-fault environment. I guess that comes out of the States to some extent. There has been a whole sea-change. People now expect, as of right, and unrealistically expect that everything is going to be perfect. Americans want to live forever and want to remain beautiful forever. I guess the Europeans will go that way – they're always 10 years behind.

Also there is an unrealism about in the sense that people don't understand science. By and large people are so ignorant about science and they don't understand the problems and the difficulties and they forget also what it was like before they had these drugs.

The folk memory is so short.

Terribly short. Of course we can cure that – haven't we got penicillins, haven't we got phenothiazines, we can do this, this and this. It is the same argument that is used by the animal liberationists and the other ecologists or the rights movements – we don't need to do it, we don't need to continue to do dissection of animals, why should we do anatomy? It's all there, it has all been done and it's all on file, on computer file no less.

What these people don't realize is that science is built by accretion of not only what other people have done but you have to learn manually from those people. Take John Vane – he passed on a little bit of his knowledge to me and hopefully I will pass on a bit of mine to my students. If you have a clear break and you no longer have that experimental connection, the practical connection, the hands-on connection, if you no longer have that then the students might as well be working on their own trying to reinvent the wheel. That's what will happen eventually. It will be like the Greeks – it will all be theory and no practice and you know what happened to the Greeks.

What about the climate though in terms of difficulties in bringing drugs to the market because they have to be whiter than white?

Inevitable. What has saved us so far is technical advances. We can now do things we couldn't do 10 years or even 5 years ago and hopefully technical advances will keep up with the demands the regulatory agencies place on us. There will still be no substitute for being smart – that's what it comes down to and it will be the smart people and the smart companies who will survive.

Select bibliography

Hughes, J., Smith, T.W., Kosterlitz, H.W., et al. (1975). Identification of two related pentapeptides from the brain opiate agonist activity. *Nature*, **258**, 577–79.

From mental illness to neurodegeneration

Let's start with how you came to be in chemistry and then with Ciba-Geigy.

Basically, my mother wanted me to be a lawyer and she wanted it so badly that probably I decided not to be a lawyer. At that time in school I had a teacher in chemistry who was somehow able to interest me in chemistry, so I went to Basel and studied chemistry. But before reaching the end of my studies, I realized that synthetic chemistry was not really what I wanted to do. When I was finished and I was looking for a job – at that time it was not really general practice to do a postdoc, you looked for a job in industry if you were a chemist – I tried to get a job which was not linked to synthetic chemistry but there were none. So I found a job with Roche in medical marketing. I was with them for a year and I was mainly involved in the marketing of CNS drugs and that raised my interest in that kind of business. After a year I felt that marketing wasn't what I wanted to do either, so I called my former biochemistry Professor at the University, who had a Department at Ciba-Geigy, and asked him whether he could offer me a job and he said 'oh yes, fine, come over'.

When was this?

This was during 1970. I had two possibilities. I could go either into what was a precursor of molecular biology – DNA biochemistry – or into CNS and because of my involvement in Roche in CNS drugs, I picked CNS and that's how I came to Ciba-Geigy with barely any knowledge of the field. What I brought with me was a solid background in analytical chemistry and, at the time, this was of interest because the methodology to determine neurotransmitters and things like that was just evolving. So I grew into that business and we did, for years actually, CNS biochemical pharmacology – determining the effects of drugs on noradrenaline turnover, release or synthesis or 5-HT turnover and so on. In Ciba-Geigy, at that time, our main area of interest was antidepressants. The second area was neuroleptics, where we actually never got a drug into the market but nevertheless in terms of research the emphasis was rather significant. So I got to work with those drugs.

About the time I entered the company, maprotiline was in its final stage before getting approved so I joined actually long after anafranil and imipramine entered the market but before the last tricyclics made it. I used to work on antidepressants up to about 10 years ago, and then the interest started to shift a little. We got into more neurological diseases, starting out actually with epilepsy. There was a programme on epilepsy and then we started a programme on Gaba-B antagonists and so I moved more and more away from antidepressants. I still kept busy with brofaromine, which needed a lot of backup work, but there weren't actually any active programmes for antidepressants any more for almost 10 years. Now I am purely working in the neurodegenerative area.

Did you join before the merger? Why did they join?

I started in 1971 about two weeks after the companies had joined. I think Geigy was in trouble actually. Geigy had been in trouble once before after the War and was then saved by a concerted action of the three others.

How much competition is there between the three companies here in Basel? It would be hard to believe that there's quite the degree of competition that there's been between some companies like, for instance, when the minor tranquillizers were in trouble, part of that trouble seems to have come from the companies that were trying to produce 5-HT-1A agonists.

There is definitely some kind of competition in the market place but still I think the market segments don't overlap too much and we don't try too much to hurt each other.

Maprotiline was about to hit the market in 1970 – how did it look at the time, because it was in a sense going to be the logical development from everything else before and this was the most specific catecholamine reuptake inhibitor.

It was in the last phase, just before production. As always in a company, there was heavy opposition against the compound inside the company, there were supporters and opponents.

And this is always for each drug.

I've never seen anything else. You see you cover yourself by being negative. When you argue in a company that a drug shouldn't be developed for this or that reason, the chances of being right are much larger. If you say, you must develop this drug because it's going to be a big success, you can be proved wrong. When you oppose and destroy a drug, you can never be proved wrong

How much of a hazard is this building up large groups of sceptics within a company?

Oh Ciba-Geigy has a pretty good record of that. We have been too hard with our drugs for 20 years and so we have never finished one since maprotiline in the CNS area, at least. I think it's a big problem. In order to get a drug to the market you have to go past a point of no return. You have to commit yourself to a decision once made and not always be questioning it after that. If something is proved toxic that's another thing but to reiterate the question whether is it really worthwhile to do it and do that every two weeks, that really inhibits development.

Maprotiline is curious in that it became for a long time the best- selling anti-depressant in parts of Europe but in other parts of the world, the UK for instance, it didn't really seem to take off. Can you account for this variation?

There may be two reasons for that. The reason which I would invoke first, is the marketing. The more you do for a drug in terms of marketing, the more it will sell. This will not necessarily positively affect the benefits, because it costs a lot more to do the marketing, but it will certainly increase the sales. The other reason may be that the Anglo-Saxon countries were the 5-HT countries and the more German-speaking and orientated countries, including the Scandinavian countries, were more catecholamine countries. It has to do with specific single researchers involved in the area. Alec Coppen was one of the dominant figures in the UK and he was pro-5-HT and Arvid Carlsson and a few other people in Europe, Norbert Matussek, were noradrenaline people. So one group preached one story and the other preached the other story and this has some impact on the practising psychiatrists.

Maprotiline led to Levoprotiline which is . . .

Oxaprotiline is a hydroxylated derivative of maprotiline. It had two enantiomers. Levoprotiline was the non-noradrenaline reuptake inhibiting enantiomer. We originally wanted to have a double-blind comparison of plus versus minus oxaprotiline, that is of 'dextroprotiline' and levoprotiline. We wanted to test the catacholamine hypothesis and this pair of enantiomers seemed ideal. This was a good idea and it would have been possible to finance it but there was a legal problem. The toxicity studies were available for the minus enanatiomer but we would have had to provide additional toxicity studies for the plus enantiomer, therefore this direct comparison couldn't happen.

The first trial that was made was levoprotiline against the racemate. There were several small trials, and one of these small trials seemed to indicate a positive effect and then it got out of control. There was a clamour in certain corners of the company – 'oh, gee, we have a breakthrough, we have something which doesn't work according to the catecholamine mechanism'. This is something totally new. From then on science had no control over it. We argued that these are limited trials, these are not placebo-controlled trials, these may be biased trials but nobody listened. It was the big thing.

Then they went into big, still poorly controlled trials in East Germany and Czechoslovakia and so on. The drug got better from one trial to the other, until it finally collapsed. Because when the double-blind trials came, no efficacy could be shown. Interestingly though, there are still a lot of clinical investigators, especially in Germany, who stubbornly say this drug is active. They saw changes in patients, which they interpreted as positive. One guy said, look this drug doesn't really affect the core symptoms of depression, but it makes those patients who sleep badly, sleep better. It makes those who have eating disorders shake off their eating disorders. It sort of takes care of the peripheral problems. In any case, it all collapsed because the pivotal trials were negative. It was sad because had we chosen the plus-enantiomer to develop, we would have ended up with a drug – not a very innovative one but at least we would have had a drug.

Roland Kuhn was involved in this, wasn't he?

Yes. Roland Kuhn tried for a long time to convince the company to continue to develop levoprotiline, because he considered it to be an active drug. He actually wrote some pretty tough letters to higher ups in the company because he felt that Ciba–Geigy was doing wrong in abandoning the development of the drug. There were others as well. It is very difficult to judge who is right and wrong because this is not a black and white story. It is definitely clear that the drug did something but what it was, nobody could really properly describe it. I think to reach registration with such a drug would have been extremely difficult. It was obvious that in a normal depressed population you couldn't reach a significant effect with the given armamentarium of clinical investigators. So to try and register that compound as an antidepressant was hopeless and nobody had a brilliant idea of what other indication we could chase.

There's a curious irony in that Kuhn would say 'well, I found the first anti-depressant and I knew it worked without clinical trials to prove it'. He was still saying in 1989 that 'all these clinical trials are a complete waste of time, what have they ever found'.

In a way, I understand this comment because the more controlled the clinical trial is, by our standards, in terms of done right by statistical considerations and things like that, the more it tends to obscure any finesses. I would believe Kuhn if he says that if he treats a small number of patients and observes them carefully that he can tell you more about a drug than a big clinical trial. The big controlled clinical trials against placebo, they are good for establishing firm data on the efficacy of the compound in a given indication but they are no good for finding an indication. When you are sure about your indication, you need to do one of those big trials to nail it down. To convince authorities and health care managers.

The next antidepressant that Ciba were involved with, was of course brofaromine. Do you want to take me through its development?

Well, I'll try not to be emotional because this for me is a kind of emotional case. I devoted a lot of time to that drug and I still think it was a grave mistake to abandon the development. We were working on 5-HT uptake inhibitors back in 1972/73.

Sorry for interrupting but that was very early to be working on 5-HT reuptake inhibitors . . . Who started the 5-HT reuptake story? Hyttel has suggested he did and Arvid Carlsson was talking about this idea back in 1969.

I think Lilly did. You see, as always, these things germinate and then eventually they get tackled and at several places at the same time. I don't know how the publication dates compare but publication dates don't tell you when they started because the publication policies of companies are very different. Some publish early, some publish late. And the same is true for patent dates. So unless you ask the people involved, you will never know. I, for our case, know that we started almost immediately after I arrived.

And why did you want to make a 5-HT reuptake inhibitor?

We happened to screen compounds for noradrenaline uptake inhibiting properties because we were still in the phase where maprotiline was still being prepared for introduction. And we hit upon a compound in the screen, which inhibited noradrenaline uptake but also inhibited serotonin uptake and MAO-A. We only found out about the MAO-A inhibition because it increased noradrenaline levels and, as a pharmacologist, when you see that your first reaction is let's see if that inhibits MAO-A. So we were there with a compound which had in similar doses, noradrenaline uptake inhibiting, serotonin uptake inhibiting and MAO-A inhibiting properties. Although it was relatively weak with respect to each single property it was a potent drug in pharmacological models. We thought wow this is just the right thing. Unfortunately this compound died in toxicity because it killed the dogs. But the series was born. The chemical structure was entirely different; it had nothing to do with tricyclics.

This was all the more interesting. So, one of the chemists, Raymond Bernasconi, was particularly productive. He produced about 300 analogues of that compound. And the next thing we hit in that chemical series were very selective and at that time very potent 5-HT uptake inhibitors. They were more potent than fluoxetine, for instance, and so we thought when we have them why shouldn't we try something with them. We had a number of candidates which dropped out one after the other but one of them, the most potent one, made it actually into early development and it was then killed because of some dubious results in clinical pharmacology studies. It was thought that it might change the blood clotting time or reduce thrombocyte numbers or something. After the compound had been killed, it was shown that it results were erroneous and brought about by a wrong manipulation but it was too late to save it. The next analogues, all of a sudden, showed again 5-HT uptake inhibitory and MAO-A inhibitory properties and at that time we said why don't we try to select MAO inhibitors – if they are selective for MAO-A and reversible they might get around the tyramine problem.

Just before we go onto that can I quickly ask you, when you found the reuptake inhibitors, did you know what you would actually use them for – it's not clear that Lilly had depression in mind for fluoxetine.

Oh, it was absolutely clear that it was depression. There was no question, because we were aware at that time of the two mainstream theories of serotonin on the one side and noradrenaline on the other side. We had taken care of noradrenaline appropriately, so why not try the other area. There was never any doubt.

So we found drugs in this series of benzofuranylpiperidines which did not show much 5-HT uptake inhibition but were pretty good as MAO inhibitors and we selected one of them which was brofaromine. At that time we were openly declared almost insane because people had these stories about the MAO inhibitors in mind. We fought a long fight to get the compound into development. It was put into Phase 1 development in 1977 and there it stayed until Peter Bieck opened this Human Pharmacology Institute in Tubingen in Germany. He started to do phase I studies of that compound and it proved to be a good MAO inhibitor and he also did some pioneering work in tyramine potentiation studies.

So it got to the end of Phase I. It looked good but clinical development was not able to take it from there. It was in Phase II for an extraordinarily long time. Eventually they managed trials of something like 12 patients a year. There was no urgency until management realized that Roche was developing moclobemide. For a certain period of time we kept alive brofaramine by saying Roche develops moclobemide so MAO inhibitors must be good and they said Ciba is developing brofarmine so MAO inhibitors must be good – so we kept each other alive. And then at one point in time, perhaps 1987/88, Roche took a decision to develop moclobemide. Until this point we were ahead and from that point on we lost because they did something and we didn't.

So the whole development phase of brofaramine was much too long and then at the end when it became clear that maybe depression wasn't the best indication for that compound, that panic disorders or OCD, or post–traumatic stress disorder or one of the major anxiety indications, was a more appropriate target for this compound, it was too late because the patent life left was so short that management considered it just not worth it. They were there with a package of clinical data which could not be used for registration and the indications that had crystallized they didn't have enough clinical trials to go for. They would have had to invest another two years or even more to do it properly and that was the end of the story of brofaramine, which I find particularly sad, because I think it was a good drug.

Why?

Well, I have spoken to a number of clinical investigators, particularly those who have used it in atypical depression or in major anxiety states, and not one of them said this drug doesn't work; on the contrary, they said we have never seen anything as powerful as that. Especially the Canadian guys, who used it first in panic disorders and it was absolutely dumbfounding. In some cases, it was almost 100% success and in many cases, it was 80% success. Most of the guys said this is the most powerful antipanic or the most powerful antisocial phobia drug they had ever seen. So from this kind of second-hand information, I believe it would have been worth developing the drug further. There was one little glimmer of hope where we thought we could get a patent for social phobia but unfortunately someone had mentioned the possible use of MAO inhibitors in social phobia in an abstract the year before and that spoilt the possibility of that. That killed it finally. That was about two years ago now.

There's actually something about this whole group of drugs that hasn't crystallized out properly. People have been saying from very early on that the MAOIs are not the same as the tricyclics. They do something different. Yes, they can get a large number of people who have got a major depressive disorder well, just as a tricyclic can, but there are some other effects — personality strengthening effects is the kind of phrase you hear.

It's very difficult to resolve. It's conceivable that they're different because most of the tricyclics at least have a large number of additional properties, for example, they are antihistaminic to various degrees, they have antiserotonergic properties which most of the MAO inhibitors don't and so the idea that they might have an overall different profile is understandable.

Are companies trapped by looking at the market size and finding that the only thing they can apparently afford to develop is an antidepressant, because it's the only thing that's got a sufficiently large market size. Then antidepressant trials all get done with instruments like the Hamilton Rating Scale, which pick up tricyclic type effects, so other drugs which may be subtly different are going to have a hard time trying to get on the market.

Well, look at how long the 5-HT uptake inhibitors took and there has been an argument for years and years that these drugs are not truly antidepressants and I don't even know whether the question has been settled yet. There are still people who say that these are 'feel good' drugs — they are not really antidepressants. I think the clinical armamentarium is just too coarse to allow fine differentiations like that.

What happened to the neuroleptic programme? Why did savoxepine not happen?

The story is almost analogous to the brofaromine story. When it finally came out that the drug was good, it was too late. So the development efforts of Ciba–Geigy during the last 20 years have not been very successful. It took too long to generate too little data of too poor quality to suffice for registration. I think they've realized that and they are trying to do something about it. It was about time. But savoxepine again is a sad story because from the evidence that we got it seemed to be a drug which relieved the positive symptoms of schizophrenia with relatively little restraint put on the patients. The interesting thing about this actually is that patients said the difference in terms of motor side effects wasn't all that great but what patients said was 'I don't have that straight jacket feeling as with haloperidol'. It was a kind of, more or less a more subtle difference in terms of mental restriction, which made it different from other neuroleptics. The plan was that it should be better with respect to extrapyramidal side effects and when that didn't turn out to be too clear, the decision was made to kill it, together with the expiration of the patent life and things like that. The Ciba–Geigy system was not able to say 'oh look we were looking for something which was better than classical neuroleptics in terms of extra pyramidal side effects. We haven't found that but we found something else'. They couldn't do that.

Sobering isn't it?

Yes well I tell you life in a pharmaceutical company can be very frustrating. I've seen a number of colleagues who had mental problems because they felt they were useless and whatever they did was for nothing.

Or seeing compounds go forward that are inferior to some of the ones worked on.

This is normal. Normally it is hardly ever the best compound, from a pharmacological point of view, which makes it. It's always the second or third best because of other properties. Maybe your best compound is not adequately metabolized or has too short or too long a half life or has this or that. The compound which finally makes it is a compromise of all those things.

How do we solve this problem that a company will only bring a drug on if it's going to be a large market share compound?

The companies will, in one way or another, have to change their philosophy. When you go for a mechanistic approach, you have to be consistent and say look I'm going for this or that mechanism but I don't know the indication yet and we will have to go for any indication where we think we can prove efficacy. We will have to do that first, irrespective of the market size and take it from there. Now if you are not willing to do that, you put too many restrictions into the system. If you say I want a mechanistic approach, we should go for something which interacts with a target protein or whatever, but it must make $300 million a year, then the restrictions are so difficult that you will hardly ever make it.

They will have to ease up on either of the two restrictions and the more logical one for me is to ease up on the financial restriction and say look we are going to try to develop a drug which acts on this mechanism and we are going to try and see what it does. Now you can't take that to the extreme either because it costs a hell of a lot of money, so you'd better have some idea of the indication in the first place but this indication need not necessarily be a big one. So an indication like petit mal, with a market size of $100 million or even less would, for me personally, be enough to start with, because it has quite often been seen that the first indication was not the last one. But it should be an easily testable indication; it should not be something like stroke which is a very difficult indication to test. It should be something with a clear endpoint, where you don't have to treat people for two or three years. But asking for both a mechanism and for a big market share reduces your options considerably.

We don't seem to have been able to decide what we really want out of this do we?

Well we want to make money. I'm speaking for the industrial manager, now. The industrial manager, at least the ones high up don't care whether you develop an antihypertensive for them which makes money or an antidepressant – all that counts is that it makes money.

Yes. The point that I'm actually trying to get at here is that there seems to be some confusion at the moment about whether we should be going down the route of producing pure and clean drugs that are acting on a particular mechanism or whether we produce drugs to treat illnesses and for 20 years or so we have been going down the route of purer cleaner drugs but with increasingly confusing results.

This is true. The least thing we could have expected, and I think something which many of us expected when we went down the way to cleaner drugs, was that we would find out which aspects of which illnesses certain mechanisms affected. We were somehow expecting illnesses to be composed of modular pieces. To give you an example, we could have expected that serotonin was affecting the mood component of depression whereas noradrenaline was controlling more the drive aspect of depression and perhaps you could argue that acetylcholine was controlling the vegetative aspects and so on.

I think we have to get away from this thinking because illnesses are not puzzles composed of different pieces. It's not like a car, which is made of wheels and a motor and a gearbox and things like that. It's not as simple because these things interact and when we hit one system directly with a drug, indirectly we induce alterations in other systems which will finally rearrange the equilibrium of the system as a whole and leave us with an altered system and from the alteration in the system you couldn't say what initiated the alterations. Likewise, it may prove wrong to try and interfere with one particular mechanism to achieve a good therapeutic effect because the system has so many possibilities to compensate and to neutralize the original impact, so that of the anticipated action of the drug very little remains. In contrast, if you block a system in different places you restrict the degrees of freedom and the system can't evade that easily.

The main driving force behind trying to get cleaner and cleaner drugs was chemistry. Because for the chemists to optimize a drug for one parameter, they considered that as a possible task. To optimize for two parameters is much more difficult and to optimize for three parameters is just impossible, at least today. So chemists have always wanted clean drugs . . . they know exactly what they have to do. I should not say nasty things about that but I can afford it in a way because I'm a chemist by formation. Chemists are simple minded, at least as far as biology is concerned. They think in boxes and as soon as things become complicated, they suspect the biologists have got it wrong. As long as chemists have the say in big companies this won't change. At present, there are companies in which chemists predominate in terms of the managerial hierarchy and there are companies where this is not so.

Could this problem get worse because all the people who now work in the various aspects of drug development are going to be molecular biologists as well and they are also thinking in . . .

It accentuates the problem because in the past decade the chemists were going for the interaction with a particular receptor. Now they are going for a clean and pure interaction with a particular receptor subtype and in two years from now they will go for the pure and clean interaction with the splicing variant of a particular subtype. So it gets smaller and smaller or from bad to worse if you want. It reminds me a bit of the attempts in the middle ages to explain the movements of the moon by all sorts of strange spirals.

And it's going to require someone like a Kepler or a Copernicus to turn everything around.

I think it's a fashion and perhaps in 10 years people will revert to the integrative view.

But will we be able to revert — because we'll be going down so far down the road of producing junior scientists now who will be in the middle management then who have been thinking in this way. Will they be able . . .?

In 10 years from now or maybe 20 years, someone will stand up and present whole-animal pharmacology as a totally new idea and there will be nobody there who remembers that it has actually been done before.

I've heard people recently come out with things that I know were around in the 1960s but they make it sound like it has just be thought up.

Yes, I occasionally see that in the literature. Stuff is published now which I know has been done before. It has not been done in exactly the same way or by the same techniques but the conclusion that was reached was quite the same and these guys weren't even quoted because the literature is too old. I think the danger of re-inventing the wheel is pretty serious. The literature is getting too vast. The old literature is hardly accessible any more, it's somewhere down in the basements.

Is there anything about this whole idea about trying to get more and more pure, more and more specific drugs that stems from people's wish to have more technical control over life, as it were? I was brought up short recently when somebody on some radio programme said that cabbages, for instance, have something like 47 different natural pesticides in them, few of which would get through the FDA, if people tried to actually extract them and get a licence for them actually as a pesticide, but yet these are what give cabbage its taste. Do we all – both us as consumers and you in industry – want things increasingly sanitized . . .?

Yes, dirty is out. It is interesting though that I've seen very recently some articles by people who have a background in the area, who have come back saying 'look, we're running down a blind alley by going for purer and purer drugs'. So the voices can be heard now but they are not being heard by the management of the pharmaceutical industry. The main driving force for this craving for pure drugs is that we want to know how it works. If something works by two or three mechanisms, how can we know which ones give what, and this is not satisfying. The other very strong point which is one I made already before is that the chemists say I can't optimize for three properties and I want to optimize. This is what I can do and so I am going to optimize. Pharmacological purity is also important when it comes to screening drugs in an *in vitro* system, using a high throughput screen. This is not possible for things that have three or four different properties. For these you will have to resort to animal models, which are not fashionable nowadays. It's slow, complicated, expensive and laborious and causes problems with the animal rights people.

So there are all the reasons why people are going for clean drugs now but whether these reasons suffice to lead to good drugs is another question. Sometimes it reminds me of the guy who had lost his purse in the night and he was actually looking under a street light and was looking for something and someone else asked him what are you doing. I lost my purse he said. Did you lose it here? No I lost it on the other side of the road. The other person said why don't you look there. Because there is light here. We may be doing something similar by going for clean drugs, I fear.

But it's tricky isn't it? You don't either want to go to the opposite extreme of saying well let's go back to herbs.

I don't think it's the question of herbs or not herbs. I think those people who do not put the emphasis so much on the cleanliness of drugs are not arguing that we should go back to herbs. You could say that they are more aware that the nervous system is more plastic and reactive and tends towards homeostasy.

But people will say that herbs are the ultimate integrative view.

Well, there are people who argue like that but I don't take that seriously because herbs are mixtures of chemicals aren't they? I think herbs are nice and herbs are perhaps good to make tea and they are also good to have a look into them for active ingredients but to eat herbs to treat my illness because I think it's better than drugs, I don't accept.

Things seem to have changed since the 1960s when you trained. Back in the 1960s when we produced the first compounds there was the feeling that nature is tricky, nature is dangerous and human beings try to control nature and using drugs is a clever way to use human intelligence to control things for the benefit of mankind. Now we've got the opposite. Nature is good . . .

Mankind can't be moderate and intermediate. They have to be extreme. The pendulum was on one side and the pendulum is now on the other side, and I think either extreme is wrong.

But is it just purely the chance swing of the pendulum or have the kind of developments over the last 20–30 years given credance to the idea that nature is good and man's efforts to tamper with nature are not so good?

Oh, we have begun to realize that what we were doing to nature wasn't doing nature or ourselves any good. But instead of bringing us back to an intermediate position and trying to control what we do, it has for some people at least swung the pendulum to the other side and now everything that man does is bad and only nature is good. But nature is neither good nor bad. Nature is nature and herbs are herbs. They are good source for finding a drug, for instance, and it's a good approach to look in Chinese herbs for a new active ingredient but that wouldn't stop me from trying to improve that ingredient by chemical manipulations.

But for some people that's almost heresy. There's an awful lot of people out there who would think that if a compound actually exists in nature that it oughtn't to be changed. It's very presumptuous to try and improve on nature.

I have no sympathy for this view at all but I accept that it exists. Why should we not try to make that stuff better than it is. There is always something which can be improved, even if its only bioavailability and pharmacokinetics. I can give you an example. There's a compound that has been isolated from a Chinese herb and the herb was used for 4000 years to treat epilepsy and hypertension. The active ingredient has now been found and it is a very complicated molecule with an extremely short half life. Why not take that compound now and make some modifications which keep its activity and increases its half life. You've got a more useful drug – what's wrong with that? I think many of the people who advocate the use of herbs in a dogmatic way are fundamentalists in a way, aren't they?

Are they?

I think they are. They believe in almost in a spiritualistic way in forces. It's comparable to homoeopathy. Our generation of natural scientists have been educated in a way which has no room for something like homoeopathy. I can't understand how things get more powerful by diluting them to the extent that you can hardly find one molecule in a bottle. This is against everything which we have learnt. We are probably so much impregnated by modern natural sciences that we will never be able to grasp that. I have serious problems with this way of thinking and I have exactly the same sort of problems with people who think that an ingredient in a herb is in any way better than the same ingredient outside the herb.

There seems to be this interaction at the moment between scientific thinking and popular culture, so that, for instance, we have these hysterias about health, about holes in the ozone layer, etc., etc. It seems as we generate knowledge and as health becomes the media event it is becoming world-wide, people are being exposed to information about holes in the ozone layer and they don't have a feel for the risks, they just get hysterical – herbs maybe seem safer.

For the non-fundamentalist and, more or less, neutral observer, it's very difficult to understand how serious a situation is. The ozone hole. You hear all sorts of messages but to know exactly how bad it is, because even the measurement data that are reported in the newspapers are very different, so we don't really have the data available to make an appropriate judgement. Again this information is used and abused by all sorts of groups for their interests and they are then distorted and communicated that way and they have an impact on the public and depending on the nature of the individual, of the public, they will react differently. They will say 'to hell, I've heard enough of this – I'm not paying attention to it anymore' or they start screaming and shouting and jumping up and down and saying 'the world is coming to an end'. To have a take-home message from such reports in the newspapers is almost impossible because you don't know what has happened to the message before, from the moment it was sent off until it got to you.

You have this uncontrolled amplification of facts and you don't know the amplication factor. By the time it comes to you, you don't know what the original message was. We used to play that telephone game when we were kids – there was a row of kids and one started to say something into the ear of the next and it went round the table and it was compared when it came back from what it was originally – that's probably what we are witnessing with the media now.

Is it a thing that needs to be controlled in some ways because the problem is if drugs are the issue – if fluoxetine is causing suicide is the issue and any expert intervenes to say well look the evidence really isn't there, the disinterested view never seems credible; besides, it's not newsworthy to say that fluoxetine isn't causing suicide.

I think with drugs it's a different issue than with the ozone hole because it's probably easier to control issues with a drug than issues on the ozone hole, so lets keep with the drugs. I think if something emerges like the question 'does fluoxetine cause suicide or not?', this is something that really affects patients who are treated with such a drug and it should be clarified as properly and as cleanly as possible and the result of this should be communicated. There is nothing worse than this situation of rumours. I think it is in the interest of the patient, the doctor, the authorities and the industry to clear up these things rather than to try and cover them up. It is also probably for the concerned company, the worst thing they can do because eventually the truth will come out and the damage will be all the greater if it took longer for the truth to come out. I don't think the industry, even in purely financial terms, has an interest in covering up things because you can't cover them up for eternity.

Let me introduce another angle on this which is a phrase I picked up from you, so I need to give you the credit for it because I've been using it ever since. This may be linked with the development of modern drugs but people now seem to feel that they are 'born with a warranty' in a way that they didn't 20 or 30 years ago. Any thoughts on the origins of this kind of feeling?

Well, I think maybe the critical event was the availability of antibiotics because until antibiotics became widely available to me and you, you could catch an infection and die. It was normal. Nobody knew anything different. The idea of being born with a warranty goes back to an incident in my childhood where I was pretty sick, I had what they called at the time a renal inflammation and I had to be in bed for six months. I complained to my doctor about having to be restricted in that way and I obviously complained so hard that he got mad and shouted at me 'do you think you have a right to be healthy'. This made a really strong impression on me and that's probably the reason why I started thinking about this warranty business.

Surgery also in this century made advances and you could rescue someone from a situation where in the last century there would have been a death. So death or illness had another value for people a hundred years or more back from now and they accepted illness and they accepted death. Whereas when the treatments became available, some hopes were raised and people expected more and more from medicine and drugs. So in one way or another, people expected that whatever happens to them someone can help them and they are terribly disappointed if they learn that in some cases this is not possible. I think this is something new. The roots are probably in the availability of treaments and the raising of hopes.

I'm absolutely sure that it's new. It's a feature of the last 15 to 20 years only I think. In this regard, did the thalidomide tragedy have much bigger, long-term effects than was ever thought at the time? It's eroded trust in all sorts of ways; it's eroded trust in the industry; it's eroded trust in the medical profession.

It showed for the first time that things can get out of control. It eroded let's say the claim of science to be true and helpful under any circumstance. I think it still has an impact – it undermines the trust and this is the thing But it hasn't detracted from most people's belief that they are born with a warranty.

No, but do you not think it's caused the belief which is the flip-side of born with a warranty that we would have been okay if some drug hadn't done something awful to us. If some outside agency hadn't done something awful to us.

Is that such a frequent phenomenon? What I often hear is another argument that is, why does the state spend so much money on research and you still haven't found a treatment against this and that. This I hear much more often than it is a drug that has done that to me and that's why I'm like this now.

Yes, but there's a feeling that if things go wrong that there has to be a reason and increasingly we feel the reason will be something man-made; it isn't just nature, it isn't just an act of God.

This is what I would call the paranoiac fundamentalist view of things but there are not many paranoiac fundamentalists. This is a small minority. People may complain about side effects but they rarely blame a drug for an illness.

Well, it's big enough to influence practice in the US. I think the feeling there is that if you go for medical treatment and things go wrong there will be a law suit.

Yes but you have to turn it the other way round. Because you can sue them and you often win, that's why you claim such things, because otherwise you couldn't sue them. So you make your story in order to retrieve money from them. Not necessarily because you believe in it.

Let me hop back. One of the points you made earlier was that when you actually entered the field first there was a more open approach towards things and now you find that the junior people working with you are theory bound.

Yes. Part of this is the almost dogmatic belief in the idea that the drug must be perfectly pure in order to be a good drug and I find that this dogmatic belief is almost scary. You can't argue with them because they would say look it doesn't make sense to look for anything other than pure compounds. Interestingly, they wouldn't really argue with you when you say if we test it out maybe you will find dirty drugs are better but they say I don't want to go for this because I have no control of it. So the control over the mechanism of action, 'knowing what you do' is more important for them, than to find a good therapeutic agent. And this reflects a sort of selfishness. It's not the patient which interests them, it's not the therapy which interests them. They want to see how it works. They want to enjoy getting it right and these are elements of a dogmatism, I think.

So where does that attitude come from? Do you think it's just the maturing of the field because when you guys went in first, things like the amine theories were fiction? They were obvious fictions − you could be sceptical about them.

None of the theories that are available now are any better than that. I would even say that at that time although it was clumsy and the bases of the theories were no good, one tried to develop a drug with a rationale. Now they go for the next clean receptor or the next clean target protein and they try to find something which interacts with it and they say 'we'll see what it does'. They don't spend a lot of time in figuring out why something could work and trying to get experimental support for the theory before they start. Now if they develop a drug, when they have a clean drug, they say now let's see what it does. Somehow research got mechanized.

Why is that so? It's difficult for me to say. It must be a product of their education at University. Perhaps the basis of this is the idea that if we try hard enough we will find out how everything works. There are no limits. And with the event of molecular biology, which is definitely a very useful technique, the expectation that everything is doable is much more common than it was. We were more aware of the limits that we have because the limits were more obvious. Young researchers nowadays think if they've got a target protein, they know it all. They are not aware of the fact that they've just got a step farther but they still don't know why interaction with this target protein causes a beneficial effect in an illness. They don't realize that from the target protein to the illness is probably a much longer way than they had from the receptor to the target protein. Maybe we were the same and we thought we knew everything if we knew the receptor but we haven't been that dogmatic − we were allowing for dirty drugs.

It's a time of change within the industry, here in Switzerland.

Not only in Switzerland. It's happening everywhere. The conditions have changed. The economic situation of health care management in the widest sense has changed. It has become overtly clear that the costs of health maintenance were rising disproportionately and something had to be done about it. There are a number of possibilities. You can investigate which are the largest cost items in the whole bill and then for each of these items think about what you can do. The largest item is definitely not the drugs. The drugs are somewhere between 10 and 15% of the total costs. But they are an easy target. You just tell those who sell the drugs how much they can ask for them and you restrict the number of drugs allowed on the market. That's relatively easy to control.

In Germany, they started three or four years ago a process of controlling drug prescription both in terms of pricing and in terms of quantities of drugs prescribed very seriously. This has led to a pretty big decrease in the market size in Germany. Other countries are following more or less rapidly. We don't know how the situation will develop in the United States. So perspectives for the pharmaceutical industry have become less predictable than they were. In any case, if you're a company manager you are probably wiser to expect a worsening of the situation than an improvement so you better take care that you are not caught on the wrong foot. And you had better slim down, as long as you can slim down in a controlled way, before you are forced to. And this is precisely what's happening.

Leading to considerable job losses?

Oh yes, especially if a merger of two larger companies like Roche and Syntex, is added in on top; this will end in major bloodshed. Not all the people who will lose their jobs have lost them already. This is a process that is ongoing now. They are determining who, and why and when – nobody knows exactly who exactly will be hit. I don't like to make forecasts like this but it is clearly possible that the number of pharmaceutical companies will diminish and only a few will remain. The weakest will drop out . . .

And is this good or bad?

Depends on your point of view. From the point of view of health care costs, it's probably good. On the other hand, from the point of view of new drugs, new developments, new ideas getting translated into possible treatments, it is probably not good because from the statistical point of view, the more people working to reach a goal by different means, the higher the chances that one of them will reach the goal. So definitely I expect that this will lead to a poorer armamentarium of drug therapy than if there were more competitors in the market place. It is also possible that if there is only a few remaining that they will even break up the market into different segments, where they are more or less alone, and there is no competition any more and this will stop any impetus to improve. So the danger that we are moving to an industrial situation which is comparable to what they had in the Eastern block before the end of the Cold War is quite real.

Allied to the current situation as regards health care generally, though, the industry seems to be less enthusiastic about mental health at the moment.

Yes and no. It is certainly true with respect to psychiatric diseases. Most of the industry had its major emphasis, at least as far as CNS research is concerned, in the psychiatric area. The reasons were probably the availability of hypotheses, whatever good they were. They stimulated ideas, they stimulated research, people have a kind of framework to operate within and that's why these theories were more or less well explored in terms of drug therapies. Two elements may have contributed to the change now. First of all the perception that neurodegenerative diseases are becoming more and more important in terms of social and economic costs. Then there is the idea that animal models for at least some of the neurodegenerative diseases are more reliable and 'better' than the animal models for psychiatric diseases. There were some ideas about mechanisms by which, for instance, the negative effects of strokes and other impairments could be controlled. So companies are shifting their resources toward the neurodegenerative area. Of course, there is also the big market that they expect to be waiting out there, which is getting bigger with increasing life expectancy.

It's also a market where small amounts of improvement will be reimbursed whereas marginal improvements in antidepressants won't be reimbursed.

Yes, it's much easier to get an antineurodegenerative drug into the market, the best example is Tacrin. Tacrin is debatable whether it has any effect at all and a compound with a comparable improvement over placebo could never be introduced for the treatment of depression but for Alzheimer's because there is no treatment, they take whatever they get and this is going to be so for some time. So it also offers a kind of perspective – they are looking to introduce drugs in a series, so that different companies can always be a little better than their predecesor and so you can make money for a while. When you are beginning to make a reasonable improvement it's harder to do better than that. The lack of pharmacotherapeutic agents is one of the major reasons why people have moved into these areas. The official version is that this is a serious problem and as an ethical company we have to do something for mankind, but the driving force is money.

An interesting possibility about the movement of companies out of the psychiatric area is that it actually may be the best thing that has ever happened because you can't work in the CNS without the work you're doing having implications for mental illness generally.

You and I know that, but the managers may not. It's good for two reasons.

It is interesting because it makes people work on different mechanisms and it may turn out that these mechanisms have some implications for psychiatric diseases as well. It may also be that some of the psychiatric diseases finally turn out to be neurodegenerative diseases and the other thing is that is may just prove beneficial to take a step back and to look at it from a different angle.

We may be in the situation of Chicken Erna, who is enclosed in a fence which is U-shaped and open at one end. On the other side of the fence, there's food and chicken Erna tries to get the food desperately and runs back and forth along the fence but it doesn't occur to it that by going through the open back side and going around the fence, it could get the food. It may well be that we have been in a similar situation with the monoamine hypotheses and receptor research on psychiatric diseases. By leaving it for a little while and coming back to it from another side, we may find alternative solutions to the problem. So turning away momentarily from psychiatric research may ultimately prove beneficial for biological psychiatric research.

It's an interesting thought, isn't it, but it does mean that the period we have been in is closing as it were?

We are definitely at a turning point, yes. Well let's not put it as dramatically as that but the way biological research in the CNS area was done is changing now – definitely. I don't think that's a bad thing. We need some changes because when a particular way of doing research continues for too long, it is self perpetuating and it will not produce anything new, so we all need a break.

Curiously, though, some of the classic mental illness drugs and in particular deprenyl have for some time pointed the way towards the neuroprotective area. So in a sense, there's a continuity there that people from outside the field may not appreciate.

It is, I think, only seemingly a continuity because the interesting things which deprenyl does don't obviously have anything to do with MAO. It's probably a coincidence that one of these old MAO inhibitors is the spearhead leading into a new area. But it's nevertheless funny and it's also funny that at least part of those people who had been involved with the old MAO stuff are now again in business with this new stuff. This is not accidental because some of the people who have been working with the MAO inhibitors were attentive enough to see other other properties of the drugs and were interested enough in the other properties to more or less change their direction of research.

But now where did the other properties come from because those of you who have been working in this area have gone on working on the neuroprotective aspects of these compounds even though the most recent clinical trials came out with fairly disappointing results. You haven't been deterred at all.

No, because nobody in the field expected major beneficial effects of anything. Everybody was happy with a small effect and I think by today's standards the effects of deprenyl in the data/top study, that is the protraction of the disease for one year, is pretty good because there's nothing better and there is no reason to assume that you cannot improve on deprenyl.

My hunch though is that the reason why you are all working on in the area regardless of a reasonably small clinical effect is that you have hunches about what's actually happening with the drug.

Well, if we had an improvement with the antidepressants it all depends on the likeliness that you can make it credible to the authorities so that they will allow you to register your drug. A marginal improvement in the antidepressant area will not lead to that but a marginal improvement in the neurodegenerative area will. That may be too cynical because we believe deprenyl's neuroprotective effect will lead to something that is more than marginally better.

Yes, but perhaps like the early amine days, if you have a marginal improvement that you can't explain you've got something of a blind alley. Whereas in this case, lots of people have theories about what's happening with deprenyl that you can build on.

With all theories of course it's better to have a theory which is plausible than none. It needs not be true but it must be plausible. You cannot sell a drug only, you have to sell a story with it. The better the story, the higher the chances of your success in getting the drug into the market. A drug faces usually its hardest time within the company. Once you have overcome the difficulties inside the company you meet less resistance outside. And so the story is good for the introductory brochure and to convince the registration authorities but the best and the most important purpose of the story to go with the compound is inside the company – to convince management that it is solid reasoning and all that sort of thing. Many drugs that got into the market based on a theory that proved unsatisfactory have proved very useful.

Politics. Talking about politics, some time back you introduced me to the idea of the little Machiavelli. How big a part of the company culture is this?

Well, a very big part I think. We are all human beings and human beings are fighting for rank order and rank order is finally what it's all about. I just don't believe those people who say that they do something for the company's sake and the louder they say it . . . there was a book published recently which was discussed in the newspapers which goes even farther than the little Machiavelli. It was written under the pseudonym, I.N.

Sider, and nobody knows who is it. It was thought that it could be a former manager of Sandoz, but it has not been confirmed. It describes the power play, the politics, in much more colourful detail. I don't think it is in English. I haven't read it yet, I just read the discussion in the newspaper and it is interesting. This journalist thought it was largely overdone, so they showed it to a guy from Sandoz, who after having read it said 'I haven't learned anything new'.

But linked into all this is the idea that companies make various decisions because the managerial people involved are looking after their careers rather than trying to develop the field.

Oh, I think it would not be realistic to say that this is not true. Maybe the non-industrial players in the game do too little to clarify certain things. For instance, we still do not know whether there are particular populations of depressed people who react specifically to one type of drug or another and whether this is reproducible from one episode to the other. They are all complaining of the Hamilton Rating Scale as an instrument to evaluate drug effects but who makes a serious effort to develop something else?

Why do you think the medical profession are doing so little?

These things are major efforts — they are not something I think that one person can do. So it's a question of getting organized, a question of getting finance. Clearly, especially at the present time, the drug industry has no interest in financing such things because they've got enough to do with financing their drug developments. So this would be in a domain where the public or the universities or whatever would have to finance that sort of thing. For some reason nobody is taking the initiative. I assume the same career thinking is involved because it is obviously a lot of work which will not lead to immediate results which can be published and so people might want to do fancier things.

In a sense, compared with 20 years ago, the psychiatric profession doesn't exist any more. When the drugs came out, they were able to dictate to the industry — these are the medical conditions that we want to treat, this is the way we want to run trials, these are the scales we want to use. But the big names in the field, the Martin Roths, the Mayer-Grosses, the Hanns Hippius's, are all moving on and not being replaced by comparably big figures and at this stage trial procedures have been globalized, they are multi-sited and the industry dictates to us, this is the protocol, this is how we do it. So the capacity for independent thought and action has decreased.

This has probably been an inevitable development because the industry had to change the procedures for clinical trials because the registration authorities asked for proof of the efficacy of drugs and the statisticians said that it has to be done this or that way to be able to reach a conclusive answer and that finally led to devising trial procedures which were devised so as to provide a clear cut answer as what was effective and what wasn't. In the end, you might argue that this is to the benefit of the patient and of the health insurance costs because it will prevent inactive drugs from entering the market, which previously you couldn't do. But I admit it ties up efforts and also available patients to an extent that makes other trials difficult but that doesn't detract from the fact that these trials are sorely needed.

What are the groups like ACNP, ECNP, CINP going to do in the new neurodegenerative world?

I think they've got to change their character. At ACNP, there is more and more neurodegenerative stuff coming in. I haven't been at the last CINP but I hear that neurodegeneration is taking more space. So I think the shift in industry will be reflected in the shift in programmes. It depends how ECNP, ACNP and CINP adapt. If they provide room for these topics there will be no need to fund new groupings. If they show resistance new groups will form, there's no question.

How long is it going to be before we have a compound to treat some of the neurodegenerative disorders? A really new compound.

Let me give you an optimistic assessment – five years from now. I think this is perhaps overly optimistic but I wouldn't be surprised if we had something with a better than marginal effect within 10 years actually in the clinic.

So at this stage you feel there are a few compounds you actually have that are going to be those compounds.

Yes. They are at an early stage and they may still fail for pretty trivial reasons and that will prolong the process.

And there will be a few more nervous breakdowns if that happens?

Well, yes, I guess so. Not from my part. I've been in so many that it doesn't hurt anymore.

25 Thomas A. Ban

They used to call it psychiatry

Chasing up the question of who discovered any of the psychotropic drugs or was responsible for the major psychopharmacologic organizations is a bit like watching Akira Kurosawa's movie 'Rashomon', in which someone is murdered and the witnesses and finally even the victim's ghost each give their version of the events and none of them tally. I had this impression very strongly after reading Towards CINP, *which you and Hanns Hippius put together. Having collected all this material, though, you are in a better position than anyone to answer the question of who was responsible for the 1957 meeting in Milan that laid the basis for the CINP?*

I don't know for sure, but probably Emilio Trabucchi. He had the necessary foresight. But, it could have been Silvio Garattini, still his first assistant at the time.

Silvio has proven his foresight — setting up the Mario Negri Institute.

There was a great need for Institutes like the Mario Negri. Universities, by and large, had lost their independence from the State and other vested interests by the 1950s. During the past decades, they have been less and less able to fulfil their role of generating unbiased information with the necessary speed about the steadily growing number of new drugs. In the absence of the necessary machinery to meet the need, education about how to use the new drugs had to be substituted by information disseminated by each company about its own product.

Recently several alternative possibilities are emerging with the capability of generating unbiased information — not just bits of information but all the information relevant to the development of a particular drug. But in the early 1960s a non-profit foundation, such as Garattini's, was the only viable alternative. It was certainly better placed than departments at the universities.

Who else were the key people in the development of CINP? What were the forces at work to produce it?

The ones who actually proposed the founding of an international organization were Corneille Radouco-Thomas, who became chairman of the Department of Pharmacology at Laval, and Wolfgang de Boor, the psychiatrist from Cologne, who just about a year before published his monograph on *Pharmacopsychology and Psychopathology*. They were the ones who picked up that psychopharmacology had come about – that an important new discipline was born.

A few exceptional psychiatrists like Pierre Deniker and Heinz Lehmann recognized right away that treatment with chlorpromazine was a qualitatively different therapy. That with the new drugs a new world was coming about. But psychiatrists in general were very slow – did not seem to be aware that the new drugs revolutionized psychiatry. So, it fell to pharmacologists, who came from the medical end, like Radouco-Thomas, to take the leading role in the founding of CINP. And the founding of CINP had to be encouraged strongly by the industry. Ciba, Geigy, Sandoz and Roche were all involved. In Milan, Ciba seemed to be the most involved.

The figure who is hard to call in all of this is Rothlin; you've probably talked to more people about his role in this than anyone else, what do you make of it?

Rothlin is one of the controversial figures. Undoubtedly, he was not just a good scientist but also a very strong person. I have the notion that without someone like him bridging the gap between academia and industry, the CINP could not have been born at that point in time. To let him have his way was the price that had to be paid. Some of the founders would have liked to set the stage for the development of CINP on a broader base. Trabucchi would have preferred to open the doors as wide as possible. But Rothlin's position prevailed and the doors were closed, open only by invitation to a few. So neither Heinz Lehmann, nor Fritz Freyhan, who played a most prominent role in the early history of American psychopharmacology, were invited to become founders of the CINP.

There seems to have been a serious clash of personalities between Herman Denber and himself.

Yes. There were clashes between Rothlin and some of the other founders as well. But, regardless of the difficulties they had with each other, the founding group represented a wide range of interests complementing each other in a very desirable way. Denber was a young psychiatrist working in a psychodynamically orientated setting in New York, who recognized the important implications for psychiatry that psychopathology can be induced experimentally. Radouco-Thomas was a young pharmacologist trained in traditional pharmacology who recognized that a new important field of pharmacology was developing. Bradley was one of the first of a new breed of neuropharmacologists. And Rothlin was the powerful former director of Sandoz who led the pharmacology laboratories of his company into the new age. It was very important to have someone of Rothlin's stature to bridge with industry because psychiatry was so slow to join in.

For me, a graduate from medical school in 1954 and then working in a junior position with patients in a large psychiatric hospital in Budapest, it was quite obvious that there was a major change. But my enthusiasm was not necessarily shared. Even towards the end of the 1950s, I found that some of my supervisors at McGill firmly believed that all that drugs like chlorpromazine can do is to render patients accessible to psychotherapy. Only gradually did they begin to change their tune by allowing for the remote possibility that the two treatments combined might be better than either one alone. And it was not before the late 1960s that some of the best-known American psychiatrists teaching at some of the best-known universities of North America were ready to accept that neuroleptics work in their own right and, in fact, work better in the treatment of schizophrenia than any other treatment so far. The same story was repeated with the antidepressants. Even at respectable universities such as Vanderbilt – the university with which I have been affiliated for the past 17 years – the idea keeps lingering on that in depression, treatment with an antidepressant and psychotherapy combined is better than either of them alone.

It is clear that even people like Roland Kuhn, with the training he had, had great problems trying to come to grips with what had happened when there was a drug which helped people who were depressed.

But he did come to grips with it rather promptly in spite of being a psychotherapist. And while his peers had difficulties even to accept the fact, he was able to recognize it. It is fascinating that some people are able to overcome their beliefs. And this is, for me, the most important thing in the case of Kuhn. His recognition of the antidepressant effect of imipramine was a key discovery, and the simple fact that he was able, in spite of his training, to accept that a chemical can affect something as intimately 'psychological' as depression, was instrumental in bringing psychiatry into the modern world. Because, if you really want to reduce things to basics, the discoveries which opened the path for the development of modern psychiatry are the discoveries of the effects of chlorpromazine, lithium, imipramine, and meprobamate. And of these four discoveries of the psychopharmacological revolution, one was his.

With all fairness to the vast array of drugs which followed, the best any of these drugs have done is to substitute one side effect for another, while creating by their rapidly growing number a tremendous turmoil for physicians, and by their steadily increasing cost a serious financial burden for patients. Because even with the impressive progress made in brain research, psychiatry has never really been able to resolve how *to go beyond just using chlorpromazine in schizophrenia and imipramine in depression.*

Could I ask you about that? In 1987 you wrote an article, which, by virtue of both its title and its content, was very different to anything that had been written before, or since — 'The Prolegomenon to the Clinical Prerequisite'. This has been one of the few efforts to go beyond just the simple giving of drugs to construct a rational basis for therapeutics. So there are two questions, first of all why were you interested to do that kind of thing but also why has the field been so slow to do it?

Well, I know why I had been interested, but I can speculate only why the field has been so slow. I had become interested because I was determined *to go beyond just using chlorpromazine in schizophrenia and imipramine in depression.* And since, in my own evaluation, one of the most important contributions of psychopharmacology was that it focused attention on the biologic heterogeneity of populations within the traditional nosologic categories, I thought that replacement of biologically heterogeneous diagnostic concepts by homogeneous ones, at least in terms of pharmacotherapeutic responsiveness, would open the possibility for a more discriminate use of psychotropics.

I waited for a long time, though, before addressing the issue and only after many years of clinical investigations with newer and newer molecules did I acknowledge that none of the new drugs was better in overall therapeutic efficacy. So by the late 1960s, I was certain that a decision must be reached about whether there is a particular population, which responds to a particular drug. And if there is such a population, to find a way to identify it.

Regarding your second question, I really don't know why the field was so slow to follow suit. Understandably, the splitting of the broadest possible population for which therapeutic effectiveness could be demonstrated was contrary to the interest of the pharmaceutical industry because it narrowed the market for their drugs. And undoubtedly the field was busy with developing a complex methodology for the detection of therapeutic efficacy and with the testing of the clinical activity of newer and newer psychotropics. But probably the single most important factor was that its attention was distracted from the seemingly trivial clinical problem of heterogeneity of a diagnostic population by the newer and newer and more and more sophisticated theories about the action mechanism of psychotropics. The issue of identifying the treatment responsive population, if any, should have been dealt with immediately after the introduction of chlorpromazine and imipramine.

How do we do it?

We have no generally accepted way. For some time, I thought that for identifying the treatment responsive population one would need to find a way to link the action mechanism of psychotropics with the pathomechanism of mental disease. And since both, mental disorders and the action mechanism of drugs, can be described to some extent in terms of conditional reflex variables, I went ahead and developed a conditioning test battery for the study of psychopathological mechanisms and psychopharmacological effects. It was of sufficient merit to win the McNeil award of the Canadian Psychiatric Association in the late 1960s. But before long I realized that what I was trying to do was far too complicated, impractical and might even be somewhat far-fetched. Therefore, after documenting what was done, I decided to move on and leave conditioning to those interested in personality and behaviour.

By that time I had the belief that mental illness starts beyond what can be learned and was very much involved with psychopharmacology. First, I had been engaged in research in which we induced psychopathology with drugs, and later on in research in which we controlled psychopathology with drugs; and since it was possible to do it in both ways, I felt that finally we could meaningfully talk about mental illness because what we were talking about was no longer just a matter of belief, but was accessible and demonstrable experimentally. And it seemed to be that psychopharmacology had also provided convenient biochemical measures which link the action mechanism of the drug with the clinical state or even the pathomechanism of the illness. There were new hopes – and great disappointments – when attempts to identify treatment responsive populations by biochemical measures yielded inconsistent findings.

At this point I realized that it is unrealistic to expect empirically derived objective measurements to replace traditional psychiatric concepts in the foreseeable future. With this in mind I turned to regression analysis to see whether the treatment responsiveness could be identified on the basis of symptoms, the elementary units of mental illness. But by doing this in a number of different studies, we found that the psychopathologic symptom profile of the ideal patient, who would have responded to the same treatment, was different from one study to another.

I don't know whether our findings would have been different if the set of psychopathologic symptoms included in the linear regression equations were not restricted to behavioural rating scale variables. I was ready to explore this by employing the symptoms listed in the AMDP, but by the time I was ready to proceed Frank Fish reported that by dividing schizophrenia on the basis of Karl Leonhard's criteria he found that unsystematic schizophrenia responds significantly better to neuroleptics than systematic schizophrenia. To pursue this line of research further, I developed a guide to Leonhard's classification of chronic schizophrenia, and later a polydiagnostic evaluation with the capability of diagnosing the same patient by diagnostic formulations derived by different methods. It is referred to as the Composite Diagnostic Evaluation System, or in brief, the CODE System. The prototype is the Composite Diagnostic Evaluation of Depressive Disorders or CODE-DD, which includes 25 conceptually different formulations relevant to the classification of depressive illness. If the treatment responsive population to imipramine or to any of the other antidepressants can be identified on the basis of currently recognized nosologic endpoints of depressive illness, it should be possible to identify it by employing CODE-DD.

You've been fairly unique in this regard. More recently there are other people who have been working on systems like OPCRIT and things like that, but they are doing it for slightly different reasons. Why do you think the field has been so lacking in interest in this exercise?

I might have been unique when I started, but I don't think that I am unique any longer. There is a considerable interest these days in the CODE System, just as much as in the OPCRIT. CODE-DD has been translated into Italian, French, Polish, Estonian and several other languages. And there is ongoing research with the CODE System in Hungary under the direction of Peter Gaszner, who was Vice President of ECNP and in Argentina under the direction of Ronaldo Ucha Udabe, who wrote one of the first texts in psychopharmacology with the late Edmondo Fisher. In fact, the Japanese have developed an even more comprehensive instrument referred to as COALA, which stands for Comprehensive Assessment List for Affective Disorders.

But I agree with you that for a long time there was little interest in psychopathology and nosology, although I would argue that this lack of interest was not restricted to the field of psychopharmacology. When psychopharmacology came about psychodynamics was the mainstream of psychiatry in the US, and a social orientation was dominant in psychiatry in the UK, and neither psychodynamically-orientated psychiatrists nor social psychiatrists had much appreciation for traditional psychopathology and nosology. Both were actually more interested in the patient and how the patient deals with the disease and adapts to society than in the disease itself. Even in Germany, interest in traditional psychopathology and nosology was minimal because it was not found to be of much use clinically. And after the introduction of the new psychotropics, people like me were so taken by psychopharmacology that we believed that we need not be bothered with psychopathology or nosology. We would have preferred to replace rather than retain the old psychopathologic and nosologic concepts, and were disappointed that none of the biologic measures was shown to be anything more than epiphenomena of the behavioural state present with the illness.

There has been a tradition in the UK, with people like Eysenck, that has been concerned to develop on these lines . . .

Eysenck's attempt to render the biologic basis of personality accessible to pharmacologic manipulation was far ahead of his time. Whether one agrees with his theory is an entirely different story. His dimensional concepts confound the abnormal with the pathological, perceiving the pathological on a continuum with the normal... presuming that psychology and psychiatry are one field in which the same language is spoken and the same laws prevail. Nevertheless, his work stimulated a great deal of interest and even today, he has followers all around the world.

During the 1960s, I was very interested in his work. But today I believe that mental illness is based on a pathologic process which produces detectable pathologic changes which become manifest in distinctive psychopathologic symptom patterns. And depending on the nature of the detectable pathologic change, there seems to be two major classes of mental disease: one with structural changes which are directly detectable by the method of pathologic anatomy, and one with functional changes in the processing of impulses, which have become indirectly detectable by the method of psychopharmacology. Not every psychiatrist, of course, would agree and some would even argue that the group without directly detectable structural changes does not fulfil Morgagni's criteria of disease. But is it not really just semantics whether it does or does not fulfil Morgagni's criteria? Regardless, psychotropic drugs have rendered the biologic substrate of these disorders accessible to pharmacological manipulation in a predictable way. And even if our residents are still taught that psychotropic drugs can only suppress symptoms without having an effect on the disease, the fact remains that responsiveness of a particular symptom to a particular drug depends on the illness in which the symptom occurs.

The field is so big now that there's no one individual or even a group of individuals who can stand back and try to put things together again. At the same time, the industry is both producing new drugs and producing entities that their drugs treat. Does the field have the capacity to analyse itself?

The field has grown tremendously, but I don't think that it is so big that it would not be possible to put it together again if the vested interests, which keep it fragmented, would permit this. The field is increasingly controlled by the industry – but the industry is not necessarily evil. Without industry the medicalization of psychiatry would be far from where it is today, and neither the diagnosis nor the treatment of mental illness would be sufficiently advanced that psychiatry could participate in an integrated health care system with the other branches of medicine. But the medicalization of psychiatry is far from being complete. One of the last major areas of resistance, the area of neuroses, was overcome during the last decade and the medicalization of the different disorders subsumed under the category of neuroses is under way. We are, of course, paying an enormous price for this by using newer and newer drugs, which are more and more expensive, yet not even proven that they are better than old psychotropics. We are using these drugs also in wider and wider populations with more and more extended indications – and we might be treating artificially created entities which, even if they can be reliably identified, one wonders to what extent fulfil criteria of disease.

But while industry, to expand its market, is rapidly progressing with the medicalization of mental illness, it is leaving behind a disorganized profession of psychiatry, struggling to find its identity with steadily decreasing financial resources. In spite of this, I believe that the field has the capacity to analyse itself because we have all the necessary prerequisites for such an analysis. After all, we do have therapeutically effective psychotropic drugs to practice psychiatry as a medical discipline. And we also have the necessary computer technologies, which would allow us to offer a reliable and accountable clinical service, to establish databases, and to process and analyse the collected data with a continuous validation of diagnostic and therapeutic knowledge.

I am fully aware, of course, that even if we have the capacity, we do not have the capability to utilize our capacity within the traditional structural organization. Psychiatrists today are consumers or solicitors of the goods used in the treatment, diagnosis and assessment of the mentally ill. And associations, collegiums and societies are increasingly becoming brokers between the pharmaceutical industry and the profession. But a multinational corporation in psychiatry, based on the model of multinational business organizations, with a network of diagnostic and treatment centres, operating with the same computerized system and feeding into the same central databank, would have the capability. Such a corporation if it remains restricted to illness could provide a worldwide service with a sufficiently reduced expense that treatment would become available and accessible to everyone who needs it. I am keenly aware that attending to the illness without taking full care of the patient does not suffice. But, regardless of what I do or don't believe in, helping patients reintegrate with society is a social obligation that neither depends upon nor requires medical training, a privilege dependent on how much the community can afford it . . .

There is a particularly tricky group of people that I would be keen to hear your response on: what about personality disorders?

I have difficulties with the concept of personality disorders. Some are exaggerations of personality traits while others might just as well be the result of a pathologic process – in the same way as anxiety disorders are slowly being seen this way. What we refer to as anxiety disorders today were labelled for long as neuroses and perceived as abnormal personalities under stress. Even in the ICD-9, neuroses and personality disorders were still lumped together. The DSM-III was the first classification which separated them. Now I would think that some personality disorders are abnormalities in the statistical sense, while others are clinical syndromes, similar to the neuroses, which have nothing to do with development.

But I must admit that I have problems even with the concept of personality. I really don't like it. If people have so much difficulty coming to any kind of agreement about what a concept means, as in the case of personality, there must be something wrong with the concept. The only reason to have concepts is to be able to communicate, and if we have problems using a concept in communicating, we might just as well throw out such a concept. And if the dismissed concept leaves a void one should replace it with one which corresponds more with the real world. Eysenck went just as far as one can go in defining personality in a scientific way, but his concept of psychopathy has no roots in reality.

Well, he had hoped that the constructs he was using would be drug sensitive. He did predict that certain drugs were going to shift people along a dimensional spectrum but that didn't work out once imipramine appeared.

Whether it did or didn't, I don't know. Theoretically, it should have insofar as at least stimulants, sedatives, and alcohol are concerned. I would be more inclined to think that the reason why no one is talking about the relationship between Eysenck's dimensions of personality and drugs is because it leads to a dead end.

Let me bring you back. You and Hanns Hippius appeared to pick up this history issue more than anyone else. Why were you interested in the history?

With the rapid growth of the field, the CINP grew into a major, politically powerful organization and has undergone several drastic changes in its leadership. Since the time of its inception CINP was a President's organiz-ation, and during their short, two-year tenure each President was given a chance to leave his imprint. The history committee was really Ole Rafael-sen's creation about 10 years ago at the San Juan congress. Hanns Hippius and I became the first members – and a few months later Ole died unexpectedly.

Hanns and I continued with the activities planned, including the recon-struction of CINP's poorly kept records. We began reviewing history through the CINP congresses which we have been having every two years. And while working on 'Thirty Years' we became aware that people who had been around when CINP was formed were aging, and felt that if we really wanted to find out not just what happened, but also how it influenced the course of events which led to what we have at present, we were getting close to our last chance. We thought that the best way of finding out was to ask each of the founders to give a brief account of their perception of the field in the mid-1950s and their perception of the field in the early 1990s. 'Psychopharmacology in Perspective', the collection of these manuscripts, was ready by the time of the Nice Congress in 1992. Soon after we began preparing the first booklet of a systematic review of the history of CINP, covering the period from the 1955 Paris Colloquium on Chlorpromazine, sponsored by Rhône-Poulenc, through the Milan Symposium, to the time of the inaugural meeting of CINP in the fall of 1957.

We are planning to continue our systematic review. There is, of course, a close relationship between the programme of CINP congresses and the history of neuropsychopharmacology. And when looking at the programme of the congresses, we could see a steadily widening gap between preclinical and clinical research – and an impasse in pharmacotherapeutic progress.

Whether feedback from psychiatry could have broken the deadlock is difficult to say. Personally, I would think that we would be far ahead in the pharmacotherapy of mental illness if Fish's findings had not been ignored and the differential responsiveness to neuroleptics between the systematic and unsystematic schizophrenias verified. I would also think that we could have cut short a lot of meaningless experimentation if it would have been clarified whether reserpine-induced psychopathology is dysphoria, a pathologic emotion, or dysthymia, a pathologic mood, and whether the anticholinergic-induced psychopathology is delirium, a clouded state of consciousness, or dementia, a disintegration of personality.

I know that it sounds like I keep saying revive good old psychopathology and nosology and all our problems in neuropsychopharmacology would be solved. But this is definitely not my position. All I am trying to say is that we should carefully examine whether psychopathology and nosology, the two basic disciplines of psychiatry, could provide biologically meaningful concepts before dismissing 100 years of psychiatric tradition. On the other hand, if none of the concepts of psychopathology and nosology turn out to be useful, which is unlikely but not impossible, I think that we would be justified in rebuilding the discipline that was called psychiatry from new, entirely different elements. The term 'psychiatry', with its link to the animal spirit, psyche, soul has become anachronistic anyway with the introduction of psychotropic drugs.

Since the 1960s there has been a growing tension between clinical psychopharmacology and neuropharmacology – and there has been also a growing tension within CINP. The organization was in place and held regular congresses every other year, alternating between one open and one closed meeting. And although each congress in its own right was a success, the different disciplines remained isolated, and the people, instead of becoming one big family became polarized into political factions and national representations. Rothlin continued as president for a second term, but Trabucchi, who was considered by many to be the real founding father of CINP, quietly withdrew after the successful first congress he organized in Rome. And the revolution was killing its own children . . . during the second CINP congress in Basel, two of the original founders, Denber and Radouco-Thomas, were pushed aside. The same happened to Phil Bradley during the Copenhagen congress. Of the original founders, only Pierre Deniker was to become President. And the tension which pervaded the business meeting in Basel continued for years.

By the early 1980s, it became evident that keeping the channels of communication open could not prevent significant differences in drug preference. Transcultural differences certainly cannot explain why maprotiline a selective norepinephrine reuptake inhibitor, is the most extensively

employed antidepressant in France, whereas fluoxetine, a selective serotonin reuptake inhibitor, is in the United States. Nor can it explain why
clozapine, a great success in Germany, is virtually not used by the Italians.
It is telling that in countries which are less prosperous and even in
prosperous countries among the poor, imipramine remains the most frequently prescribed drug in the treatment of depression and chlorpromazine
in the treatment of schizophrenia.

The history of modern pharmacotherapy in psychiatry is certainly not
a straightforward story. It is rather disturbing that D2 receptor blockade,
which, as believed for a long time is an essential prerequisite for therapeutic
effects in schizophrenia, now appears to be a curse – that D2 receptor
blockade is out and D4 receptor blockade is in without the slightest
evidence that D4 blockers are more efficacious than haloperidol or chlorpromazine.

Even the chronology of development is somewhat confounding. For
me, the psychopharmacologic revolution began with the introduction of
chlorpromazine, but the muscle relaxant mephenesin, the predecessor
of meprobamate, the first propanediol tranquillizer, and the antituberculo-
tic isoniazid, the predecessor of iproniazid, the first monoamine oxidase
inhibitor antidepressant, had already been around in the early 1950s. One
should probably start with lithium which, in the ultimate analysis, appears
to be the most important contribution insofar as pharmacotherapy in
psychiatry is concerned. And the first publication on lithium was in print
already in the late 1940s.

There was considerable delay between Cade's early report on lithium
in the late 1940s and Schou's demonstration of its therapeutic efficacy in
the mid-1950s, and an even longer delay between Schou's report and the
spread of lithium therapy in psychiatry. In fact, it took place only well
after the introduction of the first benzodiazepines in the early 1960s.
And the spread of the benzodiazepines, backed by Roche's multinational
organization, was much faster than the spread of lithium, backed by
Mogen Schou, a professor of psychiatry. But in spite of all the support
the benzodiazepines received, the shift from the propanediols to the
benzodiazepines in the control of anxiety took significantly longer in
Europe than in the United States. And even today, however effective and
safe the benzodiazepines are, the use of propanediols in Eastern Europe
and in the developing world continues.

I have no doubt that the introduction of the benzodiazepines was a
major contribution. But even if the benzodiazepines are so close to the
natural anxiolytic that mother nature created a benzodiazepine receptor
in the brain, within the framework of the psychopharmacologic revolution
the breakthrough drug in the treatment of anxiety was meprobamate.
Frank Berger's contribution cannot be sufficiently emphasized. By recognizing the relationship between muscle relaxant and anxioytic effects,
Berger revived the James – Lange theory of emotions, and rendered

anxiety accessible to scientific scrutiny. I am not surprised that of the two meetings in psychopharmacology prior to the Milan Symposium, one, the Paris meeting in 1955, dealt with chlorpromazine, whereas the other, the New York meeting in 1956, dealt with meprobamate.

Silvio Garattini would also say that drugs like meprobamate looked as important to them in the 1950s as chlorpromazine and . . .

The relative importance of these two drugs depends on the framework of psychiatry one operates in. Within the European framework, the importance of chlorpromazine is overwhelmingly greater. But the European concept is a very narrow concept which grew out from the psychoses. On the other hand within the American framework, in which psychiatry included from the very beginning alcoholism, psychopathy and neuroses, the importance of meprobamate is comparable to chlorpromazine.

One also hears very little these days about reserpine. It is almost forgotten that during the mid-1950s it looked just as important as chlorpromazine. Some of these drugs provided important bridges. Just as the propanediols provided a bridge between the barbiturates and the benzodiazepines, reserpine provided the bridge between neuropharmacology and psychopharmacology, between therapeutic effects and brain monoamines, between transmission of impulses at the synaptic cleft and processing of experience . . . It was the recognition of the importance of serotonin release in the action mechanism of reserpine in the mid 1950s that opened up the possibility of employing the pharmacologic approach in the study of the brain and in the exploration of the relationship between biochemical mechanisms and mental functions. It was the introduction of the pharmacologic approach which turned the pharmacotherapeutic rebellion into a psychopharmacologic revolution.

What about Brodie's role in all of this?

He played the most significant role. He trained most of those who created modern neuropharmacology. It was a new way of thinking, a new way of looking at things that people picked up while working for him. Julius Axelrod, who as you know was awarded the Nobel prize, started out as a technician in Brodie's laboratory, Arvid Carlsson, who was first to figure out how chlorpromazine and haloperidol works, spent some time with him in Bethesda and one could go on and on with the listing of the names. It is rather unfortunate that some of them, especially in North America, imposed themselves as authorities in psychiatry and by doing so have created insurmountable difficulties for a healthy and desirable interaction between the two disciplines. Another person who is undervalued is Nate Kline. He did some of the early clinical work with reserpine, picked out the monoamine oxidase inhibitors and had the guts to stand up for lithium's importance.

The other thing that he seems to have done that gets played down is his work in Congress that provided the funds to create the Psychopharmacology Service Center.

Yes, his testimony before a subcommittee of the US Congress in the late 1950s played an important role in it. And there are a great many other things he did. He generated the funds necessary to open a psychiatric institute in Haiti, to sponsor the annual Denghausen meetings and one could go on and on. He was a great man, regardless of how one looks at it. I don't think he got the recognition he deserved. In a certain way there are similarities with Brodie, but of course there are important differences. Kline did not train up a school. Working with Brodie stimulated people to develop the methodology which created a new science. Now, I cannot say that the same applies to Nate, but he was certainly quick in recognizing the importance of psychopharmacology. And he did it in an era when you virtually could not get into academic psychiatry in America without being psychoanalysed – when psychoanalysis was the mainstream of psychiatry, distracting attention from the possibility that the administration of a drug might correct something wrong going on in the brain. But even if Kline did not train a school, he pioneered a new way of thinking in psychiatry. It was this new way of thinking that made it possible to recognize the importance of the monoamine oxidase enzymes, and later on other genetically determined enzymes – and to develop the link between psychiatry and molecular genetics.

Is it totally impossible 10 years from now that we might rewrite the history in terms of a lesser focus on chlorpromazine because the implications on genetic . . .

Probably not rewrite, but sort of round it up . . . and give proper recognition also to the chain of events triggered by the introduction of reserpine and the monoamine oxidase inhibitors. And instead of dismissing the neurobiologic approach to complement it with a molecular genetic approach.

Why did you leave Hungary?

I was on vacation, travelling around in the Balkan countries when the Hungarian revolution began. I flew home from Belgrade when the Russian troops moved out from the city and left before the borders were shut, after the Russian tanks rolled in. I had no clear cut plans. The reason I left was simply that I wanted to see the world outside the iron curtain and was interested to learn. I left sometime in mid-November and for a period of two months was permanently on the move. But by mid-January 1957 I was in Canada, a fellow at the prestigious Montreal Neurological Institute. Whether I got my fellowship entirely on merit it is difficult to know. As a medical student I won first prize for a work I had done in collaboration with a fellow student on post-traumatic epilepsy. And Penfield apparently was or was made aware of this work. It was certainly a good start for a 27-year-old who had just arrived in the new world. But then I felt that I was really more interested in psychiatry and decided that I should complete my training.

I picked the place Heinz Lehmann was at because I had heard about his work on chlorpromazine. I went there on 1 July 1958 and within a couple of months I had been involved with him in research on phencyclidine. I also began with my work on conditioning. In those years we still had to write a thesis to get our diploma in psychiatry at McGill. And the title of my dissertation was 'conditioning and psychiatry'. I received my diploma with distinction in 1960 and my thesis was published as a monograph in 1964 with a forward by Horsley Gantt, at the time one of the last living pupils of Pavlov.

After spending a year with Heinz Lehmann at Verdun, I was ready to start working with Gerald Sarwer-Foner at the Veterans' Administration Hospital but the departmental chairman, Ewen Cameron, was looking for someone with the background I had in conditioning and psychopharmacology and I was asked whether I would be interested in working with him. I was, and after substituting for the chief resident at the Allan briefly I became Cameron's researcher for the rest of the year. And even after I had received my diploma I continued with Cameron as the junior member of his research team.

What was Cameron like?

He was an independent, goal-directed, well-organized man with exceptional administrative skills. He had studied with Henderson and worked with Eugen Bleuler and Meyer in his formative years but the Cameron I knew was definitely his own man. Strong, energetic and decisive with courage to pursue whatever he believed in. They called him 'Chief' – and he called us 'Docs' and the nurses 'Lassies'. He was the Chief, there was just no doubt about this.

In Cameron's time, the Allan was a truly eclectic place with facilities such as day hospital and speciality clinics, which were very much avant garde those days and with one of the largest and most respected training programmes with residents from all around the world. All of this was of Cameron's making. What most impressed me was that Cameron ran the largest clinical service with the most difficult patients. Every day he walked around and talked to each patient and every other day we had rounds with him when we sat around a table. I was marginally involved because I was doing the research but still participated with my research patients.

I really think that what happened later was very unfortunate and uncalled for in his case. I cannot help but wonder why it happened in such an underhanded way and after so many years since everything Cameron did was done in the open and with the knowledge of his peers. He kept the cleanest and most precise records I had ever seen with all the information given on each patient to the smallest details. He dictated his notes in front of his team in his characteristic Scottish burr and whatever he dictated was typed in the record by the next day.

Where did all the controversy come from? What did it all mean?

It is somewhat difficult to remember after so many years but over the past 30 years Cameron has been vilified by the press. The difficulties began when it came to light that one of the sources of his funding, however small, was the CIA. The project that started the controversy was part of Cameron's long-term research programme based on a mixture of psychodynamic principles and learning theory, designed for patients refractory to the traditional approaches to therapy. For Cameron, as for other dedicated researchers in the field of the time, it was never clear where treatment ended and research started. This was certainly the case for 'psychic driving', a form of psychotherapy he developed in the early 1950s. By the time I arrived to the Allan he used drugs, sleep, and sensory isolation to loosen, and depatterning to selectively erase pathologic patterns. And this is what created the problem. When Cameron left, his practices were scrutinized – but while all this took place the precarious balance at the Allan Memorial Institute shifted from eclectic to psychodynamic and in the years after the control of a small group of psychoanalysts was strengthened. It was a very closed shop, a fraternity of psychoanalysts.

I could be wrong but this is how I saw it. Cameron had been critical of psychoanalytic theory, rejected what psychoanalysis stood for. Now I am not trying to say that the Cameron affair was created by the psychoanalysts. But I do believe that Cameron's advocacy that learning might be more important in a broader sense than in the very narrow psychodynamic conceptual framework, contributed to it. It had been convenient for the psychoanalytic group to go along with what was happening and to sit back and listen to the never-ending critical appraisals of Cameron's work by different standards year after year. What is somewhat surprising is that no one ever pointed out that while Cameron's team was depatterning a patient on one bed, another team on another bed of the sleep room was busy doing anaclitic therapy – one of those therapies based on psychoanalytic theory in which adults are treated as babies.

After all, Cameron's idea to erase everything one had learned, get rid of the pathologic patterns, create a *tabula rasa* and try to rebuild things from scratch, program in new behaviour, was not as way out as some people have perceived it. And even if many people had forgotten it conveniently, Cameron had only introduced the term depatterning for a treatment which was in use, but referred to as regressive ECT by others. As you know, there were all kinds of treatments in those days – apomorphine-induced vomiting and atropine-induced toxic psychosis were considered to be therapeutic. Insulin coma, and even prolonged insulin coma therapy was still used in the treatment of schizophrenia.

Cameron was of course familiar with all the different types of treatments and to combine pharmacotherapy with psychotherapy was very much in keeping with his general approach. He adopted the concept of psychic defences from psychodynamics but treated psychic defences as if they would have a biologic substrate. But being Cameron he was impatient, looking for short cuts, trying to speed up the therapeutic process and the idea of using drugs to facilitate psychotherapy had been around for a long time. There had been psycholytic therapy, which aimed to activate unconscious, repressed memories, and psychedelic therapy, which aimed to elicit profound cosmic – mystic experiences by the administration of LSD and psilocybin – in fact this had a great many followers for many years. Abram Hoffer, a member of the pioneering team formulating the adrenochrome hypothesis in the early 1950s used psychotomimetics in the treatment of alcoholics. He, later, became well known around the world for promoting megavitamin therapy and orthomolecular psychiatry with the double Nobel laureate Linus Pauling. You know it is interesting that the two Canadian founding members of CINP were Abram Hoffer, who now lives somewhere around Victoria, and Ewen Cameron. Both of them have received excessive attention by the press over the years.

What one reads about Cameron is mainly about ethical issues. It is of course easy to agree that it is wrong to expose patients to treatment without proven efficacy, treatment which is in development, without their knowledge. But the real question is where to draw the line. Because, if one takes it literally none of the psychotherapies had data in support of their efficacy those days. I would question whether such data exist even today. And psychic driving, Cameron's brand of psychotherapy, was not sufficiently different from the rest that it would have qualified as a different kind of treatment. I spent lots of time with Cameron's patients, or at least with those assigned to me, and explained just as much about their treatment to them as I was able to comprehend myself and able to get across. And in those times, we had neither ethics committees, nor consent forms. How much attention Cameron paid to these kind of issues, which today would be dealt with by institutional review boards and ethics committees I don't know. But I do know that he felt comfortable about how things were and fully responsible for what he was doing.

Since Cameron left McGill almost 30 years have passed and during the years my frustration with him has gone. I was terribly frustrated with my work at the Allan – mainly about trivial matters, like keeping my gadgets in working order. The difficulties interfering with my activities were there day after day and influenced my attitude towards and judgement about the research but even then the rationale of the treatment, which was at the centre of the research, seemed to me at least as sound as the rationale of most other treatments in those days and Cameron's speculations were more down to earth than some of the speculations I was exposed to in the seminars I had to attend during my training.

I am now able to look at the research I was engaged with on his team without any emotional colouring and I feel that whatever was done should have been done better, in a more sophisticated way. He should have been more careful of not confounding matters by tackling too many issues together, trying to get an answer to too many questions simultaneously. There were many questions there with important theoretical implications for psychiatry – like whether the pathologic pattern could be erased by physical means. Because if pathologic patterns could not be erased by depatterning, the most drastic means that could wipe out all that was acquired after birth, it would be very unlikely that these patterns were learned and if that was the case Cameron's findings would shatter one of the basic premises on which psychodynamics was based.

Another question with important theoretical implications was the one which dealt with the nature of the disorganization induced by sensory isolation or drugs. Because if the nature of the disorganization depends on the disease and not on the person afflicted with the disease, it would imply that the disease process is independent of personality development. But Cameron was not just bluntly entering the psychological-mental sanctuary by physical means, he was also trying to render accessible to scrutiny the detectable changes, if any, displayed during therapy, by the recording of everything for which a gadget was available. The money from the CIA was spent primarily on the development and employment of objective measures. This was something he had been interested in since the early 1930s, when he wrote his text on *Objective and Experimental Psychiatry*.

I don't know whether he was aware of how sensitive an area he touched in his research. Nor do I know whether he was ready to conceptualize his own findings in the way I was doing. He never acknowledged that the answers to certain questions were already there in the notes he dictated with great regularity on his patients, in the files he was so proud of. One of the patients, whose file I am referring to, was a very severe obsessive – compulsive he depatterned. She was confused and disorientated for days, but in spite of her organic state her compulsive rituals persisted unchanged. Another schizophrenic patient remained unperturbed by prolonged sensory deprivation. She was actually better after she came out of sensory deprivation than when she entered. Such patients opened my eyes to see that some of the things I had been taught might not have been as true as I was made to believe. Whether those cases carried the same message to Cameron, it is difficult to know. He spoke little and even when he did I frequently felt that he said things tongue in cheek. By the time I could have asked him, he had passed away. Cameron died while mountain climbing – he died as he lived.

I joined Vanderbilt in 1976, and we left Montreal and moved to Nashville. Then last fall McGill's department of psychiatry had its 50th birthday. I was invited to the anniversary celebrations and, I assume in consideration of my monograph on *Psychopharmacology for the Aged*, I was assigned to a symposium on psychogeriatrics. When I went back, after being away for almost 20 years, I was struck by what I saw. The department seemed to be frozen in the state as it was in the mid 1970s. It was on my tongue to say that you may argue endlessly about the relationship between mind and body but get rid of the double standards between the biologic and the psychodynamic and get on with treating patients. I left at the end of the meeting contemplating that even if it had been right to criticize Cameron about some of the research he did, the outcome of his departure was devastating. It shifted the department into a psychodynamic mode at a time when the rest of the world was shifting in the opposite way. The department which in Cameron's time was the heart of Canadian psychiatry was struggling to adapt to the new world. I just cannot help to think that there was something else there and not just the funding from the CIA.

It was all very strange because around 1960/62, Cameron was one of the three or four big names in the world.

He was one of the Nuremberg psychiatrists and one of the psychiatrists who examined Rudolph Hess. He had been President of the American Psychiatric Association and the founding President of the World Psychiatric Association. Cameron was a hard working and creative man and this was his greatest strength. He was free of prejudices and binding beliefs and had the necessary drive to pick up and explore the possible usefulness in psychiatry of whatever new thing he picked up from the other disciplines. Most people work within someone else's framework, but Cameron had the imagination to build his own. He had arrived in Montreal, from Albany, in the early 1940s and was facing a society strongly controlled by the Catholic church. But he walked through without paying any attention to this and without ever bending his head. The clergy had no place in the psychiatric hospital insofar as Cameron was concerned. And he succeeded on his own to create the leading department of psychiatry in Canada, a department which was at that time one of the best in the world. No one in those years would have denied that Cameron was a great man. When Ellenberger arrived . . .

Cameron brought Ellenberger there?

Yes, he brought him there in the late 1950s or early 1960s. He was an eclectic and his department clearly reflected this. Regardless of what people say, he cared about his patients and he had an open mind. He was interested in everything new and tried to introduce it in his Institute. Hyden had hardly presented his theory that RNA is the molecular substrate of memory when Cameron picked it up and was ready to start with a clinical trial employing RNA as substitution therapy in elderly patients with memory impairment. He was ready to build a bridge between molecular biology and clinical psychiatry. And when existential analysis emerged, Cameron without delay hired Henri Ellenberger but he really did not know how to deal with him.

Why not?

Cameron was a pragmatic and Ellenberger was a man of books. He was expected to see patients to generate his livelihood. I assume that the time required for practice was too much of a distraction for him. He was obviously working already on the *Discovery of Unconscious*, which became a classic by the 1980s. Ellenberger was completely lost in the big machinery of the Allan and found refuge at the University of Montreal, where he became professor outside the medical field. His story reminds me of the story of Karl Jaspers who exchanged psychiatry for philosophy.

Was there anyone else he brought in like that?

There was Kral, one of the pioneers of psychogeriatrics, best known for separating benign from malignant forgetfulness. He collaborated with us in a project trying to predict therapeutic responsiveness to psychotropics by employing pharmacological load tests. He brought in Eric Wittkower, a leading psychoanalyst, who was involved with research in psychosomatics and cross-cultural psychiatry. One of the first people he brought in was Robert Cleghorn, who succeeded him at the Allan. It was actually Cleghorn's team which commissioned the work which found no memory impairment in the depatterned patients by employing the Wechsler Memory Scale. I have not seen the report but I understand that in spite of the findings Cleghorn concluded that patients might still have difficulties with remembering because there are memory problems which are not detectable by the Wechsler Memory Scale.

Why is getting funds from the CIA such a potent stick to beat people with?

Because it can be implied that CIA-funded studies were used for the development of brainwashing techniques. But of course the stick was not necessarily used. There were many distinguished scientists who got funds from the CIA. I don't really know who they were, I read about Harris Isbell, who was director of the addiction research centre in Lexington; Jolyon West, who was chairman of the department of psychiatry in Los Angeles, and Leo Hollister, one of the most prominent clinical psychopharmacologists of the United States. But there were many well-known psychologists too. I read that Hans Eysenck, Carl Rogers and Fred Skinner received funds from the CIA.

But who really knows . . . and, you know, it was never completely clear whether Cameron knew that the source of the money he received for four years or so from the Society for the Investigation of Human Ecology was the CIA. I certainly did not. But even if he had known, he would not have cared. Funds from the CIA were just as good for him as funds from anywhere else. But as you say it has been used as a stick to beat him with.

How much do you think it links up with the clash of paradigms with the analysts on one side and the biological psychiatrists on the other? Someone like Frank Ayd would say that the biological people were seen as being in league with the devil, treating people in this inhuman way – so in a sense maybe the CIA links were just the icing on the cake.

This is exactly how I see it. The CIA link helped to blow out of proportion the criticism of Cameron's work and to make biological psychiatrists look as if they were treating their patients inhumanely. You should keep in mind that the Cameron affair took place before we began with our struggle to separate facts from beliefs and hypotheses from speculations in psychiatry. Just around the time when the different approaches in psychiatry were turned into paradigms and became politicized. The two most influential paradigms were the social and the psychodynamic, one the mirror image of the other.

I felt somewhat lost those days, because paradigms were meaningless words to me. I just couldn't see why it was so important to choose whether the social creates the psychologic – my indoctrination in Hungary – or the psychologic the social – my indoctrination at McGill. Neither seemed to me to have much relevance to psychiatry but I could see that paradigms are created by social forces and that psychologizing can distract from social problems – that is, that it's the social structure which has fostered psychologizing in the US and sociologizing in the UK and that there are vested interests which have sustained the dominance of these approaches.

Absolutely. In England psychopharmacology happened outside of Oxford and Cambridge. It did not happen in the major centres.

It was the same in the United States and Canada. It was not at the Allan Memorial Institute, the primary teaching centre, and not even at the psychiatric units of the Montreal General or the Jewish General Hospitals, but at the Verdun Protestant Hospital, a kind of State Hospital, which served the poor in the English-speaking community of the city. And even at the Verdun, an ambitious Executive Director gave Dr Lehmann a hard time during the late 1950s. Fortunately, after he had been psychoanalysed, he moved away from Montreal to higher positions. But, as late as the early 1970s, another ambitious Executive Director succeeded in preventing the implementation of a programme which would have led to a rational use of psychotropics within the framework of a specially designed service structure in the hospital. Everything was in place to go ahead, but he interfered to prevent the shift in the balance between two paradigms, the psychopharmacologic and the social. I presented a brief outline of the proposed programme at the CINP Congress in Copenhagen. There was great interest, but nothing else.

In the majority of the teaching centres of Canada and the United States the psychodynamic approach remained dominant during the 1970s. I assume the same applies to the social approach in the UK. But, you know, in spite of the brutal clashes between their prominent representatives, the social and psychodynamic paradigms are quite close. Both confound the disease with how the person with the disease is interacting with the outside world. And for the drug companies it was more convenient to deal with a profession split by different approaches, entangled in paradigms fighting each other about the acceptance of psychotropic drugs, than to deal with a unified profession, ready to accept that in mental illness, pharmacotherapy is the only rational treatment. A unified profession would not have been happy to stop half-way in developing a psychotropic drug. After establishing efficacy, it would have insisted on identifying the treatment-responsive population. We would not have ended up with nearly 500 semi-finished psychotropics, but only a few with well-defined therapeutic indications.

So in a sense the industry don't want a biological psychiatry that knows what it's doing.

Right. They encouraged the interaction between psychiatry and neuro-pharmacology in a number of different ways, including the founding of organizations like the CINP, but did not pay any attention to how the different groups within psychiatry interacted with each other. The pharmaceutical industry played everything according to the rules, but never did anything beyond what was absolutely necessary to do. In spite of all their conservativism, by focusing on money and by clearly identifying their goals, the industry has been instrumental in triggering and fuelling the ongoing transformation of psychiatry into a medical discipline. This is happening because the industry has rendered pharmacotherapy accessible in the treatment of mental illness. The transformation began without the help and even in spite of the resistance of the academicians. This is why in the course of the transformation academic psychiatry has found itself floating in the air. The teaching of the treatment of mental illness has slipped out of their hands. I wonder for how long will it be possible to preserve and teach a psychiatric theory, which has nothing to do with the effective treatment of mental illness at the clinic.

In my opinion, the most important single contribution of the pharmaceutical industry was the development and introduction of a new model of operation in the form of the multinational corporation. And even if multinational corporations today exclusively serve limited business interests, they provided the basis, the foundation, for a new world. But while instrumental in the creation of a new world, multinationals act on the basis of short term planning. The pharmaceutical industry has rarely

gone beyond the generation of the minimal amount of information necessary for the registration of their drugs. And when they went beyond it
was to support marketing. I know that the companies are criticized for
this, but it is not the industry it is the profession who should be blamed.

We don't act as a profession?

You are perfectly correct and it is not the task of the industry to pull us
together. Why should they do that? After all it would be against their
own interest. But if the industry were faced with a different profession, a
profession with an identity, I'm convinced that it would act differently.

They would collaborate with psychiatry and provide the necessary
support – not generously, just as much as absolutely necessary. But they
would no longer treat the profession with handouts, the opinion leaders
of the profession as puppets and their collaborators from the profession as
'call girls'. Did you read Arthur Koestler's little book with that title? It is
about scientists who become part of the international jet set and fly from
conferences to congresses. You might find it amusing. I met Koestler
sometime during the 1970s in San Juan, while attending an ACNP meeting. He was invited by Nate Kline to participate in a panel.

A psychiatry which acted as a profession with a clearly defined identity
could have stopped the invasion of neuropharmacology, channeling away
the little money university departments of psychiatry have for teaching.
The invasion of neuropharmacologists and the enormous confusion and
shifting of priorities, created by their mere presence in departments, is
becoming a more serious problem than the invasion of anthropologists
and other social scientists had been during the psychodynamic era when
the psychoanalysts dominated the field. And, you know, neuropharmacologists in the psychiatry departments have the titles of professor of psychiatry without ever having a formal training in the field, however
unbelievable that may seem. What is even worse is that many of the
psychiatrists, because of the shifted priorities in the departments spend
their time in neuropharmacologic research instead of doing their clinical
work. Can you imagine in some departments this is even encouraged?

I might be giving you the impression that I have no appreciation for
neuropharmacology. It is really not so. I have great interest in it. And I
am obviously very much interested how the brain created the mind and
how the brain works. But this doesn't prevent me from recognizing that
research in these areas is far beyond what psychiatry deals with. I would
go even further. In the same way as I'm opposed to support research in
neuropharmacology from the budget allocated for psychiatry or the budget
of mental health, I am opposed also to the funding of brain research from
federal, state, provincial or what have you grants allocated for health and
welfare. Such grants are from the taxpayer's pocket and there are many
socially more pressing priorities than the neurosciences. I realize that I
probably belong to the small minority who believes that all the money

from the budgets of health and welfare should be spent on taking care of sick people directly and not by investing in highly sophisticated research.

I think it would be more appropriate if neuroscientists would be in Institutes like the Mario Negri, or have their own multinational corporation and we psychiatrists should also have our own – I really think that if we psychiatrists could come together and organize ourselves in a multinational corporation we could do so much more for everyone including ourselves. And we would not be at the mercy of businessmen or politicians.

To open up progress, there is a need for a change and for me a multinational corporation of psychiatry appears to be the rational next step. I have considered a number of different alternatives but none of them seemed to offer greater advantages for patients, psychiatrists, industry and even for the society we live in. In such a corporation, psychiatry could offer the least expensive and most accountable, accessible service to patients. We have all the necessary technology to provide the backbone of a multinational corporation of psychiatry. We have suitable programmes to develop the necessary software for the implementation of the same standards in diagnostic and treatment services everywhere around the world. We have the sophisticated communication systems which would allow for the delivery of centralized education programmes and we have the computer capabilities to store, process and analyse the collected data in any manner we wish. We could provide the necessary unbiased information for education to universities, feedback for planning to the companies and the statistics for the organization of mental health service to whoever is responsible for it.

Talking about tensions between psychiatry and neuroscience prompts me to ask you about your Tennessee experience. When you went there it appears to have been something of a hot bed of psychopharmacology between Fridolin Sulser and Oakley Ray. Is there any reason why this should have been the case?

While Allan Bass was chairman, the department of pharmacology of Vanderbilt became one of the tops in the United States. With the help of Frank Luton, the first qualified psychiatrist in the State, a disciple of Adolf Meyer, Bass succeeded in persuading the State of Tennessee to collaborate with Vanderbilt in founding a new kind of facility for research in neuropsychopharmacology. The idea was to have basic scientists and researchers work closely together in it. One of the buildings at the Middle Tennessee Mental Health Institute, the State Hospital serving the area, was dedicated to house the new facility and the Tennessee Neuropsychiatric Institute was opened with substantial NIMH support in the late 1960s. Bass first recruited Jim Dingell, a young pharmacologist who was studying the metabolism of imipramine, and then Fridolin Sulser, a medical doctor with industrial experience who had spent some time with Bernard Brodie at NIH. John Davis, the first clinical director of TNI, got on board somewhat later. Davis, who became well known for his book with Donald Klein on the *Diagnosis and Treatment of Psychiatric Disorders*, had David Janowsky working with him, who developed during his short stay at the TNI the cholinergic hypothesis of affective disorders.

Then it just happened that around the same time the Veterans' Administration Hospital in Nashville, which was closely affiliated with Vanderbilt, recruited Oakley Ray, a psychologist with a background in brain research. A clear thinker and excellent speaker, Oakley became one of the most popular teachers at the University, and gained an international reputation with his timely text on *Drugs, Society and Human Behaviour*. So by the time of my arrival to the TNI, a couple of years after the exodus of John Davis and his team, Tennessee was a well known center of neuropsychopharmacology. Of course, it helped Tennessee's reputation that in 1971 Earl Sutherland from Vanderbilt won the Nobel prize for his discovery of cyclic AMP.

Fridolin Sulser became one of the biggest names on the international circuit with his beta receptor down regulation hypothesis.

Sulser was already well known by the time of my arrival at the TNI. He had the reputation of a person difficult to deal with but he directed the preclinical division of TNI over many years smoothly and efficiently. He is a man with many talents – an accomplished researcher, a skilled politician, a good fund raiser and a persuasive speaker. Fridolin was always enthusiastic about the ongoing research in his laboratory and has never given up his dream to direct a research institute dedicated to neuropharmacology or molecular biology. He shifted the focus from presynaptic to postsynaptic mechanisms in the action of psychotropics – his description of postsynaptic beta receptor down regulation during treatment with antidepressants had a great impact on neuropharmacologic research.

After my arrival in Nashville, there were difficulties between Sulser and I, which unfortunately were perceived as a clash between personalities. This distracted attention from the essence of what was going on. The real issue, even if never spelled out clearly, was my position that neuropharmacology and psychopharmacology are two distinct disciplines, which must interact with each other with mutual respect but without either of the two dominating the other. For me, it was obvious that neuropharmacology, which is focused on drugs and deals with the detection of their action and the biological substrate involved in their action, is distinct from psychopharmacology, which is focused on illness and deals with the detection of which psychopathologic symptoms and the identification of which illnesses are affected by psychotropic drugs. But what was obvious to me was not obvious at all to Fridolin. He just could not accept that for psychopharmacology one needs a different training, background and maybe even a different kind of thinking. He just could not see where neuropharmacology ends and psychopharmacology begins. In retrospect

I can see that this was probably not just a blindfold – and that I probably touched one of the unspoken taboos. Because if my position had prevailed, it would have endangered the funding of neuropharmacologic research in many centres in the United States. And you know this whole issue is still not passé. Neuropharmacology is still channelling away funds from mental health and psychiatry. I hope that psychiatry will be able to put an end to this before being asked to put an end to it by the community.

Fridolin has his neurobiology laboratory these days at Vanderbilt Medical Center in the department of psychiatry. Beta receptor down regulation, a definite step in the chain of events in the brain after the administration of certain psychotropic drugs, did not provide the royal road to the understanding of the pathomechanism of depression but it was picked up by the pharmaceutical industry and turned into the pivotal test in the screening for potential 'antidepressants'. The problem with this is that it has led to us being provided with 'newer and newer antidepressants' of which one can't clearly be distinguished from the other. But of course this is far beyond Fridolin's control. It is not his fault – it is psychiatry that is to blame.

Why have the analysts here and the social psychiatrists in the UK and the purist basic scientists that work within the university framework looked down so much on any of the clinicians or basic scientists who work for the industry? It isn't as strong here as it is over in the UK, where until recently if you worked within the industry you were persona non grata. But in some respects one of the best places for people to work from recently has been within the industry.

I thought that kind of discrimination is over. It was one of the many ways to keep psychopharmacology out but it didn't succeed and we now have a steadily growing migration from academy to the industry. There are distinct advantages to working in the research departments of the drug companies. One is that your managers will provide for your support and ascertain that your research is done under optimal conditions. I don't know how it is in the UK but this is in sharp contrast to doing research at the universities in the US, where your departmental chairman and his growing entourage will expect you to provide support for their expenses and all you can expect in return is to be administered – or in everyday language to be bossed around and bugged endlessly to write applications for research grants. It's insane to spend months writing a grant application, which by the time it's approved, if it's approved, is already out of date.

And these days you have to write five applications for one that's approved.

And since everyone is busy writing new grant applications, no one is paying attention to the need for a fundamental revision of psychiatric theory and education. But the pressure to prepare grant applications can't explain the absurdity that, at a time when it is generally acknowledged that mental diseases are brain diseases, some experts in the field at some of the universities persist on keeping psychodynamics as the focal point of residency training. Nor can it explain the incredible truth that even 40 years after the introduction of chlorpromazine, some departments still refuse to accept that there was a psychopharmacologic revolution in psychiatry in the late 1950s.

There is another problem, of course, which is that by now psychopharmacology, or more precisely the pharmacotherapy of mental illness with psychotropics, is an internal part of undergraduate and postgraduate education in psychiatry but in spite of all the advances in communication technology, education in psychiatry, including education in psychopharmacology, differs from department to department and from one country to another. There is no good reason to teach pharmacotherapy differently at different universities within the same country. There is a simple, practical reason for some differences between countries because each country has its own drug regulatory agency and, however strange it is, has somewhat different psychotropic drugs available or the same drug, just across a border, may be available for different indications and in a different formulation. It's aggravating enough to have you present your passport and visa when passing the border from one country to another but to . . .

But we wouldn't have a World Cup without nations.

In a way, that's all they are good for. Tribalism in the era of multinationals – and each tribe, each university with a distinct psychiatric education and training. But seriously, mental illness is the same everywhere in the world. There is just no good reason to teach a different psychiatry in Budapest, Montreal and Nashville and if businessmen can form multinational pharmaceutical corporations which develop and market psychotropic drugs across countries, psychiatrists should be able to form multinational educational corporations which develop and disseminate educational material on how to use these drugs optimally in mental illness around the world.

Well, the argument against that would be, I guess, an ecological argument, that we've got to keep a diversity of species.

Actually I do believe in diversity, even if I recognize that mental illness restricts diversity and squeezes the diverse into stereotypes. I'm not talking about a 'brave new world' in psychiatric education. We should be listening to diversity of opinions, while communicating facts which are separated from fantasies, and theories which are separated from speculations.

Is psychopharmacology a subversive science? Compared to physics, which is theory driven, which builds large machines to demonstrate particles which physicists predict are going to be there, in psychopharmacology new drugs or machines, like PET scans, produce observations which we didn't expect were going to be there and this forces us to go back and tear up our theories rather than add to them. It's almost the opposite to physics in one sense and from that point of view, you wouldn't expect to find psychopharmacology in Oxford, Cambridge or the Maudsley in the UK or Yale or Harvard here, which like their science classical. They like their theory first and deductions from a hypothesis and they give grants when you've got that kind of grant proposal.

I never thought of psychopharmacologic research in those terms. I understand of course what you are talking about but personally I think it's wrong to label psychopharmacology a subversive science, because it appears driven exclusively by external forces to the extent that the introduction of every new drug or instrument disintegrates the old universe and opens up a new one. While undoubtedly this is the impression one gets about psychopharmacology through its most visibly promoted proponents, to define psychopharmacology as what psychopharmacologists do is begging the question.

The replacement of the cholinergic hypothesis with the catecholamine hypothesis and the catecholamine hypothesis with the indoleamine hypothesis of depression in rapid succession was undoubtedly in the interest of the drug firms. It's one of the common strategies of the pharmaceutical industry to attribute clinical relevance to pharmacological actions with psychotropics. By talking about catecholamine and indoleamine hypotheses of depression, we have undoubtedly given credibility to the marketing of antidepressants which are selective monoamine reuptake inhibitors. What's overlooked is the simple fact that all these hypotheses are actually speculations, because no one has ever identified either in terms of psychopathologic symptoms, or in terms of nosologic forms, a distinctive treatment-responsive population to any of the monoamine selective antidepressants.

We can't really say that theories have been rapidly replacing each other, because the clinical data necessary for formulating those theories have just never been there. On the other hand we have all the necessary means and orientation points for the formulation of a parsimonious psychiatric theory of mental illness, which, if proven correct in a classical way through the testing of a series of hypotheses, would bring together psychiatric theory and practice separated since the introduction of psychotropic drugs. It would also provide clinically meaningful endpoints for genetic, biochemical, physiological or pharmacological research in psychiatry. At this point the priority is to find our way to move ahead and break the deadlock in psychopharmacologic progress.

Let me get this clear, because it seems of central importance. What you are saying is when people don't respond to drugs, the industry use this as an excuse for saying we need to develop better drugs of the type we already have, and neuroscientists use it as an argument for more neuroscientific research, whereas in actual fact what should happen is more psychopathology.

Yes, in my opinion only proper psychiatric feedback can break the deadlock in pharmacotherapeutic progress. Proper psychiatric research would have identified the place of the SSRIs in the treatment of mental illness without the introduction of the ill-defined concept of serotonin spectrum disorders. Because regardless of how they are promoted the fact remains that the SSRIs are therapeutically effective only in an undefined population within any of the diagnostic groups of the alleged spectrum and in none of the diagnostic groups of the alleged spectrum is therapeutic responsiveness restricted to SSRIs. I can understand why the drug industry is trying to do everything to render such a concept acceptable, but how the profession can go along with it is above my head.

I'm even more puzzled about why the profession considers it more important to learn about the action mechanism of psychotropics than about their clinical applications. We should know it by now that the study of the action mechanism of psychotropics can't provide a royal road to the understanding of the underlying pathophysiology of nosologic concepts, because on the basis of our current knowledge none of the psychotropics we have is either selectively efficacious in a distinct psychiatric illness and/or equally effective during its different developmental stages. Neuropharmacologic research by furthering the knowledge about the action of psychotropics can lead only to the development of drugs with similar pharmacologic profiles and clinical effects to the ones we already have. I wonder why it took decades to figure out that increased affinity to D2 receptors doesn't improve the overall therapeutic efficacy of drugs in the treatment of schizophrenia and greater selectiveness to NE or 5-HT-2 receptors doesn't improve the overall therapeutic efficacy of drugs in the treatment of depression.

I don't have a crystal ball to foresee the future, but for one or another reason I have the notion that we will see more action in terms of new drug development through the manipulation of postsynaptic events and especially through the manipulation of postsynaptic receptor sites. After all it's the postsynaptic receptor which is responsible for the propagation of the electrical activity induced by the neurotransmitter released into the synaptic cleft, and it's the state of the postsynaptic receptor which, however remotely and confusingly, has some kind of relationship to the clinical state. And one should not forget that it was only after the introduction of radioactive isotope binding techniques in the late 1970s that research in this area began.

So binding technologies did make a difference?

In a way they did. They undoubtedly stimulated research to develop drugs which selectively bind to one or another receptor type or subtype. It is impressive how fast neuropharmacologists are moving in identifying newer and newer receptor types and even more impressive how fast they decipher their functional significance, which is not a simple task, because the same receptor can be linked to the inhibition of emesis in the area postrema, to the modulation of sensory input in the substantia gelatinosa, and to the regulation of anxiety in the limbic area. But when working in this fascinating area of research on the clinical side one should always keep in mind the Antaeus legend, because in the world of receptors one can get easily carried away and lose touch with Mother Earth.

Antaeus?

Antaeus was the son of Earth, a giant, who couldn't be killed while he was touching Mother Earth. According to the legend, Hercules picked him up, and when he lost touch with Mother Earth, killed him.

A few years ago I was following with great interest the work, which suggested that in obsessive – compulsive disorder there is a hypersensitivity of postsynaptic 5-HT-2 receptors with downregulation of this hypersensitivity in the course of successful treatment with an SSRI. I thought that we finally have a clinical syndrome, which is clearly linked to a particular biologic substrate and which clearly responds to a particular group of psychotropic drugs. Unfortunately neither of my expectations were fulfilled. Hypersensitivity of postsynaptic 5-HT-2 receptors turned out to be non-specific for obsessive – compulsive disorder. It was found to be present also in panic disorder. And in terms of selection of treatment, hypersensitivity of the postsynaptic 5-HT-2 receptors had no relevance whatsoever. In fact panic disorder was found to respond just as well if not better to treatment with alprazolam, a short–acting benzodiazepine, or imipramine, than to treatment with an SSRI.

There is an obvious problem in having some isolated findings here and some other isolated findings there and it's an even bigger problem, that on the basis of such isolated findings, one may decide about treatment which is not the optimal for the condition or in the best interest of the patient. The point I'm trying to make is that centrally coordinated clinical research in psychopharmacology is becoming an absolute necessity. And I just can't see the feasibility of centrally coordinated research in clinical psychopharmacology without a multinational professional corporation in psychiatry. At this point this would even be in the interest of the multinational pharmaceutical industry.

During the past decades the wealth of some of the multinationals has outgrown the wealth of some countries and at present we are seeing a rapid concentration of power in the hands of fewer and fewer companies by multinationals buying up multinationals. There are also some indications that multinationals are preparing to shift the focus of their operations from isolated products, with a product for each different medical discipline, to lines of products, with each line including a set of products for a particular discipline such as psychiatry, with different multinationals representing different lines across the world.

Of course all this is mere speculation based on very limited factual information but I have no doubt that with modern communication technology the present country- and product-based operations are becoming counterproductive and unmanageable. And since I would envisage world-wide development for the different lines of products, multinational pharm-aceutical corporations will have to shift their alliance from government to profession with a choice to deal with independent multinational pro-fessional corporations in the different medical disciplines, or set up their own multinational clinical divisions in the different areas. Both options have advantages and disadvantages. In the meantime, companies will have to continue to operate in their present mode, working with national regulatory agencies in the best way they can to ascertain the protection of their investment.

Do you think regulation has been industry-friendly? There's a good argument that can be made that we wouldn't have had the modern multinational corporation without regulation which forces smaller companies off the market.

Whether regulation is industry-friendly – personally I would think it is – depends on how you look at it. The drug companies would certainly not say that the national regulatory agencies are particularly friendly to them and I don't think that those working in the agencies would say that they are particularly friendly or unfriendly to the companies. I worked quite closely with the late Tom Da Silva, when he set up practically from scratch the CNS section of the Canadian HPB and he certainly was neither friendly nor unfriendly to the companies, but tried to set up things in a manner that his section fulfils its function by ascertaining that whatever had been agreed upon was adhered to. But then looking at it from a very different angle, the regulatory agencies in countries like the US and Canada have been as you were saying friendly to the big companies by setting the minimal standards at a level that the cost involved to get the necessary information and to prepare a submission was sufficiently high that only the big companies could afford it.

Is there a risk that the FDA-industry complex could lose contact with people on the street? This comes up in criticisms of fluoxetine, by patients' groups pointing at the whole complex of the corporations and the FDA.

I like your term FDA-industry complex. Undoubtedly fluoxetine is a rather controversial drug but its problems are really not the kind of problems that, operating within the frame of reference of the agreement between the company and the government, the FDA could do anything about. In so far as I'm concerned, fluoxetine can't make a person dangerous to others who has no potential to become dangerous, although it might make someone who is potentially dangerous become dangerous but, of course, there might be several other drugs which have a similar potential.

Let me tell you my story with fluoxetine, for which I might be on some kind of blacklist with its maker. When it was released as an anti-depressant in the US, I was on the pharmacy committee of Vanderbilt and on the basis of the information I had and with careful consideration of an excellent review from a Fellow from clinical pharmacology, I concluded that the drug was just not a sufficiently potent antidepressant that it should be put on the formulary of the medical center. In some way I was even surprised that Paul Leber, whom I very much respect, let it through just because the drug was clean on the toxicity screen even if the proof of efficacy with the required 5% level of probability was present only in a somewhat less seriously depressed population than usual.

My position after having some clinical experience with fluoxetine has not changed much in so far as fluoxetine as an antidepressant is concerned. But I must add that I wish that fluoxetine had developed clinically in a different way – even for the indication of depression because it is one of the more interesting psychotropic drugs. I'm glad that later on other indications, such as obsessive – compulsive disorder and bulimia surfaced. But then probably the most important is that the SSRIs are forcing us to face the issue of whether the use of psychotropics should be restricted to the treatment of disease or extended to the modification of behaviour, or even to render life more pleasurable.

I agree the SSRIs can't treat anyone who is depressed any more successfully than the older compounds but what they can do much more successfully is they can influence sexual behaviour – they can treat premature ejaculation, for instance. And the industry have even been out and done surveys to show that ⅓ of males have premature ejaculation problems, so there is a great deal of distress there that could be alleviated but they won't do it – at the moment anyway. They feel the consensus isn't there for that kind of social engineering at the moment.

It's one of those strange situations where business interest tones down a potential indication instead of drumming it up. But since the potential for influencing sexual behaviour is there I hope that it will not take too long that industry will bring out people from the closet with premature ejaculation as it did bring people out with agoraphobia. This is another area where, in my opinion, a multinational professional corporation could help the pharmaceutical industry a lot. Since we have the capability to do social engineering to some extent it's really just a question for how long it would take to open up for it, which might differ from country to country.

Well, there's always this curious transcultural thing. If you look at what the best selling antidepressants are in any one country, they vary widely.

I'm glad that you are bringing this up because even if there are transcultural differences which have developed through differences in diet or through inbreeding, they are skin deep and the only thing which might be influenced by them is the propensity for certain side effects. I understand that in some way it was in the interest of the drug companies to keep the possibility of transcultural differences alive but have never understood why the idea that mental patients are different from the rest of people, in this regard, had so many proponents among psychiatrists.

Some time ago one could hear it said that patients need different neuroleptic dosages in different countries. But when in the early 1980s, we conducted a study which dealt with the distribution of the different forms and subforms of schizophrenia in the hospitalized population in different countries and collected information on the dosages of neuroleptics used, we learned that the dosages used between two Japanese centres, one in the North and one in the South of Japan were greater than the difference between the dosages used between either of those centres and the centre involved in the study from the United States.

But the differences in the use of psychotropics between countries are steadily decreasing. And even if a drug is put on the market with indications which don't correspond beyond a certain point with clinical reality, there is a process which brings it closer to it, however slowly.

Dialectically?

In a way. Actually we have the necessary technology these days to develop drugs uniformly for everywhere with all the steps in the decision-making process regarding diagnosis and assessment of change captured but we are not doing it. In the same way, as in sports where we let the referee have the final say even if he is clearly wrong as shown on a video-recording, we keep in drug development a certain subjectivity. I understand of course that most people would think that's right but personally I'm unable to comprehend, even in sports, if the referee was wrong why we stick to the wrong decision when we are in a position to correct it.

It introduces the arbitrary human element, I suppose which can have its own justification.

Looking back to those early years of the 1950s, I'm always amazed how fast things moved ahead with the development of chlorpromazine. In less than a year after its synthesis, Laborit made his fundamental observations which led to the administration of the drug for the first time to psychiatric patients at Val de Grâce. Undoubtedly, the observations of Delay and Deniker were the turning point in the development of the drug but Rhône-Poulenc moved just as fast as it could, not just with the drug, but also with the development of a series of analogues.

Could you say that the companies recognized the new drugs even quicker than the professionals? They were instantly off trying to find analogues and were prepared to put money in it.

Undoubtedly! Geigy started virtually without delay with the development of imipramine, on the basis of the structural similarity between the phenothiazine and iminodibenzyl nucleus. And by 1958, Lundbeck had the first thioxanthenes. Ciba got busy with the Rauwolfia alkaloids, Roche with the hydrazine type of MAOIs and Carter Wallace with the propanediols.

While the profession was 10 years later still asking whether this was important.

Disappointing but true. It was only after the publication of the results of the Veterans' Administration Collaborative Studies in 1960, that the profession finally accepted in the United States that something important is happening in the treatment of schizophrenia. And it was only after the publication of Klerman and Cole's report in 1965 that they were ready to accept that depression might be influenced pharmacologically.

But this is part of why I was saying to you that psychopharmacology is subversive. It wasn't the recognized scientists in Oxford and Harvard who discovered all this – it was people in companies – who put their money on it.

Although I don't see psychopharmacology as a subversive science, I've the feeling that our positions are quite close. First of all, I agree with you that modern psychopharmacology was created by the drug companies and that people from the drug companies have played an important role in moving psychopharmacology ahead during the past 40 years. The difference between our positions is, that I believe that psychopharmacology at a certain point entered a stage of development in which it had become counterproductive for the drug companies to move things further, because of their business interests. And it was at that point that psychiatrists, dedicated to psychopharmacologic research, took it over and became the moving force.

Look at the psychopharmacology of schizophrenia. Psychopharmacology focused attention on the biologic heterogeneity of schizophrenia but this was obviously contrary to the interest of the drug firms. In trying to prevent the falling apart of the neuroleptic market, industry is lavishly supporting and propagating neuropharmacologic research on receptor changes in schizophrenic brains or linkages through the D_4 receptor to genetics. This kind of research is based on the assumption that schizophrenia, a concept, is one disease, whereas psychopharmacologic research should be trying to disentangle the biologic heterogeneity of schizophrenia found in clinical investigations. There is no support from industry for this kind of work done in schizophrenia and it is rather unfortunate that there is no appreciation for psychopharmacologic research in schizophrenia at the American universities.

In a steadily increasing number, the chairs in the departments are filled by psychiatrists, whom I refer to in Milovan Djilas' term as the 'new class' within psychiatry. And this 'new class' of psychiatrists by conveniently confounding neuropharmacology with psychopharmacology go along, on the basis of pragmatic considerations, with industry and neuropharmacology, perpetuating the deadlock in pharmacotherapy.

Psychiatrists of the 'new class' are ambitious, goal directed, keenly aware of the transformation psychiatry is in and they know how to pull the strings. There is a definitely laudable intention to integrate psychiatry with the rest of medicine, to replace subjective assessments by objective measures and supplement the information obtained by interview with findings derived by sophisticated instruments – indeed their determination to bring to psychiatry whatever modern technology can offer, regardless of need and price, outweighs common sense. By focusing on MRI and PET, they distract attention from the far overdue re-evaluation of psychopathology and nosology. It's pathetic but without ill will they are successfully destroying the little bit of psychiatry left in the departments after the lengthy psychodynamic era, dominated by the psychoanalysts.

If you visit one of the avant garde departments of the 'new class', you will be overwhelmed by information on ongoing research in collaboration with neuroradiologists, biochemists and other sophisticated instrumentalists. Eventually, though, you will realize that no one is engaged in psychiatric research to generate the 'clinical prerequisite' that could render the findings, with the sophisticated instrumentation, meaningful and interpretable.

In spite of all the difficulties psychopharmacology is moving ahead and, even if not without resistance, it is dragging psychiatry into the modern world. I was lucky in a way, because I had just graduated when psychopharmacology was starting in 1954 and people like Mogen Schou and Max Hamilton were just a little bit older than me – sufficiently older so that I could learn from them, while I still could get to know them, because I too was involved in what they were doing. I have been all my professional life in the Academy. I'm 65 now and the time is here to move along and try to find a way to put into practice what psychopharmacology can offer and what I have learned over the past 40 years. I have thought about writing a history of psychiatry. The title would be 'They Used to Call it Psychiatry'.

Select bibliography
Ban, T.A. (1989) CODE-DD *Composite Diagnostic Evaluation of Depressive Disorders*. JM Productions, Brentwood.

Ban, T.A. (1987) Prolegomenon to the clinical prerequisite: Psychopharmacology and the classification of mental disorders. *Prog. Neuropharm. Biol. Psychiatry*, **11**, 527–80.

Ban, T.A. (1969) *Psychopharmacology*. Williams & Wilkins, Baltimore.

Ban, T.A. (1972) *Schizophrenia. A Psychopharmalogical Approach*. Charles Thomas, Springfield.

Ban, T.A. and Hippius, H. (eds) (1994) *Towards CINP*. From the Paris Colloquium to the Milan Symposium. JM Productions, Brentwood, Tennessee.

Author index

Subject index

Printed and bound by CPI Group (UK) Ltd, Croydon, CR0 4YY

23/10/2024

01778237-0019